MEDICAL RADIOLOGY
Diagnostic Imaging

P. A. Gevenois and P. De Vuyst (Eds.)

Imaging of Occupational and Environmental Disorders of the Chest

With Contributions by

M. Akira · V. C. S. Antao · H. Arakawa · Z. A. Aziz · A. Bankier · D. E. Banks
M. W. Brauner · P.-Y. Brillet · S. Burge · A. Churg · S. J. Copley · J.-C. Dalphin · S. R. Desai
P. De Vuyst · P. Dumortier · T. Franquet · P. A. Gevenois · F. Guillon · D. M. Hansell
D. A. Lynch · N. Magy · B. Nemery · Ø. Omland · C. G. C. Ooi · J. E. Parker
A. Rask-Andersen · G. Reboux · J. A. Verschakelen

Foreword by

A. L. Baert

With 195 Figures in 289 Separate Illustrations, 47 in Color and 25 Tables

Springer

Paul De Vuyst, MD, PhD
Professor and Head
Department of Respiratory Medicine
Hôpital Erasme
Université Libre de Bruxelles
Brussels
Belgium

Pierre Alain Gevenois, MD, PhD
Professor of Radiology
Clinic of Chest Imaging
Department of Radiology
Hôpital Erasme
Université Libre de Bruxelles
Brussels
Belgium

Medical Radiology · Diagnostic Imaging and Radiation Oncology
Series Editors: A. L. Baert · L. W. Brady · H.-P. Heilmann · M. Molls · K. Sartor

Continuation of Handbuch der medizinischen Radiologie
Encyclopedia of Medical Radiology

Library of Congress Control Number: 2004116346

ISBN 3-540-21343-0 Springer Berlin Heidelberg New York
ISBN 978-3-540-21343-7 Springer Berlin Heidelberg New York

Springer is part of Springer Science+Business Media

http//www.springeronline.com

Printed in Germany

Medical Editor: Dr. Ute Heilmann, Heidelberg
Desk Editor: Ursula N. Davis, Heidelberg
Production Editor: Kurt Teichmann, Mauer
Cover-Design and Typesetting: Verlagsservice Teichmann, Mauer

Printed on acid-free paper – 21/3151xq – 5 4 3 2 1 0

Foreword

A changing industrial environment in the western world during the past decades has resulted in a considerable change in the spectrum of occupational and environmental lung disorders that we observe nowadays in medical practice. Modern radiological imaging is a important diagnostic tool for the correct management of these diseases.

This volume, unique in its concept, not only covers in a comprehensive way the imaging features of the well-known coal worker's pneumoconiosis and the severe forms of silicosis and asbestosis, but also deals extensively with the effects of new organic and inorganic materials , used in the modern chemical industry as well as with the noxious effects of cigarette smoking.

The eminently readable text is complemented by superb illustrations.

The editors, P.A. Gevenois and P. De Vuyst are well-known experts in the field. The authors of the individual chapters are outstanding specialists in the epidemiology, etiology, immunology, pathology, pathophysiology, and radiology of dust inhalation diseases. I would like to thank and to congratulate most sincerely the editors and the authors for their top-level contributions.

This superb book will be of great value for general and chest radiologists but also for pneumologists and all those active in occupational and environmental medicine. It provides them with the latest information on a very interesting medical field with an important medicosocial impact.

I am confident that it will meet the same success with the readers as many previous volumes in this series.

Leuven　　　　ALBERT L. BAERT

Introduction

Pierre Alain Gevenois and Paul De Vuyst

The spectrum of classical pneumoconiosis has changed during the past decades in industrialized countries: as a result of better control of air dust levels and reduction of workforce in large sectors of industry, the incidence of severe forms of silicosis, coal worker's pneumoconiosis and asbestosis (lung fibrosis), has decreased over time. Most incident cases of disabling pneumoconiosis result from exposures dating back several decades ago.

Parallel to the reduction of exposures in industries using natural minerals, the development of the chemical industry has led to the production of large numbers of organic and inorganic materials, including metallic alloys. More and more of these substances, including manmade organic particles, are reported as causes of interstitial lung disease in groups of exposed workers. Many different patterns of interstitial lung diseases have been reported: lung fibrosis, lung granulomatosis, giant cell pneumonitis, non specific interstitial pneumonia, chronic organizing pneumonia. Without a careful occupational history-taking and/or inquiry, all these forms may mislead the etiological diagnosis towards their respective idiopathic forms.

The major tools for diagnosis of pulmonary and pleural diseases are the imaging techniques to which this book is dedicated. Chest film reading and scoring according to the Classification established by the International Labour Office (ILO) is a standardized and wide-world used method and represents a common language between people working in this field, including in developing countries. This system facilitates for example the interpretation and comprehension of the epidemiological literature on pneumoconiosis. Many compensation systems rely on the presence of grade 1/1 or 1/0 small opacities on a plain chest film. This is however not the most sensitive to detect early changes and not the most specific one to diagnose pneumoconiosis in individuals. Indeed, the prevalence of small irregular opacities in an adult smoking population is high and the interpretation of films is subject to important inter and intra-observer variability in boundary grades, which are crucial in the acceptance of pneumoconiosis. This issue is even more important since incident cases of obvious pneumoconiosis with large opacities or high ILO grades have become exceptional. Computed tomography (CT) has largely been reported as more sensitive and more specific than chest radiograph and is thus now widely used for the diagnosis and compensation of pneumoconiosis. One of the consequences is the detection of abnormalities consistent with pneumoconiosis in patients without symptoms or lung function alterations. On the other hand, CT studies have been invaluable in the description and the distinction of the various forms of dust-related lesions, such as rounded atelectasis, diffuse pleural thickening and pleural plaques.

The majority of workers who are exposed to asbestos nowadays are end-users, in contact with asbestos still in place in buildings such as electricians, plumbers, demolition workers, asbestos removers... Most of them are self-standing workers, without any medical control or surveillance and often working without protective devices. The currently diagnosed cases are principally non malignant pleural lesions with little or no effect on lung function and the main cause of asbestos-related deaths among them is malignant mesothelioma rather than respiratory failure due to lung fibrosis. Since the incident cases of true asbestosis are rare, the development of lung fibrosis in a person with low cumulative exposure and/or low concentrations of asbestos bodies and fibers in bronchoalveolar lavage raise the possibility of idiopathic pulmonary fibrosis (IPF). Unusual exposures may however still be at the origin of severe

P. A. Gevenois, MD, PhD
Clinic of Chest Imaging, Department of Radiology, Hôpital Erasme, Université Libre de Bruxelles, Route de Lennik 808, 1070 Brussels, Belgium
P. De Vuyst, MD, PhD
Department of Respiratory Medicine, Hôpital Erasme, Université Libre de Bruxelles, Route de Lennik 808, 1070 Brussels, Belgium

diseases. Environmental exposures to tremolite asbestos have been documented in Turkish residents and migrants with burdens of fibers equal to those seen in industrial settings and subsequent asbestos-related diseases, including asbestosis.

Occupational lung diseases have also extended their links and limits. There is a clear association between silicosis or silica exposure and connective tissue disorders such as rheumatoid arthritis, systemic sclerosis and ANCA-positive vasculitides. Even "IPF" has been shown in several epidemiological studies associated with occupational exposures to metals or wood dusts. These studies beside exclude patients with asbestos or silica exposures of any importance, considering them respectively as having asbestosis or silicosis, irrespective of low cumulative exposures and/or radiological abnormalities not consistent with pneumoconiosis. The proportion of « IPF » cases with exposure to exogenous dust may be more important than previously thought. In this regard, it is interesting to note that coal miners may develop an IPF-like disease with a honeycomb pattern on thin-section CT rather than a classic coal worker's pneumoconiosis, and that these cases are now compensated in France.

Occupational agents may interact with other agents, infectious or not. Drugs can induce or trigger interstitial and/or pleural disease and this may induce confusion if these changes develop in persons with prior occupational exposure. This is particularly true for asbestos, and several cases have been reported of patients with prior asbestos exposure, who developed rapidly progressive pleural thickening or effusion, while being treated with bromocriptine for Parkinson's disease.

There is still important clinical and basic research work in occupational and environmental diseases. The research areas concern the description of new diseases due to organic and inorganic materials, nanotoxicology, mineralogical studies on the lung, genetical and immunological susceptibility to pneumoconiosis...There are indeed differences in the individual susceptibility to the adverse effects of chemicals and metals. Beryllіosis and hard metal disease may be observed after exposure to low-doses, and are known to affect only a minority of exposed workers. Important advances have been made in basic research on the immunogenetic basis of berylliosis. A human HLA class II mutated gene was found to be strongly associated with clinical berylliosis and probably with hard metal disease.

Imaging, even by CT, is crucial, but only a part of the diagnosis of occupational disease. Many patterns of interstitial lung disease, can be either idiopathic or due to an exogenous cause. Other diagnostic tools are essential. They include a careful occupational and environmental history taking, which may necessitate a visit of the house or of the workplace. Some diagnoses, especially in the field of hypersensitivity pneumonitis require sagacity worthy of Sherlock Holmes himself! They also may require mineralogical studies on bronchoalveolar lavage, immunological tests (serum precipitating antibodies, lymphocyte transformation tests...) and in some cases lung biopsy.

The diagnostic work-up in occupational and environmental lung and pleural diseases needs sometimes more than a simple chest plain film with lung function tests. In clinical practice, this can not be accepted as sufficiently accurate to confirm or refute the diagnosis of pneumoconiosis in a dust-exposed worker with interstitial lung disease. Advances in imaging, mineralogical, pathological and immunological techniques have been instrumental in describing new patterns of disease and they allow a comprehensive approach to occupational and environmental disorders. This is crucial for making a correct clinical diagnosis and for not missing treatable diseases, in the description of new patterns of diseases, and for making scientifically based expertise of difficult or litigious cases. The changing spectrum of environmental and occupational diseases makes thus essential very close collaboration between radiologists, pneumologists, occupational physicians, environmental hygiene specialists, immunologists, mineralogists, and pathologists.

Contents

Part I: The Basics for Understanding Imaging **1**

1 Epidemiology and Imaging of Dust Diseases
DANIEL E. BANKS 3

2 Responses of the Respiratory System to Inhaled Agents (Airways, Lung, and Pleura)
ANDREW CHURG, ANNA RASK-ANDERSEN, ØYVIND OMLAND,
and BENOIT NEMERY 13

2.1 Pathological Reactions to Inhaled Particles and Fibers
ANDREW CHURG 13

2.2 Bio-Aerosols and Organic Dusts
ANNA RASK-ANDERSEN and ØYVIND OMLAND 31

2.3 Chemical-Induced Lung Injury and Its Long-Term Sequelae
BENOIT NEMERY 67

3 Diagnostic Techniques
ZELENA A. AZIZ, DAVID M. HANSELL, VINICIUS C. S. ANTAO, JOHN E. PARKER,
SHERWOOD BURGE, PASCAL DUMORTIER, GABRIEL REBOUX, NADINE MAGY and
JEAN-CHARLES DALPHIN 77

3.1 Occupational and Environmental Lung Disease: The Role of Imaging
ZELENA A. AZIZ and DAVID M. HANSELL 77

3.2 ILO Classification
VINICIUS C. S. ANTAO and JOHN E. PARKER 93

3.3 Lung Function for Radiology
SHERWOOD BURGE 101

3.4 Mineralogical Analysis of Lung Samples
PASCAL DUMORTIER 115

3.5 Immunological Methods
GABRIEL REBOUX, NADINE MAGY, and JEAN-CHARLES DALPHIN 133

Part II: Imaging **159**

4 Lung Effects of Cigarette Smoking
SUJAL R. DESAI and DAVID M. HANSELL 161

5 Silicosis
CLARA GAIK CHENG OOI and HIROAKI ARAKAWA 177

6 Coal Worker's Pneumoconiosis
JOHNY A. VERSCHAKELEN and PIERRE ALAIN GEVENOIS 195

7 Asbestosis
SUSAN J. COPLEY 207

8 Non-Malignant Asbestos-Related Pleural Disorders
PIERRE ALAIN GEVENOIS and PAUL DE VUYST 223

9 Mesothelioma
ALEXANDER BANKIER and TOMAS FRANQUET 239

10 Imaging of Beryllium-Related Diseases
DAVID A. LYNCH 249

11 Hard Metal and Cobalt Disease
JOHNY A. VERSCHAKELEN and BENOIT NEMERY 257

12 Other Uncommon Pneumoconioses
MASANORI AKIRA 263

13 Hypersensitivity Pneumonitis
MICHEL W. BRAUNER, PIERRE-YVES BRILLET, and FRANÇOIS GUILLON 281

Subject Index 297

List of Contributors 301

Part I:

The Basics for Understanding Imaging

1 Epidemiology and Imaging of Dust Diseases

Daniel E. Banks

CONTENTS

1.1 Epidemiology and Imaging in Occupationally Related Lung Disease – Then and Now 3
1.2 Development of a Standardized Imaging System for Chest Radiographs 4
1.3 Reader Variability and the Diagnosis of Work-Related Lung Disease 5
1.4 What About Other Techniques for Chest Imaging? 8
1.5 What Conclusions Should be Made? 10
References 10

1.1 Epidemiology and Imaging in Occupationally Related Lung Disease – Then and Now

There are a number of reasons why one might have expected an increasing number of work-related adverse chest effects if fibrogenic dust exposures had remained unchanged compared with exposures in the past. Perhaps the most apparent and probably most important is the recognition that life expectancy has increased. In 1950, 40-year-old white men were projected to live 31.2 more years. In 2001, this same population had a projected survival of 37.3 years. All other men (non-whites) in this age group had a projected survival of 27.3 years and 32.5 years at these points in time, respectively (http://www.infoplease.com/ipa/A0005140.html).

One of the hallmarks of these work-related illnesses is the protracted latency period. This increase in projected survival times is relevant to this perspective. For example, with this increase in longevity over the past 50 years, it is reasonable to expect that workers with asbestos-related lung disease would have a longer time to, first, develop the disease and, second, progress to more severe disease. Workers at risk for mesothelioma would have a longer time period to develop this illness. In addition, this illness would have the potential to occur more frequently. Similarly, those with asbestos exposure who smoke cigarettes would have a prolonged time to develop lung cancer, even after they stopped smoking. With these data, if exposures had remained the same, these additional years of survival would result in more frequent and more severe dust-induced chest illnesses.

Yet, the picture that has developed is dramatically different. This is due to a substantial decrease (typically of several orders of magnitude) in respirable exposures. It may well be that these lessened exposures are reflected in longer survival. Although there is no prevalence of truly "representative" illness reports, several of the studies below may be considered "representative" of the decade(s) that the workers were employed and the year of publication. Selikoff, in 1965, reported on a population of asbestos workers with a 40-year latency of asbestos exposure. In this population of 121 workers, 94.2% were reported to have a radiological diagnosis of asbestosis (Selikoff et al. 1965). In a 1979 report of 359 present and retired shipyard workers with at least 10 years of exposure, 44% had parenchymal interstitial disease (Polakoff et al. 1979). More recently, in a population of electricians with at least 20 years of union membership, the prevalence of small opacities was 2.1% (Hessel et al. 1998). These reports show the dramatic decline in dust-induced lung disease.

Even at these dramatically diminished prevalence rates, we cannot dismiss the rate of occurrence of these illnesses. Although the prevalence of disease is substantially less, health issues continue to be recognized, particularly in the older or retired worker. Perhaps the most consequential of these dust diseases is asbestosis, the only major pneumoconiosis to demonstrate an increase in mortality over the past decade (Changing Patterns of Pneumo-

D. E. Banks, MD
Professor and Head, Department of Medicine, Louisiana State University Health Science Center, Shreveport, Louisiana, 71130, USA

coniosis Mortality 2004). Mortality from asbestosis peaks 40–45 years after the workers' initial occupational exposure to asbestos (Virta 2003). Since asbestos consumption increased substantially during and after World War II, with a peak in 1975 followed by a steep decrease beginning in the 1980s (Selikoff et al. 1980), asbestosis-related mortality will remain with us and perhaps even increase for another decade. Asbestos-containing materials that continue to be used in some workplaces and remain in buildings represent a potential risk for the next generation.

What happened to cause this dramatic lessening in the number of cases of dust-induced lung diseases? Regulatory agencies have become sensitized to the adverse respiratory effects of dust exposure and responded by lessening permissible exposure limits. Workers have been protected. Decisions made by governmental agencies regarding standard setting have been driven by epidemiological studies. These studies have used years of employment and dust measurements as variables and lung function tests (typically, the forced expiratory volume in one second) and chest radiography [as interpreted by the International Labor Organization (ILO) classification] as outcomes. The notion that these variables determine outcomes in a relatively predictable manner (i.e., dose dependent) is key to protecting the worker. Integrity in the collection of demographic data, lung function testing, and interpretation of chest radiographs in the standardized manner is critical to this process.

1.2 Development of a Standardized Imaging System for Chest Radiographs

There have been several sentinel events in the epidemiological studies of lung diseases in workers. These events focus on the development of a scheme to standardize the interpretation of films for the classification of pneumoconiosis. Arguably, the current system of classifying the severity of radiological simple pneumoconiosis stems from the work of Davies and Mann (1948; Oldham 1970). These investigators postulated that the number of small opacities visualized on the radiograph is the equivalent of severity of pneumoconiosis and introduced the concept of "major" categories of simple pneumoconiosis (based on profusion and extent of opacities). This notion was later incorporated into the ILO 1958 classification of the radiographs of pneumoconioses (International Labour Office 1959), in which an apparent continuum of opacities is separated into four distinct categories - from 0 to 3. Once this initiative had begun, the next steps were to relate these standardized abnormalities on the chest radiograph to demographic data. Liddell is later credited as the first to divide each major category into three subcategories (Liddell 1963).

The International Union Against Cancer (UICC) Working Group on Asbestos and Cancer in 1964 recognized the need to improve comparability and build on the 1958 classification (International Union Against Cancer 1965). In 1965, three groups met to develop a more sophisticated plan to interpret radiographs for pneumoconiosis and formulated a scheme that was to be known as the 1970 UICC/Cincinnati classification (UICC 1970). The effort to structure a meaningful program was international in scope. Working groups included: representatives of physicians from numerous countries asked by the UICC to interpret a series of chest radiographs from workers with dust disease, radiologists from the U.S. Public Health Service who were developing a scheme to interpret films of workers in asbestos manufacturing industries, and physicians keen to categorize the radiographs from workers employed at the Asbestos and Thetford mines in Quebec.

The changes from the 1958 scheme of interpretation form the basis of what is the basically the current ILO system, initially introduced as the 1970 UICC/Cincinnati classification. Changes included the division of pleural changes into "calcified" and "noncalcified," as well as changes in the manner that small opacities were described. As noted above, opacities had been categorized as major categories 0–3 in profusion. With the new scheme, a 12-point scale reflecting a series of "shades of gray" within a major category was put into place. In addition, the lung was separated into three zones for more descriptive imaging, rather than being characterized as a single entity. Finally, this new scheme separated opacities into "rounded" and "irregular" (they had previously been categorized solely as "small opacities") and then further separated irregular opacities from one size (L) into three sizes (s, t, u). Copies of "standardized" radiographs were made available from several investigators. The 1968 ILO classification system was a modification to incorporate asbestos-related diseases based in part on the UICC/Cincinnati classification system.

In 1973, Weill and Jones reported on a National Institutes of Health-sponsored workshop addressing interpretation of the chest roentgenogram (using the UICC/Cincinnati classification) as an epidemiological tool (Weill and Jones 1973). Their comments are relevant today. Overall, this working group identified problems in the interpretation of standardized radiographs. These include: (1) difficulties in distinguishing between small rounded and small irregular opacities when both are present; (2) correlating measures of profusion that accurately reflect lung function; (3) identifying the best way to use chest radiographs in assessing progression of disease; and (4) understanding how to best avoid biased readings in epidemiological surveys. They proposed several solutions: they (1) provided instructions to enable readers to distinguish small rounded from small irregular opacities; (2) developed ways to correlate profusion with lung function measurements; (3) considered small rounded and small irregular opacities as separate entities; and (4) at least in epidemiological studies, advocated the use of three (or more) readers to minimize inter-observer variability.

The 1980 ILO classification system made several changes. These included the presentation of a new set of 22 standard chest radiographs showing both round and irregular opacities, as well as large opacities. These films were used as examples of the size, shape, and profusion categories of opacities. An estimate of film quality became a part of the protocol, and the description of the pleura was more detailed (Henry 2002).

In 2000, the ILO again gave the scheme a "face lift." The standard films illustrating pleural abnormalities and 'u' shadows were replaced. Additionally, the ability to assess pneumoconiosis was to be judged on a scale from unimpeachable (+) to unusable ("u"). If not "+", then written comments are needed. A minimum width of 3 mm (previously 0–5 mm) was now required for plaques as well as for the margin to the lateral chest wall. Diaphragmatic plaques were not considered for measurement of extent, but only if absent or present. For "diffuse pleural thickening," obliteration of the costophrenic angle was recognized as necessary. New symbols for chest radiological findings were also included (Hering et al. 2003; http://www.chestx-ray.com/BReader/BReport/Compare1980_2000ver.html).

The desire to diminish variability in radiograph interpretation resulted in the formation of the Department of Labor and the National Institute for Occupational Safety and Health (NIOSH)-sponsored "B" reader program. The development of this credentialing program has been organized by NIOSH, with contractual agreements with the American College of Radiology. The goal is not only to provide standardized and reproducible interpretations of chest radiographs in workers with suspect pneumoconiosis but also to educate and teach physicians about the radiographic features of pneumoconiosis. Physicians who complete the educational program and then successfully interpret these radiographs in a manner reasonably similar to the way a series of "experts" interpreted the radiographs gain a "certificate of competence" in interpreting films (Morgan 1979; Wagner et al. 1992). This "B" reader certification can reasonably be described as challenging, with approximately half of those who take the certification test successfully completing the examination and approximately two-thirds successfully completing the re-certification examination (Wagner et al. 1992). Currently, more than 351 "B" readers are certified.

1.3 Reader Variability and the Diagnosis of Work-Related Lung Disease

To continue with the example of dust disease due to asbestos, many factors can lead to parenchymal changes on the chest radiograph that are identical to the interstitial changes of asbestosis. Explanations for these changes might include radiographic technique, aging, obesity, cigarette smoking, obstructive lung disease, as well as other interstitial lung diseases that may or may not be related to occupational exposures (Dick et al. 1992). Knowing the reason for these relatively frequently occurring "mildly abnormal" findings on the chest radiograph (i.e., category-1 irregular opacities) can be difficult.

Variability in chest radiograph interpretation for classification of the pneumoconioses was initially reported in 1949 (Fletcher and Oldham 1949), long before standardized radiographs were introduced and before the "B" reading program was initiated. Disparities in chest radiographic interpretation for pneumoconiosis are well known among physicians who testify in cases where dust-related disability is adjudicated and among the attorneys who try such cases. Yet, those who must feel the most frustrated in such cases are the workers themselves. It is difficult for the worker to understand how one "B" reader determines the worker has an advanced case of pneumoconiosis only to hear from another "B" reader that there is no evidence of dust disease of the lungs.

Despite the introduction of the "B" reader program, an attempt to introduce reproducibility into the system of radiographic interpretation, variability has continued.

In the decade of the 1970s, Reger and Morgan had 2,337 radiographs evaluated by four readers. The percentage of radiographs interpreted to have complicated coal workers' pneumoconiosis (CWP) ranged from 8.0% to 22.5%. In only 56.7% was there agreement between readers (Reger and Morgan 1970). Felson reviewed more than 55,000 radiographs from coal miners. In these films, reader variation was thought to be primarily due to: (1) poor film quality, (2) inexperience among readers with the ILO classification system, and (3) lack of familiarity with the radiographic features of CWP (Felson et al. 1973). In a review of 674 radiographs of naval dockyard workers, the inter-observer prevalence of pleural changes ranged from 14% to 30% (Sheers et al. 1978).

In the decade of the 1980s, additional concerns were expressed by investigators counting on accurate "B" readings. Parker reported that in 1985 in Minnesota, an initial reading of 566 chest radiographs found 30% of them positive for pleural changes. However, only 4% were considered positive by at least two of three readers from NIOSH interpreting the films under "blind" conditions. In this group, selective over-reading, primarily of women participating in the study, created an illusion of a generalized environmental problem (Parker et al. 1989).

In 1986, 700–750 tire workers participated in a medical screening that included posterior-anterior and right and left oblique radiographs. Of the workers, 439 (approximately 60%) were diagnosed as having abnormal chest radiographs due to inhaled asbestos. Yet, a re-reading by a panel of three "B" readers agreed that 7 (1.6%) had opacities exceeding category 0/1; 8 (1.8 %) had pleural abnormalities, and 1 (0.2%) had both. The first assessment of possible asbestos-related disease showed a prevalence rate greater than 40-fold the rate found at the re-evaluation (Reger et al. 1990).

In the decade of the 1990s, and perhaps in response to the above concerns, NIOSH scheduled a workshop addressing the "B" reader program. After considerable discussion, the workshop participants concluded that: (1) the current "B" reader program should continue; (2) in addition to re-certification every four years, ongoing quality assurance was recommended (however, no clear plan was agreed upon, or to my knowledge, initiated); and (3) within the "B" reader program, or through other approaches, the need to train other medical practitioners in the recognition of pneumoconiosis was recognized. Although not described, the authors stated that plans to improve the program were underway (Attfield and Wagner 1992). The author of an accompanying editorial noted that there was no clear consensus as to what was wrong with the program, and, thus, no clear conception of how to change it could be developed. Workshop attendees voiced support for some quality assurance of "B" readers beyond the certification–re-certification program, but no specific plan to resolve problems was thought to be free of significant problems, and no program was implemented (Balmes 1992).

Several years later, the leadership of the faculty of the Division of Respiratory Diseases Studies Group at NIOSH, the group responsible for administering the "B" reader program, addressed the concerns of variability among "B" readers (Wagner et al. 1993). The NIOSH representatives, as well as a number of others who participated in the "B" reading program, recognized that variability in chest radiographic interpretation can be very damaging to concerned parties. First, it may lead to great differences in the outcomes of epidemiological studies. Second, it can add tremendous burdens to a court system already strapped with an already great number of occupational lung disease cases. They realized that readers may disagree widely and persistently among each other when examining the same radiographs (inter-observer error) and also differ with themselves on repeated readings (intra-observer error). They opined that "the 'B' reading examination has undoubtedly contributed to control of variation among readers in the United States," yet did not reference work showing this to be the case. It is of interest to note that well-trained "lay" readers have been shown to be able to provide reliable classification of pneumoconioses (Copland et al. 1981; Peters et al. 1973).

Others have also shown problems in reproducibility of "B" reader results. Ducatman showed a large variation in the interpretation of small opacities among 23 NIOSH-certified "B" readers. To emphasize this point, he noted a 20-fold difference in the prevalence of positive findings between the readers at the two extremes (Ducatman 1991; Ross 2003).

Disagreements among readers may well be understandable when there is difficulty deciding whether a radiographic diagnosis of pneumoconiosis is truly present when the profusion of opacities is only minimally increased. Yet, it is difficult to understand situations when one "B" reader chooses category-2 profusion of small opacities, while a second "B" reader states that no increase in opacities is noted. Table 1.1 shows a head-to-head comparison between two "B" readers who interpreted the same chest radiographs of coal miners applying for disability and Black Lung benefits. Because of the great disparity between these two readings, such differences cannot be explained by the relatively subtle changes noted at the start of this section. Rather, the concern must be that one of the readers has chosen to deliberately "overread" or "underread" the radiographs.

There has been discussion regarding these disparities. To begin, disparities in chest radiograph interpretation by "B" readers has not escaped the eyes of our legal colleagues. BRICKMAN (2004) has boldly stated "'B' readers and other medical experts are misdiagnosing claimants in order to generate substantial profits. While X-ray readings and medical diagnoses do involve quite subjective judgments, since we are dealing in the aggregate with tens of thousands of X-ray readings, the huge and consistent discrepancies between 'neutral' readers and those profiting from their litigation findings cannot be attributed to 'inter-reader variability.'"

Egilman, an expert witness in areas related to asbestos-related health effects, reported irregularities on the basis of plaintiff lawyers, particularly in the undertaking of mass health "screenings" (EGILMAN 2002; EGILMAN et al. 2004). In cited examples, he reported that more money is paid for an abnormal than normal chest x-ray reading, reading sheets for radiographs less than 0/1 are not completed, and in some cases chest radiographs are "shopped around" to other B-readers until the attorney gets the desired reading. A more recent report has placed the interpretation of chest radiographs by physicians certified as "B" readers, particularly those retained by plaintiff's attorneys, under even closer scrutiny (GITLIN et al. 2004). The authors state that "reinterpretation by six independent consultants of chest radiographs read initially by 'B' readers selected by plaintiffs' counsel failed to confirm the conclusions of the initial readers. Whereas the initial readers interpreted 95.9% of the chest X-rays as positive for parenchymal abnormalities - small opacities profusion category 1/0 or higher - the consultants interpreted the same set of cases as positive in only 4.5%." The authors conclude that the magnitude of the difference in the reading of radiographs is so disparate that the data cannot be attributed to chance. In a guest editorial accompanying this article, the authors write that the report "raises considerable concern as to whether interpretations of chest radiographs rendered by B-reader radiologists acting as expert witnesses and offered as testimony in asbestos-related litigation is non-partisan and clinically accurate" (JANOWER and BERLIN 2004).

In a recent and very worrisome episode drawn from the legal experience, a judge in a consolidated case of silicosis litigants, which included 90 lawsuits from eight U.S. states involving nearly 10,000 cases, expressed serious concern about the difference in "B" reading interpretations. She called their ("B" readers contracted by the plaintiff attorneys) findings "fraudulent and stunning" (http://www.lexisone.com/news/nlibrary/m022205l.html; http://www.caller.com/ccct/editorials/article/0,1641,CCCT_840_3635211,00.html). It appears that in a series of such consolidated suits, be they related

Table 1.1. Variability in chest radiograph interpretation in coal miners by two "B" readers. *S* surface miner, *U* underground miner, *BPP* bilateral pleural plaques, *RPP* right-sided pleural plaque. Assuming a radiograph is considered positive at ILO category 1/0, then the prevalence of pneumoconiosis for reader 1 is 16/19 (84%) and for reader 2 is 3/19 (16%)

Job	Reader 1	Reader 2	Job	Reader 1	Reader 2
26 U	1/2 Q/T, BPP	0/0	10 S	1/1Q/T, BPP	0/1 S/T
15 U, 17 S	2/1 Q/T, BPP	1/1 S/T	8 U	1/1 Q/T	0/1 Q/Q
15 U	2/1 Q/T, RPP	0/1 Q/Q	3 U	1/0 Q/T	0/1 P/R
6 U	1/1 Q/T, BPP	0/0	6 U	0/0	0/0
28 U, 2 S	1/0 Q/T	0/1 Q/Q	27 S	1/1 Q/T	0/0
4 U	1/1 Q/T	0/0	13 S	1/1 Q/T	1/1 Q/T
22 U	0/0	0/0	19 U	1/2 Q/T	0/1 S/T
19 S	1/1 Q/T, BPP	0/0	12 U,15 S	0/0	0/0
15 U	1/1 Q/T	0/0	8 U	1/1 Q/T	0/1 S/T
26 S	2/1 Q/T, RPP	1/1 R/Q			

to the diagnosis of silicosis or asbestosis in workers, very often the same "B" readers are responsible for the diagnoses of pneumoconiosis (http://judiciary.senate.gov/testimony.cfm?id=1362&wit_id=3963; http://www.al.com/specialreport/mobileregister/?asbestos/seekdismissal.html).

1.4 What About Other Techniques for Chest Imaging?

If we accept that difficulties exist in the interpretation of chest radiographs for the classification of pneumoconiosis, are there more accurate imaging procedures available? Specifically, what is the role of thin-section computed tomography (CT) in screening for dust-induced interstitial fibrosis?

Early work showing relationships between asbestosis on the chest radiograph and thin-section CT was done by Katz. He showed parenchymal abnormalities consistent with asbestosis in one-third of asbestos-exposed subjects studied by CT, whereas conventional chest radiographs were abnormal in only 16% (Katz and Kreel 1979). Sperber and Mohan (1984) and Yoshimura et al. (1986) found similar results.

Aberle assessed 100 workers occupationally exposed to asbestos by chest radiograph, pulmonary function tests, and thin-section CT (Aberle et al. 1988). In 55 workers with normal chest radiographs, parenchymal abnormalities were identified in 30% using thin-section CT and considered suggestive of asbestosis in another 20%. There was a significant correlation between increasing abnormality on thin-section CT and decreasing lung volumes, consistent with a restrictive pattern. Similar thin-section CT findings were seen by Staples in asbestos-exposed persons with normal chest radiographs (Staples et al. 1989). The lung parenchyma was suggestive of asbestosis in 57 of the 169 subjects scanned. Additionally, these 57 persons had significantly different lower mean vital capacity and diffusion capacity than 76 individuals with normal thin-section CT scans.

Jarad proposed a scoring system for thin-section CT for pleural fibrosis, pleural disease, and emphysema in asbestos-related disease and tested this approach for reproducibility and inter-observer error (Jarad et al. 1992). Two readers assigned thin-section CT scan scores for fibrosis, emphysema, and pleural disease that differed by less than two categories in 96% and 92% of the scans, compared with 78% and 79% of chest radiographs. In addition, there was less intra-observer error for the thin-section CT scores than for the chest radiograph scores for all disorders.

Ameille compared the oblique chest radiograph to thin-section CT in assessing the prevalence of pleural thickening in workers exposed to low levels of asbestos (individuals employed in university buildings insulated with asbestos-containing material) (Ameille et al. 1993). Pleural thickening was recognized by right anterior oblique radiographs in 23, while thin-section CT showed only equivocal plaques in 3 and doubtful plaques in 3 others. The authors concluded that the use of oblique radiographs was not a good screening tool in this population.

Begin compared chest radiographs of long-term asbestos-exposed workers ranked either 0 or 1 by ILO category with routine thoracic CT scan (Begin et al. 1993). Even without the thin-section CT "cuts", CT scans identified significantly more irregular opacities recognized to be consistent with asbestosis than the chest radiograph, despite the absence of ILO criteria for interpretation of CT scans.

Oksa compared thin-section CT to chest radiographic, asbestos exposure and lung function variables in 21 former asbestos sprayers (Oksa et al. 1994). thin-section CT was superior to chest radiography in detecting parenchymal and pleural changes. In 12 radiographs graded category 0/0, 9 were considered to be positive using thin-section CT scan. Of the 21 sprayers, 19 had pleural plaques by thin-section CT but only 5 using chest radiograph. These authors suggest that asbestos workers with less than 1/0 ILO classification using chest radiograph should have a thin-section CT scan. Similar results were seen in the study by Neri et al. (1994). Asymptomatic shipyard workers (n=70) with "normal" chest radiographs were tested using thin-section CT. Of these, 34 were found to have pleural plaques alone, 6 had parenchymal abnormalities alone, and 13 others had both. No radiological abnormalities were shown in the remaining workers. In addition to showing that pulmonary or pleural changes due to exposure to asbestos can be detected using HRCT prior to the onset of any radiological findings, they also showed that thin-section CT findings were identified prior to the development of clinical symptoms.

Talini compared the usefulness of the thin-section CT scan to the chest radiograph in the diagnosis and assessment of the severity of silicosis (Talini et al. 1995). There was better concordance between readings for thin-section CT with pulmonary function tests and chronic bronchitis compared with the chest radiograph. Concordance for a diagnosis of silicosis between readers was higher for thin-section CT than chest radiography, yet there was no concordance between the chest radiograph and thin-section CT in the early stages of silicosis. This work did not support the hypothesis that thin-section CT is more sensitive than the chest radiograph in the early detection of silicosis.

Murray retrospectively reviewed thin-section CT scans performed at preselected levels in 49 patients exposed to asbestos (Murray et al. 1995). Two teams of thoracic radiologists evaluated: (1) all images, (2) prone images only, and (3) a single prone image through the lung bases for the presence of diffuse interstitial lung disease. A relatively high level of accuracy was obtained with a single prone scan; however, diagnostic accuracy improved to 95% or better when additional prone images were included. Using this approach, a screening study of a relatively large number of workers exposed to asbestos could be performed.

Because there is no developed standardized system for detailing asbestos-related abnormalities by thin-section CT scans, such abnormalities are usually assessed subjectively. Gamsu compared the sensitivity of a subjective semiquantitative scoring system of the extent and severity of asbestosis to a method using an accumulation of the different thin-section CT features of asbestosis in workers with histological proof of disease (Gamsu et al. 1995). He also compared the results of these two thin-section CT methods with chest radiographs in these same workers. Results showed that thin-section CT predicted asbestosis with a higher frequency than chest radiographs classified by the ILO classification and that both the subjective semiquantitative grading system and the method of using an accumulation of features of asbestosis identified using thin-section CT give similar results. Using either or both of these approaches is complementary. Importantly, the authors recognized that asbestosis can be present histologically with a normal or near normal thin-section CT.

The International Expert Meeting on Asbestos, Asbestosis, and Cancer, which took place in Helsinki in 1997, concluded that there was a need for the development of a standardized system for reporting thin-section CT scan results of asbestos-related disorders (similar to the ILO system for chest radiographs), and additional work was needed to show the specificity of lesions of the pleura identified on thin-section CT as markers of asbestos exposure (Asbestos, Asbestosis and Cancer 1997). Yet, this expert meeting concluded that "CT and thin-section CT can facilitate the detection of asbestosis and asbestos-related pleural abnormalities, as well as asbestos-related malignancies; they are not recommended as a screening tool but may be invaluable for individual clinical evaluation and research purposes."

Reliability of thin-section CT scans in detecting discrete pleural lesions was assessed in 100 volunteers employed for at least 10 years in a building with known asbestos contamination (de Raeve et al. 2001). In the first session, pleural abnormalities were detected in 13 subjects. In the second session, the scans were read again by the same radiologist and two other radiologists. The final consensus reading gave a diagnosis of pleural abnormalities in 18 subjects; 8 (44%) were detected by all three readers, 5 (28%) by two readers, and 4 (22%) by only one reader. One scan, rated normal by all readers during the second session, was reconsidered because pleural abnormalities were noted at the first reading. The intra-observer agreement for first reader was good, but the inter observer agreement between the readers was only fair to moderate in the second reading session. In conclusion, when reviewing the prevalence of pleural abnormalities in subjects with low-level exposure, the potential for a lack of consistency in reporting pleural abnormalities should be recognized.

Savranlar compared chest radiography to thin-section CT in 71 coal workers with and without early and low-grade CWP (Savranlar et al. 2004). Of the workers, 4 were excluded because of the presence of progressive massive fibrosis. Profusion categories 0/1 to 1/1 were defined as "early", and 1/2 and 2/2 were "low-grade." Discordance between the chest radiograph and thin-section CT was high. When coal miners with normal chest radiographs were compared with their own thin-section CT scans, 6 of 10 cases were positive using thin-section CT. This led these investigators to suggest that thin-section CT was a better tool to identify early pneumoconiosis.

In the recent American Thoracic Society statement, a chest film clearly showing the characteristic signs of asbestosis in the presence of a compatible history of exposure is adequate for diagnosis (American Thoracic Society 2004). Although conventional CT is superior to the chest radiograph in identifying parenchymal lesions, rounded atelectasis, and pleural plaques, this has been displaced by thin-section CT, as it is more sensitive for detecting parenchymal fibrosis. thin-section CT is perhaps most useful when readers disagree about the presence or absence of abnormalities on the chest radiograph, when chest radiographic findings are borderline, when diminished lung function is identified in association with normal chest radiographic findings, and when pleural abnormalities do not allow a clear interpretation of parenchymal markings. thin-section CT can detect early pleural thickening (i.e., 1–2 mm in thickness) with much more sensitivity than the chest radiograph.

In conclusion, there are numerous examples showing that imaging by thin-section CT scan is more sensitive than the chest radiograph for asbestos effects. However, this advantage has not clearly been shown for other dusts. Furthermore, there may well be substantial variability among thin-section CT scan interpretation even by experienced readers, particularly in the interpretation of pleural abnormalities among asbestos workers. There is no standardized protocol for the interpretation of the thin-section CT when addressing potential dust-induced effects.

The usefulness of any screening test depends on the prevalence of illness within the population, the test accuracy, the seriousness of the condition that might be recognized, patient risks, and cost. Such an assessment of parameters in the context of the use of thin-section CT for screening for dust-induced chest illnesses is beyond the scope of this report. No comments regarding screening for asbestos-related adverse health effects using thin-section CT are provided in the recent American Thoracic Society statement (American Thoracic Society 2004). Determining the role of thin-section CT scan in the screening of dust-induced chest illness is of great interest.

1.5 What Conclusions Should be Made?

Although variability in interpretation of chest radiographs has been recognized for a long time, there appears to be an increasing number of examples of "unexplainably" disparate interpretations by "B" readers. There also appears to be a temporal correlation between asbestos screening programs initiated for legal actions and the number and strength of challenges to the accuracy and integrity of the "B" reading program.

In response to the concern that medically inadequate assessments occur when asbestos screening is done for legal action, the American Association of Occupational and Environmental Clinics stated that (http://www.aoec.org/content/principles_1_3.htm#asbestos):

Screening on the basis of chest radiograph and work history alone does not provide sufficient information to make a firm diagnosis of work-related illness, assess impairment, or guide patient management. An appropriate screening program for asbestos-related lung disease includes: properly chosen and interpreted chest radiographs, reviewed within 1 week of screening; a complete exposure history; symptom review; standardized spirometry; and physical examination. Timely physician disclosure of the results to the patient, appropriate medical follow-up, and patient education are essential. Omission of these features in the asbestos-screening process falls short of the standard of care and ethical practice in occupational health. Perhaps key to the above protocol is the formation of a physician–patient relationship.

Is there a way to guarantee integrity of data collection by the care providers in this process? The standards for lung-function testing are widely available and can be objectively implemented. Yet, it appears that the accuracy of interpretation of radiographs by "B" readers is much more difficult to monitor. Perhaps there are ways to better guarantee the accuracy of a single "B" reader between the re-certification examinations (currently required every 4 years). Any such plan would likely require more frequent monitoring of radiograph interpretation. Perhaps the best first step would be for the leadership of NIOSH to begin a discourse regarding these critical concerns.

Independent of the potential loss of credibility in the interpretation of radiographs in medical disability court cases, without our ability to depend on the integrity of "B" readings, the accurate measurement of dust effects on the radiograph may be lost. If this were to occur, the development of new or changes in existing dust standards essential to protect worker lung health may be at risk.

References

Aberle DR, Gamsu G, Ray CS (1988) High-resolution CT of benign asbestos-related diseases: clinical and radiographic correlation. AJR 151:883-891

Ameille J, Brochard P, Brechot JM et al (1993) Pleural thickening: a comparison of oblique chest radiographs and high-resolution computed tomography in subjects exposed to low levels of asbestos pollution. Int Arch Occup Environ Health 64:545-548

American Thoracic Society (2004) Diagnosis and initial management of nonmalignant diseases related to asbestos. Am J Respir Crit Care Med 170:691-715

Asbestos, Asbestosis, and Cancer (1997) The Helsinki criteria for diagnosis and attribution. Scand J Work Environ Health 23:311-316

Attfield MD, Wagner GR (1992) A report on a workshop on the National Institute for Occupational Safety and Health B reader certification program. J Occup Med 34:875-878

Balmes JR (1992) To B-read or not to B-read. J Occup Med 34:885-886

Begin R, Ostiguy G, Filion R et al (1993) Computed tomography in the early detection of asbestosis. Br J Ind Med 50:689-609

Brickman L (2004) On the theory class's theories of asbestos litigation: the disconnect between scholarship and reality 31. Pepperdine Law Review 33:42

Changing patterns of pneumoconiosis mortality United States 1968-2000 (2004) MMWR Weekly 53:627-632 http://www.cdc.gov/mmwr/index.html

Copland L, Burns J, Jacobsen M (1981) Classification of chest radiographs for epidemiological purposes by people not experienced in the radiology of pneumoconiosis. Br J Ind Med 38:254-261

Davies I, Mann KJ (1948) Proc 9th Int Congress Industrial Med, Bristol, John Wrights, pp 769-772

De Raeve H, Verschakelen JA, Gevenois PA et al (2001) Observer variation in computed tomography of pleural lesions in subjects exposed to indoor asbestos. Eur Respir J 17:916-921

Dick JA, Morgan WKC, Muir DFC et al (1992) The significance of irregular opacities on the chest roentgenogram. Chest 102:251-260

Ducatman AM (1991) Variability in the interpretation of radiographs for asbestosis abnormalities: problems and solutions. Ann NY Acad Sci 643:108-120

Egilman D, Rankin Bohme S (2004) Attorney-directed screenings can be hazardous. Am J Ind Med 45:305-307

Egilman D (2002) Asbestos screenings. Am J Ind Med 42:163

Felson B, Morgan WKC, Bristol LJ et al (1973) Observations on the results of multiple readings of chest films in coal workers' pneumoconiosis. Radiology 109:19-23

Fletcher DM, Oldham PD (1949) The problem of consistent radiological diagnosis in coalminers' pneumoconiosis. Br J Ind Med 6:168-183

Gamsu G, Salmon CJ, Warnock ML, Blanc PD (1995) CT quantification of interstitial fibrosis in patients with asbestosis: a comparison of two methods. AJR 164:63-68

Gitlin JN, Cook LL, Linton OW et al (2004) Comparison of "B" readers interpretation of chest radiographs for asbestos related changed. Acad Radiol 11:843-856

Henry DA (2002) International Labor Office classification system in the age of imaging: relevant or redundant. J Thor Imag 17:179-188

Hering KG, Jacobsen M, Bosch-Galethe E et al (2003) Further development of the International Pneumoconiosis classification - from ILO 1980 to ILO 2000 / German Federal Republic version. Pneumologie 57:576-584

Hessel PA, Melenka LS, Michaelchuk D et al (1998) Lung health among electricians in Edmonton, Alberta, Canada. J Occup Environ Med 40:1007-1012

International Labour Office (1959) Meeting of experts on the international classification of radiographs of the pneumoconioses. Occup Safety Hlth 9:2

Janower ML, Berlin L (2004) 'B' readers' radiographic interpretations in asbestos litigation: is something rotten in the courtroom? Acad Radiol 8:841-842

Jarad NA, Wilkinson P, Pearson MC et al (1992) A new high resolution computed tomography scoring system for pulmonary fibrosis, pleural disease, and emphysema in patients with asbestos related disease. Br J Ind Med 49:73-84

Katz D, Kreel L (1979) Computed tomography in pulmonary asbestosis. Clin Radiol 30:207-213

Morgan RH (1979) Proficiency examination of physicians for classifying pneumoconiosis chest films. AJR Am J Roentgenol 132:803-808

Murray KA, Gamsu G, Webb WR et al (1995) High-resolution computed tomography sampling for detection of asbestos-related lung disease. Acad Radiol 2:111-115

Neri S, Antonelli A, Boraschi P et al (1994) Asbestos-related lesions detected by High-Resolution CT scanning in asymptomatic workers. Specificity, relation to the duration of exposure and cigarette smoking (in Italian). Clin Ter 145:97-106

Oksa P, Suoranta H, Koskinen H et al (1994) High-resolution computed tomography in the early detection of asbestosis. Int Arch Occup Environ Health 65:299-304

Oldham PD (1970) Numerical scoring of radiological simple pneumoconiosis. Inhaled Particles 2:621-632

Parker DL, Bender AP, Hankinson S et al (1989) Public health implications of the variability in the interpretation of "B" readings for pleural changes. J Occup Med 31:775-780

Peters WL, Reger RB, Morgan WKC (1973) The radiographic categorization of coal workers' pneumoconiosis by lay readers. Environ Res 6:60-67

Polakoff PL, Horn BR, Scherer OR (1979) Prevalence of radiographic abnormalities among northern California shipyard workers. Ann NY Acad Sci 330:333-339

Reger RB, Cole WS, Sargent EN, Wheeler PS (1990) Cases of alleged asbestos-related disease: a radiologic re-evaluation. J Occup Med 32:1088-1090

Reger RB, Morgan WKC (1970) On the factors influencing consistency in the radiographic diagnosis of pneumoconiosis. Am Rev Respir Dis 102:905-915

Ross RM (2003) The clinical diagnosis of asbestosis in this century requires more than a chest radiograph. Chest 124:1120-1128

Savranlar A, Altin R, Mahmutyazicioglu K (2004) Comparison of chest radiography and high-resolution computed tomography findings in early and low-grade coal worker's pneumoconiosis. Eur J Radiol 51:175-180

Selikoff IJ, Churg J, Hammond EC (1965) The occurrence among insulation workers in the United States. Ann NY Acad Sci 132:139-155

Selikoff IJ, Hammond EC, Seidman H (1980) Latency of asbestos disease among insulation workers in the United States and Canada. Cancer 46:2736-2740

Sheers G, Rossiter CE, Gilson JC et al (1978) U.K. naval dockyards asbestos study: radiological methods in the surveillance of workers exposed to asbestos. Br J Ind Med 35:195-203

Sperber M, Mohan KK (1984) Computed tomography - a reliable diagnostic modality in pulmonary asbestosis. Comput Radiol 8:125-132

Staples CA, Gamsu G, Ray CS, Webb WR (1989) High resolution computed tomography and lung function in asbestos-exposed workers with normal chest radiographs. Am Rev Respir Dis 139:1502-1508

Talini D, Paggiaro PL, Falaschi F et al (1995) Chest radiography and high resolution computed tomography in the evaluation of workers exposed to silica dust: relation to functional findings. Occup Environ Med 52:262-247

UICC (1970) Cincinnati classification of the radiographic appearances of pneumoconioses. A cooperative study by the UICC committee. Chest 58:57-67

Virta RL (2003) Worldwide asbestos supply and consumption trends from 1900 to 2000: US Geological Survey Open-File Report 03–83. Reston, Virginia: U.S. Department of the Interior US Geological Survey. Available at http://pubs.usgs.gov/of/2003/of03-083/of03-083.pdf

Wagner GR, Attfield MD, Kennedy RD et al (1992) The NIOSH B reader certification program. An update report. J Occup Med 34:879-884

Wagner GR, Attfield MD, Parker JE (1993) Chest radiography in dust-exposed miners: promise and problems, pitfalls and imperfections. Occup Med 8:127-141

Weill H, Jones R (1975) The chest roentogram as an epidemiologic tool: report of a workshop. Arch Environ Health 30:435-439

Yoshimura H, Hatakeyama M, Otsuji H et al (1986) Pulmonary asbestosis: CT study of curvilinear shadow. Radiology 158:653-658

2 Responses of the Respiratory System to Inhaled Agents

ANDREW CHURG, ANNA RASK-ANDERSEN, ØYVIND OMLAND, and BENOIT NEMERY

2.1 Pathological Reactions to Inhaled Particles and Fibers

ANDREW CHURG

CONTENTS

2.1.1 Introduction 13
2.1.2 Lesions Caused by Metals and Related Compounds 13
2.1.3 Coal Workers' Pneumoconiosis and Related Diseases 17
2.1.4 Silicosis and Other Diseases Caused by Crystalline Silica 19
2.1.4.1 Pathological Features 19
2.1.5 Disease Caused by Non-Asbestos Silicates 20
2.1.6 Asbestos-Related Disease 21
2.1.6.1 Benign Asbestos-Induced Pleural Disease 22
2.1.6.2 Asbestosis 24
2.1.6.3 Carcinoma of the Lung 25
2.1.7 Man-Made Mineral Fibers 26
References 27

2.1.1 Introduction

This chapter describes and illustrates the gross and microscopic features of pathological reactions to inhaled particles and fibers. In assembling such a chapter, one needs to make a decision about whether to classify pathological reaction patterns on a generic basis (for example, diffuse interstitial fibrosis) and then list the agents that might produce such a pattern or to describe patterns seen in response to specific agents. I have adopted the latter approach here, but it is important to recognize that many of the pathological reaction patterns described can be seen with a variety of agents. More details, including descriptions of entities too uncommon to be included here, can be found in CHURG and GREEN (1998), ROGGLI et al. (2004) and CHURG et al. (2005a).

A. CHURG, MD
Department of Pathology, University of British Columbia, 2211 Wesbrook Mall, Vancouver, BC V6T 2B5, Canada

2.1.2 Lesions Caused by Metals and Related Compounds

Metals and related compounds (metal salts, metal oxides) as well as metal fumes (primarily welding fumes) produce a variety of lesions (Table 2.1.1) (KELLEHER et al. 2000). However, there is considerable variation in the frequency with which specific lesions are found with particular agents. For example, macules are seen with many different dusts; whereas, relatively few dusts produce interstitial fibrosis, and many of the reports of interstitial fibrosis are of questionable validity (see below and CHURG and GREEN 1998). Some dusts, such as hard metal and beryllium, operate through immunological mechanisms and produce quite different and fairly distinctive lesions; these are described at greater length.

Table 2.1.1. Dusts that commonly produce macules

Metals	Non-metallic dusts
Aluminum	Most non-asbestos silicates
Antimony	Coal
Barium („Baritosis:“)	Cigarette smoke
Iron („Siderosis“)	Particulate air pollutants
Lanthanum and other rare earths	
Tin („Stannosis“)	
Titanium dioxide	
Welding fumes	
Zirconium	

A *dust macule* is theoretically defined as a nonpalpable nonfibrotic grossly pigmented lesion that microscopically consists of dust, either free or in macrophages, around small airways and vessels (WRIGHT and CHURG 1998 and Fig. 2.1.1). Many metals and related compounds produce dust macules (Table 2.1.1); however, macules may also be seen with exposure to non-metallic dusts, particularly silicates. When macules are found on pathological

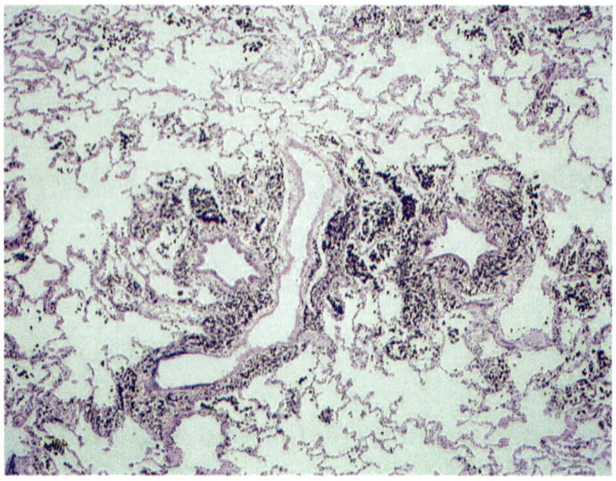

Fig. 2.1.1. Dust macule from the lung of a welder. Note the darkly pigmented dust (iron) that has accumulated in the center of the lobule around the small airways and vessels. There is no significant fibrosis associated with this lesion

examination, or corresponding rounded opacities are present on radiographic examination, specific disease names can be used. For example, in those with iron exposure, the process is called siderosis and, with tin exposure, stannosis. Dusts that produce macules are always more radiodense than air or lung tissues, so that macules appear as fine rounded opacities (simple pneumoconiosis), generally more prominent in the upper zones, on chest radiographs.

On gross examination, dust macules appear as colored "spots" in the centers of the lobules (Fig. 2.1.1); similar (un-named) collections of dust frequently extend along the interlobular septa and pleural lymphatics, and, thus, radiographs may also show Kerley B lines, reflecting collections of dust along interlobular septa. In addition to metals, many other types of dust (coal, silica, silicates, and even cigarette smoke) also produce macules. The exact color of the macule depends on the nature of the dust, and, in fact, the most common macule is the collection of black pigment seen in the centers of lobules in cigarette smokers and many city dwellers, the latter from inhaled particulate air pollutants. Some dusts can produce macules with specific colors, including the red-brown lesions found in hematite (iron ore) miners, the black macules seen in coal miners (Section 2.1.3), the grey lesions caused by tin, and the while macules in those exposed to the paint pigment, titanium oxide.

Macules were originally defined to separate these lesions, which were thought to be nonfibrotic "blemishes" of little functional impact, from the heavily collagenized nodules of silicosis (Wright and Churg 1998), a form of pneumoconiosis that was believed to produce major functional impairment. For this reason, dusts producing only macules were originally considered to be "inert." However, more recent studies have shown that, although macules may initially have little associated fibrosis, with time and/or continued dust accumulation, considerable fibrosis may occur and that, with sufficient exposure, no dust is truly inert. Many dusts that produce macules can also cause fibrosis of the walls of the small airways, presumably as a reaction to the dust accumulating in and around the airways, and the airways may become so distorted and fibrotic as to be almost unrecognizable (Fig. 2.1.2). In addition, enlarged airspaces frequently develop around the fibrotic small airways (Fig. 2.1.2), a process termed focal emphysema.

Focal emphysema is in many ways similar to the centrilobular emphysema seen in cigarette smokers, and it is likely that the combination of distorted small airways and focal emphysema is responsible for the finding of airflow obstruction that is now recognized as a consequence of high levels of dust exposure in some individuals (Churg et al. 1985; Wright et al. 1992; Churg and Wright 2003; Becklake 1985, 1989a,b; Oxman et al. 1993; Garshick et al. 1996; Dimich-Ward et al. 1996). It should be emphasized, however, that the usual cause of airflow obstruction is cigarette smoking and that only a small minority of dust exposed workers appear to develop clinically significant airflow obstruction as a result of the dust (Garshick et al. 1996; Guidotti 1998). It is possible that cigarette smoke and dusts interact in

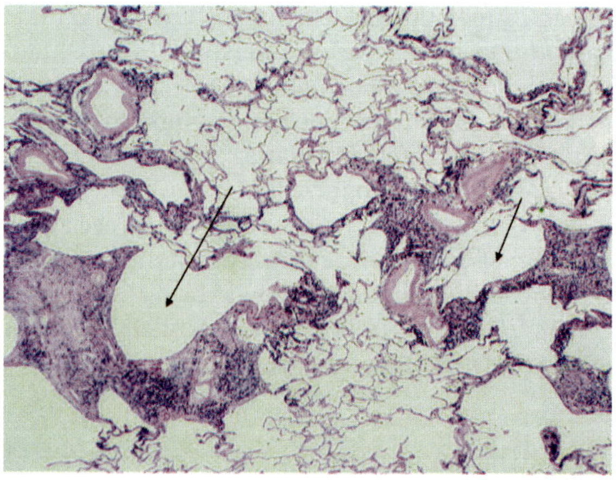

Fig. 2.1.2. Fibrotic macule from the lung of a hematite (iron-ore) miner. In contrast to figure 2.1.1, there is both marked fibrosis and focal emphysema (*arrows*). Lesions of this type may cause airflow obstruction

this regard, since both agents produce lesions in the same location.

Interstitial fibrosis: diffuse interstitial fibrosis is an uncommon finding in workers exposed to metals and related compounds. Because diffuse interstitial fibrosis is a fairly common disease in the general population, it is unclear in many instances whether dust exposure is really the cause of the lesions in a given individual. This is true of the few case reports of workers exposed to rare earths (Vocaturo et al. 1983), copper (so-called "vineyard sprayer's lung" (Villar 1974; Pimental and Marques 1969), and dental technician's pneumoconiosis, a condition seen in workers who make dental prostheses using chromium, cobalt, molybdenum, beryllium, or nickel (Nayebzadeh et al. 1999). Chest roentgenographs have been reported as showing reticulonodular infiltrates; the few pathological specimens have been claimed to resemble berylliosis, silicosis, and hard metal disease (Rom et al. 1984; Brancaleone et al. 1998; Kronengberger et al. 1981; Carles et al. 1978).

However, true diffuse interstitial fibrosis does appear to occur with exposure to beryllium (see below), aluminum (rarely), cobalt/hard metal (see below), silicon carbide (Funahashi et al. 1984; Masse et al. 1986), and probably in a few individuals exposed to very large amounts of iron, particularly from welding (Kelleher et al. 2000). For aluminum, silicon carbide, and iron, the major pathological findings are a combination of diffuse interstitial fibrosis and huge amounts of dust. Inhaled iron particles can be separated from endogenous iron because the former become ferruginated; i.e., they are phagocytized by macrophages and coated with an iron-containing protein that stains with the usual Prussian blue iron stain. In contrast, the inhaled iron particles themselves do not stain with ordinary histochemical stains for iron.

Hard Metal Disease and Disease Caused by Cobalt: Hard metal (cemented tungsten carbide with cobalt) is an extremely hard synthetic compound used in tool bits, drills, and bearings that operate in conditions requiring strength and rigidity at high temperatures (Coates and Watson 1971; Bech et al. 1962). Hard metal is prepared by heating finely divided tungsten and carbon to form tungsten carbide; then cobalt and sometimes other metals are added, and the mixture is fused at a high temperature to form the final product. The fabrication process generates a very fine dust (Coates and Watson 1971; Bech et al. 1962). While most cases of hard metal disease have been described in production workers, disease is also found in those who file or grind hard metal tools for actual use, for example, in some saw mill workers (Kennedy et al. 1995). The sensitizing agent is not the tungsten carbide but the cobalt, and cobalt can be extracted from the metal by liquid lubricants used to cool the work piece; thus, aerosolized coolants are also a source of disease (Sjogren et al. 1980; Cugell 1992). A disease clinically and morphologically identical to hard metal disease has been reported in diamond polishers who use a polishing agent containing cobalt but not hard metal (Demedts et al. 1984).

Hard metal exposure can produce adult respiratory distress syndrome, contact dermatitis, occupational asthma, a syndrome resembling extrinsic allergic alveolitis (hypersensitivity pneumonia), and a distinctive form of interstitial fibrosis (Cugell 1992; Cirla 1994; Chiappino 1994; Migliori 1994). Pathological descriptions exist only for the interstitial fibrosing process, and here the typical picture is that of interstitial fibrosis and interstitial inflammation that is predominantly centrilobular in distribution, accompanied by a desquamative interstitial pneumonia or a giant cell interstitial pneumonia-like picture (Fig. 2.1.3). Giant cells are not seen in every case but when present may be extremely large (Fig. 2.1.3) (Coates and Watson 1971; Davison et al. 1983). Early disease confined to the centrilobular regions appears as ground glass nodules on thin-section computed tomography. With continued exposure, the process spreads, linking centrilobular regions (Fig. 2.1.3). Honeycombing and diffuse severe fibrosis may be seen in very advanced cases.

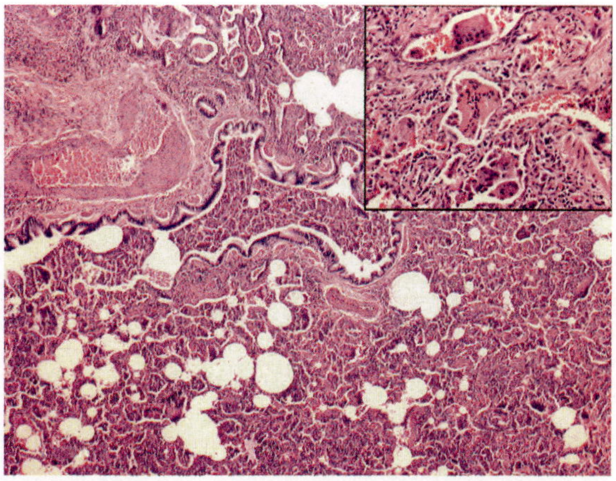

Fig. 2.1.3. Hard metal disease. The lower power view shows fairly advanced diffuse interstitial inflammation and fibrosis with numerous airspace macrophages and giant cells. The inset shows several very large giant cells

The histological picture in classic cases is diagnostic. Black particulate material is sometimes seen in macrophages and giant cells but is never abundant. When the history of exposure is uncertain, tungsten particles can usually be demonstrated by energy dispersive X-ray spectroscopy of histological sections or dissolved tissue, and their presence confirms the diagnosis, since tungsten is never found as a background atmospheric contaminant in the general population. Particles of cobalt may also be found but are less common because cobalt is soluble in tissue fluid (Coates and Watson 1971; Bech et al. 1962; Davison et al. 1983).

Berylliosis: Beryllium and beryllium alloys are used in a variety of applications requiring lightness, strength, and high resistance to fatigue. While berylliosis was prevalent in industries using beryllium prior to 1950 (Sprince 1986), most cases are now seen in workers in the few factories that produce beryllium alloys (Kelleher et al. 2000). Because berylliosis is a form of hypersensitivity reaction, disease may be seen not only in those handling or machining beryllium-containing materials but also in those in the same factory who have no direct contact.

Beryllium disease occurs in acute and chronic forms. Acute berylliosis is a form of adult respiratory distress syndrome and for all practical purposes is no longer seen, since it only occurs with high exposure.

Chronic berylliosis is a systemic granulomatous disease in which the lung is the primary target, and morphologically it is identical to sarcoidosis. Microscopically, one finds noncaseating granulomas that tend to follow the bronchovascular bundles (Fig. 2.1.4). As is true of sarcoidosis, the granulomas may coalesce to produce nodular lesions that gradually scar. In advanced cases, diffuse interstitial fibrosis and honeycombing may be observed (Churg and Colby 1998; Freiman and Hardy 1970). As is true of sarcoid, beryllium granulomas may also be found in hilar lymph nodes and in extrapulmonary sites, including the skin, liver, spleen, pancreas, kidney, adrenals, bone marrow, muscle, and central nervous system (Churg and Colby 1998). There is contradictory evidence for an increased risk of lung cancer in those with beryllium exposure (Saracci 1991; Levy et al. 2002; Hayes 1997; Steenland et al. 1996).

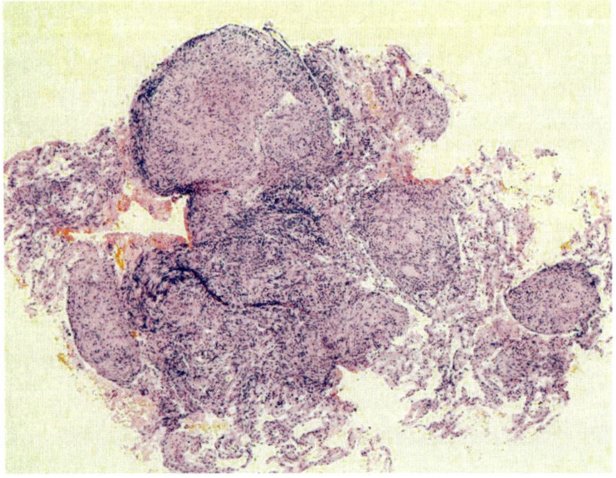

Fig. 2.1.4. Berylliosis. This image is from a transbronchial biopsy and shows several noncaseating granulomas. Histologically this appearance is identical to sarcoidosis

A good history of exposure is important in making the diagnosis. Beryllium lymphocyte proliferation testing (blast transformation and proliferation of a patient's peripheral blood lymphocytes on exposure to beryllium compounds) is valuable as an adjunct to diagnosis and for population screening (Jones and Williams 1983; Kelleher et al. 2000); however, while these tests show beryllium sensitization, it is as yet unclear whether they necessarily indicate the presence of disease. A variety of chemical techniques are available for documenting the amount of beryllium in lung tissue and urine (Churg and Colby 1998), and beryllium particles can also be demonstrated in paraffin tissue sections using atmospheric thin window energy dispersive X-ray spectroscopy (Butnor et al. 2003).

Lung Cancer: Lung cancer has been accepted or proposed to be associated with exposure to a variety of metals and other inhaled dusts (reviewed in Hayes 1997; Steenland et al. 1996) (Table 2.1.2).

Table 2.1.2. Agents producing carcinoma of the lung in humans

Agent
Accepted/probable carcinogens/exposures
Asbestos
Arsenic
Beryllium
Chromates
Chloromethyl ether
Nickel
Radon and radon daughters
Silica
Smelting (arsenic exposure)
Possible carcinogens/exposures
Aluminum pot-room work
Cadmium
Foundry work
Iron mining
Silicon carbide manufacture
Welding

Many of these associations are controversial. From the point of view of pathological examination, there is usually nothing that would indicate that a particular lung cancer is associated with a particular occupational exposure, and questions of attribution are purely epidemiological. Although arguments have been made about specific locations within the lung or specific histological cell types being indicators of particular causative agents, careful review has shown that neither location nor cell type have any value in assigning causation (Ives et al. 1983; Churg 1994a). The one exception is the presence of asbestosis, which strongly associates a lung cancer with asbestos exposure (Section 2.1.6).

2.1.3 Coal Workers' Pneumoconiosis and Related Diseases

The diseases associated with coal mining are listed in Table 2.1.3, a compilation from a large US autopsy population called the National Coal Workers Autopsy Study (Green 1998). Coal workers' pneumoconiosis (CWP), which encompasses simple and complicated forms, is the most commonly diagnosed condition; the process is considered "complicated pneumoconiosis" or "progressive massive fibrosis" when there are pathological or radiographic lesions greater than 1 cm in diameter. Rounded opacities smaller than this size are termed "simple CWP" (Merchant et al. 1986; Parkes 1982; Lapp and Parker 1992; Love and Miller 1982; Attfield and Hodous 1992). This distinction can be of clinical significance: miners with only simple CWP tend to have minimal functional abnormalities, although a small percentage appears to develop clinically significant airflow obstruction. In contrast, miners with complicated CWP (progressive massive fibrosis or PMF) often have pulmonary impairment, and PMF may be associated with premature death (Cochrane 1962; Ortmeyer et al. 1974).

Table 2.1.3. Types of pneumoconiosis found in the National Coal Workers Autopsy Study, 1971-2000 (From Green 1998)

Lesion	Percentage of cases
Macules	46%
Macules plus focal emphysema	36%
Micronodules	19%
Complicated pneumoconiosis	6%
Silicosis	13%

Pleural and Lymphatic Changes: As is true of other dusts, coal-mine dust accumulates in the sub-pleural connective tissues, interlobular septa, and pleural lymphatics in coal miners. The pleural surfaces are often deeply black pigmented, with pigmentation usually greatest in the upper zones of the lung. The peribronchial, hilar, and associated lymph nodes are generally enlarged and densely black on cut surface. Silicotic nodules are commonly observed in lymph nodes in coal miners, typically in the absence of silicotic nodules in the parenchyma (Green et al. 1989). This does not constitute silicosis, which requires the presence of silicotic nodules in the parenchyma.

Coal Dust Macules: Coal dust macules are the most common finding in CWP and are similar to macules associated with other types of dust in that they consist of pigmented lesions ranging in size from 0.5 mm to 6 mm in diameter centered on respiratory bronchioles. They are frequently associated with surrounding focal emphysema (Figs. 2.1.5, 2.1.6). The density of the macules is greatest in the upper zones of the lung but may involve all regions. Microscopically, the coal dust macule is composed of coal dust-containing macrophages and free coal particles in the walls of respiratory bronchioles (Fig. 2.1.6). Over time, the macules become more collagenized (fibrotic). Focal emphysema is seen in both smoking and non-smoking miners, and some require the combination of macules and focal emphysema for a diagnosis of simple CWP (Kleinerman et al. 1979).

Coal Dust Nodules: Coal dust nodules are usually seen in lungs with numerous macules. They tend to be upper zonal and may be centered on respira-

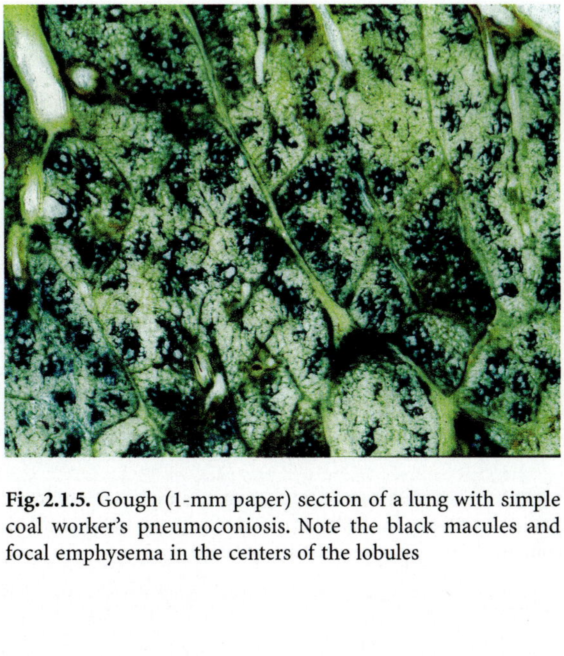

Fig. 2.1.5. Gough (1-mm paper) section of a lung with simple coal worker's pneumoconiosis. Note the black macules and focal emphysema in the centers of the lobules

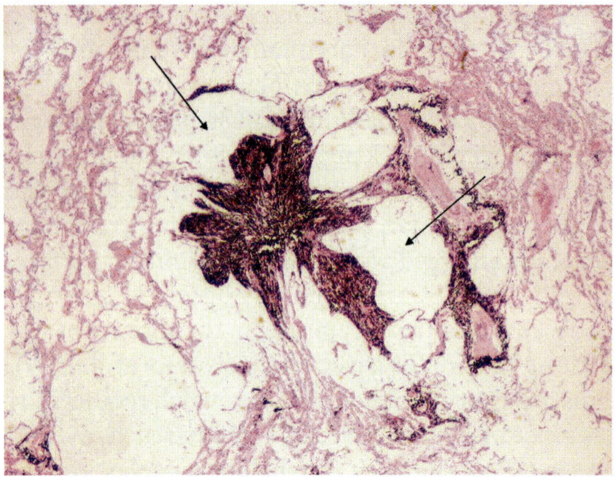

Fig. 2.1.6. Microscopic image of a coal dust macule from a case of simple coal worker's pneumoconiosis. Although the macule represents a fibrotic and distorted respiratory bronchiole, it is impossible to see the underlying airway in this advanced lesion. Focal emphysema is also present (*arrows*)

tory bronchioles; however, they are also frequently seen in the interlobular septa and in the subpleural and peribronchial connective tissues. Nodules are usually distinctly firm to palpation. They tend to have rounded borders and a collagenized center; the greater the silica content, the greater the tendency for the nodules to show concentrically arranged collagen (Fig. 2.1.7). In fact, coal dust nodules probably represent a form of mixed dust fibrosis (coal plus silica).

Progressive Massive Fibrosis: PMF or complicated CWP typically appears on a background of severe simple CWP. PMF lesions are most commonly observed in the upper and posterior portions of the lung and are usually bilateral. They may be round, oval, or irregular and tend to obliterate anatomic boundaries, leading to destruction of the bronchovascular structures and obliteration of interlobular fissures. On cut section, the typical lesion is rubbery to hard, dark black in color (Fig. 2.1.8), and may show cavities of varying sizes containing semi-fluid black contents that can scintillate due to the presence of cholesterol crystals.

Microscopically, PMF lesions show free coal dust, extensive collagen, and macrophages. Necrosis and cavitation are common. Residual outlines of coal dust or silicotic nodules may be observed, although some lesions appear to have little underlying structure. The fibrosing process tends to contract, so that large portions of a lobe may end up as relatively small CWP lesions, and one can often find distorted airways and vessels that disappear into the fibrotic masses; this phenomenon leads to both airflow obstruction, restriction, and pulmonary hypertension.

Rheumatoid Pneumoconiosis (Caplan's Syndrome): Rheumatoid pneumoconiosis occurs in miners with circulating rheumatoid factor but not necessarily evidence of arthritis. It is also seen in workers exposed to silica (Caplan et al. 1962). Radiographic examination typically shows rapidly enlarging, circumscribed nodules ranging in size

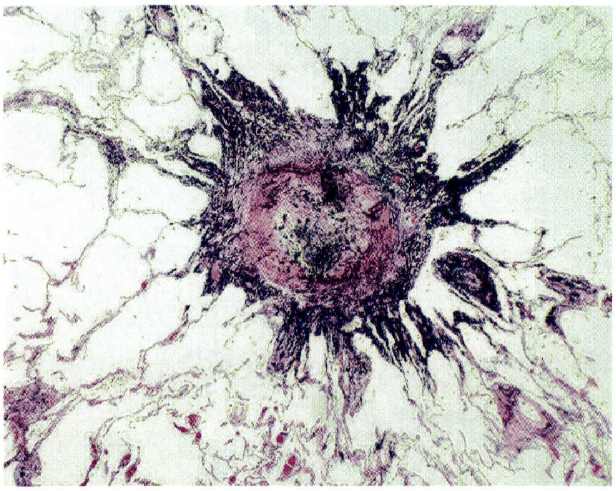

Fig. 2.1.7. Coal dust nodule from a case of simple coal worker's pneumoconiosis. The lesion is rounded with partially whorled collagen in the center and an irregular periphery

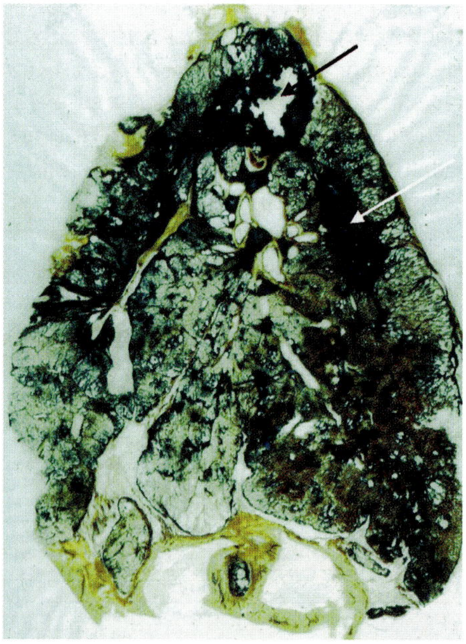

Fig. 2.1.8. Gough (1-mm paper) section of a lung from a worked with complicated coal worker's pneumoconiosis (progressive massive fibrosis). The *arrows* show two large lesions. The lesion in the apex has partially cavitated

from 0.3 cm to 5.0 cm in diameter. Grossly, the nodules are paler and more yellow than PMF lesions and show concentrically arranged dark and light pigmented bands. They may also show central cavitation and calcification.

Microscopically, rheumatoid pneumoconiotic lesions are similar to rheumatoid nodules occurring in the lungs of non-occupationally exposed individuals, except for the presence of rings of coal dust, frequently around the periphery. The central zone is eosinophilic and necrotic, and there is usually a layer of palisaded fibroblasts and macrophages (WAGNER and McCORMICK 1967). It is crucial to rule out infections, particularly tuberculosis, before making a diagnosis of rheumatoid pneumoconiosis.

Silicosis in Coal Workers: Silicotic nodules in the parenchyma are fairly common in coal miners (Table 2.1.3) and are morphologically similar to those seen in silicosis of other causes (Section 2.1.4)

2.1.4 Silicosis and Other Diseases Caused by Crystalline Silica

Silica is silicon dioxide, SiO_2, and "silicosis" is caused by inhalation of crystalline silica. Silicosis has existed for thousands of years and has been found in Egyptian mummies. In industrial times, the disease has been associated with mining, stone cutting, grinding, and sandblasting, although a variety of other occupations are also at risk (GIBBS and WAGNER 1998; CDC/NIOSH 1994; GRAHAM et al. 1991; DUMONTET et al. 1991; O'DONNELL et al. 1991; CAHILL et al. 1992; GROBBELAAR and BATEMAN 1991; NORBOO et al. 1991; BAR-ZIV and GOLDBERG 1974; WHITE et al. 1991). There are several different mineralogical forms of silica that are associated with human disease: these include quartz, tridymite, and cristobalite (GIBBS and WAGNER 1998). There is some suggestion in the literature that cristobalite is more dangerous than other forms of crystalline silica, but this is not clearly established. Amorphous silica, for example, diatomaceous earth, is not by itself pathogenic; however, on calcining, diatomaceous earth is converted to cristobalite. Despite dust restrictions, cases of silicosis are still encountered in industrialized countries; in some third world countries, the incidence of silicosis in some traditional occupations such as grinding is extremely high. Silicosis (and probably high levels of silica exposure as well) predispose one to mycobacterial infections.

2.1.4.1 Pathological Features

Chronic Silicosis: Table 2.1.4 lists the pathological reactions produced by exposure to silica. Simple silicosis (i.e., nodular lesions less than 1 cm in diameter) constitute by far the most common disease. Simple silicotic nodules are rounded, distinctly fibrous lesions (Figs. 2.1.9, 2.1.10) that are sharply demarcated from the surrounding lung parenchyma and that may be pale green, grey, or blue, or, if there is co-exposure to another dust, more distinct pigments. Silicotic nodules are more common in the upper and posterior regions of the lung and are often found scattered in the visceral pleura, the latter often referred to as "candle wax" lesions (CRAIGHEAD et al. 1988). Microscopically, mature simple silicotic nodules show concentrically arranged, whorled bundles of mature hyalinized collagen with variable calcification in the central region (Fig. 2.1.10). The nodule

Table 2.1.4. Pathological reactions to silica

Acute silicosis (silicoproteinosis)
Chronic silicosis
Simple silicosis (nodules)
Complicated pneumoconiosis (massive fibrosis)
Rheumatoid pneumoconiosis (Caplan's syndrome)
Lung cancer*

*Disputed association

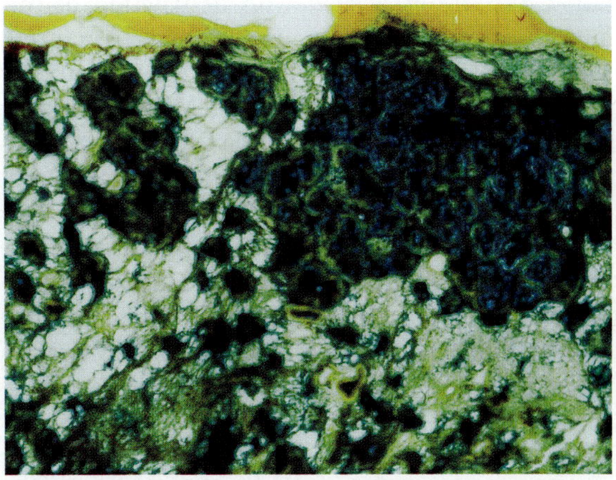

Fig. 2.1.9. Gough (1-mm paper) section of a lung from a worker with simple and complicated silicosis. Note the numerous individual round silicotic nodules. The large lesion on the right is greater than 1 cm in diameter and, thus, represents complicated silicosis. This lesion has formed by conglomeration of individual silicotic nodules

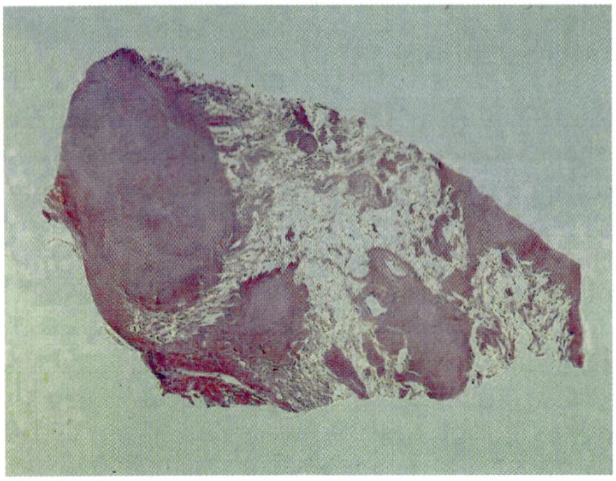

Fig. 2.1.10. Microscopic view of simple silicotic nodules. Note the general sharp borders and eosinophilic centers, the latter indicating the presence of collagen

is usually surrounded by a more cellular periphery, consisting of dust-containing macrophages, fibroblasts, reticulin, and occasional lymphocytes. Polarizing microscopy usually shows poorly birefringent particles consistent with quartz both within the hyalinized nodule and at the periphery; however, silica polarizes poorly in ordinary tissue sections, and, in some instances, the individual particles are below the limit of resolution of the light microscope.

Silicotic PMF or complicated pneumoconiosis consists of lesions with a diameter of 1 cm or more (International Labour Office 1980) (Fig. 2.1.9). As is true with CWP, PMF is usually bilateral and upper to mid-zonal. PMF lesions may undergo cavitation and are associated with destruction of the lung parenchyma and bronchovascular structures. Marked distortion of the adjacent lung is seen due to fibrotic contraction of the lesion. Microscopically, silicotic PMF lesions almost always form on a background of simple pneumoconiosis and, in fact, consist of agglomerated simple silicotic nodules (Fig. 2.1.9).

Accelerated Silicosis and Silicoproteinosis (Acute Silicosis): Classical chronic silicosis takes many years to decades to manifest. However, some patients develop more rapid disease. In accelerated silicosis, there are more cellular nodules that may have a more granulomatous appearance. These consist of histocytic cells enmeshed in a variable amount of mature and immature collagen and reticulin. Hyalinization and circular orientation of the collagen fibers may be seen but are not as well developed as in classic chronic silicosis.

Acute silicosis, or silicoproteinosis, is caused by exposure to high concentrations of freshly fractured silica, usually with very small particle size. Silicoproteinosis has been described in tunnelers, silica flour workers, sand blasters, rock drillers, and workers in the ceramic industry (Davis 1986; Craighead et al. 1988; Gibbs and Wagner 1998). Microscopically, it is characterized by the accumulation of granular proteinaceous fluid containing cholesterol clefts and dense macrophage remnants in the alveolar spaces. Polarization microscopy usually reveals large numbers of weakly birefringent silica particles. A mild chronic inflammatory infiltrate is frequently present. Early silicotic nodules may be seen as well. Most reported cases of acute silicosis have been fatal.

Rheumatoid Pneumoconiosis: Rheumatoid pneumoconiosis or Caplan's syndrome is seen in workers with silica exposure as well as those with coal exposure. Apart from the presence of coal pigment in the lesions in coal workers, the conditions are quite similar in their pathological and radiological appearances (Section 2.1.3).

Emphysema: It has been suggested that there is an association of exposure to high levels of silica and/or silicosis and the development of emphysema, independent of cigarette smoking. However, this idea is controversial (Becklake et al. 1987; Hnizdo et al. 1991, 2000; Hnizdo and Vallyathan 2003; Sharma et al. 1991; Wyndam et al. 1986; Hessel et al. 1990; Cowie and Mabema 1991; Hnizdo 1992).

Silicosis and Lung Cancer: The possible relationship between silica exposure or silicosis and lung cancer is an extremely controversial issue that has yet to be adequately resolved. The International Agency for Research in Cancer classified silica as a group-1 human carcinogen in 1997 (IARC 1997). Epidemiological studies have shown fairly consistently that the presence of radiographic silicosis is associated with an excess incidence of lung cancer, even after accounting for the effects of cigarette smoking (Kurihara and Wada 2004). Whether silica exposure in the absence of silicosis confers an increased risk is much less certain; some studies have found such an association, but others have not (Hughes et al. 2001; McDonald et al. 2001b; Kurihara and Wada 2004).

2.1.5 Disease Caused by Non-Asbestos Silicates

Mineralogy: Silicates consist of silica groups with a cation, such as magnesium, aluminum, etc. Examples of silicate minerals are commonly encountered: talc, mica, vermiculite, and kaolin. Silicates are ubiquitous in the environment, and, in fact, approximately one-third of all mineral species are silicates. They are a constituent of soil, road dust, and building materials and constitute a major component of suspended particulates in the airborne environment. Silicate minerals are used in a large number of industrial processes ranging from paper, paint, drugs, and drilling muds to ceramics and cosmetics. Asbestos fibers are also silicates; however, their fibrous shape confers somewhat different biological properties, and, hence, they are considered separately in section 2.1.7.

Most silicate minerals are highly birefringent and can be easily detected in tissue sections with polarizing microscopy; indeed, the presence of large numbers of highly birefringent particles in histological sections should always raise a question of silicate exposure. Silicates may form ferruginous bodies in tissue sections; that is, silicate particles to which the lung has added a gold-colored iron protein coating, and these can serve as a guide to the nature of the underlying dust (see Churg and Green 1998 for illustrations).

Pure exposures to silicates are relatively uncommon, and many no longer occur; for example, talc is no longer used as a mold-release agent in rubber tire manufacture, a process that, in the past, sometimes led to talcosis (Fig. 2.1.11). In most instances, the lung diseases produced by the (nonasbestos) silicates appear to be relatively benign and only occur in workers exposed to high concentrations of dust over a prolonged period of time; however, diffuse interstitial fibrosis and progressive massive fibrosis, although uncommon, are associated with serious pulmonary disability.

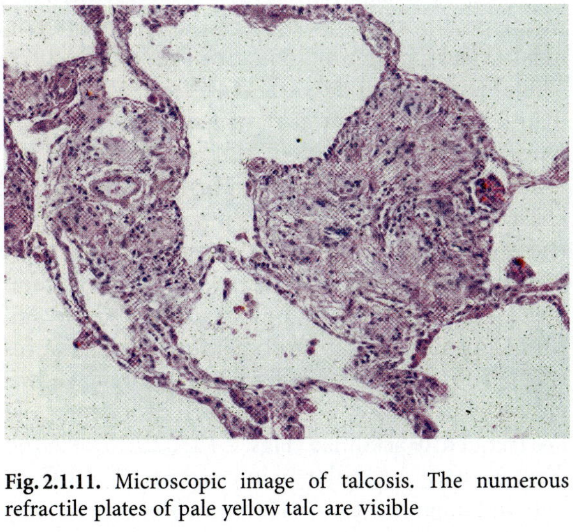

Fig. 2.1.11. Microscopic image of talcosis. The numerous refractile plates of pale yellow talc are visible

Pathological Reactions to Silicate Minerals: Pure silicate exposures can produce a variety of pathological reactions (Table 2.1.5) (Green and Churg 1998), and there is considerable variability from mineral to mineral in regard to the frequency of the reactions observed. Macules are probably the most common finding and are similar to the lesions seen with metal and coal exposure, i.e., collections of dust and dust-laden macrophages around the small airways and vessels. As with metals and coal, silicate macules may become fibrotic. Granulomas are collections of silicate particles that evoke giant cell reactions; when large, these are termed nodules. Diffuse interstitial fibrosis caused by silicate exposure is uncommon but is generally readily recognized because of the presence of innumerable birefringent particles; the classic example of diffuse fibrosis caused by silicates is talcosis (Fig. 2.1.11). Progressive massive fibrosis appears as generally bilateral mid to upper zone mass lesions that microscopically contain collagen and huge numbers of silicate particles. Talc, mica, and kaolin have been reported to cause pleural fibrosis.

Table 2.1.5. Pathological reactions to silicate minerals

Macules
Granulomas
Nodules
Progressive massive fibrosis
Diffuse interstitial fibrosis
Pleural fibrosis

2.1.6 Asbestos-Related Disease

Mineralogy: Asbestos is a name for a set of naturally fibrous silicate minerals. Asbestos minerals have been used because of their high tensile strength, high heat resistance, resistance to chemical attack, and ability to be woven into cloth (Dupres et al. 1984). These properties vary by asbestos fiber type. There are six accepted types of asbestos fibers: namely, chrysotile, amosite, crocidolite, anthophyllite, tremolite, and actinolite. These fibers can be separated into two broad mineralogical groups: chrysotile or amphiboles, the latter including amosite, crocidolite, tremolite, actinolite, and anthophyllite. Table 2.1.6 lists the diseases caused by asbestos. While Table 2.1.6 is correct in broad outline, there are considerable discrepancies in the ability of the different types of asbestos fiber to cause particular diseases, in part based on the chemistry and stability of the fibers (Morgan et al. 1977; Hume and Rimstidt 1992; Churg 1994b; Hodgson and Darnton 2000; McDonald 1990). Chrysotile, for example, only produces malignant pleural mesothelioma at extremely high exposure levels and does not produce peritoneal mesothelioma at all. Amosite and crocidolite are potent mesothelial carcinogens and also cause asbestosis and lung cancer at lower exposures than are required for chrysotile (Hodgson and Darnton 2000; McDonald 1990; Churg et al. 1989, 1990; EPA 2003). The conditions under which a particular type of fiber causes a particular disease are complex and are beyond the scope of this chapter. A variety of tumors not listed in Table 2.1.6 have also been postulated to be caused by asbestos: these include carcinomas of the digestive tract, larynx, kidney, ovary, and lymphomas. These associations are not generally accepted, and these tumors are not discussed here.

Table 2.1.6. Diseases caused by asbestos

Nonneoplastic pleural disease
Pleural effusions
Pleural fibrosis
Pleural plaques
Rounded atelectasis
Nonneoplastic parenchymal disease
Asbestosis
Carcinoma of lung (when asbestosis is present)
Malignant mesothelioma of pleura and peritoneum

Asbestos Bodies: Asbestos occurs in the lung in two forms. Most of the mineral is present as the bare or uncoated fiber, the form in which it was inhaled. However, a minority of fibers acquire a gold-colored iron protein coating in the lung and are then referred to as asbestos bodies. Asbestos bodies are one form of ferruginous body, i.e., exogenous particles and fibers that are coated by macrophages (Churg and Green 1998; Churg and Warnock 1981; Crouch and Churg 1984). Because of the iron protein coating, ordinary histochemical iron stains are an excellent and sensitive method of detecting asbestos bodies in tissue sections. The presence of asbestos bodies in ordinary histological sections is required for the diagnosis of asbestosis using pathological material, but it should be appreciated that, by themselves, asbestos bodies are only markers of exposure. In and of themselves, they do not constitute a disease.

2.1.6.1 Benign Asbestos-Induced Pleural Disease

Terminology: As shown in Table 2.1.6, asbestos induces several different types of benign lesions of the pleura; some authors have referred to the benign pleural lesions as "pleural asbestosis," an incorrect and confusing usage, since asbestosis by definition refers only to asbestos-induced parenchymal fibrosis.

Epidemiological Features: Clinical studies (Gaensler and Kaplan 1971; Epler et al. 1982) indicate that there is a time sequence in the development of asbestos-related pleural disease. Within the first 10 years of exposure, asbestos effusion is relatively common, while pleural fibrosis and pleural plaques are rare. Thereafter, the frequency of fibrosis and plaques increases, although new effusions may still occur (Rudd 1996; Gaensler and Kaplan 1971; Epler et al. 1982). This sequence supports the notion that fibrosis, and possibly plaques as well, are the organized residua of old effusions.

Clinical and pathological features: Asbestos effusion is defined by: (1) a history of exposure to asbestos; (2) pleural effusion, often hemorrhagic; (3) no other disease that would cause pleural effusion; and (4) no malignancy developing in the pleura within 3 years (Gaensler and Kaplan 1971; Epler et al. 1982; Rudd 1996). Many asbestos effusions are asymptomatic; however, in some instances patients present with pleuritic pain, dyspnea, or hemoptysis and show the usual findings associated with an effusion (Gaensler and Kaplan 1971; Epler et al. 1982; BTTA 1972). Microscopically, biopsies of benign asbestos effusions show a combination of fibrin and organizing pleuritis.

In most patients, pleural plaques and pleural fibrosis are asymptomatic, and the disease is essentially an incidental finding noted by the radiologist or pathologist (Sargeant et al. 1977; Solomon et al. 1979, 1984; Begin et al. 1984; Aberle et al. 1988). Pleural plaques appear grossly as flattened or knobbed very hard, commonly calcified, sharply circumscribed lesions on the diaphragmatic (Figs. 2.1.12, 2.1.13) or chest wall pleura and rarely on the visceral pleura (Roberts 1971; Solomon et al. 1979). In contrast, diffuse pleural fibrosis primarily affects the visceral pleural, where it appears grossly as a thickened and fibrotic pleura, often with obliteration of the fissures (Fig. 2.1.14). Microscopically, pleural plaques show a very typical "basket weave" pattern of collagen and are frequently acellular (Figs. 2.1.13, 2.1.15). Pleural fibrosis often is similar in appearance to the findings in benign asbestos effusion; older lesions may

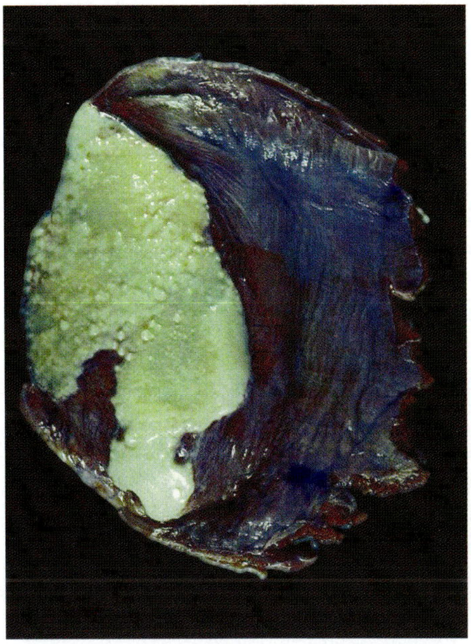

Fig. 2.1.12. Pleural plaque. In this instance, the lesion is situated on the diaphragm, which has been excised at autopsy. Note the typical smooth and knobbly surface. From CHURG and GREEN (1998), used with permission

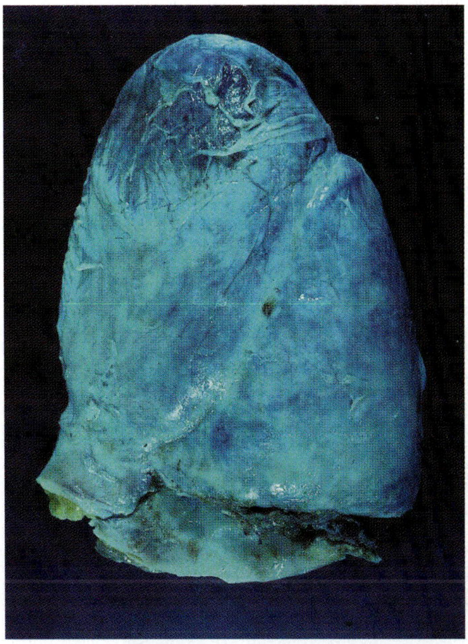

Fig. 2.1.14. Diffuse pleural fibrosis caused by asbestos exposure. Note the thickened pleura and the obliterated fissure. From CHURG and GREEN (1998), used with permission

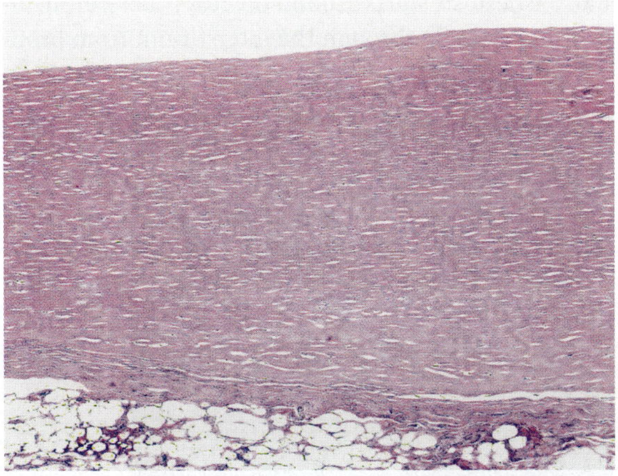

Fig. 2.1.13. Microscopic appearance of a pleural plaque showing the typical basket-weave pattern of collagen

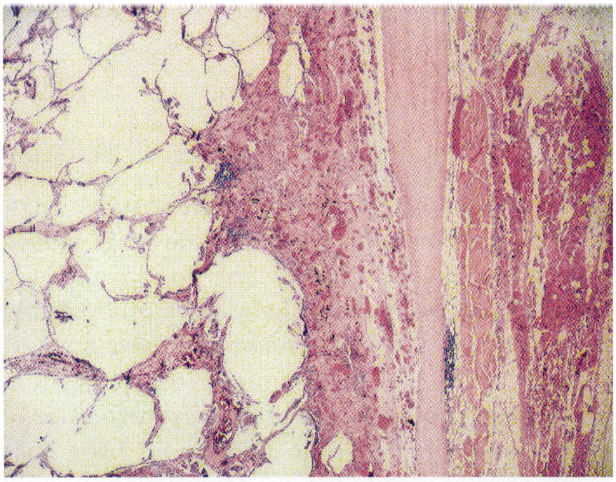

Fig. 2.1.15. Microscopic image showing a pleural plaque (*P*) overlying diffuse asbestos-induced pleural fibrosis (*F*). The visceral and parietal pleurae have fused, and chest wall muscle is visible at the right side of the image

be paucicellular (Fig. 2.1.15). It is not uncommon to find both plaques and pleural fibrosis in the same patient, and, in these instances, the visceral and parietal pleurae are commonly fused by the prior inflammatory process (Fig. 2.1.15).

Rounded atelectasis is a form of scarring of the pleural with contraction to form a pseudo-mass in the underlying lung (HILLERDAL 1989; MINTZER and CUGELL 1982; HILLERDAL and HEMMINGSSON 1980). On gross examination, lungs with rounded atelectasis show an area of retraction of the lung tissue immediately under a fibrosed pleura or pleural plaque. Often there is obvious distortion of the surrounding lung in a more or less semi-circular fashion (Fig. 2.1.16). The histological findings are those of pleural fibrosis and/or pleural plaque.

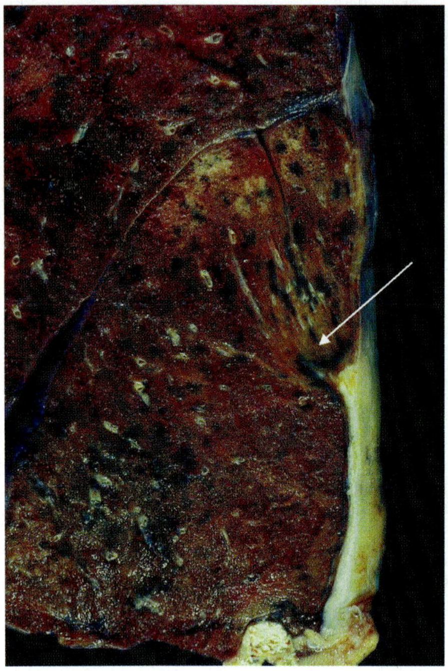

Fig. 2.1.16. Rounded atelectasis. The lesion is caused by pleural scar forming under a plaque with traction and twisting of the underlying lung (*arrow*) to produce a radiographically visible lesion. From Churg and Green (1998), used with permission

2.1.6.2 Asbestosis

Definition and Epidemiology: Asbestosis is bilateral diffuse interstitial fibrosis of the lungs caused by the inhalation of asbestos fibers and is the only condition to which the label "asbestosis" should be applied (ATS 1986; Harber and Smitherman 1991). It is clear from epidemiological studies that the asbestosis is only seen after heavy exposure to asbestos and that there is a threshold fiber dose below which asbestosis is not seen. This threshold dose is in the range of 25–100 fiber/cc per year, with amosite- or crocidolite-induced asbestosis appearing at the low end of the range and chrysotile-induced asbestosis requiring doses of 100 fiber/cc per year or more (Dupres et al. 1984; Brown 1994; Weill 1994; Jacobson et al. 1995). This requirement for a history of high exposure should be kept in mind in diagnosing asbestosis, since it is clear that the disease is frequently overcalled on plain chest films (Gitlin et al. 2004).

Clinical and Pathological Features: Patients with asbestosis usually are clinically similar to those with usual interstitial pneumonia and present with shortness of breath, dry cough, and Velcro rales at the lung bases on inspiration; a restrictive pattern of pulmonary function with small lung volumes, and decreased diffusing capacity is seen in more advanced cases (ATS 1986; Harber and Smitherman 1991; Murphy et al. 1978; Medical Advisory Panel 1982). Most cases of asbestosis can be diagnosed on clinical and historic data, and biopsy is usually reserved for instances in which the clinical features are atypical or the history is obscure.

On gross examination, lungs with asbestosis frequently show diffuse visceral pleural fibrosis, which, as noted, is a separate disease. On cut section, asbestosis shows bilateral diffuse interstitial fibrosis most marked in the lower zones and most severe in the periphery, with relative sparing of the central portions of the lung (Fig. 2.1.17) (Hourihane and McCaughey 1966; Hinson et al. 1973; Craighead et al. 1982). In advanced disease, honeycombing is present. From the point of view of morphology, the gross appearance of asbestosis is not specific and can be exactly mimicked by usual interstitial pneumonia.

Microscopic diagnosis of asbestosis requires (a) diffuse interstitial fibrosis and (b) the presence of asbestos bodies in ordinary 5-μm paraffin sections (Hourihane and McCaughey 1966; Hinson et al. 1973; Craighead et al. 1982; Churg and Green 1998). Early asbestosis starts around the respiratory bronchioles and spreads through the interstitium from bron-

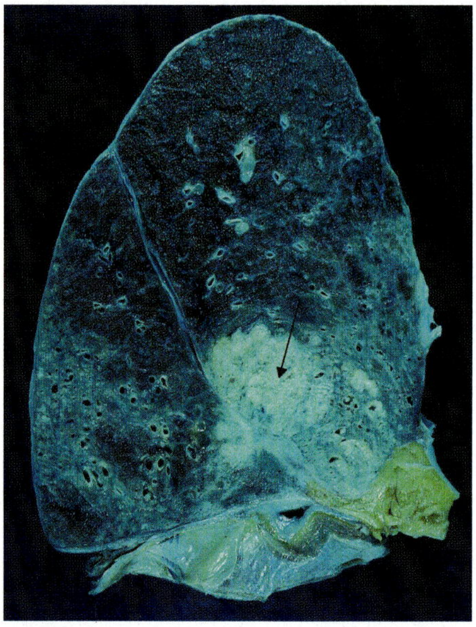

Fig. 2.1.17. Autopsy lung showing asbestosis (diffuse interstitial fibrosis) in the lower zones, along with a large lung cancer (*arrow*). The presence of asbestosis allows one to attribute the lung cancer to asbestos exposure. From Churg and Green (1998), used with permission

chiole to bronchiole; however, in my opinion, fibrosis of the walls of the respiratory bronchioles and alveolar ducts represents a nonspecific reaction to many mineral dusts and is not asbestosis (reviewed in CHURG and WRIGHT 2003). Thus, true interstitial fibrosis must be seen to allow a diagnosis of asbestosis.

In well-established disease, the interstitial process appears as patchy to more confluent diffuse dense interstitial fibrosis, which is paucicellular (Fig. 2.1.18). Asbestosis is often described as microscopically similar to usual interstitial pneumonia. With severe disease, areas of honeycombing are present. Although advanced disease often bears some microscopic resemblance to usual interstitial pneumonia, fibroblast foci are rare in asbestosis. As well, some cases show a more even distribution of fibrosis that mimics nonspecific interstitial pneumonia.

It has been suggested (CRAIGHEAD et al. 1982) that one should observe at least two asbestos bodies in tissue sections before rendering a diagnosis of asbestosis to avoid overdiagnosing asbestosis because of asbestos bodies created by background asbestos exposure to the general population. However, ROGGLI and PRATT (1983) calculated that, at least in North America, the chance of finding an asbestos body from background exposure in an ordinary standard-sized tissue section is on the order of 1% and then only if the section is stained for iron and minutely examined. Thus, the finding of even a single asbestos body in a histological section usually indicates high-level exposure to asbestos and, in the presence of a suitable pattern of diffuse interstitial fibrosis, allows the diagnosis of asbestosis (Fig. 2.1.19). Iron stains are extremely helpful in detecting bodies and should always be used if bodies are not visible in routine preparations.

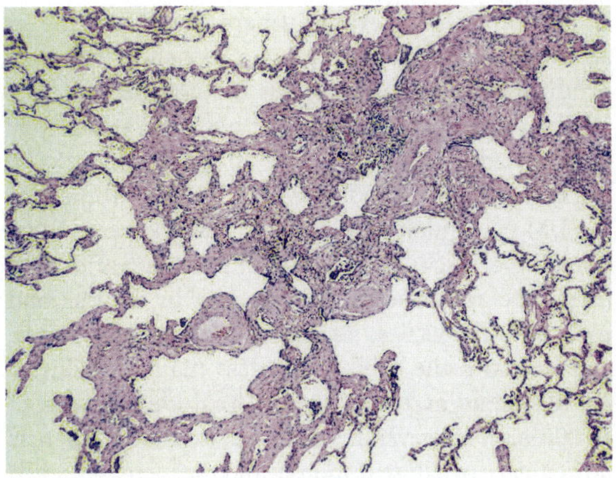

Fig. 2.1.18. Microscopic view of a case of relatively mild asbestosis. Note the pattern of paucicellular diffuse interstitial fibrosis. Asbestos bodies cannot be seen at this low magnification

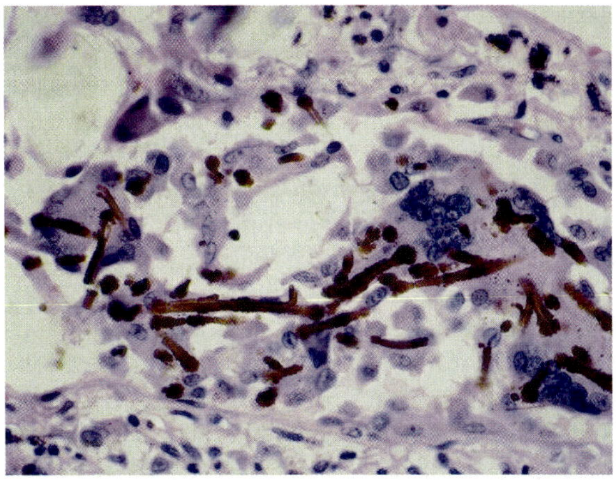

Fig. 2.1.19. Asbestos bodies from another case of asbestosis. Both diffuse interstitial fibrosis and asbestos bodies are required for the pathological diagnosis of asbestosis

As is true of most forms of diffuse interstitial fibrosis (ATS/ERS 2002), transbronchial biopsies are totally unsuitable for diagnosing asbestosis. At a minimum, a large open or thoracoscopic biopsy is required.

2.1.6.3 Carcinoma of the Lung

Epidemiological considerations: Epidemiological studies have established a definite relationship between heavy asbestos exposure and an excess risk of lung cancer (MCDONALD 1980, 1990; HEALTH EFFECTS INSTITUTE 1991; MCDONALD and MCDONALD 1986; EPA 2003). However, the exact relationship between asbestos exposure and the development of lung cancer is controversial. Three schools of thought exist: (1) any exposure to asbestos, no matter how low, increases risk; (2) only a relatively high-level exposure, an exposure in the range that produces asbestosis, increases risk; and (3) only asbestosis itself increases risk (BROWNE 1986a,b; CHURG and Wright 1993; ROGGLI et al. 1994; WEISS 1999; JONES et al. 1996). A detailed discussion of the rationale behind these theories can be found in CHURG and GREEN (1998) and CHURG et al. (2005a). My belief is that only the presence of asbestosis conveys an increased risk, and, therefore, I attribute a lung cancer to asbestos exposure only when there is clinical or pathological evidence of asbestosis (Fig. 2.1.17).

Considerable effort has been devoted in the literature to the proposition that asbestos-associated lung cancers are of a particular histological cell type or have a particular location in the lung. Unfortunately, careful examination of the literature shows that there are no consistent differences in tumor location between tumors arising in workers with asbestos exposure compared with ordinary cigarette smokers (KANNERSTEIN and CHURG 1972; WHITWELL et al. 1974; KARJALAINEN et al. 1993; AUERBACH et al. 1984; JOHANNSON et al. 1992; BRODKIN et al. 1997; LEE et al. 1998; WEISS 2000). Similarly, although individual reports may claim that one cell type or another predominates, there are no consistent differences in histological type between cancers arising in cigarette smokers and workers with asbestos exposure (KANNERSTEIN and CHURG 1972; WHITWELL et al. 1974; KARJALAINEN et al. 1993; AUERBACH et al. 1984; JOHANNSON et al. 1992; BRODKIN et al. 1997; LEE et al. 1998; WEISS 2000; DE KLERK et al. 1996; CHURG 1985 and reviewed in IVES et al. 1983; CHURG 1994a). To make matters more complicated, there has been a secular increase in the frequency of adenocarcinomas and a decrease in the frequency of squamous carcinomas; the former are now the most frequent single type of lung cancer in the US in non-asbestos-exposed cigarette smokers of both sexes (IVES et al. 1983; CHURG 1994a).

Malignant Mesothelioma: As is true of carcinoma of the lung, the exact relationship of malignant mesothelioma and asbestos exposure is complicated (reviewed in CHURG and GREEN 1998; EPA 2003; CHURG et al. 2005a,b). The important issue of differences between chrysotile and amphiboles has been mentioned above.

From the point of view of pathology, malignant mesotheliomas are tumors of the serosal membranes and, thus, surround the lung when they arise in the pleural cavity and surround the abdominal viscera when they arise in the peritoneal cavity (Fig. 2.1.20). Histologically, mesotheliomas show a wide variety of patterns but basically can be broken down into epithelial, sarcomatous, and mixed epithelial and sarcomatous forms. A variety of special immunochemical stains are frequently helpful in making the diagnosis of malignant mesothelioma. Extensive reviews of the pathological requirements for the diagnosis of mesothelioma can be found in CHURG and GREEN (1998) and CHURG et al. (2005a,b).

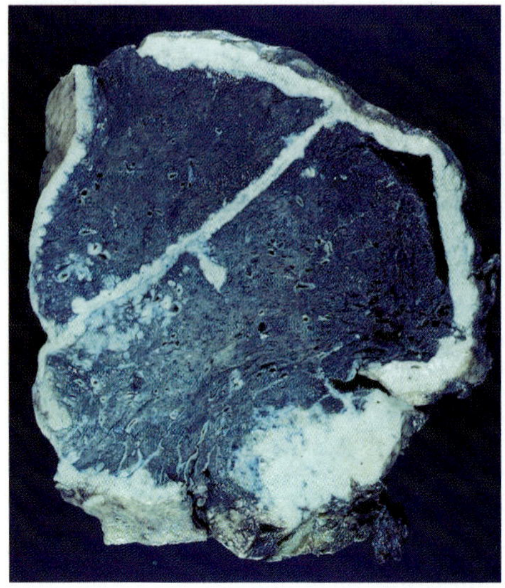

Fig. 2.1.20. Diffuse malignant mesothelioma of the pleura showing the characteristic pattern of tumor surrounding the lung. Tumor also grows down the major fissure

2.1.7 Man-Made Mineral Fibers

Mineralogy: Man-made mineral fibers (MMVF, also called synthetic vitreous fibers) are amorphous silicates that can be separated into several types, including fiberglass (glass wool, glass filaments), rock and slag wool, referred to in the US as "mineral wool," and refractory ceramic fibers. MMVF are used primarily for thermal and acoustic insulation, industrial textiles, specialized filters, and as reinforcing agents. Although inoculation studies in which large numbers of these fibers introduced into the pleural or pericardial cavity of laboratory animals cause malignant mesotheliomas (HESTERBERG and HART 2001), there is no evidence that these fibers cause mesotheliomas in humans (BOFFETTA et al. 1997; MARSH et al. 2001a,b). Refractory ceramic fibers do produce pleural fibrosis in humans (COWIE et al. 2001). Refractory ceramic fibers are fibrogenic in animal models, but there is no evidence that they produce parenchymal fibrosis in humans.

The question of lung cancer has been extensively investigated in very large-scale (approximately 25,000 workers in Europe and more than 32,000 workers in the US) epidemiological studies. There appears to be a small increase in lung cancer deaths that varies with fiber type and process: it is greatest in the slag and rock wool industries, less in the glass wool industry, and lowest in the continuous glass filament industry (HESTERBERG and HART 2001; DOLL 1987; MARSH et al. 2001a,b). However, in most of these studies, there is no evidence of a dose response, and the increases are in some instances nonsignificant when local lung cancer rates are used for comparisons (MARSH et al. 2001a,b), suggesting that the apparent increases may be not real.

References

Aberle D, Gamsu G, Ray CS, Feuerstein IM (1988) Asbestos-related pleural and parenchymal fibrosis detected with high-resolution CT. Radiology 166:729-734

American Thoracic Society (1986) Diagnosis of nonmalignant diseases related to asbestos. Am Rev Respir Dis 134:363-368

ATS/ERS (2002) International Multidiscplinary consensus classification of the idiopathic interstitial pneumonias. Am J Respir Crit Care Med 165:277-304

Attfield MD, Hodous TK (1992) Pulmonary function of U.S. coal miners related to dust exposure estimates. Am Rev Respir Dis 145:605-609

Auerbach O, Garfinkel VA, Joubert L (1984) Histologic type of lung cancer and asbestos exposure. Cancer 54:3017-3021

Bar-Ziv J, Goldberg GM (1974) Simple siliceous pneumoconiosis in Negev bedouins. Arch Environ Health 29:121-126

Bech AO, Kipling MD, Heather JC (1962) Hard metal disease. Br J Indust Med 19:239-252

Becklake MR (1985) Chronic airflow limitation: its relationship to work in dusty occupations. Chest 88:608-617

Becklake MR (1989a) Occupational exposures: evidence for a causal association with chronic obstructive pulmonary disease. Am Rev Respir Dis 140:S85-S91

Becklake MR (1989b) Occupational pollution. Chest 96:372S-378S

Becklake MR, Irwig L, Kielkowski D, Webster I, de Beer M, Landau S (1987) The predictors of emphysema in South African gold miners. Am Rev Respir Dis 135:1234-1241

Begin R, Bergeron D, Cantin A, Berthiaume Y, Peloquin S, Bisson G, Lamoureux G (1984) Radiographic assessment of pleuropulmonary disease in asbestos workers: postero-anterior, four view films, and computed tomograms of the thorax. Br J Indust Med 41:373-383

Boffetta P, Saracci R, Andersen A, Bertazzi PA, Chang-Claude J, Cherrie J, Ferro G (1997) Cancer mortality among man-made vitreous fiber production workers. Epidemiology 8:259-268

Brancaleone P, Weynand B, De Vuyst P, Stanescu D, Pieters T (1998) Lung granulomatosis in a dental technician. Am J Ind Med 34:628-631

Brodkin CA, McCullough J, Stover B, Balmes J, Hammar S, Omenn GS, Checkoway H, Barnhart S (1997) Lobe of origin and histologic type of lung cancer associated with asbestos exposure in the carotene and retinol efficacy trial (CARET). Am J Indust Med 32:582-591

Browne K (1986a) A threshold for asbestos related lung cancer. Br J Indust Med 43:556-558

Browne K (1986b) Is asbestos or asbestosis the cause of the increased risk of lung cancer in asbestos workers. Br J Indust Med 43:145-149

Browne K (1994) Asbestos-related disorders. In: Parkes WR (ed) Occupational lung disorders, 3rd edn. Butterworth-Heinemann, Oxford, pp 411-504

British Thoracic and Tuberculosis Association and the Medical Research Council Pneumoconiosis Unit (1972) A survey of pleural thickening: its relation to asbestos exposure and previous pleural disease. Environ Res 5:142-151

Butnor KJ, Sporn TA, Ingram P, Gunasegaram S, Pinto JF, Roggli VL (2003) Beryllium detection in human lung tissue using electron probe X-ray microanalysis. Modern Pathol 16:1171-1177

Cahill BC, Harmon KR, Shumway SJ, Mickman JK, Hertz MI (1992) Tracheobronchial obstruction due to silicosis. Am Rev Respir Dis 145:719-721

Caplan A, Payne RB, Withey JL (1962) A broader concept of Caplan's Syndrome related to rheumatoid factors. Thorax 17:205-212

Carles P, Fabre J, Pujol M, Duprez A, Bollineilli R (1978) Pneumoconioses complexes chez les prothesistes dentaires. Poumon Coeur 34:189-192

CDC/NIOSH (1994) Work-related lung disease surveillance report, 1994. DHHS (NIOSH) number 94-120, Aug 1994

Churg A (1985) Lung cancer cell type and asbestos exposure. JAMA 253:2984-2985

Churg A (1993) Asbestos, asbestosis, and lung cancer. Modern Pathol 6:509-511

Churg A (1994a) Lung cancer cell type and occupational exposure. In: Samet JM (ed) Epidemiology of lung cancer. Dekker, New York, pp 413-436

Churg A (1994b) Deposition and clearance of chrysotile asbestos. Ann Occup Hyg 38:625-634

Churg A, Colby TV (1998) Diseases caused by metals and related compounds. In: Churg A, Green FHY (eds) Pathology of occupational lung disease, 2nd edn. Williams and Wilkins, Baltimore, pp 77-128

Churg A, Green FHY (1998) Pathology of occupational lung disease, 2nd edn. Williams and Wilkins, Baltimore

Churg A, Warnock ML (1981) Asbestos and other ferruginous bodies. Their formation and clinical significance. Am J Pathol 102:447-456

Churg A, Wright JL (2003) Bronchiolitis caused by occupational and ambient atmospheric particles. Semin Respir Crit Care Med 24:577-584

Churg A, Wright JL, Wiggs B, Pare PD, Lazar N (1985) Small airays disease and mineral dust exposure. Am Rev Respir Dis 131:139-143

Churg A, Wright JL, DePaoli L, Wiggs B (1989) Mineralogic correlates of fibrosis in chrysotile miners and millers. Am Rev Respir Dis 139:891-896

Churg A, Wright J, Wiggs B, DePaoli L (1990) Mineralogic parameters related to amosite asbestos induced fibrosis in man. Am Rev Respir Dis 142:1331-1336

Churg A, Myers J, Tazelaar H, Wright JL (2005a) Thurlbeck's pathology of the lung, 3rd edn. Thieme Medical Publishers, New York, pp 769-862

Churg A, Cagle PT, Roggli VL (2005b) Tumors of the serosal membranes. Fascicles series IV. American Registry of Pathology, Washington DC (in press)

Chiappino G (1994) Hard metal lung disease: clinical aspects. Sci Total Environ 150:65-68

Cirla AM (1994) Cobalt-related asthma. Sci Total Environ 150:85-94

Coates EO, Watson JHL (1971) Diffuse interstitial lung disease in tungsten carbide workers. Ann Intern Med 75:709-716

Cochrane AL (1962) The attack rate of PMF. Br J Indust Med 19:52-62

Cowie RL, Mabema SK (1991) Silicosis, chronic airflow limitation, and chronic bronchitis in South African gold miners. Am Rev Respir Dis 143:80-84

Cowie HA, Wild P, Beck J, Auburtin G, Peikarski C, Massin N, Cherre JW (2001) An epidemiological study of the respiratory health of workers in the European refractory ceramic fiber industry. Occup Environ Med 58:800-810

Craighead JE, Abraham JL, Churg A, Green FHY, Seemayer TE, Vallyathan V, Weill H (1982) The pathology of asbestos-associated diseases of the lungs and pleural cavities: diagnostic criteria and proposed grading schema. Arch Pathol Lab Med 106:544-596

Craighead JE, Kleinerman J, Abraham JL, Gibbs AR, Green FHY, Harley RA, Rüttner JR, Vallyathan V, Juliano EB (1988) Diseases associated with exposure to silica and non-fibrous silicate minerals. Arch Pathol Lab Med 112:673-720

Crouch E, Churg A (1984) Ferruginous bodies and the histologic evaluation of dust exposure. Am J Surg Pathol 8:109-116

Cugell DW (1992) The hard metal diseases. Clin Chest Med 13:269-279

Davis GS (1986) The pathogenesis of silicosis. Chest 89:166S-169S

Davison AG, Haslam PL, Corrin B, Coutts II, Dewar A (1983) Interstitial lung disease and asthma in hard-metal workers: bronchoalveolar lavage, ultrastructural, and analytical findings, and results of bronchial provocation tests. Thorax 38:119-128

Demedts M, Gheysens B, Nagels J, Verbeken E, Lauweryns J, ven der Eeckhout A (1984) Cobalt lung in diamond polishers. Am Rev Respir Dis 130:130-135

De Klerk NH, Musk AW, Eccles JL, Hansen J, Hobbs MST (1996) Exposure to crocidolite and the incidence of different histological types of lung cancer. Occup Environ Med 53:157-159

Dimich-Ward H, Kennedy S, Chan-Yeung M (1996) Occupational exposures and chronic obstructive pulmonary disease. Can Respir J 3:133-140

Doll R (1987) Symposium on MMMF, Copenhagen, Oct 1986: overview and conclusions. Ann Occup Hyg 31:805-819

Dumontet C, Biron F, Vitrey D (1991) Acute silicosis due to inhalation of a domestic product. Am Rev Respir Dis143:880-882

Dupres JS, Mustard JF, Uffen RJ (1984) Report of the Royal Commission on Matters of Health and Safety Arising from the Use of Asbestos in Ontario. Toronto, Queen's Printer for Ontario

EPA (2003) Technical support document for a protocol to assess asbestos-related risk. EPA Documejnt 9345.4-06

Epler GR, McLoud TC, Gaensler EA (1982) Prevalence and incidence of benign asbestos pleural effusion in a working population. JAMA 247:617-622

Freiman DG, Hardy HL (1970) Beryllium disease. The relation of pulmonary pathology to clinical course and prognosis based on a study of 130 cases from the US Beryllium Case Registry. Hum Pathol 1:25-44

Funahashi A, Schlueter DP, Pintar K, Siegesmund KA, Mandel GS, Mandel NS (1984) Pneumoconiosis in workers exposed to silicon carbide. Am Rev Respir Dis 129:635-640

Garshick E, Schenker MB, Dosman JA (1996) Occupationally induced airways obstruction. Med Clin North Am 80:851-878

Gaensler EA, Kaplan AI (1971) Asbestos pleural effusion. Ann Intern Med 74:178-191

Gibbs AR, Wagner JC (1998) Diseases due to silica. In: Churg A, Green FHY (eds) Pathology of occupational lung disease, 2nd edn. Williams and Wilkins, Baltimore, pp 209-234

Gitlin JN, Cook LL, Linton OW, Garrett-Mayer E (2004) Comparison of "B" readers' interpretations of chest radiographs for asbestos related changes. Acad Radiol 11:843-856

Graham WGB, Ashikaga T, Hemenway D, Weaver S, O'Grady RV (1991) Radiographic abnormalities in Vermont granite workers exposed to low levels of granite dust. Chest 100:1507-1514

Green FHY (1998) Coal workers' pneumoconiosis and pneumoconiosis due to other carbonaceous dusts. In: Churg A, Green FHY (eds) Pathology of occupational lung disease, 2nd edn. Williams and Wilkins, Baltimore, pp 129-208

Green FHY, Churg A (1998) Diseases due to non-asbestos silicates. In: Churg A, Green FHY (eds) Pathology of occupational lung disease, 2nd edn. Williams and Wilkins, Baltimore, pp 235-276

Green FHY, Althouse R, Weber KC (1989) Prevalence of silicosis at death in underground coal miners Am J Ind Med 16:605-615

Grobbelaar JP, Bateman ED (1991) Hut lung: a domestically acquired pneumoconiosis of mixed aetiology in rural women. Thorax 46:334-340

Guidotti T (1998) Attribution of chronic airways disease to occupational dust exposures. Appl Occup Environ Hyg 13:576-588

Harber P, Smitherman J (1991) Asbestosis: diagnostic dilution. J Occup Med 33:786-793

Hayes RB (1997) The carcinogenicity of metals in humans. Cancer Causes Control 8:371-385

Health Effects Institute (1991) Asbestos in public and commercial buildings: a literature review and synthesis of current knowledge. Health Effects Institute, Cambridge MA

Hessel PA, Sluis-Cremer GK, Hnizdo E (1990) Silica exposure, silicosis and lung cancer: A necropsy study. Br J Ind Med 47:4-9

Hesterberg TW, Hart GA (2001) Synthetic vitreous fibers: a review of toxicology research and its impact on hazard classification. Crit Rev Toxicol 31:1-53

Hillerdal G (1989) Rounded atelectasis. Clinical experience with 74 patients. Chest 95:836-841

Hillerdal G, Hemmingsson A (1980) Pulmonary pseudotumours and asbestos. Acta Radiol Diag 21:615-620

Hinson KFW, Otto H, Webster I, Rossiter CE (1973) Criteria for the diagnosis and grading of asbestosis. In: Bogovski P, Gilson JC, Timbrell V, Wagner JC (eds) Biological effects of asbestos. Pergamon, Oxford, pp 54-579

Hnizdo E (1992) Loss of lung function associated with exposure to silica dust and with smoking and its relation to disability and mortality in South African gold miners. Br J Ind Med 49:472-479

Hnizdo E, Vallyathan V (2003) Chronic obstructive pulmonary disease due to occupational exposure to silica dust: a review of epidemiological and pathological evidence. Occup Environ Med 60:237-243

Hnizdo E, Sluis-Cremer K, Abramowitz J (1991) Emphysema type in relation to silica dust exposure in South African gold miners. Am Rev Respir Dis 143:1241-1247

Hnizdo E, Murray J, Davison A (2000) Correlation between autopsy findings for chronic obstructive airways disease and in-life disability in South African gold miners. Int Arch Occup Environ Health 73:235-244

Hodgson JT, Darnton A (2000) The quantitative risks of mesothelioma and lung cancer in relation to asbestos exposure. Ann Occup Hyg 44:565-601

Hourihane DO'B, McCaughey WTE (1966) Pathological aspects of asbestosis. Postgrad Med 42:613-622

Hughes JM, Weill H, Rando RJ, Shi R, McDonald AD, McDonald JC (2001) Cohort mortality study of North American industrial sand workers. II. Case-referent analysis of lung cancer and silicosis deaths. Ann Occup Hyg 45:201-207

Hume LA, Rimstidt JD (1992) The biodurability of chrysotile asbestos. Am Mineral 77:1125-1128

IARC Working Group on the Evulation of Carcinogenic Risks to Humans (1997) Silica, some silicates, coal dust and para-aramid fibrils. IARC Monogr Eval Carcinogenic Risks to Humans 68:1-475

International Labor Office (1980) Guidelines for the use of the International classification of radiographs of the pneumoconiosis, rev edn. International Labor Office, Occupational Safety and Health, series no 22 (Ref Revision 80). International Labor Office, Geneva

Ives JC, Buffler PA, Greenberg D (1983) Environmental associations and histopathologic patterns of carcinoma of the lung. Am Rev Respir Dis 128:195-209

Jacobsson K, Stromberg U, Albin M, Welinder H, Hagmar L (1995) Radiological changes in asbestos cement workers. Occup Environ Med 52:20-27

Johannson L, Albin M, Jakobsson K, Mikoczy Z (1992) Histological type of lung carcinoma in asbestos cement workers and matched controls. Br J Indust Med 49:626-630

Jones WW, Williams WR (1983) Value of beryllium lymphocyte transformation tests in chronic beryllium disease and in potentially exposed workers. Thorax 38:41-44

Jones RN, Hughes JM, Weill H (1996) Asbestos exposure, asbestosis, and asbestos-attributable lung cancer. Thorax 51 [Suppl 2]:59-515

Kannerstein M, Churg J (1972) Pathology of carcinoma of the lung associated with asbestos exposure. Cancer 30:14-21

Karjalainen A, Anttila S, Heikkila L, Kyyronen P, Vainio H (1993) Lobe of orogin of lung cancer among asbestos exposed patients with or without diffuse interstitial fibrosis. Scand J Work Environ Hlth 19:102-107

Kelleher P, Pacheco K, Newman LS (2000) Inorganic dust pneumonias: the metal-related parenchymal disorders. Environ Hlth Perspect 108 [Suppl 4]:685-696

Kennedy SM, Chan-Yeung M, Marion S, Lea J, Teschke K (1995) Maintenance of stellite and tungsten carbide saw tips. Occup Environ Med 52:185-191

Kleinerman J, Green FHY, Harley R, Taylor G, Laqueur W, Pratt P, Wyatt S, Naeye R (1979) Pathology standards for coal workers' pneumoconiosis. Arch Pathol Lab Med 103:375-431

Kronenberger H, Morgenroth K, Tuengerthal S (1981) Pneumoconiosis in dental technicians: Clinical, physiological, radiological, and histological findings. Am Rev Respir Dis 123:127

Kurihara N, Wada O (2004) Silicosis and smoking strongly increase lung cancer risk in silica-exposed workers. Ind Health 42:303-314

Lapp NL, Parker JE (1992) Coal workers' pneumoconiosis. Clin Chest Med 13:243-251

Lee BW, Wain JC, Kelsey KT, Wiencke JK, Christiani DC (1998) Association of cigarette smoking and asbestos exposure with location and histology of lung cancer. Am J Respir Crit Care Med 157:748-755

Levy PS, Roth HD, Hwang PM, Powers TE (2002) Beryllium and lung cancer: a reanalysis of a NIOSH cohort mortality study. Inhal Toxicol 14:1003-1015

Love RG, Miller BG (1982) Longitudinal study of lung function in coal miners. Thorax 37:193-197

Marsh GA, Youk AO, Stone RA, Buchanich JM, Gula MJ, Smith TJ, Quinn MM (2001a) Historical cohort study of US man-made vitreous fiber production workers. I. 1992 fiberglass cohort follow-up. J Occup Environ Med 43:741-758

Marsh GA, Gula MJ, Youk AO, Buchanich JM, Churg A, Colby TV (2001b) Historical cohort study of US man-made vitreous fiber production workers. II. Mortality from mesothelioma. J Occup Environ Med 43:757-768

Masse S, Begin R, Cantin A (1986) Pathology of silicon carbide pneumoconiosis. Modern Pathol 1:104-108

McDonald JC (1980) Asbestos and lung cancer: has the case been proven? Chest 78:374-376

McDonald JC (1990) Cancer risks due to asbestos and man-made fibers. Rec Res Cancer Res 120:122-133

McDonald JC, McDonald AD (1986) Epidemiology of asbestos-related lung cancer. In: Antman K, Aisner J (eds) Asbestos-related malignancy. Grune and Stratton, New York, pp 57-79

McDonald JC, Armstrong BG, Edwards CW, Gibbs AR, Lloyd HM, Pooley FD, Ross DJ, Rudd RM (2001a) Case-referent survey of young adults with mesothelioma. I. Lung fiber analyses. Ann Occup Hyg 45:513-518

McDonald AD, McDonald JC, Rando RJ, Hughes JM, Weill H (2001b) Cohort mortality study of North American industrial sand workers. I. Mortality from lung cancer, silicosis and other causes. Ann Occup Hyg 45:193-199

Medical Advisory Panel to the Asbestos International Association (1982) Criteria for the diagnosis of asbestosis and considerations in the attribution of lung cancer and mesothelioma to asbestos exposure. Int Arch Occup Environ Hlth 49:357-361

Merchant JA, Taylor G, Hodous TK (1986) Coal workers' pneumoconiosis and exposure to other carbonaceous dusts. In: Merchant JA, Boehlecke BA, Taylor G, Pickett-Harner M (eds) Occupational respiratory diseases. US Department HHS, PHS, NIOSH, publication no 86-102, pp 329-384

Migliori M, Mosconi G, Michetti G, Belotti L, D'Adda F, Leghissa P, Musitelli O, Cassina G, Motta T, Seghizzi P (1994) Hard metal disease: eight workers with interstitial lung fibrosis due to cobalt exposure. Sci Total Environ 150:187-196

Mintzer RA, Cugell DW (1982) The association of asbestos-induced pleural disease and rounded atelectasis. Chest 81:457-460

Morgan A, Davies P, Wagner JC, Berry G, Holmes A (1977) The biological effects of magnesium-leached chrysotile asbestos. Br J Exp Pathol 58:465-473

Murphy RLJ, Gaensler EA, Ferris BG, Fitzgerald M, Solliday N, Morrisey W (1978) Diagnosis of "asbestosis." Observations from a longitudinal survey of shipyard pipe coverers. Am J Med 65:488-498

Nayebzadeh A, Dufresne A, Harvie S, Begin R (1999) Mineralogy of lung tissue in dental laboratory technicians' pneumoconiosis. Am Ind Hyg Assoc J 60:349-353

Norboo T, Angchuk PT, Yahya M, Kamat SR, Pooley FD, Corrin B, Kerr IH, Bruce N, Ball KP (1991) Silicosis in a Himalayan village population: role of environmental dust. Thorax 46:341-343

O'Donnell AE, Mappin FG, Sebo TJ, Tazelaar H (1991) Interstitial pneumonitis associated with "crack" cocaine abuse. Chest 100:1155-1157

Ortmeyer CE, Costello J, Morgan WKC, Sweckers S, Peterson MR (1974) The mortality of Appalachian coal miners. Arch Environ Health 29:67-72

Oxman AD, Muir DCF, Shannon HS, Stock SR, Hnizdo E, Lange HJ (1993) Occupational dust exposure and chronic

obstructive pulmonary disease: a systematic overview of the evidence. Am Rev Respir Dis 148: 38-48
Parkes WR (1982) Pneumoconiosis due to coal and carbon. In: Parkes WR (ed) Occupational lung disorders. Butterworth-Heinemann, London, pp 175-232
Pimental JC, Marques F (1969) Vineyard sprayer's lung: a new occupational disease. Thorax 24:678-688
Roberts GH (1971) The pathology of parietal pleural plaques. J Clin Pathol 24:348-353
Roggli VL, Pratt PC (1983) Numbers of asbestos bodies on iron-stained sections in relation to asbestos body counts in lung tissue digests. Human Pathol 14:355-361
Roggli VL, Hammar SP, Practt PC, Maddox JC, Legier J, Mark EJ, Brody A (1994) Doses asbestos or asbestosis cause carcinoma of the lung. Am J Indust Med 26:835-838
Roggli VL, Oury TD, Sporn TA (2004) Pathology of asbestos-associated diseases, 2nd edn. Springer, Berlin Heidelberg New York
Rom WN, Lockey JE, Lee JS, Kimball AC, Band KM (1984) Pneumoconiosis and exposures of dental laboratory technicians. Am J Public Health 74:1252-1257
Rudd RM (1996) New developments in asbestos-related pleural disease. Thorax 51:210-216
Saracci R (1991) Beryllium and lung cancer. JNCI 83:1362-1363
Sargeant EN, Jacobson G, Gordonson JS (1977) Pleural plaques: a signpost of asbestos dust inhalation. Semin Roentgenol 12:287-297
Sharma SR, Pande JN, Verma K (1991) Effect of prednisolone treatment in chronic silicosis. Am Rev Respir Dis 143:814-821
Sjogren I, Hillerdal G, Andersson A, Zetterstrom O (1980) Hard metal lung disease: Importance of cobalt in coolants. Thorax 35:653-659
Solomon A, Sluis-Cremer GK, Goldstein B (1979) Visceral pleural plaque formation in asbestosis. Environ Res 19:258-264
Solomon A, Sluis-Cremer GK, Thomas RG, Wright VMF (1984) Calcified plaques on mediastinal pleural reflections associated with asbestos dust exposure: four case reports. Am J Indust Med 6:53-57
Sprince NL (1986) Beryllium disease in occupational respiratory diseases. In: Merchant JA (ed) US Department of Health and Human Services (NIOSH), publication no 86-102, pp 385-400
Steenland K, Loomis D, Shy C, Simonsen N (1996) Review of occupational lung carcinogens. Am J Indust Med 29:474-490
Villar T (1974) Vineyard sprayer's lung. Clinical aspects. Am Rev Respir Dis 110:545-555
Vocaturo G, Colombo F, Zanoni M, Rodi F, Sabbioni E, Pietra R (1983) Human exposure to heavy metals. Rare earth pneumoconiosis in occupational workers. Chest 83:780-782
Wagner JC, McCormick JN (1967) Immunological investigations of coal workers' pneumoconiosis. J R Coll Phys (Lond) 2:49-56
Weill H (1994) Asbestos cement manufacturing. Ann Occup Hyg 38:533-538
Weiss W (1999) Asbestosis: a marker for the increased risk of lung cancer among workers exposed to asbestos. Chest 115:536-549
Weiss W (2000) Asbestosis and lobar site of lung cancer. Occup Environ Med 57:358-360
White NW, Chetty R, Bateman ED (1991) Silicosis among gemstone workers in South Africa: Tigers-eye pneumoconiosis. Am J Ind Med 19:205-213
Whitwell F, Newhouse MD, Bennett DR (1974) A study of the histological cell types of lung cancerin workers suffering from asbestosis. Br J Indust Med 31:298-303
Wright JL, Churg A (1998) Diseases caused by gases and fumes. In: Churg A, Green FHY (eds) Pathology of occupational lung disease, 2nd edn. Williams and Wilkins, Baltimore, pp 57-76
Wright JL, Cagle P, Churg A, Colby TC, Myers J (1992) Disease of the small airways. Am Rev Respir Dis 146:240-262
Wyndham CH, Bezuidenhout BN, Greenacre MJ, Sluis-Cremer GK (1986) Mortality of middle aged white South African gold miners. Br J Ind Med 43:677-684

2.2 Bio-Aerosols and Organic Dusts

Anna Rask-Andersen and Øyvind Omland

CONTENTS

2.2.1 Spectrum of Respiratory Effect *32*
2.2.2 Extrinsic Allergic Alveolitis *32*
2.2.2.1 Etiology *33*
2.2.2.2 Epidemiology *34*
2.2.2.3 Pathogenesis *36*
2.2.2.4 Clinical Aspects *36*
2.2.2.4.1 Symptoms *36*
2.2.2.4.2 Physical Examination *37*
2.2.2.4.3 Laboratory Findings *37*
2.2.2.4.4 Lung Function Tests *37*
2.2.2.4.5 Radiological Findings *38*
2.2.2.4.6 Histopathology *38*
2.2.2.4.7 Immunoserological Studies *38*
2.2.2.4.8 Diagnostic Methods *39*
2.2.2.5 Differential Diagnosis *40*
2.2.2.6 Treatment *41*
2.2.2.7 Prognosis *41*
2.2.2.8 Prevention *41*
2.2.3 Organic Dust Toxic Syndrome *42*
2.2.3.1 Etiology *42*
2.2.3.1.1 Terminology *44*
2.2.3.2 Epidemiology *44*
2.2.3.3 Pathogenesis *46*
2.2.3.4 Clinical Aspects *47*
2.2.3.4.1 Symptoms *47*
2.2.3.4.2 Physical Examination *48*
2.2.3.4.3 Laboratory Findings, Lung Function Tests, Histopathology *48*
2.2.3.5 Differential Diagnosis *49*
2.2.3.6 Treatment *50*
2.2.3.7 Prognosis *50*
2.2.3.8 Prevention *50*
2.2.4 Asthma *50*
2.2.4.1 Definition *50*
2.2.4.1.1 Occupational Asthma *50*
2.2.4.1.2 Outdoor Air Pollution and Asthma *51*
2.2.4.2 Etiology and Epidemiology *51*
2.2.4.2.1 Risk Factors Outside Occupation *51*
2.2.4.2.2 Occupational Exposure *52*
2.2.4.3 Pathogenesis *52*
2.2.4.4 Clinical Aspects *53*
2.2.4.4.1 Symptoms *53*
2.2.4.4.2 Physical Examination *53*
2.2.4.4.3 Laboratory Findings *53*
2.2.4.4.4 Lung Function Tests *53*
2.2.4.4.5 Radiological Findings *53*
2.2.4.4.6 Histopathology *54*
2.2.4.5 Diagnostic Methods and Differential Diagnosis *54*
2.2.4.5.1 Diagnosis Methods of Occupational Asthma *54*
2.2.4.6 Treatment *54*
2.2.5 Chronic Obstructive Pulmonary Disease *54*
2.2.5.1 Definition *54*
2.2.5.2 Occupational COPD *54*
2.2.5.3 Outdoor Air Pollution and COPD *55*
2.2.5.4 Etiology and Epidemiology *55*
2.2.5.4.1 Risk Factors Outside Occupation *55*
2.2.5.4.2 Occupational Exposure *55*
2.2.5.5 Pathogenesis *56*
2.2.5.6 Clinical Aspects *56*
2.2.5.6.1 Symptoms *56*
2.2.5.6.2 Physical Examination *56*
2.2.5.6.3 Laboratory Findings *57*
2.2.5.6.4 Lung Function Tests *57*
2.2.5.7 Radiological Findings *57*
2.2.5.8 Histopathology *57*
2.2.5.8.1 Diagnostic Methods and Differential Diagnosis *57*
2.2.5.8.1 Diagnosis Methods of Occupational COPD *57*
2.2.5.9 Treatment *58*
2.2.6 Prevention *58*
2.2.6.1 Primary Prevention *58*
2.2.6.2 Secondary and Tertiary Prevention *59*
2.2.6.3 Initiating Preventive Activities *59*
2.2.7 Conclusion *59*
References *59*

A bio-aerosol is a suspension in gas of solid or soluble particles of biological origin. Airborne and settled particles of biological origin are often referred to collectively, in the field of occupational hygiene, as organic dust. Bio-aerosol and organic dust exposures may vary qualitatively as well as quantitatively from one occupation or one environment to another. In some bio-aerosol or organic dust exposures, the exposure is primarily biological in origin, but a sig-

A. Rask-Andersen, MD, PhD
Department of Medical Sciences, Occupational and Environmental Medicine, University Hospital, 751 85 Uppsala, Sweden
Ø. Omland, MD, PhD
Department of Environmental and Occupational Medicine, Aalborg Hospital, Århus University Hospital and Institute of Public Health, University of Århus, University Park Building 260, Vennelyst Boulevard 6, 8000 Århus C, Denmark

nificant portion may also be inorganic or mineral in origin, i.e., field dust exposure in farming. In certain types of farming, such dust may contain biologically active material such as silica (LEE et al. 2004), but this chapter is focusing on the potential health effects caused by the organic portion in bio-aerosols and organic dusts.

2.2.1 Spectrum of Respiratory Effect

Respiratory health effects are well-recognized problems after exposure to bio-aerosols and organic dusts. A number of different symptoms and diseases sometimes overlapping each other may affect subject after such exposure. In this chapter, the following illnesses are described:

- Extrinsic allergic alveolitis, also known as hypersensitivity pneumonitis (HP)
- Organic dust toxic syndrome
- Asthma
- Chronic obstructive pulmonary disease (COPD)

Historical Notes

The hazardous effects of inhalation of organic dust has already been reported, in 1555, in Olaus Magnus' masterpiece *Historia de gentibus septentrionalibus*, a history of the northern peoples (OLAUS et al. 1996). In the chapter entitled "Threshing during the winter time," Olaus Magnus described how the dust may damage the vital organs of the threshers. Olaus Magnus emphasized that the dust is so fine that it will almost unnoticeably penetrate into the mouth and accumulate into the throat. If this is not quickly dealt with by drinking fresh ale, the thresher may never again or only for a short period eat what he had threshed, according to Olaus Magnus.

Bernardino Ramazzini reported symptoms from the respiratory tract in flax and hemp carders as well as in sifters and measurers of grain (RAMAZZINI 1700). This reference is often cited incorrectly in terms of date since the second edition of 1713 was translated into English in 1940. In this second edition, Ramazzini added some chapters, but the chapters on organic-dust-induced symptoms were included already in the first edition of *De morbis artificum* published in 1700.

In Iceland, reports appeared during the 18th and 19th centuries concerning a disease called "heysótt" caused by moldy hay (ELIASSON 1982). Despite all knowledge from different countries, however, the danger of exposure to moldy material in farming was forgotten, until it was rediscovered and described by Campbell in 1931 (CAMPBELL 1932). Pepys introduced the name extrinsic allergic alveolitis in 1967 (PEPYS 1967). In the US, the term "extrinsic hypersensitivity pneumonitis" is preferred, since the disease is not only restricted to the alveoli and the parenchyma of the lung, but also affects the small airways. During the 1980s, researchers started to realize that mold dust exposure could also cause benign short-term febrile attacks that could be mistaken for allergic alveolitis, which is a severe lung disease with risk of sequelae. In 1985, it was decided to call these benign febrile attacks caused by inhalation of organic dust the Organic dust toxic syndrome (ODTS) (DOPICO 1986).

Asthma is one work-related respiratory tract disease that may affect farmers and was described for the first time in 1924 (CADHAM 1924). In an analysis of data from the European Community Respiratory Health Survey (ECRHS), the highest risk of asthma attributed to occupation was found for farmers (KOGEVINAS et al. 1999). Other organic dust exposure are also well known risk factors for asthma development (SIGSGAARD and SCHLUNSSEN 2004). A higher prevalence of chronic bronchitis and chronic airflow obstruction has been documented among certain farming populations, such as grain and animal feed workers, than in control subjects.

2.2.2 Extrinsic Allergic Alveolitis

Extrinsic allergic alveolitis or HP is an immunologically mediated inflammatory lung disease in the lung parenchyma induced by the inhalation of either organic or inorganic antigens and characterized by hypersensitivity to the antigens (BOURKE et al. 2001). The prototype for the disease and the most widespread form of allergic alveolitis in the world is farmer's lung disease, caused by inhalation of mold dust from hay, straw or grain. However, allergic alveolitis may be associated with a variety of occupations and exposures (SCHATZ and PATTERSON 1983). The disease is usually named colorfully after the environment in which it occurs and has been reported after over 30 different occupations and environments (ANDO and SUGA 1997). Dust of moldy bagasse thus gives rise to bagassosis, moldy redwood dust to sequeosis (after *Sequoia sempervirens*), dust of moldy cork to suberosis (Cork oak, *Quercus suber*), aerosols from contaminated humidifiers to humidifier lung and so on (Table 2.2.1). Humidifier lung is another type of allergic alveolitis. As working practices change, some syndromes are eradicated, but new etiological agents are recognized and new types of allergic alveolitis are constantly reported. Outbreaks of allergic alveolitis (and asthma) among industrial metal-grinding machinists working with water-based metalworking fluids have frequently been associated with high levels of mycobacteria in the metalworking fluids.

Regardless of the causative agents or its environmental setting, the pathogenesis and clinical manifestations of the disease are similar. This suggests that the sequence of immunopathological events involved in allergic alveolitis is common to all exposures. Usually the disease is caused by inhalation of dust from bacteria and fungi, but inhalation of proteins can also cause allergic alveolitis, for example in bird-fancier's lung, which is due to a serum factor in bird droppings. Inhalation of certain chemical substances, for example isocyanates (Carroll et al. 1996), and intake of certain drugs, for example the antiarrhythmic agent amiodarone, can cause a similar disease (Akoun et al. 1984). Only allergic alveolitis caused by inhalation of bio-aerosols is dealt with in this chapter.

2.2.2.1 Etiology

Extrinsic allergic alveolitis occurs in response to repeated inhalation of a wide variety of organic dusts such as animal proteins, microorganism products and chemical compounds (Girard et al. 2004). These antigens are small enough to reach the alveolar space (<3 μm in diameter). The exposure appears in occupational, home or recreational environments. The first cases of farmer's lung disease described by Campbell in 1932 were associated with moldy hay (Campbell 1932). In the 1960s, Pepys discovered that sera from patients with farmer's lung contained precipitating antibodies against extract from moldy hay (Pepys et al. 1962). Lacey and Lacey found a high concentration of mold dust in the air surrounding persons working with moldy hay (Lacey and Lacey 1964). In 1963, Gregory demonstrated that "farmer's lung hay" had been heated spontaneously during maturation (Gregory and Lacey 1963). In studies during the following year, the same group of researchers found that the antigens in moldy hay were thermophilic molds and actinomycetes, especially *Micropolyspora faeni* (nowadays called *Saccharopolyspora rectivirgula*) and to a lesser extent *Thermoactinomyces* (Pepys and Jenkins 1965; Pepys et al. 1963). Depending on the climate and farming methods, however, there are differences between countries in the flora of the microorganisms in moldy hay (Terho and Lacey 1979). Only about two-thirds of farmers with allergic alveolitis have antibodies to classical farmer's lung antigen (Girard et al. 2004).

In Swedish studies during the 1940s, one of the agents responsible for farmer's lung disease was found to be moldy grain, which was threshed by stationary threshers indoors in barns (Törnell 1946; Bexell and Edfeldt 1949). Moldy straw can also cause the disease (Rask-Andersen 1989b). In Iceland, moldy hay is a major problem, partly as a result of the damp climate and partly because of the manner in which the hay is stacked (Eliasson 1982). In Sweden, forest areas often form part of the farm estates. When oil became expensive during the energy crisis of the 1970s, farmers began to use wood chips for heating purposes. Wood chips stored in stacks easily became moldy and soon gave rise to a new type of allergic alveolitis – wood chips disease. Similar exposure occurs in the paper-mill industry, where large piles of wood chips are stored outside the factories. There have been cases of allergic alveolitis (paper mill worker's lung) in such factories, for example among mechanics repairing technical equipment inside these piles of wood chips (Lindesmith et al. 1988). In Japan, the most common kind of allergic alveolitis is caused by inhalation of seasonal mold that contaminates the home environment (Ando et al. 1991).

Exposure to many birds such as pigeons, parakeets and chicken can cause bird-fancier's lung. Pigeon breeder's disease (PBD) is one of the most common clinical forms of allergic alveolitis and is caused by inhalation of various pigeon-derived materials. Pigeon intestinal mucin has been identified as a major antigen in PBD (Todd et al. 1991). This antigen is a high-molecular-weight glycoprotein comprising 70–80% carbohydrate with a heavily glycosylated protein core and is resistant to degradation (Todd et al. 1991; Calvert et al. 1999).

A characteristic feature of allergic alveolitis is that symptoms occur in a few exposed persons (1–15%) (Bourke et al. 2001; Girard et al. 2004). Not all subjects who are exposed to the antigens associated with allergic alveolitis produce antibodies or develop disease, and individual characteristics may play a role in the development of the disease. During the last couple of years, it has become clear that genetic differences among individuals may be very important in determining the outcome of exposure (Schuyler 2001). Evaluation of major histocompatibility complex (MHC) class-II alleles and tumor necrosis factor alpha (TNF-alpha) promoter suggests that genetic factors located within the MHC region contribute to the development of PBD (Camarena et al. 2001). From case reports of children falling ill with allergic alveolitis, it is known that one-quarter of the cases had a family history of allergic alveolitis, usually involving a sibling or parent with the same exposure (Fink et al. 2005). Environmental cofactors such as virus infections might also be present to trigger the development of the disease (Fink et al. 2005).

Allergic alveolitis can affect an exposed person at any age. Since 1960, 95 cases of allergic alveolitis in children have been communicated in the literature (Fink et al. 2005). The youngest reported case described the onset of symptoms at 8 months. Of the cases, 59% were males and 25% had a family history of HP, usually involving a sibling or parent with the same exposure. Both sexes can be afflicted with allergic alveolitis, but it occurs most commonly in men (Emanuel and Kryda 1983). In Finland, there is higher incidence of farmer's lung disease among women, which is due to fact that Finnish farmers' wives take care of the cattle (Terho et al. 1983).

Farmer's lung has been called a disease of nonsmokers (Warren 1977; Dalphin et al. 1993), like certain inflammatory diseases such as sarcoidosis and ulcerative colitis (Douglas et al. 1986). In healthy farmers, precipitating antibodies to mold antigens are found in a higher frequency among nonsmokers than among smokers (Gruchow et al. 1981; Cormier and Belanger 1985). A reason for this may be changes in the local immunological system in the lungs of smokers (Holt and Keast 1977; Andersen et al. 1982). In mice, nicotine exposure decreases the pulmonary inflammatory response by virtue of its anti-TNF-α effect (Blanchet et al. 2004). Despite that smoking may have a beneficial effect on some inflammatory diseases, it can absolutely not be recommended for prevention. The risks of other devastating and common clinical sequelae of tobacco abuse are overwhelming compared with the low risk of allergic alveolitis, which can be easily prevented in other ways, namely by exposure control. Also, when allergic alveolitis does occur in smokers, it promotes an insidious and more chronic form of the disease and worsens the clinical outcome (Ohtsuka et al. 1995).

There is no overrepresentation of atopy among patients with farmer's lung disease – on the contrary there are fewer atopic subjects among these patients than expected (Hargreave 1973), for the probable reason that an atopic patient with asthma has bronchial hypersensitivity and cannot tolerate the high exposure to dust associated with farmer's lung disease. As early as the 1930s, Campbell drew attention to the fact that the hay that caused respiratory symptoms gave rise to dense clouds of "white" or "hay" dust (Campbell 1932).

There have been reports of a decreased susceptibility to PBD in pregnant women (Chapela et al. 1985). In 17% of 67 women with this disease, the disease was manifested after delivery. It is believed that changes in the immune system during pregnancy cause a relatively hyporeactive condition in the mother, protecting the fetus against rejection. The same mechanism is also operative during pregnancy in rheumatoid arthritis, systemic lupus erythematosus and other connective tissue diseases.

Animals can also be affected with allergic alveolitis and there have been reports of positive precipitins to mold antigens in cattle and horses (Wilkie and Nielsen 1981; Asmundsson et al. 1983).

Examples of allergic alveolitis caused by inhalation of bio-aerosols and organic dusts are listed in Table 2.2.1

2.2.2.2 Epidemiology

Prevalence rates vary widely among countries and are influenced by factors such as climatic, seasonal and geographical conditions; local customs; smoking habits; and differing work practices and processes (Bourke et al. 2001). The first study of the incidence of farmer's lung disease was carried out by Staines and Forman (1961) in three areas of Great Britain. A questionnaire was sent to general practitioners and consultants, and they were asked to report cases of farmer's lung disease. The incidence figures were calculated to be 11.5 per 100,000 of the farmer population in East Anglia, 73.1 per 100,000 in South West England and 193.1 per 100,000 in Wales. A correlation with the summer rainfalls was noted, with an increasing number of farmer's lung cases after a wet spring and rainy summer. Boyd recorded a prevalence of 110 per 100,000 of the farming population in the county of Caithness in Scotland in 1971 (Boyd 1971). This figure was based on the number of

Table 2.2.1. Common forms of allergic alveolitis caused by bio-aerosols and organic dusts

Disease	Antigen source	Probable antigen
Farmer's lung disease	Moldy hay, straw or grain	Thermophilic actinomycetes
		Saccharopolyspora rectivirgula (Micropolyspora faeni)
		Thermoactinomyces vulgaris
		Aspergillus species
Mushroom worker's disease	Moldy compost and mushrooms	Thermophilic actinomycetes
		S. rectivirgula
		T. vulgaris
		Aspergillus species
		Mushroom spores
Suberosis	Moldy cork	Penicillium species
Wood trimmer's disease	Contaminated wood trimmings, at times in sawmills	Rhizopus species
		Mucor species
Pigeon breeder's disease (bird-fancier's lung)	Pigeon droppings	Altered pigeon serum (probably IgA)
	Pigeon bloom (derived from feathers)	
	Pigeon intestinal mucin	
Japanese summer-type hypersensitivity pneumonitis	House dust	Trichosporon cutaneum
		Cryptococcus albidus
Metal-working fluid hypersensitivity pneumonitis	Contaminated metal-working fluid	Pseudomonas species?
		Acinetobacter species?
		Mycobacterium species?

patients referred to hospital and therefore probably included more severe forms of the disease. In a study by Grant (1972) in Scotland, the prevalence of farmer's lung disease was estimated to be 86 per 1,000 in Orkney and Ayrshire and 23 per 1,000 in East Lothian. The diagnosis was based on questionnaires only. Of the farmers, 48 were suspected to have farmer's lung and most of them underwent radiological examination of the lungs, pulmonary function tests and precipitin tests. The majority of the patients had normal results in these tests, which implies that these cases did not fulfill the diagnostic criteria for allergic alveolitis as suggested in 1985 (doPico 1986; Terho 1986). Other authors, using similar investigation methods, have found similar prevalence figures. In 1976, Pether and Greatorex (1976) reported a prevalence of about 23 per 100,00 of the farming population in Somerset, Great Britain. Madsen et al. (1976) noted a history typical of farmer's lung syndrome in 3.9% of the farmers in Utah, United States. Only 13% had precipitating antibodies to *Saccharopolyspora rectivirgula* (formerly *Micropolyspora faeni*) and 28% had abnormal spirograms (Madsen et al. 1976). Katila found a prevalence of farmer's lung of 4% in a Finnish study based on questionnaires reported in 1979 (Katila 1979). Farmer's lung disease was considered to be present if a farmer stated that he had experienced recurrent fever in association with farm work. Recurrent fever was defined as fever with respiratory symptoms occurring three or more times a year during the last 3 years. Of the farmers, 12 were diagnosed as having farmer's lung disease and only 1 had restrictive lung function impairment; 4 had antibodies against *Thermoactinomyces vulgaris*. In a questionnaire study in the French Doubs province, the prevalence of clinical farmer's lung was 1.4% (Dalphin et al. 1993).

Although there is a rather high prevalence of farmer's lung disease when based solely on symptoms reported in questionnaires, it is a rare disease when strictly defined. In 1986, Terho et al presented a Finnish study of the incidence of hospital-diagnosed and clinically confirmed cases of farmer's lung. They found that in 1980 there were 186 new cases of farmer's lung disease in Finland and that in 1981 there were 153. About two-thirds of the patients were women. The mean annual incidence rate of farmer's lung among the entire farming population was 44 per 100,000 persons.

Farmer's lung disease is associated with dairy farming, as shown in a Finnish study, where the highest incidence of this condition has been found in regions with dairy farming (Terho et al. 1980b). The cases of farmer's lung disease occur during October to April, when stored hay is used to feed cattle and the farmers are exposed to mold on repeated occasions daily during the indoor cattle-feeding period (Hapke et al. 1968; Terho et al. 1980b). There is also a yearly variation in the incidence of farmer's lung correlated to rainfall and farming methods (Staines and Forman 1961; Grant et al. 1972; Terho et al. 1983; Vohlonen et al. 1987).

Great differences in the incidence of farmer's lung disease among countries have been thought to depend on variations in climate and farming methods. This is partly true, but the high incidence figures reported by some investigators might be explained by the criteria used for diagnosing farmer's lung, which has meant that cases of ODTS have been included in this condition.

In a clinical study of pigeon breeders in the Canary Islands, the prevalence of PBD was 8% (Rodriguez de Castro et al. 1993) compared with 10.4–31% in Scotland (Banham et al. 1986; Bourke et al. 1989).

It has to be pointed out that allergic alveolitis cannot be diagnosed on questionnaires only since the diagnosis is based on a combination of clinical, radiological and functional findings together with an evaluation of the exposure. Questionnaires are suitable for screening to detect suspected cases. If the patient has seen a doctor, medical records have to be collected and evaluated. If the patient has not sought medical care, it is impossible to diagnose allergic alveolitis retrospectively. In conclusion, large surveys relying upon questionnaires of symptoms and measurement of precipitating antibodies often overestimate the prevalence of allergic alveolitis and correlate poorly with more comprehensive assessments of extrinsic allergic alveolitis based on patients undergoing comprehensive investigations in the hospital; the latter underestimate the true prevalence (Bourke et al. 2001).

2.2.2.3 Pathogenesis

The pathogenesis of allergic alveolitis has been the subject of investigations, but most of the mechanisms involved in the pathogenesis of HP remain incompletely understood (Girard et al. 2004). After Pepys discovered the precipitating antibodies to mold antigens, he suggested that the histopathological changes in the lung in allergic alveolitis were those of an Arthus, or "immune complex"-mediated reaction (type III). This Arthus reaction would explain the appearance of symptoms and clinical signs 4–8 h after antigen exposure and account for the transient presence of neutrophils in bronchoalveolar lavage (BAL) fluid after antigen exposure (Schatz and Patterson 1983). Various arguments have been raised against this theory and greater emphasis has been placed on the role of cell-mediated immune responses. Lack of vasculitis in biopsy material provides strong evidence against an Arthus (type-III) form of allergic tissue injury (Reyes et al. 1982).

Actually, the disease does not fit neatly with one of the four types of allergic reaction. The nature of inflammatory events reflects the stage of the disease. Following inhalation of antigen, a complex formed by soluble antigens and IgG antibodies triggers the complement cascade, and alveolar macrophage activation is induced resulting in an increase of macrophages (Girard et al. 2004). These cells secrete cytokines and chemokines that attract neutrophils in alveoli and small airways (Patel et al. 2001). The number of T-lymphocytes is also increase with a predominance of the CD8+ T-lymphocyte subset resulting in a decrease in the CD4+/CD8+ ratio (in contrast to sarcoidosis there, the reverse is seen) (Girard et al. 2004). Different upregulating mechanisms results in a stronger interaction between macrophages and T cells and a more effective antigen-presenting capacity (Girard et al. 2004). In conclusion, the pathogenesis involves many immunological processes, and recent findings shed light on some of the mechanism, but many concepts remain unclear in this complex immunological disease (Girard et al. 2004).

2.2.2.4 Clinical Aspects

2.2.2.4.1 Symptoms

Cough, dyspnea and fever are the most common symptoms in allergic alveolitis and they have their onset or become worse 4–6 h after exposure to moldy material. The cough may be dry or there may be sputum production. The dyspnea may become so severe that the patient is unable even to walk across a room.

In 1953, Fuller suggested that farmer's lung disease occurred in three different phases (Fuller 1953):

Phase one. The acute attack is characteristically rapid in onset, with a rise in temperature on the evening of the day of exposure. The fever lasts for only 2 days or 3 days and is accompanied by an irritating cough. A few rhonchi and crepitations may be heard. Frontal headache, lassitude and marked anorexia are usually present and can persist for several days after all the chest symptoms have disappeared. A radiograph may show nothing abnormal after a single exposure to moldy material.

Phase two. The symptoms experienced during this phase are increasing breathlessness with a short dry cough. Sputum is sparse and mucopurulent. The patients also complain of feeling shivery at night after exposure to hay dust. On examination, the patient will be breathless, even when undressing, and cyanotic. Crepitations are heard over the lower lobes, and fine alveolar mottling is seen on the chest X-ray. If the patient is removed from contact with dusty hay or straw, he will be quite free from symptoms in 3 months or 4 months.

Phase three. The symptoms and signs in this phase do not differ from those in other forms of pulmonary fibrosis. The patient has exertional dyspnea and, if he comes into contact with moldy material, he will suffer recurrence of the symptoms. There is no clubbing or cyanosis. On the chest X-ray, there are signs of fibrosis in the upper zones of both lungs with emphysema at the bases.

In general the phases suggested by Fuller have been used in a slightly different manner by other authors (Fuller 1953). Three forms are often referred to rather than phases. Often the acute form of allergic alveolitis has been used as a term for more fulminant cases of allergic alveolitis.

The symptoms of what is now often named the organic dust toxic syndrome (ODTS) are very similar to those described by Fuller as phase one of allergic alveolitis. The patients have fever and shivering with an onset 4–8 h after exposure to moldy material. Influenza-like muscular aching, cough, headache and difficulty in breathing occur. Even if the acute symptoms of ODTS can be quite fulminant, the functional changes with a few exceptions are not so pronounced as in allergic alveolitis and, in contrast to the latter disease, the symptoms last only a few days (Emanuel et al. 1975; Pratt and May 1984; Rask-Andersen 1989a).

2.2.2.4.2 Physical Examination

Basal crepitating rales on auscultation of the lungs is a typical clinical finding in allergic alveolitis. In severe cases, the patient may have dyspnea at rest and labial cyanosis.

2.2.2.4.3 Laboratory Findings

Both in allergic alveolitis and in the ODTS there is a leukocytosis with an increase in segmented neutrophil cells (Emanuel and Kryda 1983; Rask-Andersen 1989a, b). The erythrocyte sedimentation rate (ESR) is usually increased. In allergic alveolitis, serum electrophoresis shows signs of light activity with an increase in gammaglobin, haptoglobin and alpha-antitrypsin (Vergnon et al. 1983).

The serum IgE level and the eosinophil count are typically normal, since atopy is not a feature of allergic alveolitis (Salvaggio and Karr 1979).

Angiotensin converting enzyme (ACE) in serum is not usually elevated in allergic alveolitis (McCormick et al. 1981; Tewksbury et al. 1981; Vergnon et al. 1983) in contrast to that in sarcoidosis (Lieberman 1975). However, in some cases of allergic alveolitis, it can be increased (Konig et al. 1981).

Both positive rheumatoid factor (Schatz and Patterson 1983), 1983) and positive antinuclear factor may be found in allergic alveolitis (Tukiainen et al. 1980). Tukiainen et al. (1980) also found hypocalciuria in some patients. Total plasma lactate dehydrogenase is elevated in acute phases of allergic alveolitis (Rask-Andersen 1989b; Matusiewicz et al. 1993).

2.2.2.4.4 Lung Function Tests

Most of the patients with allergic alveolitis show decreased lung function with a typical restrictive pattern (Rankin et al. 1962; Bishop et al. 1963; Williams 1963; Hapke et al. 1968). Obstructive changes have been described, however (Pepys and Jenkins 1965; Warren et al. 1978; Bourke et al. 1989). In addition, there is a decrease in the diffusion capacity (the transfer factor of the lung for carbon monoxide: TL,CO) due to the inflammatory infiltration in the alveolar septa (Williams 1963; Seal et al. 1968; Warren et al. 1978). Lung compliance is reduced, i.e., the lung is stiffer than normal (Williams 1963; Warren et al. 1978). Abnormal function of the small airways has been reported (Warren et al. 1978), as has trapped air (non-ventilated lung volume), which may be caused by small airways occlusion due to bronchiolitis (Sovijarvi et al. 1980). Nitrography has shown an elevation of the alveolar plateau (Rankin et al. 1962). The oxygen tension (PaO) in blood is generally decreased at rest in the acute stage of farmer's lung. However, the typical restrictive pattern in pulmonary function testing may be transient and is not always present.

Bronchial hypersensitivity to inhaled histamine has been observed in one-quarter of patients with farmer's lung during the acute phase of the disease and in one-fifth after rechallenge some months later (Monkare et al. 1981). In a study in Belgium, bronchial hyperreactivity was found in 50% of patients with farmer's lung disease (Freedman and Ault 1981).

2.2.2.4.5 Radiological Findings

In the early stages of allergic alveolitis, the chest radiographs may be normal or may show various degrees of reticulonodular interstitial infiltrates at both lung bases (Ando and Suga 1997). A meta-analysis of available reports showed that only 80% of subjects with acute HP had abnormal chest radiographs (Hodgson et al. 1989).

The typical pattern of the chest X-ray in allergic alveolitis is one of diffuse, fine, nodular shadows, either general or predominantly in the bases. During the early stages in particular, the changes can be so discrete that they are difficult to detect, but widespread patchy opacities may also be seen (Mindell 1970). There are cases of allergic alveolitis with a normal chest X-ray, despite serious lung function disturbances with severe hypoxemia and diffusion impairment (Arshad et al. 1987). In chronic cases, diffuse interstitial fibrosis may be observed, often in the upper parts of the lungs (Hapke et al. 1968).

Thin-section computed tomography (CT) scanning of the chest has proved to be a remarkably sensitive tool for detecting early interstitial changes in acute allergic alveolitis. Upper lobe predominant, hazy bronchocentric "ground-glass" nodular opacities with air-trapping are typical findings (Lynch et al. 1992).

2.2.2.4.6 Histopathology

Allergic alveolitis is characterized by an interstitial and alveolar inflammation. In 1982, Reyes et al. (1982) published a histopathological review of 60 cases of farmer's lung disease. They reported that an interstitial alveolar infiltrate, consisting of plasma cells, lymphocytes and, occasionally, eosinophils was present in 100% of the cases. Granulomas were observed in 70%. In up to two-thirds of the cases, there was an interstitial fibrosis, but this was usually not severe. A mild form of bronchiolitis obliterans was noted in 50% of the cases. Vasculitis did not appear to be a feature of this condition. Emanuel and Kryda (1983) found that foreign body material, either refringent or non-refringent, could be present and Seal et al. (1968) reported that foreign body giant cells could occur in the granulomas. In chronic cases, Seal and colleagues (1968) observed infiltrates of lymphocytes in the alveolar septa, which were thickened with collagen deposit.

Heino et al. (1982) performed an electron microscopic study of the airways in those with farmer's lung disease and found cell destruction even at a level as high as the carina. The ciliated cells were affected most, showing a picture resembling that of bronchitis. Owing to the damage to the epithelium, superficial afferent nerves could be susceptible to irritation, inducing bronchial hyperreactivity.

2.2.2.4.7 Immunoserological Studies

In the early 1960s, Pepys et al. (1963) discovered that a high percentage of patients with farmer's lung disease had precipitating antibodies of IgG type against mold antigens. Precipitins against *Saccharopolyspora rectivirgula* (*Micropolyspora faeni*) were found in 87% of sera from patients with this disease. In other types of allergic alveolitis, also, there are circulating antibodies against the antigens related to the disease, and antibodies belonging to the IgA and IgM classes have been detected (Patterson et al. 1976). However, some patients with allergic alveolitis lack circulating antibodies against the responsible antigen (Hapke et al. 1968; Roberts et al. 1976). The precipitin test lacks specificity for the disease, because there are also perfectly healthy asymptomatic exposed and "unexposed" persons who have positive precipitating antibodies against antigens (Roberts et al. 1976; Schatz et al. 1977). Therefore, a positive precipitating antibody test only confirms that the patient has been exposed to an offending antigen and is not useful as a screening method for farmer's lung disease, although it can support a diagnosis of allergic alveolitis in a particular case (Fink et al. 1971; Cormier and Belanger 1985).

It is important to have the right panel of antigens for Farmer`s lung tests, since the species of bacteria and fungi can vary in different countries, depending on weather conditions. Terho in Finland has suggested that the antigen panel should contain at least *T. vulgaris, M. faeni* and some fungi from the *Asp. Glaucus* group, e.g., *Asp. umbrosus.*

The precipitating antibodies can be detected using several different methods (Moser 1979). The Ouchterlony agar gel double immunodiffusion method is mostly used (Ouchterlony 1958). The precipitins can still be positive 10 years after the farmer has left the farm (33%), but they are correlated to whether or not the farmer has left the farm (Braun et al. 1979).

2.2.2.4.8 Diagnostic Methods

The diagnosis of allergic alveolitis is based on a series of nonspecific clinical symptoms. As in medicine in general, the history is the most important diagnostic aid. It is very important to ask about exposure to offending antigens in patients with symptoms compatible with allergic alveolitis. To ask about a patient's occupation is one of the basic questions a doctor should ask his patient, as pointed out centuries ago in 1700 by Ramazzini. It is also very important to carefully analyze the symptoms. When did they appear in relation to the exposure? Several other important key facts (Fink et al. 2005) should always be included in the history, such as:

1. Circumstances surrounding the onset of the clinical manifestations
2. Their severity and persistence
3. Temporal relationships between relevant exposures and disease exacerbation
4. The clinical course of disease

Basal crepitating rales on auscultation of the lungs is a typical clinical finding in allergic alveolitis. In severe cases, the patient may have dyspnea at rest and labial cyanosis. Chest radiography is an important examination in cases of suspected allergic alveolitis. However, the changes may be difficult to detect and it is valuable to have an experienced roentgenologist view the radiographs. It must be kept in mind that the chest X-ray may be normal in some cases of farmer's lung disease.

Lung function tests are also of diagnostic value in allergic alveolitis and, if possible, should be carried out in all cases. It is useful to follow the lung function during the recovery phase. The preferable methods are static and dynamic spirometry and measurement of the diffusion capacity of carbon monoxide (DLCO). The latter is the most sensitive test and the capacity can still be reduced after the chest X-ray has become normalized (Tukiainen et al. 1980; Kokkarinen et al. 1993).

In smaller hospitals, there may be no possibilities of performing lung function tests, at least not of the advanced kind. However, measurement of arterial oxygen tension (PaO_2) in arterial blood samples is generally possible even in small hospitals and is a very useful diagnostic method.

Routine blood tests with measurement of hemoglobin, white blood cell count and ESR are of no help in the differential diagnosis, since the ESR and white blood cell reactions are similar to those in infectious diseases.

Skin tests with extracts of moldy hay have not been generally considered of diagnostic value (Pepys and Jenkins 1965; Freedman et al. 1981), although some authors have stated that skin tests are easy and effective in the diagnosis of farmer's lung disease and better than the precipitin test in distinguishing patients with farmer's lung from asymptomatic farmers (Morell et al. 1985). In doubtful cases, lung biopsy is a useful diagnostic method. However, it is not suitable for routine diagnosis, as it may cause complications.

Analysis of BAL fluids might provide useful supportive data in the diagnosis of allergic alveolitis and usually reveals intense lymphocytosis of predominantly CD8+ T-suppressor cells (Patel et al. 2001). On the contrary, in sarcoidosis, BAL fluid usually demonstrates CD4+ T-helper cell lymphocytosis (Sharma and Fujimura 1995).

Provocation with moldy material is not a routine diagnostic method. Some authors warn about the danger of provocation tests, as they entail risk of permanent impairment of the lung function with recurrent episodes of allergic alveolitis; moreover, deaths from single exposure have been reported (Barrowcliff and Arblaster 1968). Also, it is hard to distinguish between allergic alveolitis and ODTS induced by mold dust provocation.

Several different diagnostic criteria for extrinsic allergic alveolitis have been proposed and all have significant problems that limit their utility (Fink et al. 2005). In a study of a total of 661 patients from seven countries, who had lung disease for which HP was considered possible, a panel of clinical experts used the combined savvy of as the final arbiter of classification (Lacasse et al. 2003; Morris 2003). The patients' clinical histories, physical examinations and laboratory studies were incorporated into a stepwise logistic regression model to quantify the degree to which each feature predicted the assigned clinical diagnosis. This model was derived retrospectively in a 400-patient cohort and validated prospectively in a separate cohort of 261 patients. Six significant predictors of HP were found (Table 2.2.2). The probability of HP ranged from 0% in patients with none of these features to 98% in patients with all six. Not surprisingly, exposure to a known offending antigen – present in 97% of the patients and 33% of the control subjects – was the strongest predictor with an odds ratio of 38.8 [95% confidence interval (CI) 11.6–129.6]. The area under the receiver operating characteristic curve was 0.93 (95% CI 0.90–0.95).

Table 2.2.2. Diagnostic criteria of extrinsic allergic alveolitis (Lacasse et al. 2003)

Exposure to a known offending antigen
Positive precipitating antibodies to the offending antigen
Recurrent episodes of symptoms
Inspiratory crackles on physical examination
Symptoms occurring 4 to 8 hours after exposure
Weight loss

2.2.2.5 Differential Diagnosis

Infectious lung diseases, of both virological and bacteriological origin, have to be ruled out in cases of suspected allergic alveolitis and ODTS. An analysis of the history and the pattern of the chest X-ray changes may be helpful, as may serological, virological and bacteriological tests.

Sarcoidosis is another differential diagnosis that may be difficult to distinguish from allergic alveolitis, as the two diseases have features in common. For example, sarcoidosis affects non-smokers more than smokers, and the chest X-ray patterns may look alike, but bilateral hilar lymphomas are not seen in allergic alveolitis. In sarcoidosis, there is an acute stage and a chronic stage with pulmonary fibrosis, just as in allergic alveolitis. The lung biopsy changes in allergic alveolitis and sarcoidosis may be difficult to separate, but there is little alveolitis in sarcoidosis and the granulomas are found at the locations of the lymphatics in the periphery of the lobules and in the bronchovascular sheath (Reyes et al. 1982). In farmer's lung disease, alveolitis is the predominant lesion, and this is associated with centrilobular granulomas and mild bronchiolitis obliterans. In allergic alveolitis there are generally no granulomas in other organs, as are found in sarcoidosis. However, there have been reports about association between farmer's lung and granulomas in the spleen (Terho et al. 1980a; Venho et al. 1982), celiac disease (Robinson 1976; Turton et al. 1983) and jejunal villous changes (Robinson et al. 1981). Analysis of BAL fluids might provide useful supportive data in the diagnosis of allergic alveolitis and usually reveals intense lymphocytosis of predominantly CD8+ T-suppressor cells (Patel et al. 2001). On the contrary, in sarcoidosis, BAL fluid usually demonstrates CD4+ T-helper cell lymphocytosis (Sharma and Fujimura 1995).

In the end stage of allergic alveolitis, it is impossible to discriminate the condition from that caused by idiopathic lung fibrosis. However, there may be unknown agents responsible for this "idiopathic" lung fibrosis (Snider 1986). Several authors have, for example, reported cases of allergic alveolitis due to mold exposure in domestic environments. A correct diagnosis of allergic alveolitis can be difficult to settle in such cases (Patterson et al. 1981; Torok et al. 1981; Kawai et al. 1984; Jacobs et al. 1986). If the history is carefully analyzed, there should be no trouble in differentiating between occupational asthma and allergic alveolitis, as asthma usually has an immediate onset after the exposure.

In allergic bronchopulmonary aspergillosis, another differential diagnosis against allergic alveolitis, there may be fever, pulmonary infiltrates and antibodies to Aspergillus. Moreover, Aspergillus may cause allergic alveolitis in some patients and aspergillosis in others. In aspergillosis, however, eosinophilia and elevated total serum IgE levels are found and the exposure circumstances are different. Schatz and Patterson reviewed the major features of aspergillosis, asthma and allergic alveolitis in 1983.

2.2.2.6 Treatment

The best treatment for allergic diseases is to remove the patient from contact with the offending allergen. That might be easy in the case of allergic alveolitis caused by hobby activities, but difficult in other situations. For most farmers, there are, for example, many financial, educational and psycho-social reasons that make it extremely difficult to discontinue farming.

Cortisone has been used for many years in the treatment of allergic alveolitis and has been found to reduce IL-8 synthesis, a chemotactic factor from T cells and neutrophils (Denis 1995). Cortisone treatment seems to hasten the disappearance of radiological changes and should be given to severely ill patients to ameliorate symptoms, but no apparent benefit is derived from long-term treatment (Monkare 1983; Monkare et al. 1985). The cortisone treatment should be given for about 2 months (Tukiainen et al. 1980).

In a study of 30 patients with farmer's lung disease, inhaled disodium cromoglycate did not prevent exacerbation in two patients and produced no significant changes in respiratory symptoms in the others (Monkare et al. 1982).

2.2.2.7 Prognosis

If the exposure to mold dust ceases – for example, if the farmer is admitted to hospital – the symptoms usually subside fairly rapidly. The lung function impairment may, however, persist for a longer time (Williams 1963; Rankin et al. 1967). The more severe the attack, the greater the chance of permanent lung function impairment (Hapke et al. 1968). Repeated exposure to moldy hay and subsequent recurrent episodes of farmer's lung disease were found to carry a more serious prognosis in a study by Barbee et al. (1968), who reported that 5 of 50 patients died as a result of their lung disease during an average of 6 years of follow-up. Fatal cases after single acute exposure to moldy hay have occurred (Barrowcliff and Arblaster 1968). Braun et al. (1979) found a death rate of 9.2% in those with farmer's lung disease. The average length of farmer's lung disease at the time of death in that study was 17 years. In Barbee's study, 30% of 44 patients were dyspnoeic on exertion as a sequela of farmer's lung disease. The most striking and consistent physiological abnormality in the symptomatic patients was a decreased DLCO, and Barbee recommends that patients with farmer's lung should be followed up with serial measurements of DLCO. Thus, 70% of the farmers in Barbee's study did not have any persistent symptoms and were able to continue their farm work.

Monkare (1984) followed up 93 patients with farmer's lung disease for a mean period of 8.6 months (Monkare 1984). After this period, 49% of the patients still showed impaired DLCO. Those undergoing corticosteroid treatment no longer showed impaired DLCO, although corticosteroid treatment did not diminish the appearance of radiological fibrosis and had no obvious effect on the recovery of lung function in patients with an initially low DLCO value. In 96% of the patients, the course of the disease was reversible. During the follow-up, 13% experienced exacerbations and they had a more serious prognosis regarding pulmonary function than the others. Respiratory symptoms were reported by 39% of the patients.

In another Finnish study, PaO_2 improved most rapidly; the improvement in forced vital capacity (FVC) was slower, and the recovery of DLCO took the longest time. No patient had been diagnosed with asthma at the time of the diagnosis of farmer's lung disease, but asthma was later diagnosed in 7 of 101 patients during the 5-year follow-up (Kokkarinen et al. 1993).

Mean FVC improved significantly for up to 1 year. In mean DLCO, there was improvement for up to 2 years. Mean PaO_2 rose to its maximum within 1 month of the initial examination and did not change significantly thereafter. In conclusion, the pulmonary function of FL patients improved for up to 2 years after the initial acute episode.

In general, in a Canadian study with follow-up of 61 patients, Cormier found that 5 years or more after the acute episode, the pulmonary function in subjects who had continued farm work was no worse than that in subjects who had ceased all contact with the barn (Cormier and Belanger 1985). They recommended that patients with farmer's lung should continue farming, take all possible preventive measures, have regular evaluations of pulmonary function and consult a doctor at the slightest suspicion of recurrence.

2.2.2.8 Prevention

The most important measure in preventing allergic alveolitis (and ODTS) is the avoidance of antigen exposure. This can be accomplished in several ways. The best way is to change the farming methods. However, owing to climatic conditions and weather variations, some cases of mold growth are unavoidable even if the equipment is adequate. If the farmer is forced to handle moldy material, he should use a respirator. In some cases, the farmer is forced to change his or her occupation, but the advice in this matter is a very delicate task which should be undertaken by specialists in pulmonary and occupational medicine. Information about the dangers of mold exposure is also important in preventing disease.

2.2.3 Organic Dust Toxic Syndrome

The ODTS is an acute, febrile, noninfectious, flu-like, short-term reaction that can be produced by inhalation of bio-aerosols and organic dusts. The symptoms are influenza-like and dominated by fever and chills. It is often associated with myalgias, cough, headache and chest discomfort. Physical examination, chest X-ray and pulmonary function usually reveals nothing abnormal. Precipitins to mold or bacteria are often absent, but a polymorphonuclear leukocytosis is common as is tolerance to the causative agent after repeated exposure. Clustering of cases is not uncommon. Except in rare cases with underlying lung disease, the condition is of a benign nature and is self-limiting, with no reported sequelae. No treatment is required if the exposure is terminated. The condition is quite common.

Similar febrile conditions may also appear after inhalation of other agents, namely metals and combustion products of polymers as well as highly reactive chemicals used in polymer production. There is striking resemblance between these febrile conditions regardless of the different nature of the causative exposure. Independent of the exposure, the symptoms and signs as well as the course and duration of the illnesses are almost identical. Even BAL findings are similar in febrile reactions caused by different exposures. There is evidence that the pathogenesis might be the same and, therefore, the term *inhalation fever* was coined as an embracing term for all febrile reactions to inhalation of noxious substances. The term *inhalation fever* was originally used in 1978 in the Lancet in an editorial as a heading to describe the febrile and constitutional symptoms of metal fume fever, byssinosis and humidifier fever but nobody paid any further attention to the term until it was proposed as a unifying term for febrile reactions to inhalation of noxious substances in 1992 (Anonymous 1978; Rask-Andersen and Pratt 1992).

Historical Notes

Febrile illnesses after exposure to dust in the textile industry have long been well-known symptoms where natural fibers are used. The so-called mill fever, Monday fever or gin fever follows the exposure to dusty cotton in cotton mill workers, while engaged in the initial stages of cotton processing. Identical illnesses occur in workers inhaling jute, soft hemp, kapok and flax dust (Parkes 1982). The latter is called heckling fever. Acute illness was reported among rural mattress makers using low grade, stained cotton (Neal et al. 1942). The condition was caused by inhalation of gram-negative, rod shaped bacteria.

Another account of a febrile syndrome after exposure to organic dust was published in 1960 by Plessner, who described *Le fièvre du canard*, duck fever (Plessner 1960). Workers were affected by fever after cleaning feathers to produce down. Exposure to bird proteins in bird droppings may also cause ODTS. In 1959, humidifier fever was reported for the first time (Pestalozzi 1959). During the years, a number of other exposures to bio-aerosols have also been reported to cause febrile syndromes such as exposure to mold dust in farming and sawmills, grain dust in grain elevators, endotoxin in sewage handling, garbage plants and swine confinement buildings, etc. (Manfreda and Warren 1984).

2.2.3.1 Etiology

ODTS has been reported from a variety of environments where workers are at risk of exposure to bio-aerosols and organic dust (Pestalozzi 1959; Emanuel et al. 1975; Lundholm and Rylander 1983; Pratt and May 1984; Rask-Andersen 1989a,b; Malmros et al. 1992). There has been no report of specific organisms being more prone to cause ODTS than others as has been reported in allergic alveolitis. Probably a number of organisms may cause ODTS. All the exposures that can cause allergic alveolitis can possibly also cause ODTS as, for example, illustrated by agents in farming such as moldy hay, moldy straw and moldy grain, well-known for causing allergic alveolitis.

ODTS in farming is frequently associated with one specific job done on a single occasion, such as moving moldy corn or cleaning silos or granaries, and shoveling moldy grain or moldy hay. These jobs are of a limited duration but the exposure is often extreme. A concentration of up to 10^{10} spores/m^3 has been observed in worst case measurements of dust causing ODTS (Malmberg et al. 1993). In allergic alveolitis, the exposure to mold dust is also high, even if less than that in ODTS (in the range 10^9 spores/m^3). The exposure that results in allergic alveolitis is often repeated for weeks during work tasks that the farmer performs every day, e.g., distribution of moldy straw as bedding. Moldy grain was the most common cause of ODTS in a study of Swedish farmers. In a cross-sectional survey of 1,706 New Zealand farmers, symptoms of ODTS were reported frequently by people who worked on an orchard, by horse breeders and by those who reported working with the grain mill (Kimbell-Dunn et al. 2001).

Several authors have reported ODTS after work with moldy silage after working with opening of "capped" silos (Emanuel et al. 1975; May et al. 1986). Moldy silage has not been associated with allergic alveolitis, perhaps because uncapping of silos is a job that is done on a single occasion and not repeated for days or weeks.

During the 1970s, due to increasing prices of oil, wood chips for heating purposes were introduced. In wood chips that have been stored under damp conditions, there can be substantial mold growth. There have been several reports of both allergic alveolitis and ODTS caused by moldy wood chips (Rask-Andersen 1989a, b). In the US, employees at a municipal golf course became ill with ODTS after manually unloading a trailer full of moldy wood chips (Anonymous 1986). There is also a potential risk of exposure to moldy wood chips in the paper pulp industry (Kryda et al. 1989).

In Scandinavian sawmills, there are problems with mold growing on wood as well. Previously, the sawn timber was dried outside in timber yards in Swedish sawmills. To speed up the process, drying in kilns was introduced some decades ago. The temperatures in these kilns are ideal for growth of thermotolerant and thermophilic fungi and, to prevent mold growth, chemicals were sprayed all over the board. However, the use of chemicals was banned in the 1970s because of the cancer risk. When the dried mold-contaminated wood is handled in the trimming department, the workers might be exposed to mold dust. Cases of both ODTS and allergic alveolitis have been reported in wood trimmers (Belin 1980; Rask-Andersen et al. 1994). In North America, the timber is also dried in kilns but at a higher temperature. The microorganisms are then killed and there are no problems with mold. However, if higher temperatures were to be used when drying Scandinavian timber, it might crackle and get warped.

Grain fever – flu-like feverish episodes in the evening after handling grain – is a familiar condition to grain elevator workers and in harbor workers loading and unloading grain from ships (Warren et al. 1974; Cockcroft et al. 1983; Manfreda and Warren 1984). Usually, these grains have not been visibly moldy, although some reports pointed out the increased probability of grain fever after exposure to moldy grain (Manfreda and Warren 1984). ODTS has also been described among Chinese rice-granary workers (Ye et al. 1998). From swine confinement buildings, there are reports of flu-like complaints after exposure to dust that does not appear to be moldy (Donham 1990). In the mill fever appearing in workers in the card rooms in the cotton industry, there are no reports of mold dust exposure. Dust exposure studies reveal that inhaled lipopolysaccharides (endotoxins) arising from gram-negative microorganisms play a role in the mill fever (Rylander and Lundholm 1978; Castellan et al. 1984). Febrile attacks in swine confinement buildings and sewage workers are also believed to be caused by endotoxin (Lundholm and Rylander 1983; Donham 1990). In a Danish waste sorting plant, ODTS was suspected in 3 of 15 employees. Measurements showed high levels of bacteria and endotoxin in the air (Malmros et al. 1992). It has been shown that exposure levels of endotoxin at a level between 0.5 μg/m^3 and 1 μg/m^3 cause fever (Rylander 1987). Much lower concentrations of exposure are required to cause bronchoconstriction, dry cough and upper airway symptoms.

A survey of 28 employees in a mushroom-growing plant in an old mine closed down for mining revealed that four subjects – three men and one woman – had suffered febrile attacks related to work that were typical of ODTS (Rask-Andersen, unpublished data). The exposure causing the fever was cleaning out the beds in which the mushrooms were cultivated. The beds consisted of a mixture of half horse manure and half compost material. Water from the mine was used for irrigation and there were problems with mold growth on the surface of the beds. In this mushroom-growing plant, the women were picking the mushrooms while the men were working with the beds. Actually, half of the six men working in the plant had experienced febrile attacks in relation to work. One women, a mushroom picker, was diagnosed with asthma. After the water used for irrigation was exposed to ultraviolet rays, the mold problems diminished substantially. In a Japanese study of 69 mushroom workers who produce *Hypsizigus marmoreus* (Bunashimeji), six had experienced ODTS (Tanaka et al. 2002). In a case report, fever, myalgia and marked dyspnea was reported 12 h after shoveling composted wood chips and leaves (Weber et al. 1993).

Humidifier mist is another example of an exposure that can cause both inhalation fever and allergic alveolitis. The associated illnesses are termed humidifier fever and humidifier lung, respectively (Baur et al. 1988). In humidifier fever; several different microorganisms have been suspected as causative agents, in particular thermophilic *Actinomycetes, Flavobacteria, Aspergilli* and other fungi, as well as algae (Baur et al. 1988).

During the late 1970s, an outbreak in southern Sweden of repeated symptoms typical of inhalation fever, starting 4 h after a hot bath, involved 56 persons, nearly all of whom lived in an area supplied with water from the same source (Atterholm et al. 1977). The causal agent, which was never identified, was found to enter the body by inhalation. Similar symptoms were also reported after sauna or bathing in 100 people living in a small community in Finland (Muittari et al. 1980). The water source of the community was a small lake and it was found that the water was contaminated with several bacteria, fungi and algae. Water inhalation provocation tests produced the same kind of symptoms.

It is possible that patients with ongoing allergic alveolitis might get superimposed attacks of ODTS or inhalation fever, but the clinical course of allergic alveolitis will then go on to be quite different from inhalation fever. However, the multitude of non-immunological and immunological mechanisms involved in the pathogenesis of allergic alveolitis also give rise to symptoms such as fever and myalgia after acute exposures. One of our patients was in hospital to be observed because of farmer's lung disease. He was sent home over the weekend. During that time, he and two neighbors cleaned out a barn with 15-year-old grain. Our patient experienced an acute severe exacerbation of his condition and the other two got typical ODTS. From case histories, it seems as if these episodes of fever and exacerbation in patients with allergic alveolitis occur after exposure to especially heavy mold dust on a single occasion, in contrast to the daily lower grade mold dust exposure repeated for weeks that is said to be typical of allergic alveolitis. Often these exacerbations bring the patient to hospital, which might explain why some of the laboratory findings are similar in ODTS/inhalation fever and allergic alveolitis. It has been shown that inhalation of moldy hay induce symptoms and increase the number of circulating neutrophils both in patients with allergic alveolitis and in controls. However, in patients with an acute episode of farmer's lung disease, the neutrophils are primed for an enhanced respiratory burst and may thereby damage the lung (Larsson et al. 1988; Vogelmeier et al. 1993).

2.2.3.1.1 Terminology

To say that the terminology of work-related febrile attacks has been confusing is an understatement. Previously, all the names mentioned above as well as a variety of other names have been used for the condition – colorful names that give a hint about the exposure and environment causing these febrile illnesses (Table 2.2.3). During the second half of the 1970s and beginning of the 1980s, several investigators realized that there were cases of illnesses caused by inhalation of mold dust that did not fit into the general pattern of allergic alveolitis. Terms such as "Precipitin negative farmer's lung", "pulmonary mycotoxicosis" and "silo unloader's syndrome" were used for these reactions (Edwards et al. 1974; Emanuel et al. 1975; Pratt and May 1984). Following a symposium held in 1985, in an attempt to try to make the confusion less, it was decided to call these febrile attacks caused by inhalation of organic dust the *ODTS* (doPico 1986). However, this term is not quite suitable to use for humidifier fever since that condition is caused by inhalation of mist not by dust.

2.2.3.2 Epidemiology

ODTS is probably a common condition across all exposures but was not the subject of epidemiological studies until the 1980s. The lack of interest is probably because of the limited duration and relatively non-serious nature of ODTS and because tolerance to repeated exposure often occurs (Taylor 1986). However, although fever tolerance develops, the exposure might still be annoying. Other reactions induced by exposure to fumes and dusts might remain resulting in a higher frequency than expected of chronic respiratory disorders in populations with

Table 2.2.3. Inhalation fever after exposure bio-aerosols and organic dusts (RASK-ANDERSEN 1996)

Exposure	Name
Mist	
Mist from humidifiers contaminated with microorganisms	Befeuchterfieber (Humidifier fever)
	Monday morning fever
Contaminated tap water	Bath water fever
Steam from water in a sauna bucket	Sauna taker's disease
Organic dust	Organic dust toxic syndrome (ODTS)
Moldy silage	Precipitin test negative farmer's lung
	Atypical farmer's lung
	Pulmonary mycotoxicosis
	Silo-unloader's syndrome
Grain dust in grain elevators	Grain fever
Moldy grain, hay or straw in farming	No specific name
Sewage sludge	No specific name
Moldy wood chips	No specific name
Moldy board in trimming departments of sawmills	Wood trimmer's disease
Mold dust from composts used for mushroom cultivation	No specific name
Moldy oranges	No specific name
Moldy books in a museum	No specific name
Work in animal confinement buildings	No specific name
Plucking duck	La fièvre de canard (Duck fever)
Stained cotton	Mattress-maker's fever
Work in the cotton mill	Cardroom fever
	Factory fever
	Gin fever
	Monday fever
	Mill fever
	Weaver's cough
Flax dust	Heckling fever
Hemp dust	Hemp fever
Jute dust	Mill fever
Probably all other exposures that might cause allergic alveolitis for many of the different types	No specific name for the febrile conditions (although there are names of allergic alveolitis)

these kinds of exposures. Episodes of ODTS indicate that working conditions are poor. The association of ODTS and chronic respiratory diseases has to be studied further, and persons at risk of developing chronic respiratory disorders have to be identified.

There are difficulties in studying ODTS since there is no test available to detect prior episodes of this condition. Investigators must rely on questionnaire information – seeking a history of work-related febrile illness, often years in the past. In the Swedish studies of ODTS in farmers and wood trimmers, a key question as follows was used: *Have you had attacks of fever and chills in relation to your work that do not seem to be caused by common cold or influenza?* (MALMBERG et al. 1988). If the subject answered yes to this question, he was asked to answer a number of attendant questions on symptoms, exposure, time-relation, severity, duration etc. This question has a very high sensitivity but the specificity is lower. The specificity can be increased by follow-up interviews. One surprising finding in our studies of farmers was that the incidence of ODTS increased throughout the years and was highest during the last couple of years, probably due to memory lapses, which illustrates that the information sometimes is remote (RASK-ANDERSEN 1989a).

Another difficulty in studying the epidemiology of ODTS is that doses and exposure differ a lot because of the complexity of the occupational environments in which this group of conditions occurs (TAYLOR 1986). There is also variability in the content of fumes and dusts. It appears that if only the exposure is high enough all individuals are affected by inhalation fever, illustrated by clustering of cases (PRATT and MAY 1984; BRINTON et al. 1987).

ODTS may affect all age groups, including children who have been exposed while working with their parents (GATZEMEIER 1981). Grain fever was more common in nonsmokers in a study of 1200 farmers and farmers' wives in Manitoba, Canada (MANFREDA et al. 1986).

Some individuals get ODTS only once, while others have recurrent attacks. Of 80 farmers with ODTS, 44% had one episode, the remaining had two attacks or more often several years apart (RASK-ANDERSEN 1989a). In studies of grain workers, a few reported over 100 episodes of grain fever during their work life (DOPICO et al. 1984). In studies of farmers and wood trimmers, there have also been some persons that have reported a similar frequency of attacks, although maybe not exceeding 100 (RASK-ANDERSEN 1989a).

While cases of allergic alveolitis occur almost exclusively during the indoor feeding season for cattle, ODTS may affect farmers at any time of the year depending on work task although the condition is most common during the fall (PRATT and MAY 1984; RASK-ANDERSEN 1989b). The clustering effect of ODTS has been noted by several authors reporting cases of ODTS after work in silos with moldy silage (Emanuel et al. 1975; Pratt and May 1984; Rask-Andersen 1989b). In principal farmer's lung disease often only affects one person on a farm even if other individuals are exposed. In the largest outbreak of ODTS ever reported, 55 of 67 exposed persons (82%) fell ill after a mean latency period of 9.4 h after a hay party at a college fraternity (Brinton et al. 1987).

ODTS after organic dust exposure is common in farmers. After two large Swedish studies, it was concluded that approximately every tenth Swedish farmer had experienced ODTS (cumulated incidence) (Malmberg et al. 1985, 1988). Similar figures (13.6–15%) have also been reported from Finland and Canada (Warren et al. 1987; Husman et al. 1990). The prevalence of acute febrile episodes in swine growers is 10–30% (Donham 1990).

In contrast, in the two Swedish studies as well as in other Finnish studies, the yearly incidence of allergic alveolitis was, when strictly diagnosed, low, ranging from 0.2 to 0.4 per thousand in the farming population (Malmberg et al. 1985, 1988; Terho et al. 1987). Surprisingly, in a Scottish study from the 1970s, the prevalence of allergic alveolitis was much higher (2.3–8.6%; Grant et al. 1972). However, the diagnosis of allergic alveolitis was based only on questionnaires in many of the cases in that study. It is unknown how many of the cases really fulfilled the modern diagnostic criteria of allergic alveolitis having chest X-ray abnormalities and decreased pulmonary function (Terho 1986). Actually, a prevalence of allergic alveolitis of 2–8% could in reality have been an incidence of ODTS after organic dust exposure and would be consistent with the Swedish and Finnish findings (Grant et al. 1972; Terho et al. 1987; Malmberg et al. 1988). In the US, an annual prevalence among American farmers of 20–30%, compared with a lifetime prevalence of 1–2% for HP and 5–12% for occupational asthma has been reported (Kline and Hunninghake 2001).

In questionnaire surveys in Swedish saw mills, 10–20% of wood trimmers had reported ODTS but allergic alveolitis was rare (Belin 1980; Rask-Andersen et al. 1994). Of randomly selected working male controls aged 19–65 years, 3% had experienced febrile attacks in one Swedish study (Rask-Andersen et al. 1994). Among the controls with febrile illnesses, there were some farmers and some welders who probably had had typical inhalation fever. The others might have given an incorrect answer to the question. One case of allergic alveolitis was found among the controls as well as in the wood trimmers.

In a cross-sectional survey in a Turkish cellulose plant, among 109 reed workers exposed to reed dust and 78 unexposed office workers, ODTS symptoms were only reported by the reed workers (23.9%) (Coplu et al. 2005).

Published reports vary with regard to how frequently grain fever occurs, probably due to differences in definitions and to difficulties in measurement as well as differences in exposure. Grain fever was reported by 33% of grain scoopers, while 1.4% of grain elevator workers in Thunder Bay, Canada, reported grain fever (Kleinfeld 1974; Broder et al. 1979).

Mill fever in the cotton industry is common, especially among new employees. Prevalences of 6–7% have been reported (Schilling et al. 1955; Werner 1955). In a cottonseed oil mill, one study reported prevalences in new workers ranging from 10% to 50% (Ritter and Nussbaum 1944).

Even for allergic alveolitis caused by bird protein, the prevalence varies from one series to another. As early as 1959, duck fever was being reported but, otherwise, there did not seem to be much distinction between febrile illnesses and allergic alveolitis caused by this exposure (Plessner 1960). It is possible that some authors have included cases of ODTS in their series of PBD if the diagnosis is based on questionnaires. In a study from the Canary Islands, 8% were reported to have allergic alveolitis, a prevalence that is unexpectedly high (Rodriguez de Castro et al. 1993).

2.2.3.3 Pathogenesis

Despite the fact that ODTS is common, the exact mechanisms involved in the pathogenesis are unknown. The fact that there is also often uncertaintyas to the exact etiological agents causing ODTS helps to explain why it is hard to clarify the mechanisms involved in the pathogenesis. It is obvious that ODTS might be caused by a number of different agents. Despite the difficulties, many hypotheses of the pathogenesis have been suggested involving immune-complex, interleukins, TNF, activation of macrophages and complement (Wintermeyer et al. 1997; Spurzem et al. 2002). Findings during recent years indicate that inhalation fever is caused by an acute pulmonary inflammatory cellular response involving a network of cytokines.

Since even non-sensitized individuals not previously exposed to the agents are affected by ODTS, no allergy mechanisms are involved. Precipitins to thermophiles are usually negative in ODTS and there is no evidence that antibodies are involved in the mechanisms of the condition (Emanuel et al. 1975; Pratt and May 1984; Rask-Andersen 1989a).

In the 1970s, the name pulmonary mycotoxicosis was used for ODTS after uncapping silos, but it has not been possible to identify any significant mycotoxin concentrations in dust causing this syndrome (Emanuel et al. 1989; May et al. 1989). Endotoxin has been found in the cotton industry as well as in swine and poultry confinement buildings, but a Swedish study found no dose–response relationship when investigating endotoxin levels in dust causing ODTS in farmers (Rask-Andersen et al. 1989). Neither could any endotoxin be found in the trimming departments of Swedish sawmills. Only three kinds of mold grow in this environment – *Aspergillus fumigatus, Rhizopus rhizopodiformis* and *Paecillomyces varioti* – and these species do not generate endotoxin.

It has been shown by several groups that the pathogenesis of ODTS involves the induction of a peripheral blood leukocytosis and airway neutrophilia (Emanuel et al. 1975, 1989; Lecours et al. 1986). In an animal model for ODTS in the guinea pig, animals were exposed to airborne cotton dust for 6 h; a febrile response occurred by 5 h and lasted for several hours. Concurrent with this response was a change in pulmonary function, which consisted of rapid shallow breathing with airflow limitation during exhalation. Evaluation of BAL indicated a neutrophilic inflammation of the lung and increased amounts of TNF, with a peak 3 h after exposure (Griffiths-Johnson et al. 1991).

In an epidemic of acute fever, respiratory-tract symptoms and muscle pain, starting 4 h after a hot bath, involving 56 persons, the mean C-reactive protein value was 54 mg/l (ref. value <3) (Atterholm et al. 1977). In a study of volunteers, an inflammatory response to weighing pigs was also shown in all exposed individuals, although only some experienced a febrile reaction (Malmberg and Larsson 1993). In a study of three volunteers who developed ODTS after using wood chip mulch dust, a marked elevation in neutrophil percentage in their BAL fluid (range 10–57%) was noted. When these three subjects underwent control BAL fluid measurements, the postexposure comparison demonstrated increased BAL proinflammatory cytokine and neutrophil levels consistent with the theory that cytokine networking in the lung may mediate ODTS (Wintermeyer et al. 1997).

In a study of acute-phase reactants in rabbits exposed to an aerosol of fungal spores, haptoglobin analysis was compared with depressions in PaO_2 following challenge. It was found in three experiments that none of seven rabbits with an augmented haptoglobin level prior to challenge demonstrated a decrease in PaO_2 after aerosol challenge. Perhaps that finding could explain some of the mechanisms in the development of tachyphylaxis (Baseler and Burrell 1981).

2.2.3.4 Clinical Aspects

2.2.3.4.1 Symptoms

During the actual exposure inducing ODTS, there might be some preliminary symptoms with irritation in the throat and a dry irritation cough. The constitutional symptoms come on after a latent interval approximately 4–8 h after the original exposure, usually in late afternoon or early evening. The symptoms are dominated by fever and shivering. The fever has a gradual increase, followed in most cases by a shivering attack and sweating. A temperature as high as 41°C has been reported. The fever and chills often go with additional symptoms such as myalgia, headache, general malaise, cough and chest discomfort (May et al. 1986; Rask-Andersen 1989a; Spurzem et al. 2002). Some persons get a feeling of irritation or oppression retrosternally. Severe dyspnea is not common. Instead some persons have a sense of discomfort in the chest especially on taking a deep breath (Rask-Andersen 1989a). These respiratory symptoms as well as the other additional symptoms do not occur in all cases. Severity of the condition varies significantly. There are milder reactions without fever after dust exposure. Some workers just report that they feel cold and tired after exposure to fume or dust but have no fever. In a study of volunteers weighing pigs, an inflammatory response was also shown in all exposed individuals although only some experienced a febrile reaction (Malmberg and Larsson 1993). Perhaps there is some kind of threshold in the extent of the exposure that has to be overcome to induce fever. The symptoms resolve 24–48 h after termination of exposure, followed by complete recovery.

Tolerance or Tachyphylaxis

The reaction includes an unexplained tolerance effect, in which symptoms lessen with repeated daily exposure but are much worse on return to work after a break, such as a weekend. Thus, the condition has been called Monday-morning fever and such an effect has been described in mill fever, humidifier fever and in saw mill workers affected by fever (MERCHANT 1987; BAUR et al. 1988). Actually, wood trimmers felling ill on Mondays have been accused of having hangovers after the weekend.

There have been speculations that mainly those workers starting working in swine confinement buildings experienced the flu-like episodes of inhalation fever (MALMBERG and LARSSON 1993). There have been similar reports from the grain industry in North America (DOPICO et al. 1984). Swedish researchers were actually warned of the danger of the work by swine confinement workers when the researchers as volunteers were weighing pigs. Subsequently, the project leader himself fell ill with typical inhalation fever, thus giving an excellent opportunity to study BAL fluid and bronchial responsiveness in inhalation fever (MALMBERG and RASK-ANDERSEN 1993).

2.2.3.4.2 Physical Examination

There are usually no physical signs (PRATT and MAY 1984; RASK-ANDERSEN 1989a). However, if the patient has high fever, there might be an increased pulse rate and possibly respiratory rate. Physical examination usually reveals few abnormalities except that minor rales can be heard in some cases (EMANUEL et al. 1975; PRATT and MAY 1984; RASK-ANDERSEN 1989a).

In the literature, there are a few case reports of more severe ODTS reactions. In one report, a 68-year-old smoker and farmer who became ill after cleaning out a grain bin was found to be hypoxic with combined respiratory acidosis and metabolic alkalosis (pH 7.45, $_{p}CO_2$ 45, $_{p}O_2$ 58) (SIGURDARSON et al. 2004). The patient was hospitalized and treated with supplemental oxygen, steroids and antibiotics. He gradually improved although oxygen continued to be needed over the next 3 months. Spirometry showed a fixed airflow obstruction with a forced expiratory volume in 1 s (FEV_1) of 1.35 (34% predicted), FVC of 3.06 (60% predicted) and FEV1/FVC ratio of 44% with no significant response to bronchodilators. Lung volumes showed hyperinflation, while DLCO was well preserved at 82% predicted. The patient probably had preexisting (though undiagnosed) COPD. The case demonstrates that, in patients with underlying lung disease, ODTS may present as a cause of exacerbation and that recovery may be prolonged and complicated. In another case report, a 52-year-old male was reported to have developed fever, myalgia and marked dyspnea 12 h after shoveling composted wood chips and leaves. Inspiratory crackles, hypoxemia and bilateral patchy pulmonary infiltrates were seen (WEBER et al. 1993).

2.2.3.4.3 Laboratory Findings, Lung Function Tests, Histopathology

An increased sedimentation rate as well as a leukocytosis with an increased number of segmented white blood cells is common (RASK-ANDERSEN 1989a; SPURZEM et al. 2002; SEIFERT et al. 2003). Farmer's lung precipitins are usually negative in ODTS (EMANUEL et al. 1975; PRATT and MAY 1984; RASK-ANDERSEN 1989a). However, precipitins to wood mold antigens are often positive in workers in the trimming departments of sawmills, even in workers who had never had ODTS (BELIN 1980; RASK-ANDERSEN et al. 1994). A positive precipitin test is thus a sign of exposure not of disease.

There is no association between atopy and ODTS (MANFREDA et al. 1986). The moldy material that causes ODTS gives rise to dense clouds of dust. One would expect that subjects with atopy and allergic asthma would not be affected by ODTS. Because of bronchial hyperresponsiveness, they probably can't stand the high levels of mold dust required to induce ODTS.

The chest radiograph, blood gases and pulmonary function tests are usually normal (MAY et al. 1986). In some cases, however, there may be transient changes that in principle return to normal within 24 h (EMANUEL et al. 1975, 1989; PRATT and MAY 1984; RASK-ANDERSEN 1989a). Decreases both in lung volumes as well as in diffusion capacity (DL_{CO}) and PaO_2 have been reported, but most subjects fail to show interstitial infiltrates and a restrictive breathing pattern. Maybe transient decreases in the pulmonary function would be seen in more cases if repeated spirometries were done. Many patients might not be investigated until the spirometry had returned to normal. It is also possible that patients might have decreased lung volumes even if the volumes are within the predicted values. Usually, it is not known what the lung volumes are before the exposure, and the patient's original lung volume might be over 100% of the predicted value.

In the previously mentioned study of volunteers weighing pigs, one of six subjects developed typical ODTS (MALMBERG and LARSSON 1993). Two experienced malaise, drowsiness and a fainting sensation, but temperature changes of less than 1°C. Bronchial responsiveness increased in all subjects within 6 h (more than three doubling steps difference in a methacholine test compared with pre-exposure values). In another study, in which farmers with ODTS were interviewed, it was quite common that the farmers reported an increased general sensitivity to dust after the febrile attack (RASK-ANDERSEN 1989a). This could be an expression for increased bronchial responsiveness after the febrile attack. Other researchers have had similar impressions, but in a study from upstate New York increased bronchial hyperresponsiveness was not found in a follow-up study of ten farmers (MAY et al. 1990).

As mentioned before, there are a few reports in the literature of more severe cases of febrile reaction after organic dust exposures. A woman who was 41 years of age developed pulmonary edema after massive fungal inhalation at an orange storehouse (YOSHIDA et al. 1989). BAL fluid showed 96% alveolar macrophages, 3% lymphocytes and 1% neutrophils. A transbronchial lung biopsy in the same patient disclosed a hyperemic tracheobronchial tree but almost nothing abnormal in the alveoli and the interstitium. Lung biopsy in two farmers with severe ODTS revealed a multifocal process with exudates, neutrophils and histiocytes in bronchiole, alveoli and interstitium, and large numbers of fungal spores. Species of mesophilic and thermophilic actinomycetes and of *Aspergillus* and *Penicillium fungi* were recorded in the lavage fluid (EMANUEL et al. 1989). In a Japanese case report, a 60-year-old man was admitted to the hospital because of fever, coughing and dyspnea that developed after he entered a silo that had been filled with chips of wood in the preceding 3 months (NAGAI et al. 1998). A chest X-ray film revealed bilateral ground-glass shadows. Histological study of the lung showed a multifocal acute process; the alveoli and interstitial areas contained many fungal hyphae and spores. Serological reactions were negative to ten antigens known to induce HP. The patients recovered quickly without steroid therapy. In three cases of ODTS, bilateral alveolar and interstitial infiltrates on chest roentgenograms were seen (PERRY et al. 1998). Two patients became hypoxemic and required mechanical ventilation, but recovered completely with high-dose steroids. Histological examination showed acute and organizing diffuse alveolar damage in two biopsy specimens and an acute bronchopneumonia in the third. No patient had residual functional deficits or chest radiographic abnormalities.

2.2.3.5 Differential Diagnosis

Patients are often seen by general practitioners and it is important not to forget ODTS in the differential diagnosis of workers with unclear fever. Clinically, it is important to differentiate ODTS from other diseases to avoid unnecessary medication. A thorough occupational history is important for the diagnosis of ODTS, since it is an exclusion diagnosis made on clinical grounds with no specific test currently available. People who are unaware of the hazard sometimes think that they are developing a cold or influenza, and tend to attribute their symptom to this, especially as the illness may not start until they have finished work and returned home. The rapid recovery tends to confirm their belief. Hence it is not uncommon for employees not to seek assistance until they had more than one attack. Probably a lot of cases of ODTS go undiagnosed. In a Swedish study, 23 of 80 farmers affected by ODTS consulted a doctor (RASK-ANDERSEN 1989a). The Swedish farmers were familiar with the condition's benign nature and didn't seek medical care. If they did, they sometimes knew more about the condition than their physicians.

In some cases, it might be hard to differentiate ODTS and allergic alveolitis. They might actually represent parts of a spectrum of responses to complex organic dusts rather than completely distinct clinical entities. Probably many cases of benign short-term febrile attacks caused by inhalation of bio-aerosols have been misdiagnosed as allergic alveolitis both in single cases and epidemiological studies. This can explain some of the high prevalences of farmer's lung disease reported in the 1970s that other groups have not been able to confirm (GRANT et al. 1972; TERHO et al. 1987; MALMBERG et al. 1988). Other differential diagnoses are chemical toxic pneumonitis, asthma and infectious diseases, e.g., virus infections such as influenza. It is important to realize that, from knowledge of the history, someone who is naive to an exposure (a newly hired employee, e.g., doing a dirty job of shoveling chips) <u>cannot</u> have allergic alveolitis because they have not been sensitized. In allergic alveolitis, but usually not in ODTS, there are also decreased blood gases, chest X-ray changes, and decreased pulmonary function according to the diagnostic criteria by Terho (1986). As evident after the presentation of the clinical picture in ODTS, there is some overlapping between ODTS and allergic alveolitis. A time criterion may perhaps be added to the diagnostic criteria of allergic alveolitis. Allergic alveolitis is a severe lung disease going on for weeks or months.

2.2.3.6 Treatment

ODTS is with a few exceptions of a benign nature, self-limiting and of a short duration. No specific treatment is required in the absolute majority of cases. If exposure stops, the symptoms subside spontaneously in 12–48 h (Emanuel et al. 1975; Pratt and May 1984; Rask-Andersen 1989a; Seifert et al. 2003). The patient should be immediately removed from contact with the causative exposure, placed at rest in bed, if needed, and treated symptomatically. Analgesics and fever-decreasing agents give symptomatic relief. The administration of oxygen in severe cases has also been recommended.

2.2.3.7 Prognosis

There are no reported sequelae in ODTS. However, long-term follow-ups are needed. Extensive investigations have revealed no effects in respiratory function, gas exchange or exercise capacity in farmers who have experienced ODTS, in some cases repeated attacks (Malmberg et al. 1985); neither does grain fever lead to fibrosis or permanent disability (Manfreda and Warren 1984). However, in Finland, farmers' wives who had experienced ODTS had more chronic bronchitis than others (Husman et al. 1990). Also, in a questionnaire study of 7496 farmers from four European countries, ODTS was a major predictor of chronic bronchitis (Radon et al. 2003). Prospective studies on the association between ODTS and COPD and other chronic respiratory symptoms are needed.

2.2.3.8 Prevention

Previously, when the differences between allergic alveolitis and ODTS were not realized, workers had been unnecessary forced to change occupation because of attacks of fever. However, there is no need to change occupation because of ODTS. Instead, good working practice is important to avoid further episodes. Inhalation of bio-aerosols and organic dust can be prevented by adequate exhaust ventilation and the application of local exhaust ventilation to the source. In farming, the development of mold should be avoided by using the correct farming methods. However, owing to climatic conditions and weather variations, some instances of mold growth are unavoidable even if the equipment is adequate. A new technique might also introduce new risks. If a worker is forced to handle moldy material or work in the presence of toxic fumes, he should use a respirator in order to avoid unnecessary illness. Availability of information about the danger of inhaling mold dust or toxic fumes is also important in preventing disease.

2.2.4 Asthma

2.2.4.1 Definition

Asthma is an ill-defined disease and there is no consensus as to whether asthma is a disease in its own right or is a clinical variant in a continuum of symptoms of chronic non-specific lung disease (Fletcher 1976), with bronchial hyperreactivity and allergy as predisposing factors. Asthma might be described as a chronic inflammatory disease in the airways where several cells are activated. Repeated episodes of inflammation will, in those predisposed, result in wheeze, breathlessness, chest congestion and cough, especially at night and early in the morning. Usually the symptoms are associated with variable airway obstruction, which is most often reversible, either spontaneously or in response to treatment. Existing unspecific bronchial hyperreactivity will increase due to inflammation (National Heart Lung and Blood Institute 1991).

2.2.4.1.1 Occupational Asthma

The disease is characterized by variable airflow limitation and/or bronchial hyperresponsiveness due to causes and conditions attributable to a particular environment, and not to stimuli encountered outside the workplace (Bernstein 1999).

2.2.4.1.2 Outdoor Air Pollution and Asthma

Substances of the air pollution, such as diesel particles, ozone, SO_2 and NO_x, have been associated with asthma and have been found to be a risk factor in childhood asthma. Studies have shown that these substances can induce and worsen symptoms in subjects already suffering from asthma (Bascom et al. 1996a, b).

2.2.4.2 Etiology and Epidemiology

The prevalence of asthma is high, between 2.9% and 7.2% at least in Scandinavian populations (Ulrik and Lange 1994; Pallasaho et al. 1999), and several published studies indicate an increasing occurrence of the disease. Population-based incidence studies have found an incidence between 20 pr.10^5 pr. year and 250 pr.10^5 pr. year (McWhorter et al. 1989; Yunginger et al. 1992; Kivity et al. 1995; Fishwick et al. 1997; Milton et al. 1998). Asthmatics rarely die from their disease, but there is some indication of an increase in mortality (Desideri et al. 1997). Several risk factors associated with asthma have been described.

2.2.4.2.1 Risk Factors Outside Occupation

Gender and age. Asthma incidence is highest during the first years of life, and is highest in boys. The gender ratio changes during adolescence to an incidence that is higher in females between 15 years and 50 years. Later in life, the ratio changes in favor of males (Yunginger et al. 1992).

Atopy. To become sensitized, an exposure to allergens is imperative, and data suggest that there is an increased risk of becoming sensitized with increasing exposure (Lau et al. 1989). There is a strong correlation between aged standardized IgE concentration and asthma, and the time of debut of the disease in all age classes (Burrows et al. 1989, 1991), and atopy alone might increase the risk of asthma by 30% (Pearce et al. 1999).

Host factors. Genetic factors most probably influence both the atopic constitution and the specific airway disease at least. Twin studies have suggested the heritability of asthma to be 36–75% (Koppelman et al. 1999). An increasing number of studies have identified linkages between specific areas of the genome that contain candidate genes as well as markers for different phenotypes. Generally, the reproducibility of the findings has been low, and this might indicate that the genetic contribution to the etiology of asthma is of additive nature and represented by several gene polymorphisms.

Early life. The findings in studies regarding associations between fetal growth and atopic diseases have been conflicting. Some have found a protective effect, others have observed increased risk (Leadbitter et al. 1999; Brooks et al. 2001).

Nutrition. Like the fetal growth on asthma, data regarding breastfeeding and asthma are conflicting with no unequivocal support of a protective effect. Breast milk contains fatty acids and mediators that might enhance asthma and wheezing in children. In several studies, obesity has been found to increase the risk of asthma, especially among women (Somerville et al. 1984; Schwartz and Weiss 1990; Shaheen et al. 1999). Constituents of nourishment such as vitamin C and E, selenium and magnesium have in some studies been inversely associated with asthma.

Sibship size. Several studies have demonstrated an inverse relationship between sibship size and hayfever, atopic eczema and sensitization in childhood. Data are less clear regarding childhood asthma and family size. Recent studies have found a protective effect for developing asthma in childhood of having more than one older brother in the family (Ball et al. 2000), while previous studies have shown no protective effect of a large family (Rona et al. 1999).

Infections. Data of the effect of early-life infections and respiratory infections in particular on asthma are not all supportive of an inverse relationship, although studies from different parts of the world have found a protective effect (Anderson 1974; Flynn 1994; von Mutius et al. 1994; Ball et al. 2000; Matricardi et al. 2000).

Growing up on farms. Several studies from different countries (Switzerland, Austria, Germany, Finland, Sweden, Denmark, Norway, Australia) have shown a protective effect of growing up on a farm toward asthma, especially on farms with livestock. The protective effect from the farming environment might be the endotoxin exposure from the animal housings (Riedler et al. 2001).

Indoor air pollution and passive smoking. Maternal smoking seems to increase the risk of childhood asthma, and data suggest that passive smoking from parents in the homes increases the risk of childhood asthma by 13–37% (Strachan and Cook 1998). A major risk factor from the indoor environment is exposure to house dust mites, and a dose–response relationship has been described (Peat and Li 1999). Indoor dampness and fungal spores have also been shown to increase the risk of childhood asthma.

Smoking. Smoking seems to have an influence on asthma. Both incidence studies (Larsson 1995) and prevalence studies (Vesterinen et al. 1988; Omland et al. 1999) have shown an association with asthma, although others (Lundback 1998) have failed to find such an association.

2.2.4.2.2 Occupational Exposure

The risk of asthma attributable to occupation has been investigated by several authors, and the findings indicate an attributable risk between 3% and 21% (Heederik et al. 1989; Viegi et al. 1991, 1994; Ng et al. 1994; Kogevinas et al. 1996, 1999; Sunyer et al. 1998). The data are based on both incidence and prevalence data. More that 250 substances have been identified as causes of occupational asthma (OA) (Chan-Yeung and Malo 1994). Data from the ECRH survey suggest that there is an increased risk of asthma in farmers, painters, plastic workers, cleaners, spray painters and agricultural workers, regardless of gender, and for farmers and cleaners among countries (Kogevinas et al. 1999).

Organic dust. Exposure to organic dust is very common and is a causal as well as aggravating factor for asthma. Finnish data indicate that organic dust might be responsible for as much as 60% of the total amount of occupational asthma (Karjalainen et al. 2000). In Table 2.2.4, organic dust exposures and types of asthma are listed.

2.2.4.3 Pathogenesis

Two different types of occupational asthma are described depending on latency period from start of exposure to start of symptoms.

1. Exposure to agents with immunological potential nearly always induces OA with a latency period. This is the most frequent kind of OA, and is usually caused by exposure to high-molecular-weight agents (e.g., flour, animal dander; >1 kDa). Less frequent OA is induced by exposure to low-molecular-weight agents (<1 kDa) binding to proteins forming complexes that might result in an IgE response. IgE-mediated OA often results in an immediate (histamine release) or a delayed (eosinophil) response with leukotriene release response (Mapp et al. 1994). However, low-molecular-weight agents primarily induce

Table 2.2.4. Common occupations and type of organic dust causally related to occupational asthma (Sigsgaard and Schlunssen 2004)

Occupations	Agents	IgE mediated	Non-IgE mediated
Farmers, veterinarians, animal dander	Animal urine or dander	++	++
	Grain dust	++	++
	Endotoxin		++
	Storage mites	++	
	Fungi, molds	+	++
Swine breeding	Swine dander	+	++
	Endotoxin		++
Wood workers, carpenters, saw mill workers	Western red cedar	+	++
	Other wood dust (pine, iroko, oak, etc.)	+	++
	Endotoxin		++
	Fungi, molds	+	++
Bakers, food workers	Flour	++	++
	Amylase	++	
	Storage mites, cockroach	++	
Waste handlers	Endotoxin		++
	Fungi, molds	+	++
Sewage workers	Endotoxin		++
	Fungi, molds	+	++
Health care workers	Latex	++	
Cotton workers	Endotoxin		++

++: Common mechanism, + Rare mechanism. From 48

OA through receptors other than IgE. Bacteria, molds, isocyantes and metals are able to activate a membrane-bound receptor and start the inflammatory cascade with release of cytokines. The toll-like receptor is, for some of the microbiological agents, identified as the cell surface receptor. For most of the low-molecular-weight agents, the receptors have not yet been identified (BASU and FENTON 2004).

2. Exposure to agents with no immunological potential usually results in OA with no latency period. This irritant-induced asthma most often occurs after single (RADS) or multiple incidents of high exposure.

2.2.4.4 Clinical Aspects

2.2.4.4.1 Symptoms

Shortness of breath, wheezing and cough are the classical triad of asthmatic symptoms. The symptoms are often most prevalent at night or early in the morning and may be episodic or daily depending on the severity of the disease. Association between symptoms and exposure to allergens, irritants, exercise and viral infections often occurs. The classical symptoms might not be present, especially in subjects with poor perception of breathlessness (VEEN et al. 1998).

2.2.4.4.2 Physical Examination

Wheeze may or may not be present during a forced expiration. In mild asthma, there will be diffuse wheezing, good diaphragmatic motion and only a slightly elevated pulse and respiration rate. In moderate asthma, the pulse and respiration rates are more elevated, the wheeze is diffuse and the diaphragmatic motion will be moderate. Severe asthma is characterized by tachycardia and tachypnea, cyanosis, and signs of fatigue. Wheeze might not be present because of severe airflow limitation with complete airway closure.

2.2.4.4.3 Laboratory Findings

Tests for sensitization to airborne allergens are of great importance. The allergens can induce airway inflammation and, if sensitized, the allergens can prolong bronchial hyperresponsiveness and by cessation of exposure increase the severity of the disease (PLATTS-MILLS et al. 1982). The allergens can be identified using traditional bioassay in allergy skin tests or by means of in vitro assay in radio allergosorbent test (RAST) or enzyme-linked immunosorbent test (ELISA). Blood pO_2 and pCO_2 are usually normal, but with increasing severity of the disease, hypoxemia and CO_2 retention can occur.

2.2.4.4.4 Lung Function Tests

Central in the diagnosis and treatment of the disease is lung function testing. Using simple methods, these tests enable confirmation of the diagnosis, assessment of the severity of the disease and monitoring of the effect of the treatment given. The FEV_1 and peak expiratory flow (PEF) are the most sensitive tests for airflow limitation and the most widely used. In mild to moderate asthma in remission, lung function tests are usually normal or slightly reduced. In more severe asthma with pronounced airflow obstruction, there can be a reduction in maximum expiratory flow, an increase in residual volume and functional residual capacity, and a decrease in vital capacity (WOOLCOCK et al. 1971).

Bronchial Hyperresponsiveness.
Almost all patients with asthma will, from time to time, experience hyperresponsiveness of the airways. Although not always present, it is a major finding in those with asthma and, when demonstrated, it serves as an important tool to both the diagnosis and the severity of the disease. However, bronchial hyperresponsiveness is not specific to asthma. The reaction can be associated with COPD, cystic fibrosis, left cardiac failure, and up to 15% of a population can be bronchial hyperreactive without any other signs or symptoms of asthma. The simplest and most common way of performing the unspecific challenge is by exercise or by inhaling methacholine or histamine using standardized protocols.

2.2.4.4.5 Radiological Findings

Chest radiography does not play a central part in the diagnostic efforts, although a radiograph is included in the diagnostic procedure mainly to exclude other pulmonary causes and diseases. Hyperinflation and increased peribronchial tissue density are common findings.

2.2.4.4.6 Histopathology

Cellular and structural changes involving both the airways and lung parenchyma occur in asthma. In the airways, the dominating cells infiltrating the wall are CD4 lymphocytes, eosinophils and mast cells. Structural changes involve increased smooth muscle mass, hypertrophy of mucous glands and goblet-cell hyperplasia (Carroll et al. 1996). Alveolar infiltration of eosinophils and CD4 lymphocytes in nocturnal asthma and alveolar infiltration of neutrophils in severe steroid-dependent asthma have been described. Destruction of alveolar walls, as frequently seen in COPD, is uncommon in asthma (Dunnill et al. 1969).

2.2.4.5 Diagnostic Methods and Differential Diagnosis

The presence of wheeze, breathlessness and cough, especially at night or early in the morning, strongly suggests the diagnosis of asthma. PEF measurements (with a 24-h variation) of less than 20% and an improvement in PEF of 60 l/min or more after inhalation of a β-adrenergic agonist is regarded to be diagnostic of asthma. Plain chest radiography enables exclusion of differential diagnoses such as lung infection, pleural effusion, vascular abnormalities and other processes that compress trachea or main bronchi, bronchiectasis, bronchiolitis and left ventricular failure. Using reversible tests and/or serial PEF measurements, COPD as the main differential diagnosis can be excluded.

2.2.4.5.1 Diagnosis Methods of Occupational Asthma

In the clinical evaluation of subjects actively participating in the work force and with newly diagnosed asthma, thoughts should be included regarding occupation and exposure. Of great importance is an occupational history with quantitative and qualitative data regarding exposure. Second to the diagnosis would be to look for a temporo-spatial distribution of symptoms and lung function indicative of an occupational origin to the disease. Serial PEF measurements during both working periods and free time are of great use. If not previously performed, tests for IgE-mediated disease and unspecific bronchial hyperresponsiveness would be the third step. A specific challenge test using occupational exposure agents would, as a final diagnostic step, secure a proper diagnosis. The specific challenge is usually not necessary to ensure the diagnosis.

2.2.4.6 Treatment

The major principle in the pharmacological treatment of asthma is to control the chronic inflammation and to relieve symptoms due to airflow obstruction. Several regimes are available, but a systematic presentation of these is beyond the scope of a description of asthma associated with occupation and environment. Exposure to sensitizing agents from the workplace is the most important factor in occupational asthma. Early diagnosis and removal from exposure is associated with a good prognosis, with fewer symptoms, cessation of lung function impairment and reduced use of medication.

2.2.5 Chronic Obstructive Pulmonary Disease

2.2.5.1 Definition

During recent years, several consensus statements have been proposed (American Thoracic Society 1995; Siafakas et al. 1995; Pauwels et al. 2001). The COPD is characterized by slowly progressive, most often irreversible, airflow obstruction. Signs and symptoms of chronic bronchitis and/or emphysema are usually present. The airflow obstruction is at most related to abnormal inflammatory reaction in the bronchi to toxic gasses or particles.

2.2.5.2 Occupational COPD

There is no well-established definition of the disease, but occupational COPD might be characterized by slowly progressive airflow obstruction mainly due to exposure to toxic gasses or particles from a particular occupational environment and not to exposures outside the workplace.

2.2.5.3 Outdoor Air Pollution and COPD

Outdoor air pollution is not regarded as a cause of the disease, rather as a factor related to worsen the status of the disease.

2.2.5.4 Etiology and Epidemiology

Based on a spirometric definition, 5–15% of an adult population will have COPD, and the prevalence of the disease, according to the World Health Organization (WHO), is expected to increase to the fifth most frequent cause of death world wide by the year 2020. About 50% of patients are alive 10 years after the time of diagnosis, and more than one-third die of respiratory failure. Several risk factors have been described, especially tobacco.

2.2.5.4.1 Risk Factors Outside Occupation

Tobacco. Cigarette smoking is by far the most well-established environmental risk factor for COPD.

Cigarette smokers have an increased prevalence of lung symptoms, increased loss in lung function and increased risk of death compared with non-smokers (US Department of Health and Human Services 1984).

Outdoor air pollution. Although industrialized air pollution in cities in the Western world has decreased substantially during the last 40–50 years, the air pollutant load still exists and is not negligible. Central substances in the air pollution are diesel particles, ozone and particulate air pollution called PM_{10}. Several studies have shown a negative effect of the exposure on respiratory health, with an increased risk of hospital admission due to exacerbation of COPD, decrements in lung function and mortality (MacNee and Donaldson 2002).

Host factors. Genetic factors seem to influence the development of COPD (Molfino 2004). The most important is the Z-deficiency type of α_1-antitrypsin, with increased risk of panlobular emphysema. Other gene factors might have an association with COPD, but data are premature. Bronchial hyperreactivity and disturbed growth of the lungs are associated with the disease.

Others. Indoor air pollution, infections and low economical status are factors associated with COPD (Siafakas et al. 1995).

2.2.5.4.2 Occupational Exposure

Most of the knowledge of associations between occupation and COPD are based on epidemiological studies in population and working groups at risk. About 15–20% of the COPD cases are reported associated with occupational exposure (Viegi and Di Pede 2002).

Inorganic dust. Associations between exposure to inorganic dust and COPD/chronic bronchitis have been described in several studies, with increased risks for coal miners, gold miners, in miners exposed to zinc, copper and nickel, in workers exposed to quartz, asbestos and cadmium, and in tunnel- and construction workers.

Organic dust.

Confinement building exposure. Farmers are exposed to a mixture of irritating gases such as NH_3, H_2S, NO_x and organic and inorganic dusts. Among never-smoking farmers working in animal confinement buildings, there was a significant association between total dust exposure and COPD (adjusted OR 6.6; 95% CI 1.10–39.5 in the highest exposure group) (Monso et al. 2004). In swine farmers and confinement workers, associations have been found between increased risk of chronic bronchitis, impact on lung function and endotoxin exposure (Zejda et al. 1994). In 8 of 12 cross-sectional studies in farmers with a control group, baseline FEV_1 was significantly reduced among farmers with livestock (swine and dairy) and potato production. Longitudinal studies indicate an increased yearly loss in FEV_1 of 20–40 ml in swine confinement workers, while farmers with dairy and grain production do not, to the same extent, have increased loss in FEV_1 (Omland 2002).

Grain dust. No studies have been published in grain-exposed workers where COPD has been the outcome, but studies in Canadian grain workers have shown a significant association between grain dust exposure and reduction in FEV_1 in non-smokers, ex-smokers and in smokers (Pahwa et al. 2003).

Cotton dust. Workers exposed to cotton dust have been shown to have an increased annual loss in FEV_1, and data from a recent published 15-year longitudinal cohort study are supportive of a development chronic airway obstruction among the exposed, although there was no evidence of a direct dose–response relationship to endotoxin or total dust exposure (Christiani et al. 2001).

Wood dust. Most studies in wood-dust-exposed workers have focused on associations with asthma, but published data from cross-sectional and in longitudinal studies have found, from dose–response curves, an increased frequency of chronic respiratory symptoms and lower/increased decline in lung function among those exposed (Liou et al. 1995; Noertjojo et al. 1996).

2.2.5.5 Pathogenesis

The pathological changes of smoking-induced COPD are a mixture of emphysema and small airway disease, and smoking also causes an increased annual decline in FEV_1 in 20% of regular smokers (Fletcher and Peto 1977). Why only a few of the smokers develop clinically significant COPD is not known, but genetically mediated differences in the inflammatory response might play a central role. A threefold risk of airflow obstruction in current or ex-smokers and in children of patients with COPD with no plasma deficiency of $'\alpha_1$-antitrypsin has been demonstrated; and polymorphisms on genes coding for glutathione-S1-transferase and epoxide hydrolase, and tumor necrosis- $'\alpha$ are genetic variations that might explain the observed differences in risk (Silverman et al. 1988). The inflammation in COPD is characterized by an increased number of neutrophils, granulocytes, macrophages, and especially CD-8 positive lymphocytes initiating the liberation of mediators such as leukotriene B_4, interleukin 8 and tumor necrosis-$'\alpha$. Besides inflammation, oxidative stress and imbalance in lung elastin and elastases are involved in the development of COPD. When the balance between oxidants and antioxidants shifts toward oxidants, oxidative stress occurs (Sies and Cadenas 1985). Several studies have found increased oxidative stress in smokers and in patients with COPD (Rahman and MacNee 1996; Repine et al. 1997). Oxidative stress induces direct oxidation of several molecules leading to cell dysfunction, cell death and damage of the extracellular matrix and can act as a pre-inflammatory stimulus. Data are suggestive of an enhancing effect of the oxidative stress to transcription of several genes that regulate the influx of macrophages. Elastin is the principle component of elastic fibers, and the protein and the degradation of the elastic fibers in the lungs is associated with the development of emphysema. The elastic fibers are present around the alveolar ducts, in the opening of the alveoli and in the alveolar wall. The degradation of elastin is caused by proteolytic activity and, in emphysema, disruption and degradation of elastin have been demonstrated (Werb et al. 1982; Fukuda et al. 1989). Human and animal studies have shown that in smoking-induced emphysema, proteinases from macrophages and neutrophils might be involved in the degradation (Betsuyaku et al. 1999).

Little is known of the effect on the lungs of environmental exposures other than smoking. There is some evidence that exposure to cadmium, coal and silicia (Törnell 1946; Bexell and Edfeldt 1949; Terho and Lacey 1979) can cause emphysema, and the risk of developing COPD due to occupational exposure is greater when exposed to dust than to gas and fumes (Krzyzanowski et al. 1986; Xu et al. 1992).

2.2.5.6 Clinical Aspects

2.2.5.6.1 Symptoms

Cardinal symptoms are breathlessness, cough and sputum production. Most of the patients suffer all the symptoms (Burrows et al. 1965). Breathlessness develops gradually throughout the years – at the start, this is present during hard physical exercise and in connection with lower lung infections, and later during mild physical exercise and at rest. Breathlessness at night is seldom a symptom in COPD. The intensity of the breathlessness in COPD is best related to changes in end-expiratory pressure (O'Donnell et al. 1997). Cough and sputum production are most frequent in the morning and during the winter. The sputum tends to increase in relation to lung infection, changing from a colourless to a more purulent appearance. The cough threshold seems to be normal, at least in mild COPD (Choudry and Fuller 1992). Some patients have wheeze and chest tightness or tenderness, and COPD patients with hypoxemia and CO_2-retention often suffer from headache, difficulties in concentration and fatigue.

2.2.5.6.2 Physical Examination

Most patients seek the physician because of breathlessness when FEV_1 is reduced to about 1.5 l. The clinical presentation can vary a lot from (a) the "pink puffer" appearance with profound breathlessness, the hyperinflated, barrel-shaped thorax, a tendency to hyperventilation and being skinny to (b) the "blue bloater" appearance with minor breathlessness, being less hyperinflated, and showing cyanosis of the lips, normal or increased body weight and edema of the legs. On auscultation, COPD patients with emphysema will have an enlarged border of the lungs, horizontal situated costae, a tendency to costal respiration, prolonged expiration and decreased intensity of the vesicular breath sound with or without crackles or rales. Crackles or rales might be the only finding in a COPD patient with no emphysema.

2.2.5.6.3 Laboratory Findings

Blood samples will usually show normal values for blood pO_2 and pCO_2, but with increasing progression in the disease hypoxemia and CO_2-retention can occur. In these COPD patients, cor pulmonale is commonly present (MacNee 1994). Of the COPD patients, 1–2% will have a reduced plasma α_1-antitrypsin concentration.

2.2.5.6.4 Lung Function Tests

The airflow limitation will be mirrored by a reduction in the FEV_1/FVC ratio, FEV_1 and expiratory flow. In patients with symptomatic COPD, and especially with emphysema, the diffusion capacity (*T*L,CO, Kco) is reduced. Reduction in Kco is associated with the severity of the emphysema assessed by CT scanning (Gould et al. 1991). Static lung volumes, TLC and RV will be normal or increased. The severity of the airflow limitation in COPD is graded arbitrarily by the reduction in FEV_1:

Mild: FEV_1 ≥80% of predicted
Moderate: FEV_1 30–79% of predicted
Severe: FEV_1 <30% of predicted

2.2.5.7 Radiological Findings

Plain chest radiograph will usually be normal (Simon et al. 1973). In emphysema, low diaphragms, an increase in the retrosternal airspace, a reduction in size and number of peripheral pulmonary vessels, and areas of transradiency are found. Using thin-section CT scanning, it is possible to distinguish between different types of emphysema. While centrilobular emphysema is prominent in the upper zones, the panlobular type is diffuse throughout the lung zones (Kuwano et al. 1990).

2.2.5.8 Histopathology

Structural changes such as atrophy, focal squamous metaplasia and ciliary abnormalities in the epithelium in the central airways have been described. The major cellular component is the CD8+ T-lymphocytes in both the central and peripheral airways (O'Shaughnessy et al. 1997). Besides CD8+ T lymphocyte infiltration in the peripheral airways, increased smooth muscle thickness occurs. The main morphological form and degree of emphysema can be demonstrated, but the techniques are time consuming, and CT scan pictures seem to be a better way to demonstrate changes in vivo (Gould et al. 1988).

2.2.5.8.1 Diagnostic Methods and Differential Diagnosis

If subjects with breathlessness, cough and sputum production have airflow limitation, COPD is the probable diagnosis, especially with a positive history of exposure to tobacco and/or exposure to other environmental air pollutants mainly of occupational origin. By excluding lung infection, pleural effusion and cardiomegaly by means of plain chest radiography, and excluding asthma using reversible tests, the diagnosis of COPD is quite clear. Λ_1-antitrypsin deficiency, bronchiectasis, ciliar dyskinesis and cystic fibrosis should be excluded, especially in younger subjects.

2.2.5.8.1 Diagnosis Methods of Occupational COPD

The first step in diagnosis is a systematic and chronological occupational history with registration of all employments with job title, name of the workplace and the kind of industry. Acute episodes of respiratory symptoms in relation to previous and/or present exposures might be of value, especially if others at the workplace and with the same exposure have experienced symptoms of the same kind. Then for each employment a quantitative description of the air pollution (dust, gases, fumes) present is needed. Both direct and bystander exposure are of importance, together with information on job task and the use of respiratory protective equipment. Quantitative data regarding the exposure are not always available, but will if present be of importance. Access to previous and present hygiene measurements together with visits to the workplaces will increase the strength of the argument to a denial or an acceptance of a causal association between exposure and disease.

2.2.5.9 Treatment

The major goal is to reduce the speed of the excessive fall in lung function and, thus, prolong the time to invalidity and death. Cessation of exposure, primarily to smoking but also to occupation, is the only treatment that is able to do so. The majority of the available treatment is symptomatic and aims to reduce the breathlessness by reducing the airway obstruction, ease the cough and sputum production, and to fight the bacterial infections. Several regimes are available, but a systematic presentation of these is beyond the scope of a description of COPD associated with occupation and environment.

2.2.6 Prevention

Since most of the occupational and environmental diseases of the lungs are mainly caused by exposures, there is a major task in reducing the exposures to levels that do not initiate lung diseases. Although looking for subjects with increased risk of developing lung diseases is of importance, our primary concern ought to be a search for exposures in occupations and in the environment that induces inflammatory changes in the respiratory tract or induces sensitization in order to identify and reduce agents at risk. All aspects of prevention (primary, secondary, and tertiary) are useful in the work to avoid or reduce the severity of occupational and environmental lung diseases. Smoking cessation is not described in this section.

2.2.6.1 Primary Prevention

Primary prevention includes all activities to avoid diseases occurring in healthy individuals. The foundation for primary preventive work is reliable risk estimates, and established dose–response relationships between exposure and disease.

In occupational settings, data have been published that demonstrate allergens, that the concentration of exposure is associated with the number of subjects that become sensitized or develop asthma especially for exposure to high-molecular-weight allergens (Baur et al. 1998). In studies among bakers (Houba et al. 1998), in subjects working with laboratory animals, (Hollander et al. 1996) and in subjects exposed to latex (Hunt et al. 2002), dose–response relationships between exposure and sensitization or symptoms have been established. Besides exposures to high-molecular-weight allergens, exposures to low-molecular-weight allergens also have demonstrated a dose–response relationship between exposure and asthma, in subjects exposed both to wood dust from Western Red Cedar and to isocyanates (Tarlo et al. 1997; Brooks et al. 2001). Dose–response relationships have also been established between exposures and allergic alveolitis (Malmberg et al. 1993). In a study among Swedish farmers, exposure to microorganisms was associated with the disease. Few studies have focused on COPD and exposure to organic dust, but a recent published study in never-smoking animal farmers found a dose–response relationship between exposure to organic dust and COPD (Monso et al. 2004). The adjusted OR for COPD was 6.6 (95% CI 1.10–39.5) in the highest exposure group (<9.4–76.7 mg/m^3 total dust).

Several environmental factors might influence upon the risk of developing allergic diseases. In particular, indoor exposure to environmental tobacco and airborne allergens have been studied, and the majority of data suggest a dose–response relationship between exposure to house dust mites and cat allergens and sensitization towards the same allergens; further there is an association between sensitization and the development of allergic airway symptoms, especially in children with a disposition to allergy (Celedon et al. 2002; Bornehag et al. 2003). There seems to be an association between indoor environmental tobacco smoking and asthma or asthma symptoms. Studies indicate an especially significant association between maternal smoking and asthmatic bronchitis/asthma in the child, showing a dose–response relationship between severity of the symptoms and the intensity of the exposure (Strachan and Cook 1998). As opposed to the negative effect of maternal smoking, breastfeeding during the first months of life seems to protect against the development of asthma and reduces the prevalence of asthmatic bronchitis and asthma in childhood (van Odijk et al. 2003).

2.2.6.2 Secondary and Tertiary Prevention

Secondary prevention deals with initiatives including early diagnosis and medical treatment in subjects with a disease in order to prevent symptoms and further progression, and the purpose of tertiary prevention is closely connected. Tertiary prevention tries to impede further deterioration in patients with chronic disease. There is data to support that early recognition of occupational asthma and consequent elimination of relevant exposure has a positive effect on the prognosis of the disease (Vandenplas et al. 2003). As in asthma, cessation of exposure is of great importance for the prognosis of allergic alveolitis and COPD. Classical methods for this kind of intervention would be surveillance programs in workers at risk by means of questionnaire, spirometry and a test for IgE-mediated sensitization. Besides a reduction in exposure to sensitizing agents, a reduction in exposure to irritant exposure should be borne in mind. Environmental exposure to tobacco smoke triggers symptoms of asthma, and increases the severity of symptoms and the need for medication. As in occupational settings, reduction of allergen exposure in the domestic area seems to have a significant influence of the disease control, especially to house dust mite exposure (Asher et al. 2000).

Several studies have analyzed associations between outdoor air pollution and respiratory diseases (Ackermann-Liebrich 2000). Agents such as sulfur dioxide, nitrogen dioxide, particulate matter including ultrafine particles, and ozone have been shown to have an affect on the lungs. Daily variation in particulate matter, sulfur dioxide and nitrogen dioxide are associated with exacerbation of symptoms, increased use of medication in asthmatic subjects, increased hospital admission and mortality, especially for respiratory diseases. Long-term exposure to air pollutants seems to be related to a small negative effect on lung function and symptoms of bronchitis. Despite small effects, particulate matter and nitrogen dioxide from urban air have been related to increased mortality.

2.2.6.3 Initiating Preventive Activities

Although several studies have been published supporting an assumption of a beneficial effect of primary or secondary prevention, there is no strong support from well-designed randomized, prospective intervention studies that prevention has significantly reduced the incidence of occupational or environmental respiratory lung diseases. It is not known whether the preventive efforts to reduce allergic occupational lung diseases have reduced the incidence of the diseases, and no data exist regarding COPD and occupation (Cullinan et al. 2003).

However, it seems reasonable to support any activity that reduces occupational and environmental exposure to sensitizing and irritant agents, and inert aerosols and dust. Exposure to environmental tobacco smoke in early life ought to be avoided, and breastfeeding should be encouraged for the first 4–6 months of life.

2.2.7 Conclusion

Although it has been known for centuries that bioaerosols and organic dust can cause severe hazards for the respiratory tract, it stills remains a serious problem. Let us end by citing Bernardino Ramazzini again – "If you find that work seriously affects your health, it is very wise to change occupation. Money is worthless, if you loose the most valuable of all, your health."

References

Ackermann-Liebrich U (2000) Outdoor air pollution. Eur Respir Mon 15:400–411

Akoun GM et al. (1984) Amiodarone-induced hypersensitivity pneumonitis. Evidence of an immunological cell-mediated mechanism. Chest 85(1):133–5

American Thoracic Society (1995) Standards for the diagnosis and care of patients with chronic obstructive pulmonary disease. Am J Respir Crit Care Med 152(5 Pt 2):S77–121

Anderson HR (1974) The epidemiological and allergic features of asthma in the New Guinea Highlands. Clin Allergy 4(2):171–183

Andersen P et al. (1982) Serum antibodies and immunoglobulins in smokers and nonsmokers. Clin Exp Immunol 47(2):467–473

Ando M and M. Suga (1997) Hypersensitivity pneumonitis. Curr Opin Pulm Med 3(5):391–395

Ando M et al. (1991) Japanese summer-type hypersensitivity pneumonitis. Geographic distribution, home environment, and clinical characteristics of 621 cases. Am Rev Respir Dis 144(4):765–769

Anonymous (1978) Inhalation fevers. Lancet 1(8058):249–250

Anonymous (1986) Acute respiratory illness following occupational exposure to wood chips–Ohio. MMWR Morb Mortal Wkly Rep 35(30):483–490

Arshad M, Braun SR, Sunderrajan EV (1987) Severe hypoxemia in farmer's lung disease with normal findings on chest roentgenogram. Chest 91(2):274–275

Asher I et al. (2000), Prevention of allergy and asthma:interim report. Allergy 55(11):1069–1088

Asmundsson T, Gunnarsson E, Johannesson T (1983) "Haysickness" in Icelandic horses:precipitin tests and other studies. Equine Vet J 15(3):229–232

Atterholm I et al. (1977) Unexplained acute fever after a hot bath. Lancet 2(8040):684–686

Ball TM et al. (2000) Siblings, day-care attendance, and the risk of asthma and wheezing during childhood. N Engl J Med 343(8):538–543

Banham SW et al. (1986) Relationships between avian exposure, humoral immune response, and pigeon breeders' disease among Scottish pigeon fanciers. Thorax 41(4):274–278

Barbee RA et al. (1968) The long-term prognosis in farmer's lung. Am Rev Respir Dis 97(2):223–231

Barrowcliff DF and Arblaster PG (1968) Farmer's lung:a study of an early acute fatal case. Thorax 23(5):490–500

Bascom R, Bromberg P, Costa D (1996a) State of the art:health effects of air pollution; part I. Am J Respir Crit Care Med 153:3–53

Bascom R, Bromberg P, Costa D (1996b) State of the art:health effects of air pollution; part II. Am J Respir Crit Care Med 153:477–498

Baseler MW and Burrell R (1981) Acute-phase reactants in experimental inhalation lung disease. Proc Soc Exp Biol Med 168(1):49–55

Basu S and Fenton MJ (2004) Toll-like receptors:function and roles in lung disease. Am J Physiol Lung Cell Mol Physiol 286(5):L887–892

Baur X et al. (1988) Humidifier lung and humidifier fever. Lung 166(2):113–124

Baur X, Chen Z, Liebers V (1998) Exposure-response relationships of occupational inhalative allergens. Clin Exp Allergy 28(5):537–544

Belin L (1980) Clinical and immunological data on "wood trimmer's disease" in Sweden. Eur J Respir Dis Suppl 107:169–176

Bernstein IL (1999) Asthma in the workplace. 2nd edn. Dekker, New York. XIX, pp 742

Betsuyaku T et al. (1999) Neutrophil granule proteins in bronchoalveolar lavage fluid from subjects with subclinical emphysema. Am J Respir Crit Care Med 159(6):1985–1991

Bexell E and Edfeldt O (1949) Mögelsvampinfektion under tröskningsarbete. Svenska Läkartidningen 46(2):2433

(1996) Biopsy-confirmed hypersensitivity pneumonitis in automobile production workers exposed to metalworking fluids – Michigan, 1994-1995. MMWR Morb Mortal Wkly Rep 45(28):606–610

Bishop JM, Melnick SC, Raine J (1963) Farmer's Lung:studies of pulmonary function and aetiology. Q J Med 32:257–278

Blanchet MR, Israel-Assayag E, Cormier Y (2004) Inhibitory effect of nicotine on experimental hypersensitivity pneumonitis in vivo and in vitro. Am J Respir Crit Care Med 169(8):903–909

Bornehag CG et al. (2003) Pet-keeping in early childhood and airway, nose and skin symptoms later in life. Allergy 58(9):939–944

Bourke SJ et al. (1989) Obstructive airways disease in non-smoking subjects with pigeon fanciers' lung. Clin Exp Allergy 19(6):629–632

Bourke SJ et al. (2001) Hypersensitivity pneumonitis:current concepts. Eur Respir J Suppl 32:81s–92s

Boyd DH (1971) The incidence of farmer's lung in Caithness. Scott Med J 16(5):261–262

Braun SR et al. (1979) Farmer's lung disease:long-term clinical and physiologic outcome. Am Rev Respir Dis 119(2):185–191

Brinton WT et al. (1987) An outbreak of organic dust toxic syndrome in a college fraternity. JAMA. 258(9):1210–1212

Broder I et al. (1979) Comparison of respiratory variables in grain elevator workers and civic outside workers of Thunder Bay, Canada. Am Rev Respir Dis 119(2):193–203

Brooks AM et al. (2001) Impact of low birth weight on early childhood asthma in the United States. Arch Pediatr Adolesc Med 155(3):401–406

Burrows B et al. (1965) Chronic obstructive lung disease. II. Relationship of clinical and physiologic findings to the severity of airways obstruction. Am Rev Respir Dis 91:665–678

Burrows B et al. (1989) Association of asthma with serum IgE levels and skin-test reactivity to allergens. N Engl J Med 320(5):271–277

Burrows B et al. (1991) Findings before diagnoses of asthma among the elderly in a longitudinal study of a general population sample. J Allergy Clin Immunol 88(6):870–877

Cadham FT (1924) Asthma due to grain rusts. JAMA 83(27)

Calvert JE et al. (1999) Pigeon fanciers' lung:a complex disease? Clin Exp Allergy 29(2):166–175

Camarena A et al. (2001) Major histocompatibility complex and tumor necrosis factor-alpha polymorphisms in pigeon breeder's disease. Am J Respir Crit Care Med 163(7):1528–1533

Campbell JM (1932) Acute symptoms following work with hay. BMJ 2:1143–1444

Carroll N et al. (1996) Airway structure and inflammatory cells in fatal attacks of asthma. Eur Respir J 9(4):709–715

Castellan RM et al. (1984) Acute bronchoconstriction induced by cotton dust:dose-related responses to endotoxin and other dust factors. Ann Intern Med 101(2):157–163

Celedon JC et al. (2002) Exposure to cat allergen, maternal history of asthma, and wheezing in first 5 years of life. Lancet 360(9335):781–782

Chan-Yeung M and Malo JL (1994) Aetiological agents in occupational asthma. Eur Respir J 7(2):346–371

Chapela R et al. (1985) [Effect of pregnancy and the puerperium on the development of extrinsic allergic alveolitis]. Allergol Immunopathol (Madr) 13(4):305–309

Choudry NB, and Fuller RW (1992) Sensitivity of the cough reflex in patients with chronic cough. Eur Respir J 5(3):296–300

Christiani DC et al. (2001) Longitudinal changes in pulmonary function and respiratory symptoms in cotton textile workers. A 15-yr follow-up study. Am J Respir Crit Care Med 163(4):847–853

Cockcroft AE et al. (1983) Grain exposure–symptoms and lung function. Eur J Respir Dis 64(3):189–196
Coplu L et al. (2005) Lung health in workers exposed to reed dust. Respir Med 2005. 99(4):421–428
Cormier Y and Belanger J (1985) Long-term physiologic outcome after acute farmer's lung. Chest 87(6):796–800
Cullinan P, Tarlo S, Nemery B (2003) The prevention of occupational asthma. Eur Respir J 22(5):853–860
Dalphin JC et al. (1993) Prevalence and risk factors for chronic bronchitis and farmer's lung in French dairy farmers. Br J Ind Med 50(10):941–944
Denis M (1995) Proinflammatory cytokines in hypersensitivity pneumonitis. Am J Respir Crit Care Med 151(1):164–169
Desideri M et al. (1997) Mortality rates for respiratory disorders in Italy (1979-1990). Monaldi Arch Chest Dis 52(3):212–216
Donham KJ (1990) Health effects from work in swine confinement buildings. Am J Ind Med 17(1):17–25
Dopico GA et al. (1984) Epidemiologic study of clinical and physiologic parameters in grain handlers of northern United States. Am Rev Respir Dis, 130(5):759–765
doPico GA (1986) Health effects of organic dusts in the farm environment. Report on diseases. Am J Ind Med 10(3):261–265
Douglas JG et al. (1986) Sarcoidosis:a disorder commoner in non-smokers? Thorax 41(10):787–791
Dunnill MS, Massarella GR, Anderson JA (1969) A comparison of the quantitative anatomy of the bronchi in normal subjects, in status asthmaticus, in chronic bronchitis, and in emphysema. Thorax, 24(2):176–179
Edwards JH, Baker JT, Davies BH (1974) Precipitin test negative farmer's lung-activation of the alterative pathway of complement by mouldy hay dusts. Clin Allergy 4:379–388
Eliasson O (1982) Farmer's lung disease:a new historical perspective from Iceland. J Hist Med Allied Sci 37(4):440–443
Emanuel DA, Wenzel FJ, Lawton BR (1975) Pulmonary mycotoxicosis. Chest 67(3):293–297
Emanuel DA and Kryda MJ (1983) Farmer's lung disease. Clin Rev Allergy 1(4):509–532
Emanuel DA, Marx JJ, Ault BJ (1989) Organic dust toxic syndrome (pulmonary mycotoxicosis) – a review of the experience in central Wisconsin. In: Dosman JA and Cockcroft DW (eds) Principles of health and safety in agriculture. CRC Press, Boca Raton, pp 72–75
Fink JN et al. (1971) Precipitins and the diagnosis of a hypersensitivity pneumonitis. J Allergy Clin Immunol 48(3):179–181
Fink JN et al. (2005) Needs and opportunities for research in hypersensitivity pneumonitis. Am J Respir Crit Care Med 171(7):792–798
Fishwick D et al. (1997) Occupational asthma in New Zealanders:a population based study. Occup Environ Med 54(5):301–306
Fletcher CM (1976) The natural history of chronic bronchitis and emphysema :an eight-year study of early chronic obstructive lung disease in working men in London. Oxford University Press, Oxford, New York. XIX, p 272
Fletcher C and Peto R (1977) The natural history of chronic airflow obstruction. BMJ 1(6077):1645–1648
Flynn MG (1994) Respiratory symptoms, bronchial responsiveness, and atopy in Fijian and Indian children. Am J Respir Crit Care Med 150(2):415–420
Freedman PM and Ault B (1981) Bronchial hyperreactivity to methacholine in farmers' lung disease. J Allergy Clin Immunol 67(1):59–63
Freedman PM et al. (1981) Skin testing in farmers' lung disease. J Allergy Clin Immunol 67(1):51–58
Fukuda Y et al. (1989) Morphogenesis of abnormal elastic fibers in lungs of patients with panacinar and centriacinar emphysema. Hum Pathol 20(7):652–659
Fuller CJ (1953) Farmer's lung:a review of present knowledge. Thorax 8(1):59–64
Gatzemeier U (1981) [Acute exogenous allergic alveolitis–6 cases after loading mouldy barley]. Prax Klin Pneumol 35(9):400–402
Girard M, Israel-Assayag E, Cormier Y (2004) Pathogenesis of hypersensitivity pneumonitis. Curr Opin Allergy Clin Immunol 4(2):93–98
Gould GA et al. (1988) CT measurements of lung density in life can quantitate distal airspace enlargement – an essential defining feature of human emphysema. Am Rev Respir Dis 137(2):380–392
Gould GA et al. (1991) Lung CT density correlates with measurements of airflow limitation and the diffusing capacity. Eur Respir J 4(2):141–146
Grant IW et al. (1972) Prevalence of farmer's lung in Scotland: a pilot survey. BMJ 1(799):530–534
Gregory PH and Lacey ME (1963) Mycological examination of dust from mouldy hay associated with farmer's lung disease. J Gen Microbiol 30:75–88
Griffiths-Johnson DA, Ryan LK, Karol MH (1991) Development of an animal model for organic dust toxic syndrome. Inhalation Toxicol 3:405–417
Gruchow HW et al. (1981) Precipitating antibodies to farmer's lung antigens in a Wisconsin farming population. Am Rev Respir Dis 124(4):411–415
Hapke EJ et al (1968) Farmer's lung. A clinical, radiographic, functional, and serological correlation of acute and chronic stages. Thorax 23(5):451–468
Hargreave FE (1973) Extrinsic allergic alveolitis. Can Med Assoc J 108(9):1150–1154
Heederik D et al. (1989) Chronic non-specific lung disease and occupational exposures estimated by means of a job exposure matrix:the Zutphen Study. Int J Epidemiol 18(2):382–389
Heino M et al. (1982) An electron-microscopic study of the airways in patients with farmer's lung. Eur J Respir Dis 63(1):52–61
Hodgson MJ, Parkinson DK, Karpf M (1989) Chest X-rays in hypersensitivity pneumonitis:a metaanalysis of secular trend. Am J Ind Med 16(1):45–53
Hollander A, Doekes G, Heederik D (1996) Cat and dog allergy and total IgE as risk factors of laboratory animal allergy. J Allergy Clin Immunol 98(3):545–554
Holt PG and Keast D (1977) Environmentally induced changes in immunological function:acute and chronic effects of inhalation of tobacco smoke and other atmospheric contaminants in man and experimental animals. Bacteriol Rev 41(1):205–216
Houba R, Heederik D, Doekes G (1998) Wheat sensitization and work-related symptoms in the baking industry are preventable. An epidemiologic study. Am J Respir Crit Care Med 158(5 Pt 1):1499–1503
Hunt LW et al. (2002) Management of occupational allergy to natural rubber latex in a medical center:the importance

of quantitative latex allergen measurement and objective follow-up. J Allergy Clin Immunol 110[2 Suppl]:S96–106
Huovinen E et al. (1999) Incidence and prevalence of asthma among adult Finnish men and women of the Finnish Twin Cohort from 1975 to 1990, and their relation to hay fever and chronic bronchitis. Chest 115(4):928–936
Husman K et al. (1990) Organic dust toxic syndrome among Finnish farmers. Am J Ind Med 17(1):79–80
Jacobs RL et al. (1986) Hypersensitivity pneumonitis caused by Cladosporium in an enclosed hot-tub area. Ann Intern Med 105(2):204–206
Karjalainen A et al. (2000) Incidence of occupational asthma by occupation and industry in Finland. Am J Ind Med 37(5):451–458
Katila M-L (1979) Respiratory disease in a farming population: a sero-epidemiological survey of farmer's lung and chronic nonspecific lung disease among dairy farmers in Eastern Finland Kuopio. 93
Kawai T, Tamura M, Murao M (1984) Summer-type hypersensitivity pneumonitis. A unique disease in Japan. Chest 85(3):311–317
Kimbell-Dunn MR et al. (2001) Work-related respiratory symptoms in New Zealand farmers. Am J Ind Med 39(3):292–300
Kivity S et al. (1995) The characteristics of bronchial asthma among a young adult population. Chest 108(1):24–27
Kleinfeld M (1974) A comparative clinical and pulmonary function study of grain handlers and bakers. Ann N Y Acad Sci 221:86–96
Kline JN, Hunninghake GW (2001) Hypersensitivity pneumonitis and eosinophilic pneumonias. In: Braunwald E, Fauci AS, Kasper DL, Hauser SL, Longo DL, Jameson JL (eds) Harrison's principles of internal medicine, 15th edn. McGraw Hill, New York
Kogevinas M et al. (1999) Occupational asthma in Europe and other industrialised areas:a population-based study. European Community Respiratory Health Survey Study Group. Lancet 353(9166):1750–1754
Kogevinas M et al. (1996) The risk of asthma attributable to occupational exposures. A population-based study in Spain. Spanish Group of the European Asthma Study. Am J Respir Crit Care Med 154(1):137–143
Kokkarinen JI, Tukiainen HO, Terho EO (1993) Recovery of pulmonary function in farmer's lung. A five-year follow-up study. Am Rev Respir Dis 147(4):793–796
Konig G, Baur X, Fruhmann G (1981) Sarcoidosis or extrinsic allergic alveolitis? Respiration 42(3):150–154
Koppelman GH, Los H, Postma DS (1999) Genetic and environment in asthma:the answer of twin studies. Eur Respir J 13(1):2–4
Kryda M, Emanuel DA, Marx JJ (1989) Hypersensitivity pneumonitis due to Aspergillus fumigatus in papermill workers. In: Principles of health and safety in agriculture. Dosman JA and Cockcroft DW (eds), CRC Press, Boca Raton, p 80
Krzyzanowski M, Jedrychowski W, Wysocki M (1986) Factors associated with the change in ventilatory function and the development of chronic obstructive pulmonary disease in a 13-year follow-up of the Cracow Study. Risk of chronic obstructive pulmonary disease. Am Rev Respir Dis 134(5):1011–1019
Kuwano K et al. (1990) The diagnosis of mild emphysema. Correlation of computed tomography and pathology scores. Am Rev Respir Dis 141(1):169–178
Lacasse Y et al. (2003) Clinical diagnosis of hypersensitivity pneumonitis. Am J Respir Crit Care Med 168(8):952–958
Lacey J and Lacey ME (1964) Spore concentrations in the air of farm. buildings. Trans Br Mycol Soc 47:547–552
Larsson K et al. (1988) Exposure to microorganisms, airway inflammatory changes and immune reactions in asymptomatic dairy farmers. Bronchoalveolar lavage evidence of macrophage activation and permeability changes in the airways. Int Arch Allergy Appl Immunol 87(2):127–133
Larsson L (1995) Incidence of asthma in Swedish teenagers: relation to sex and smoking habits. Thorax 50(3):260–264
Lau S et al. (1989) High mite-allergen exposure increases the risk of sensitization in atopic children and young adults. J Allergy Clin Immunol 84(5 Pt 1):718–725
Leadbitter P et al. (1999) Relationship between fetal growth and the development of asthma and atopy in childhood. Thorax 54(10):905–910
Lecours R, Laviolette M, Cormier Y (1986) Bronchoalveolar lavage in pulmonary mycotoxicosis (organic dust toxic syndrome). Thorax 41(12):924–926
Lee K et al. (2004) Personal exposures to inorganic and organic dust in manual harvest of California citrus and table grapes. J Occup Environ Hyg 1(8):505–514
Lieberman J (1975) Elevation of serum angiotensin-converting-enzyme (ACE) level in sarcoidosis. Am J Med 59(3):365–372
Lindesmith LA, Fink KN, Horvath EP (1988) Occupational medicine:principles and practical applications. Zenz C (ed) Year Book Medical Publishers, Chicago 15:226
Liou SH et al. (1996) Respiratory symptoms and pulmonary function in mill workers exposed to wood dust. Am J Ind Med 30(3):293–299
Lundback B (1998) Epidemiology of rhinitis and asthma. Clin Exp Allergy 28[Suppl 2]:3–10
Lundholm M and Rylander R (1983) Work related symptoms among sewage workers. Br J Ind Med 40(3):325–329
Lynch DA et al. (1992) Hypersensitivity pneumonitis:sensitivity of high-resolution CT in a population-based study. AJR Am J Roentgenol 159(3):469–472
MacNee W (1994) Pathophysiology of cor pulmonale in chronic obstructive pulmonary disease. Part One. Am J Respir Crit Care Med 150(3):833–852
MacNee W and Donaldson K (2002) Air pollution and COPD: mechanisms. Eur Respir Rev 12:297–302
Madsen D et al (1976) The prevalence of farmer's lung in an agricultural population. Am Rev Respir Dis 113(2):171–174
Malmberg P and Larsson K (1993) Acute exposure to swine dust causes bronchial hyperresponsiveness in healthy subjects. Eur Respir J 6(3):400–404
Malmberg P et al. (1985) Exposure to microorganisms, febrile and airway-obstructive symptoms, immune status and lung function of Swedish farmers. Scand J Work Environ Health 11(4):287–293
Malmberg P et al (1988) Incidence of organic dust toxic syndrome and allergic alveolitis in Swedish farmers. Int Arch Allergy Appl Immunol 87(1):47–54
Malmberg P, Rask-Andersen A, Rosenhall L (1993) Exposure to microorganisms associated with allergic alveolitis and febrile reactions to mold dust in farmers. Chest 103(4):1202–1209
Malmberg P and Rask-Andersen A (1993) Organic dust toxic syndrome. Semin Respir Med 14:38–48

Malmros P, Sigsgaard T, Bach B (1992) Occupational health problems due to garbage sorting. Waste Manag Res 10:227–234

Manfreda J and Warren CP (1984) The effects of grain dust on health. Rev Environ Health 4(3):239–267

Manfreda J et al. (1986) Acute symptoms following exposure to grain dust in farming. Environ Health Perspect 66:73–80

Mapp CE et al. (1994) Mechanisms and pathology of occupational asthma. Eur Respir J 7(3):544–554

Matricardi PM et al. (2000) Exposure to foodborne and orofecal microbes versus airborne viruses in relation to atopy and allergic asthma:epidemiological study. BMJ. 320(7232):412–417

Matusiewicz SP et al. (1993) Plasma lactate dehydrogenase: a marker of disease activity in cryptogenic fibrosing alveolitis and extrinsic allergic alveolitis? Eur Respir J 6(9):1282–1286

May JJ et al. (1986) Organic dust toxicity (pulmonary mycotoxicosis) associated with silo unloading. Thorax 41(12):919–923

May JJ, Pratt DS, Stallones L (1989) A study of dust generated during silo opening and its physiologic effects on workers. In: Principles of health and safety in agriculture. Dosman JA and Cockcroft DW (eds) CRC Press, Boca Raton, pp 76–79

May JJ et al. (1990) Organic dust toxic syndrome:a follow-up study. Am J Ind Med 17(1):111–113

McCormick JR et al. (1981) Serum angiotensin-converting enzyme levels in patients with pigeon-breeder's disease. Chest 80(4):431–433

McWhorter WP, Polis MA, Kaslow RA (1989) Occurrence, predictors, and consequences of adult asthma in NHANESI and follow-up survey. Am Rev Respir Dis 139(3):721–724

Merchant JA (1987) Agricultural exposures to organic dusts. Occupational Medicine:State of the Art Review 2:409–425

Milton DK et al. (1998) Risk and incidence of asthma attributable to occupational exposure among HMO members. Am J Ind Med 33(1):1–10

Mindell HJ (1970) Roentgen findings in farmer's lung. Radiology 97(2):341–346

Molfino NA (2004) Genetics of COPD. Chest 125(5):1929–1940

Monkare S (1983) Influence of corticosteroid treatment on the course of farmer's lung. Eur J Respir Dis 64(4):283–293

Monkare S (1984) Clinical aspects of farmer's lung:airway reactivity, treatment and prognosis. Eur J Respir Dis Suppl 137:1–68

Monkare S et al. (1981) Bronchial hyperreactivity to inhaled histamine in patients with farmer's lung. Lung 159(3):145–151

Monkare S et al. (1982) Does disodium cromoglycate prevent exacerbation of farmer's lung? Allergy 37(3):217–218

Monkare S, Ikonen M, Haahtela T (1985) Radiologic findings in farmer's lung. Prognosis and correlation to lung function. Chest 87(4):460–466

Monso E et al. (2004) Chronic obstructive pulmonary disease in never-smoking animal farmers working inside confinement buildings. Am J Ind Med 46(4):357–362

Morell F, Orriols R, Molina C (1985) Usefulness of skin test in Farmer's lung. Chest 87(2):202–205

Morris DG (2003) Gold, silver, and bronze:metals, medals, and standards in hypersensitivity pneumonitis. Am J Respir Crit Care Med 168(8):909–910

Moser F (1979) [Extrinsic allergic alveolitis:farmer's lung. A propos of a case]. Rev Med Suisse Romande 99(3):121–148

Muittari A et al (1980) An epidemic of extrinsic allergic alveolitis caused by tap water. Clin Allergy 10(1):77–90

Nagai K et al. (1998) [Pulmonary disease after massive inhalation of Aspergillus niger]. Nihon Kokyuki Gakkai Zasshi 36(6):551–555

National Heart Lung and Blood Institute (1991) National Asthma Education Program. Expert Panel on the Management of Asthma, Guidelines for the diagnosis and management of asthma. Bethesda, Md.:National Asthma Education Program, Office of Prevention, Education, and Control, National Heart, Lung, and Blood Institute, National Institutes of Health. XIII, p 136

Neal P, Schneitter R, Cominita P (1942) Report on acute illness among rural mattress-workers using low grade, stained cotton. JAMA 119:1074–1082

Ng TP et al. (1994) Risks of asthma associated with occupations in a community-based case-control study. Am J Ind Med 25(5):709–718

Noertjojo HK et al. (1996) Western red cedar dust exposure and lung function:a dose–response relationship. Am J Respir Crit Care Med 154(4 Pt 1):968–973

O'Donnell DE et al. (1997) Qualitative aspects of exertional breathlessness in chronic airflow limitation:pathophysiologic mechanisms. Am J Respir Crit Care Med 155(1):109–115

Ohtsuka Y et al. (1995) Smoking promotes insidious and chronic farmer's lung disease, and deteriorates the clinical outcome. Intern Med 34(10):966–971

Olaus M, Granlund J, Foote PG (1996) Historia de gentibus septentrionalibus, Romae 1555 = Description of the Northern peoples, Rome 1555. Abridged and augm. ed. 1996, London, Eng.:The Hakluyt Society. v

Omland O (2002) Exposure and respiratory health in farming in temperate zones – a review of the literature. Ann Agric Environ Med 9(2):119–136

Omland O et al. (1999) Lung status in young Danish rurals:the effect of farming exposure on asthma-like symptoms and lung function. Eur Respir J 13(1):31–37

O'Shaughnessy TC et al. (1997) Inflammation in bronchial biopsies of subjects with chronic bronchitis: inverse relationship of CD8+ T lymphocytes with FEV1. Am J Respir Crit Care Med 155(3):852–857

Ouchterlony O (1958) Diffusion-in-gel methods for immunological analysis. Prog Allergy 5:1–78

Pahwa P et al. (2003) Longitudinal decline in lung function measurements among Saskatchewan grain workers. Can Respir J 10(3):135–141

Pallasaho P et al. (1999) Increasing prevalence of asthma but not of chronic bronchitis in Finland? Report from the FinEsS-Helsinki Study. Respir Med 93(11):798–809

Parkes WR (1982) Occupational lung disorders. 2nd edn. Butterworths, London. XV, p 529

Patel AM, Ryu JH, Reed CE (2001) Hypersensitivity pneumonitis:current concepts and future questions. J Allergy Clin Immunol 108(5):661–670

Patterson R et al. (1976) Antibodies of different immunoglobulin classes against antigens causing farmer's lung. Am Rev Respir Dis 114(2):315–324

Patterson R et al. (1981) Hypersensitivity lung disease presumptively due to Cephalosporium in homes contaminated by sewage flooding or by humidifier water. J Allergy Clin Immunol 68(2):128–132

Pauwels RA et al. (2001) Global strategy for the diagnosis, management, and prevention of chronic obstructive pulmonary disease. NHLBI/WHO Global Initiative for Chronic Obstructive Lung Disease (GOLD) Workshop summary. Am J Respir Crit Care Med 163(5):1256–1276

Pearce N, Pekkanen J, Beasley R (1999) How much asthma is really attributable to atopy? Thorax 54(3):268–272

Peat JK and Li J (1999) Reversing the trend:reducing the prevalence of asthma. J Allergy Clin Immunol 103(1 Pt 1):1–10

Pepys J (1967) Hypersensitivity against inhaled organic antigens. J R Coll Physicians Lond 2(42–8)

Pepys J and Jenkins PA (1965) Precipitin (F.L.H.) test in farmer's lung. Thorax 20:21–35

Pepys J et al. (1963) Farmer's Lung. Thermophilic actinomycetes as a source of "farmer's lung hay" antigen. Lancet 41:607–611

Pepys J, Riddel R, Citron KM (1962) Precipitins against extracts of hay and molds in the serum of patients with farmer's lung, aspergillosis, asthma, and sarcoidosis. Thorax 17:366

Perry LP et al. (1998) Pulmonary mycotoxicosis:a clinicopathologic study of three cases. Mod Pathol 11(5):432–436

Pestalozzi C (1959) [Febrile group diseases in a carpentry shop caused by inhalation of moisture from air humidifiers contaminated with molds.]. Schweiz Med Wochenschr 89:710–713

Pether JV and Greatorex FB (1976) Farmer's lung disease in Somerset. Br J Ind Med 33(4):265–268

Platts-Mills TA et al. (1982) Reduction of bronchial hyperreactivity during prolonged allergen avoidance. Lancet 2(8300):675–678

Plessner M (1960) [A disease of feather sorters:duck fever.]. Arch Mal Prof 21:67–69

Pratt DS and May JJ (1984) Feed-associated respiratory illness in farmers. Arch Environ Health 39(1):43–48

Radon K et al. (2003) [Respiratory diseases in European farmers-II. Part of the European farmers' project]. Pneumologie 57(9):510–517

Rahman I and MacNee W (1996) Oxidant/antioxidant imbalance in smokers and chronic obstructive pulmonary disease. Thorax 51(4):348–350

Ramazzini B (1700) de Morbis Artificum Diatriba. Editio secunda. Modena. 2 pt. in 1

Rankin J et al. (1962) Farmer's lung:physiopathologic features of the acute interstitial granulomatous pneumonitis of agricultural workers. Ann Intern Med 57:606–626

Rankin J et al. (1967) Pulmonary granulomatoses due to inhaled organic antigens. Med Clin North Am 51(2):459–482

Rask-Andersen A (1989a) Organic dust toxic syndrome among farmers. Br J Ind Med 46(4):233–238

Rask-Andersen A (1989b) Allergic alveolitis in Swedish farmers. Ups J Med Sci 94(3):271–285

Rask-Andersen A (1996) Inhalation fever. In: Harber P, Schenker M, Balmes J (eds) Occupational and environmental respiratory disease. Mosby, St. Louis, Mo. pp 243–258

Rask-Andersen A and Pratt DS (1992) Inhalation fever:a proposed unifying term for febrile reactions to inhalation of noxious substances. Br J Ind Med 49(1):40

Rask-Andersen A, Malmberg P, Lundholm M (1989) Endotoxin levels in farming:absence of symptoms despite high exposure levels. Br J Ind Med 46(6):412–416

Rask-Andersen A et al. (1994) Inhalation fever and respiratory symptoms in the trimming department of Swedish sawmills. Am J Ind Med 25(1):65–67

Repine JE, Bast A, Lankhorst I (1997) Oxidative stress in chronic obstructive pulmonary disease. Oxidative Stress Study Group. Am J Respir Crit Care Med 156(2 Pt 1):341–357

(1998) Respiratory health hazards in agriculture. Am J Respir Crit Care Med 158(5 Pt 2):S1–S76

Reyes CN et al. (1982) The pulmonary pathology of farmer's lung disease. Chest 81(2):142–146

Riedler J et al. (2001) Exposure to farming in early life and development of asthma and allergy:a cross-sectional survey. Lancet 358(9288):1129–1133

Ritter WL and Nussbaum MA (1944) Occupational illness in cotton industries. Miss Doctor 22:96–99

Roberts RC, Zais DP, Emanuel DA (1976) The frequency of precipitins to trichloroacetic acid-extractable antigens from thermophilic actinomycetes in farmer's lung patients and asymptomatic farmers. Am Rev Respir Dis 114(1):23–28

Robinson TJ (1976) Letter: coeliac disease and diffuse lung disease. BMJ 1(6025):1593

Robinson TJ et al. (1981) Jejunal villous changes associated with farmer's lung. Postgrad Med J 57(673):697–701

Rodriguez de Castro F et al. (1993) Relationships between characteristics of exposure to pigeon antigens. Clinical manifestations and humoral immune response. Chest 103(4):1059–1063

Rona RJ, Hughes JM, Chinn S (1999) Association between asthma and family size between 1977 and 1994. J Epidemiol Community Health 53(1):15–19

Rylander R (1987) The role of endotoxin for reactions after exposure to cotton dust. Am J Ind Med 12(6):687–697

Rylander R, Lundholm M (1978) Bacterial contamination of cotton and cotton dust and effects on the lung. Br J Ind Med 35(3):204–207

Salvaggio JE and Karr RM (1979) Hypersensitivity pneumonitis; state of the art. Chest 75[2 Suppl]:270–274

Schatz M and Patterson R (1983) Hypersensitivity pneumonitis–general considerations. Clin Rev Allergy 1(4):451–467

Schatz M, Patterson R, Fink J (1977) Immunopatholgenesis of hypersensitivity pneumonitis. J Allergy Clin Immunol 60(1):27–37

Schilling RS et al. (1955) An epidemiological study of byssinosis among Lancashire cotton workers. Br J Ind Med 12(3):217–227

Schuyler M (2001) Are polymorphisms the answer in hypersensitivity pneumonitis? Am J Respir Crit Care Med 163(7):1513–1514

Schwartz J and Weiss ST (1990) Dietary factors and their relation to respiratory symptoms. The Second National Health and Nutrition Examination Survey. Am J Epidemiol 132(1):67–76

Seal RM et al. (1968) The pathology of the acute and chronic stages of farmer's lung. Thorax 23(5):469–489

Seifert SA et al. (2003) Organic dust toxic syndrome:a review. J Toxicol Clin Toxicol 41(2):185–193

Shaheen SO et al. (1999) Birth weight, body mass index and asthma in young adults. Thorax 54(5):396–402

Sharma OP and Fujimura N (1995) Hypersensitivity pneumonitis:a noninfectious granulomatosis. Semin Respir Infect 10(2):96–106

Siafakas NM et al. (1995) Optimal assessment and management of chronic obstructive pulmonary disease (COPD). The European Respiratory Society Task Force. Eur Respir J 8(8):1398–1420

Sies H and Cadenas E (1985) Oxidative stress:damage to intact cells and organs. Philos Trans R Soc Lond B Biol Sci 311(1152):617–631

Sigsgaard T and Schlunssen V (2004) Occupational asthma diagnosis in workers exposed to organic dust. Ann Agric Environ Med 11(1):1–7

Sigurdarson ST, Donham KJ, Kline JN (2004) Acute toxic pneumonitis complicating chronic obstructive pulmonary disease (COPD) in a farmer. Am J Ind Med 46(4):393–395

Silverman EK et al. (1998) Genetic epidemiology of severe, early-onset chronic obstructive pulmonary disease. Risk to relatives for airflow obstruction and chronic bronchitis. Am J Respir Crit Care Med 157(6 Pt 1):1770–1778

Simon G et al. (1973) Relation between abnormalities in the chest radiograph and changes in pulmonary function in chronic bronchitis and emphysema. Thorax 28(1):15–23

Snider GL (1986) Interstitial pulmonary fibrosis. Chest 89[3 Suppl]:115S–121S

Somerville SM, Rona RJ, Chinn S (1984) Obesity and respiratory symptoms in primary school. Arch Dis Child 59(10):940–944

Sovijarvi AR et al. (1980) Trapped air in extrinsic allergic alveolitis. Respiration 40(2):57–64

Spurzem JR, Romberger DJ, Von Essen SG (2002) Agricultural lung disease. Clin Chest Med 23(4):795–810

Staines FH and Forman JAS (1961) A survey of farmer's lung. J R Coll Gen Pract 4:351–382

Strachan DP and Cook DG (1998) Health effects of passive smoking. 6. Parental smoking and childhood asthma: longitudinal and case-control studies. Thorax 53(3):204–212

Sunyer J et al. (1998) Pulmonary ventilatory defects and occupational exposures in a population-based study in Spain. Spanish Group of the European Community Respiratory Health Survey. Am J Respir Crit Care Med 157(2):512–517

Tanaka H et al. (2002) Workplace-related chronic cough on a mushroom farm. Chest 122(3):1080–1085

Tarlo SM et al. (1997) Assessment of the relationship between isocyanate exposure levels and occupational asthma. Am J Ind Med 32(5):517–521

Taylor G (1986) Acute systemic effects of inhaled occupational agents. In: Merchant JA and Boehlecke BA (eds) Occupational respiratory diseases. National Institute for Occupational Safety and Health. Cincinnati, Ohio. pp 607–625

Terho EO (1986) Diagnostic criteria for farmer's lung disease. Am J Ind Med 10:329

Terho EO and Lacey J (1979) Microbiological and serological studies of farmers' lung in Finland. Clin Allergy 9(1):43–52

Terho EO et al. (1980a) Myopericarditis associated with farmer's lung. BMJ 281(6234):197

Terho EO, Lammi S, Heinonen OP (1980b) Seasonal variation in the incidence of farmer's lung. Int J Epidemiol. 9(3):219–220

Terho EO, Heinonen OP, Lammi S (1983) Incidence of farmer's lung leading to hospitalization and its relation to meteorological observations in Finland. Acta Med Scand 213(4):295–298

Terho EO et al. (1987) Incidence of clinically confirmed farmer's lung in Finland and its relation to meteorological factors. Eur J Respir Dis Suppl 152:47–56

Tewksbury DA et al. (1981) Angiotensin-converting enzyme in farmer's lung. Chest 79(1):102–104

Todd A, Coan RM, Allen A (1991) Pigeon breeders' lung:pigeon intestinal mucin, an antigen distinct from pigeon IgA. Clin Exp Immunol 85(3):453–458

Törnell E (1946) Thresher's lung. Fungoid disease resembling tuberculosis and morbis Schaumann. Acta Med Scand 125:191

Torok M, de Weck AL, Scherrer M (1981) [Allergic alveolitis as a result of mold on the bedroom wall]. Schweiz Med Wochenschr 111(25):924–929

Tukiainen P et al. (1980) Farmer's lung:needle biopsy findings and pulmonary function. Eur J Respir Dis 61:3–11

Turton CW et al. (1983) Red cell folate levels, food antibodies and reticulin antibodies in farmer's lung–is there an association with coeliac disease? Br J Dis Chest 77(4):397–402

Ulrik CS and Lange P (1994) Decline of lung function in adults with bronchial asthma. Am J Respir Crit Care Med 150(3):629–634

US Department of Health and Human Services (1984) The health consequences of smoking:chronic obstructive lung disease. A report of the Surgeon General., P.H.S. US Department of Health and Human Services, Office on Smoking and Health (ed). US Department of Health and Human Services, Rockville, Maryland

van Odijk J et al. (2003) Breastfeeding and allergic disease:a multidisciplinary review of the literature (1966-2001) on the mode of early feeding in infancy and its impact on later atopic manifestations. Allergy 58(9):833–843

Vandenplas O, Toren K, Blanc PD (2003) Health and socioeconomic impact of work-related asthma. Eur Respir J 22(4):689–697

Veen JC et al. (1998) Impaired perception of dyspnea in patients with severe asthma. Relation to sputum eosinophils. Am J Respir Crit Care Med 158(4):1134–1141

Venho KK et al. (1982) Splenic granulomas in Farmer's lung disease. An extrapulmonary manifestation of extrinsic allergic alveolitis. Acta Med Scand 211(5):413–414

Vergnon JM et al. (1983) [Angiotensin converting enzyme at different stages of extrinsic allergic alveolitis. Serum and alveolar study]. Bull Eur Physiopathol Respir 19(5):439–445

Vesterinen E, Kaprio J, Koskenvuo M (1988) Prospective study of asthma in relation to smoking habits among 14,729 adults. Thorax 43(7):534–539

Viegi G and Di Pede C (2002) Chronic obstructive lung diseases and occupational exposure. Curr Opin Allergy Clin Immunol 2(2):115–121

Viegi G et al. (1991) Respiratory effects of occupational exposure in a general population sample in north Italy. Am Rev Respir Dis 143(3):510–515

Viegi G et al. (1994) Risk factors for chronic obstructive pulmonary disease in a north Italian rural area. Eur J Epidemiol 10(6):725–731

Vogelmeier C et al. (1993) Activation of blood neutrophils in acute episodes of farmer's lung. Am Rev Respir Dis 148(2):396–400

Vohlonen I et al. (1987) Prevalence and incidence of chronic bronchitis and farmer's lung with respect to the geographical location of the farm and to the work of farmers. Eur J Respir Dis Suppl 152:37–46 von Mutius E et al. (1994) Prevalence of asthma and atopy in two areas of West and East Germany. Am J Respir Crit Care Med 149(2 Pt 1):358–364

Warren CP (1977) Extrinsic allergic alveolitis:a disease commoner in non-smokers. Thorax 32(5):567–569

Warren P, Cherniack RM, Tse KS (1974) Hypersensitivity reactions to grain dust. J Allergy Clin Immunol 53(3):139–149

Warren CP, Tse KS, Cherniack RM (1978) Mechanical properties of the lung in extrinsic allergic alveolitis. Thorax 33:315–321

Warren CP, Holford-Strevens V, Manfreda J (1987) Respiratory disorders among Canadian farmers. Eur J Respir Dis Suppl 154:10–14

Weber S et al. (1993) Organic dust exposures from compost handling: case presentation and respiratory exposure assessment. Am J Ind Med 24(4):365–374

Werb Z et al. (1982) Elastases and elastin degradation. J Invest Dermatol 79[Suppl 1]:154s–159s

Werner GC (1955) [Allergic edematous bronchiolitis; statistical survey on asthma caused by textile plant dust.]. Arch Mal Prof 16(1):27–45

Wilkie BN and Nielsen K (1981) Bovine hypersensitivity pneumonitis and reaginic antibody. Adv Exp Med Biol 137:693–709

Williams JV (1963) Pulmonary function studies in patients with farmer's lung. Thorax 18:255–263

Wintermeyer SF et al. (1997) Pulmonary responses after wood chip mulch exposure. J Occup Environ Med 39(4):308–314

Woolcock AJ et al. (1971) Lung volume changes in astham measured concurrently by two methods. Am Rev Respir Dis 104(5):703–709

Xu X et al. (1992) Exposure-response relationships between occupational exposures and chronic respiratory illness:a community-based study. Am Rev Respir Dis 146(2):413–418

Ye TT et al. (1998) Respiratory symptoms and pulmonary function among Chinese rice-granary workers. Int J Occup Environ Health 4(3):155–159

Yoshida K, Ando M, Araki S (1989) Acute pulmonary edema in a storehouse of moldy oranges: a severe case of the organic dust toxic syndrome. Arch Environ Health 44(6):382–384

Yunginger JW et al. (1992) A community-based study of the epidemiology of asthma. Incidence rates, 1964–1983. Am Rev Respir Dis 146(4):888–894

Zejda JE et al. (1994) Respiratory health status in swine producers relates to endotoxin exposure in the presence of low dust levels. J Occup Med 36(1):49–56

2.3 Chemical-Induced Lung Injury and Its Long-Term Sequelae

Benoit Nemery

CONTENTS

2.3.1 Introduction and Scope *67*
2.3.2 Deposition of Inhaled Chemicals in the Respiratory Tract *67*
2.3.3 Inhalation Fever *68*
2.3.4 Acute Chemical Pneumonitis *70*
2.3.4.1 Irritant Gases and Organic Chemicals *70*
2.3.4.2 Metallic Compounds *72*
2.3.4.3 Complex Mixtures *72*
2.3.5 Pathology of Toxic Pneumonitis and the Issue of "Organizing Pneumonia" *73*
2.3.6 Possible Sequelae of Acute Inhalation Injury *73*
2.3.7 Subacute Toxic Pneumonitis *74*
References *75*

2.3.1 Introduction and Scope

Although many respiratory diseases are caused by chemicals, they will not all be discussed here. Thus, lung disorders caused by tobacco smoking will not be addressed, even though tobacco smoke contains hundreds of irritant, toxic and carcinogenic chemicals and even though smoking is the most common cause of toxic damage to the airways and the lung parenchyma. Similarly, although mineral dusts and fibers are also "chemicals", the pneumoconioses and other long-term disorders that result from chronic occupational exposures to these agents will not be covered. The effects of exposure to urban air pollutants resulting from traffic, industrial activities and domestic heating will not be addressed either.

The focus of this chapter will be on the acute or subacute respiratory health effects – and their possible long-term sequelae – of exposures to high amounts of chemicals and pollutants. Such exposures are generally accidental, and they occur mainly in the workplace, but they may also occur at home or in the community, for instance, as a result of fires and explosions, volcanic eruptions, industrial disasters (e.g. Bhopal in 1984) and accidents involving trains or trucks transporting chemicals, as well as warfare or terrorism.

A great variety of substances can cause inhalation injury. The toxic compounds may be in a gaseous state, or they may consist of aerosols of liquid or solid particles. Chemicals causing lung injury may be simple gases (oxygen, ozone, carbon monoxide, sulphur dioxide, etc.), inorganic compounds in liquid or vapour form (sulphuric acid, nitric acid, etc.), simple or complex minerals (silica, cement, asbestos, man-made vitreous fibers, etc.), metallic agents (mercury, zinc, iron, steel, alloys) or composite materials (hard metal, ceramics), simple organic agents of natural or synthetic origin (acetic acid, acrolein, benzene, toluene diisocyanate, plastic monomers, pesticides, therapeutic drugs, etc.), complex synthetic materials (plastics), mixtures of organic chemicals such as fuels or their combustion products (aliphatic hydrocarbons, polycyclic aromatic hydrocarbons, etc.) and complex biological agents (vegetable, animal or microbial products, such as cellulose, enzymes, lipopolysaccharides, etc.). Most often, exposures are to mixtures of many diverse chemicals, which may be present as gases and particles, thus forming aerosols, as is the case with burning wood, plastics or other materials.

This contribution is a shortened and updated version of a book chapter (Nemery 2002), in which specific references can be found.

2.3.2 Deposition of Inhaled Chemicals in the Respiratory Tract

The site and severity of the respiratory damage caused by inhaled compounds depend mainly on the nature of the agent and the amount inhaled (Schwartz

Benoit Nemery, MD, PhD
Research Unit of Lung Toxicology, Laboratory of Pneumology and Division of Occupational, Environmental and Insurance Medicine, K. U. Leuven, Herestraat 49, 3000 Leuven, Belgium

1987). As a general rule, gaseous irritants that have a high solubility in water mainly affect the upper respiratory tract, causing rhinitis, pharyngitis, laryngitis, tracheitis or bronchitis. Such water-soluble irritants are easily trapped in the aqueous surfaces of the upper respiratory tract and the eyes, where they cause rapid irritation, thus, leading the subject to avoid further exposure. In contrast, poorly water-soluble gases are not so well scrubbed by the upper respiratory tract, and they can more easily reach the deep lung, where they may lead to pulmonary oedema, usually after a latency of several hours. Moreover, as they cause much less sensory irritation, significant exposure to such gases may be tolerated without much trouble and may even go relatively unnoticed. Consequently, such insoluble gases are more hazardous. Gases of intermediate solubilities mainly affect the upper respiratory tract and large bronchi, but high or prolonged exposures to these agents may also injure the lung and cause chemical pneumonitis. The latter may, in fact, also occur when massive quantities of highly water-soluble gases are inhaled.

With aerosols, the degree of penetration into the respiratory tract depends mainly on the size of the particles, with the smallest particles (<5 μm aerodynamic diameter) having the greatest probability of reaching the distal airways and alveoli. Such small particles are often produced by combustion processes or by condensation of vapours. The particles may be toxic by themselves (e.g. cadmium oxide, CdO), or they may carry irritants, such as sulphates or aldehydes adsorbed onto soot particles.

Chemical-induced lung injury may also be caused by routes other than inhalation. Thus, the lungs may be damaged by the aspiration of ingested liquids, such as solvents or fuels. Some chemicals, most notably agrichemicals such as paraquat or cholinesterase inhibitors, may cause lung injury following ingestion or dermal absorption. Toxic pneumonitis may also result from inhaling or injecting illegal drugs (Wesselius 1997) or as a side effect from various drugs, but this will not be covered here.

Toxic lung injury may have various clinical presentations, which, for convenience, are separated here into three main categories. A first category concerns relatively mild, febrile reactions, collectively known as inhalation fevers. The second category is that of acute chemical pneumonitis with non-cardiogenic pulmonary oedema, which follows a single or brief exposure to a toxic agent. The third category covers subacute or chronic pulmonary inflammation, resulting from a more or less prolonged exposure to pneumotoxic agents.

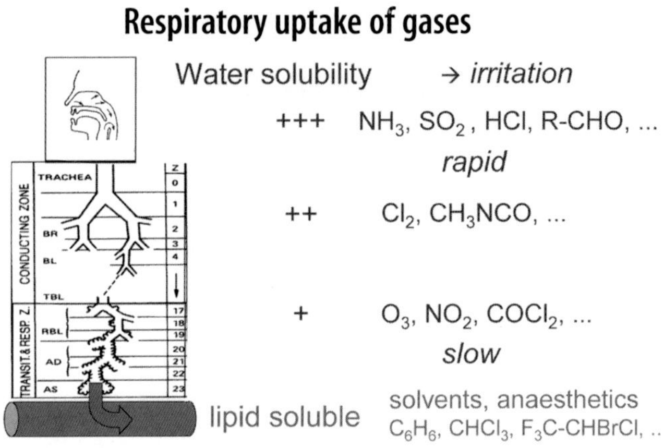

Fig. 2.3.1. The site of uptake of gases depends on their water solubility (+++ high; ++ intermediate; + low). Water soluble gases usually cause rapide sensory irritation; poorly water soluble gases cause little sensory irritation but may lead to delayed pulmonary edema.

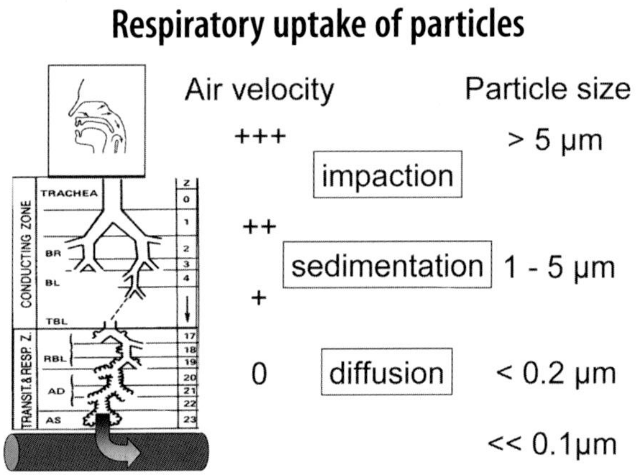

Fig. 2.3.2. The site of deposition of particles depends on air velocity (0 to +++) and particle size. Larger particles are deposited mainly in the upper respiratory tract; smaller particles may reach the bronchioli and alveoli.

2.3.3 Inhalation Fever

Inhalation fever is the name given to cover a group of flu-like clinical syndromes, such as metal fume fever, polymer fume fever and the organic dust toxic syndrome (ODTS) (Rask-Andersen 1992). The term "inhalation fever" is of relatively recent creation, and for a while it competed with the term "toxic alveolitis". There are arguments in favour of both terms, because the former emphasizes the clinical presentation and relatively benign nature of the condition, whereas the latter indicates the (presumed) main site of the toxic (i.e. non-allergic) inflammatory reaction. It seems, however, that the more clinical term has been preferred by most authors, probably because toxic alveolitis suggests a much more dramatic condition than is usually the case.

Metal fume fever is an old syndrome that is quite well known, not so much by doctors, but by those who are especially at risk of suffering from it, such as welders or other workers in metal trades (Blanc 1993). The most frequent and best documented cause of metal fume fever is that caused by heating zinc. Zinc fumes, which oxidize to fine particles of zinc oxide (ZnO), are produced, for instance, when zinc is smelted to make alloys, when zinc-containing scrap metal is molten, when metal surfaces are sprayed with zinc or when galvanized steel is welded or cut. Metal fume fever occurs when the fumes are not properly exhausted, which is often the case when these jobs are done in enclosed spaces. Both freshly formed zinc fumes and fine zinc oxide dust have the ability to cause metal "fume" fever.

The fumes of many other metals are said to cause metal fume fever too, but this seems not to have been satisfactorily documented, except for magnesium and copper.

ODTS is caused by the inhalation of large quantities of agricultural and other dusts of biological origin (Rask-Andersen 1996). Such bio-aerosols are often heavily contaminated with microorganisms that produce toxins (e.g. bacterial endotoxin, mycotoxins), which are believed to contribute to the pathogenesis of the syndrome. The syndrome is also known by various other names, such as mycotoxicosis.

Polymer fume fever is a less common cause of inhalation fever (Shusterman 1993). It occurs after exposure to the fumes that are produced when fluorine-containing polymers, such as polytetrafluoroethylene (PTFE), also known as Teflon, are heated above 300°C. This may occur when such polymers are extruded or machined or when welding metals that are covered with a PTFE layer. PTFE may also be used as a tape and also be sprayed, e.g. as a mould-release agent, and pyrolysis of this PTFE may occur in a burning cigarette, which explains why polymer fume fever occurs mainly in workers who smoke at work. Although polymer fume fever has only been well described after exposure to the fumes of fluorine-containing polymers, it may possibly occur after exposure to fumes evolving from heating other plastics.

The clinical features of the inhalation fevers are best described as those of a beginning influenza. The actual exposure may or may not have been experienced as irritant or troublesome to the eyes and respiratory tract. Then 4–8 h after the exposure, the subject begins to feel unwell, with fever, chills, headaches, malaise, nausea and muscle aches. In the case of metal fume fever, there may be a metallic taste in the mouth. Respiratory symptoms are usually mild and consist mainly of cough and/or sore throat, but occasionally subjects may have more severe responses with dyspnoea. The body temperature may rise as high as 39–40°C, but there are also less full-blown inhalation "fevers", even without fever, but with malaise, headache or systemic symptoms.

In general, chest auscultation and chest X-ray are normal, but in the more severe cases, which are more likely to seek medical attention, crackles may be heard, and there may be transient infiltrates on chest X-ray. (In the latter circumstances, one would be justified to challenge the diagnosis of inhalation fever and consider that there is a real chemical pneumonitis). Although pulmonary function is often within normal limits, reductions in vital capacity and FEV_1 are perhaps more common than generally accepted; in severe cases there may be a decrease in transfer factor and arterial hypoxaemia. Increased peripheral blood leukocytosis, with a rise in neutrophils, is a consistent finding until 24 h after the exposure; other blood tests should be normal, except, probably, for indices of an inflammatory response. Bronchoalveolar lavage studies have shown very pronounced and dose-dependent increases in polymorphonuclear leukocytes on the day after exposure to zinc fumes or organic dust.

The pathogenesis of metal fume fever and ODTS is considered to be based on a non-specific, i.e. non-allergic, activation of macrophages or pulmonary epithelial cells with local and systemic release of pyrogenic and chemotactic mediators. The mechanism of polymer fume fever is unknown, and the exact components of the fume that cause the toxicity are also unknown. It has been shown that the heating rate of PTFE influences the type and quantity of thermal decomposition products, some of which appear to be extremely toxic.

In principle, inhalation fever is a self-limited syndrome, and recovery normally takes place after a night's rest. Tolerance exists against re-exposures occurring shortly after a bout of metal fume fever or ODTS, but it seems that this feature is less typical of polymer fume fever.

The most important thing to say with regard to the diagnosis of inhalation fevers is that physicians must know the existence of such reactions and the circumstances in which they occur. The diagnosis rests essentially on the exposure history and the clinical condition, and when these clearly point to inhalation fever, no sophisticated investigations are required. However, it is important not to confuse inhalation fever with other more serious conditions, including chemical pneumonitis, which in its early phases could be mistaken for inhalation fever. One should also be aware that fumes of heated polymers, including fluorinated polymers, may be extremely hazardous and lead to severe pulmonary injury. Obviously, a differential diagnosis must also be made with various types of infectious pneumonias or with acute extrinsic allergic alveolitis (EAA), in which fever, malaise and systemic symptoms occur. This is particularly relevant in the case of exposure to bioaerosols, which is a common cause of acute EAA.

2.3.4 Acute Chemical Pneumonitis

The response to acute chemical injury in the respiratory tract is rarely compound specific. Following exposure to water-soluble irritants, there may be pronounced signs of upper airway irritation, with severe cough, hoarseness, stridor or wheezing, retrosternal pain, discharge of bronchial mucus, possibly with blood, mucosal tissue and soot. Death may occur as a result of laryngeal oedema. If the lung parenchyma is also involved, non-cardiogenic pulmonary oedema may develop over the course of several hours. It is important to realize that victims of serious inhalation accidents may feel perfectly well and walk into the infirmary or an emergency room, or even go home following the inhalation, and then experience progressive dyspnoea, shallow breathing, cyanosis, frothy pink sputum and eventually ventilatory failure. A clinical picture of adult respiratory distress syndrome (ARDS) may, thus, develop gradually over 4–72 h, even after a period of clinical improvement. In the days that follow, severe acute inhalation injury, pulmonary infectious complications may also occur.

Depending on the circumstances of the accident, there may be thermal or chemical facial burns, as well as signs of mucosal irritation and oedema, and even haemorrhage and ulcerations in the air passages. Auscultation of the chest may or may not be abnormal, with wheezing, rhonchi or crepitations. Pulmonary function can be used to monitor ambulatory subjects who have been exposed. Arterial blood gases show varying degrees of hypoxaemia and respiratory acidosis, depending on the severity of the injury. The chest radiograph is usually normal if only the conducting airways are involved, but there may be signs of peribronchial cuffing. After exposure to deep lung irritants, the chest radiograph is unremarkable in the first hours after presentation, but signs of interstitial and alveolar oedema may become visible, and, with time, patchy infiltrates, areas of atelectasis and even "white lungs" may develop. These changes may be due to tissue damage and organization, or they may reflect superimposed infectious (broncho)pneumonia.

As indicated above, a large number of inhaled agents can cause inhalation injury (Table 2.3.1). In the following paragraphs, specific categories of chemicals are briefly highlighted.

Table 2.3.1. Possible causes of toxic pneumonitis

Irritant gases:
High water-solubility: NH_3, SO_2, HCl, etc.
Moderate water-solubility: Cl_2, H_2S, etc.
Low water-solubility: O_3, NO_2, $COCl_2$, etc.
Organic chemicals:
Organic acids: acetic acid, etc.
Aldehydes: formaldehyde, acrolein, etc.
Isocyanates: methylisocyanate (MIC), toluene diisocyanate (TDI)
Amines: hydrazine, chloramines, etc.
Tear gas (CS) and mustard gas
Organic solvents, including some leather treatment sprays
Some agrichemicals (paraquat, cholinesterase inhibitors)
Metallic compounds:
Mercury vapours
Metallic oxides: CdO, V_2O_5, MnO, Os_3O_4, etc.
Halides: $ZnCl_2$, $TiCl_4$, $SbCl_5$, UF_6, etc.
$Ni(CO)_4$
Hydrides: B_2H_5, LiH, AsH_3, SbH_3
Complex mixtures:
Fire smoke
Pyrolysis products from plastics
Solvent mixtures
Spores and toxins from microorganisms

2.3.4.1 Irritant Gases and Organic Chemicals

In general, gases with high water solubility, such as ammonia (NH_3), sulphur dioxide (SO_2), hydrochloric acid (HCl), formaldehyde (HCHO), acetic acid (CH_3COOH), which also have good warning properties, only cause mild upper airway irritation, unless the exposure concentration (or duration) has been considerable. Massive inhalation accidents include explosions or accidents in mines or chemical installations causing the release of, for instance, SO_2 or NH_3 (from refrigeration installations).

The same considerations apply to chlorine (Cl_2), hydrogen sulphide (H_2S) or methyl isocyanate (CH_3CNO), which have intermediate water solubilities. Accidental release of chlorine is probably one of the most frequent causes of inhalation injury, not only in industry but also in the community as a result of transportation accidents or the use of chlorine for the disinfection of swimming pools (Das 1993). An important cause of inhalation in the domestic setting is that which results from the mixing of bleach (NaClO) with acids, thus leading to the release of gaseous chlorine, or with ammonia, thus leading to the release of volatile chloramines (including trichloramine, NCl_3) (Olson 1993). Interesting case histories of severe pneumonias, which were not immediately recognized as being of toxic origin, have been reported in (elderly) ladies who had done their cleaning in a too enthusiastic fashion (Reisz 1986). Hydrogen sulphide (H_2S), which is formed by the putrefaction of organic material in sewage drains, manure pits or ship holds and is also a frequent contaminant in the petrochemical industry, has special properties as an irritant gas because not only does it cause mucosal irritation, but it also leads to chemical asphyxia by mechanisms that are somewhat similar to those of cyanide. Victims who survive massive inhalation of H_2S may exhibit (haemorrhagic) pulmonary oedema, as well as pneumonia in the days following the event (Reiffenstein 1992). Methyl isocyanate (CH_3CNO, MIC) has gained notoriety as the chemical that caused the highest number of casualties in a single accident, when it was released from a tank in a pesticide factory in Bhopal, India, in December 1994 (Dhara 1995). MIC caused intense eye and upper airway irritation, but it may also lead to pulmonary oedema.

As indicated above, the poorly water-soluble gases are the most hazardous because they are hardly noticed, and they can penetrate down to the distal airways and cause delayed non-cardiogenic pulmonary oedema. The best-known examples of such gases are nitrogen dioxide (NO_2), ozone (O_3) and phosgene ($COCl_2$). NO_2 is a reddish-brown gas, heavier than air, and is often incorrectly referred to as "nitrous fumes". It may be encountered in a wide variety of occupational settings. A well-known risk in agriculture is that of "silo filler's disease" (Douglas 1989) (not to be confused with "silo unloader's syndrome", which is a form of the organic toxic dust syndrome). Silo filler's disease occurs because NO_2 is produced within a few days of fermentation of the silage, thus posing a risk of fatal inhalation injury for anyone entering the silo. Fatally high quantities of NO_2 may also be produced when special jet fuels explode, when tanks of nitric acid (HNO_3) explode, when materials containing high quantities of nitrogen are burned in fires or when nitric acid reacts with metals, wood or other cellulose materials. Outbreaks of acute respiratory illness in players and spectators attending ice hockey matches have been attributed to NO_2 as a result of malfunctioning ice resurfacing machines. Phosgene (carbonyl chloride) is a well-known cause of pulmonary oedema, since it was used in chemical warfare during the first world war. This chemical is used in chemical syntheses, notably in the manufacture of isocyanates, and it may be produced by thermal or ultraviolet decomposition of chlorine-containing chemicals, such as methylene chloride or trichloroethylene.

Some chemicals are made intentionally to cause respiratory irritation. The most common lacrimating agents, known as tear gases (although they are in fact aerosol-dispersed chemicals), used in riot control operations or as personal anti-harassment weapons, are *ortho*-chlorobenzylidene malononitrile (CS) and 2-chloroacetophenone (CN). The action of these agents is usually short-lived and limited to the mucous membranes of the eyes and upper respiratory tract, but their use in confined spaces (e.g. prison cells) may lead to more serious lung damage. Lung-damaging chemical warfare agents include the choking agents (chlorine, phosgene, diphosgene, and chloropicrin) and the vesicants (or blister agents). Mustard gas (sulphur mustard) caused severe bronchopulmonary damage in soldiers during the Iran–Iraq war (Willems 1989).

Exposure to organic solvents is only rarely a cause of toxic pneumonitis. However, acute exposure to very high concentrations of solvent vapours in confined spaces (e.g. in chemical tanks) may be a cause of chemical pneumonitis and pulmonary oedema, often in victims who have been unconscious. Pneumonia and respiratory distress syndrome caused by loss of alveolar surfactant may also result from the aspiration of intentionally (e.g. by "fire eaters") or unintentionally (e.g. from siphoning petrol) ingested solvents or fuels.

A special mention should also be given to cases of severe acute respiratory illness caused, generally in the domestic environment, by acute exposure in confined spaces to fluorocarbon-containing water-proofing sprays and leather conditioners (Burkhart 1996).

Some agrichemicals may cause toxic pneumonitis after non-inhalatory exposure. The best known of these agents is the herbicide paraquat, which exerts a selective toxicity for the pulmonary epithelium and causes either multi-organ failure or a delayed pulmonary fibrosis, depending on the dose, after ingestion or, more rarely, after dermal exposure (Bismuth 1995). Poisoning by cholinesterase inhibitors, such as the organophosphate or carbamate insecticides, is also associated with significant respiratory symptoms such as bronchospasm, bronchorrhea, respiratory depression and sometimes also (delayed) pulmonary oedema (Tsao 1990).

2.3.4.2 Metallic Compounds

In general, the principles governing the site and type of damage caused by inhaled agents also apply to metallic compounds, many of which may cause lung injury (Nemery 1990). Metallic compounds may be inhaled as fumes (i.e. generally as oxides), very fine particles or as salts. It is important to realize that many metals also exert their toxicity in non-pulmonary organs.

Cadmium-pneumonitis is perhaps the best-documented example of metal-induced acute pneumonitis, and accidental cases still occur. Cadmium is a by-product of the zinc and lead industry. It is used in metal plating and in special alloys, as well as in the production of batteries, pigments and plastic stabilizers. From a practical point of view, it is important to be aware that cadmium may be liberated, often unknowingly to the worker, from the welding or burning of cadmium-containing alloys and cadmium-plated metal, from the use of hard solders or from the smelting of zinc or lead (or scrap metal), which often contain significant levels of contaminating cadmium. As with other pneumotoxic agents, exposure to toxic levels of cadmium fumes does not necessarily lead to immediate respiratory symptoms, but symptoms of pneumonitis may start many hours after the exposure. Severe chemical pneumonitis may also result from exposure to high levels of mercury vapours. Several fatalities or severe pulmonary involvement have been reported as a result of the refining of gold or silver (using amalgams) in confined spaces.

The embolization of droplets of metallic mercury in the pulmonary circulation following the deliberate injection or accidental inoculation of mercury leads to a peculiar pattern of small very radiodense dots on the chest radiograph. This condition does not appear to be associated with either pulmonary or systemic manifestations of disease.

Vanadium pentoxide (V_2O_5) may be present in significant quantities in slags from the steel industry (ferrovanadium) and, because some fuel oils contain high quantities of vanadium, in furnace residues from oil refineries or in soot from oil-fired boilers. Dust containing V_2O_5 may cause upper and lower airway irritation: rhinitis with sneezing and nosebleeds, pharyngitis, acute tracheobronchitis with cough, wheeze and (possibly) airway hyperreactivity ("boilermakers' bronchitis"), as well as possibly bronchopneumonia.

The older literature also indicates that exposure to high levels of oxides of beryllium, cobalt, manganese and osmium may cause airway irritation and even bronchopneumonia. However, new technologies, such as those involving the thermal spraying of metals, may also prove to be particularly hazardous.

Cases of ARDS, some with a protracted course, have been reported in military or civilian personnel accidentally exposed to smoke bombs that liberate zinc chloride ($ZnC1_2$).

Accidental exposure, e.g. as a result of explosions, burst pipes or leaks in chemical plants, to antimony trichloride ($SbCl_3$) and pentachloride ($SbCl_5$), zirconium tetrachloride ($ZrCl_4$), titanium tetrachloride ($TiCl_4$) and uranium hexafluoride (UF_6), may also lead to severe and even fatal inhalation injury. Nickel carbonyl [$Ni(CO)_4$] is a volatile liquid of very high toxicity for the lungs and brain. Lithium hydride (LiH), phosphine (hydrogen phosphide, PH_3, used as a doping agent for the manufacture of silicon crystals, or released from aluminium phosphide grain fumigants or zinc phosphide rodenticides), hydrogen selenide (SeH_3) and diborane (B_2H_5, used as high energy fuel) have also been reported to cause acute inhalation injury with, possibly, pulmonary oedema (Cordasco 1973).

2.3.4.3 Complex Mixtures

Probably one of the commonest causes of toxic pneumonitis is smoke inhalation caused by domestic, industrial or other fires. Respiratory morbidity is often the major complication in burn victims. It may be caused by direct thermal injury (particularly if hot vapours have been inhaled), but more generally the lesions are caused by chemical injury (Loke 2000). The composition of smoke is highly complex and variable, depending on the materials that are involved and the stages of the fire. The toxic components of smoke are numerous and involve gaseous asphyxiants (CO, HCN) and irritants, as well as particulates. Of particular concern are conditions that involve the burning or pyrolysis (e.g. caused by overheating) of plastics, such as polyurethanes, polyacrylates and other polymers that are known to give off numerous, generally poorly characterized but potentially highly toxic chemicals.

2.3.5 Pathology of Toxic Pneumonitis and the Issue of "Organizing Pneumonia"

The pathology of acute toxic pneumonitis is that of diffuse alveolar damage with epithelial disruption, interstitial and alveolar oedema, haemorrhage and formation of hyaline membranes and, depending on the stage of the lesions, varying degrees of infiltration by polymorphonuclear leukocytes, hyperplasia of the alveolar and bronchiolar epithelium and interstitial or intra-alveolar fibrosis. Understandably, only few human pathology reports of acute toxic pneumonitis are available, except from autopsies of the most fulminant cases.

One of the difficult issues is that of chemical-induced organizing pneumonia (OP) or (BO)OP (bronchiolitis obliterans organizing pneumonia), as it is called by some. This entity, which has fairly distinct clinical, functional and radiological features (Cordier 2000) essentially consists pathologically of the presence of (polyps of) granulation tissue in the bronchiolar and alveolar lumen. It is often stated that OP may result as a late or delayed consequence of the inhalation of toxic substances. However, the body of evidence linking toxic exposures to the development of (BO)OP is not very large. Irritant-induced (BO)OP only constitute a minority of the originally described cases of BOOP (Douglas 1994). Almost all published instances of (alleged) irritant-induced (BO)OP have been attributed to single, generally poorly characterized inhalatory exposures. The inhalation of NO_2 is the best-documented cause of bronchiolitis obliterans. Following resolution of the acute pulmonary oedema caused by massive exposure to NO_2, a relapse in the clinical condition may occur after 2–6 weeks with dyspnoea, cough, fine crackles, a radiographic picture of miliary nodular infiltrates, arterial hypoxaemia and a restrictive or mixed impairment, with low diffusion capacity. The site of cellular damage caused by NO_2 is the centriacinar region, and the relapse phase has been attributed to bronchiolar scarring with peribronchiolar and obliterating fibrosis of the bronchioli. It is not clear whether these instances of (BO)OP result from the "normal" repair of a particularly severe form of epithelial injury (i.e. with disruption of the basement membrane) or whether they result from an abnormal pattern of cellular proliferation in this critical region of the lung. Besides NO_2, other agents reported to cause bronchiolitis obliterans in humans have included SO_2 and poorly defined fumes of plastic fires, cleansing agents and trichloroethylene degradation products (phosgene?), as well as cocaine smoking and even mycotoxins. In several of these anecdotal reports, the diagnosis of BO has been inferred mainly from clinical and functional criteria, without the distinct radiological appearance of (BO)OP, let alone its pathological features, and it is not always certain that these are all instances of toxic (BO)OP. In some instances, most notably after inhalation of water-soluble agents (SO_2 and NH_3), the disease appears to consist of a constrictive bronchiolitis obliterans, rather than the "classical" organizing BO.

It could be argued that any severe chemical injury to the epithelium of the bronchiolo-alveolar region has the potential to be followed by organizing pneumonia with obliterating bronchiolitis, which may or may not be so labelled. It follows that in clinical cases of "cryptogenic" organizing pneumonia, one should always evaluate seriously the possibility of an underlying toxic cause for the condition. This is particularly true in view of the occurrence of outbreaks of organizing pneumonia such as the "Ardystil syndrome" (see below).

2.3.6 Possible Sequelae of Acute Inhalation Injury

Following acute inhalation injury, there is often complete recovery. However, this is certainly not always the case. The experience with ARDS caused by aetiologies other than acute inhalation injury suggests that a substantial proportion of patients recover with more or less severe dyspnoea and functional impairment, often a reduced diffusing capacity. However, it is still not well known whether and how frequently pulmonary fibrosis occurs after diffuse lung injury of toxic origin. The possible occurrence of residual lesions in the airways is better documented, even though the evidence is also often based on single instances only. Thus, various chronic sequelae, such as constrictive bronchiolitis, bronchiectases, and other bronchial lesions, such as strictures or polyps, have been reported to result from acute inhalation injury, depending on the severity of the initial damage and perhaps also depending on treatment modalities, although very little hard data, let alone controlled studies, are available regarding the latter issue.

Moreover, even in the absence of structural sequelae, which may be identified by imaging studies or through bronchoscopy, or in the absence of significant defects in basal spirometry, a state of permanent non-specific bronchial hyperreactivity may be observed. This condition of adult-onset, non-allergic asthma has been named "reactive airways dysfunction syndrome" (RADS) (Brooks 1985, Nemery 1996) and occurs in a number of survivors of (severe) airway injury. The incidence and mechanisms giving rise to post-inhalation asthma and irritant-induced asthma still remain to be elucidated. Recent observations in fire fighters and other personnel involved in rescue operations during and following the collapse of the World Trade Center on 11 September 2001 suggest that RADS may occur in a high proportion of exposed subjects even without the occurrence of clinically serious injury (Banauch 2003, Nemery 2004).

An important, but in practice often neglected, aspect concerns the documentation of the lesions and their severity in victims of inhalation injury. This then leads to difficult medicolegal problems when victims seek compensation, sometimes many months or years after the event. It is, therefore, important that physicians treating victims in the early days after the incident document accurately the clinical condition and all relevant data in these patients. Documentation of the damage by bronchoscopy and high resolution computed tomography may be justified. Repeated measurements of ventilatory function and arterial blood gases must be carried out, and victims of acute inhalation injury should never be discharged without a comprehensive assessment of their pulmonary function.

2.3.7 Subacute Toxic Pneumonitis

The concept of "subacute toxic pneumonitis" is not standard. The term "subacute" is used here to indicate both the pattern of exposure (as is done in toxicology) and the clinical presentation of the disease. Thus, subacute toxic pneumonitis refers to conditions of toxic lung injury in which the onset of the disease is not so sudden as that caused by an accidental exposure, and where the exposure itself consists of repeated peaks or a more prolonged exposure over weeks to months. There are not many published examples of such situations.

The alveolar proteinosis caused by heavy exposure to silica ("acute silico-proteinosis") and possibly by other agents (Blanc 1992) would qualify for this entity. Similarly, some instances of exogenous lipoid pneumonitis seem to correspond well to the concept of subacute toxic pneumonitis. The pulmonary haemorrhagic syndrome associated with exposure to trimellitic anhydride and, possibly, to methylene diphenyl diisocyanate is also a potential form of toxic response; but, in this instance, the role of specific immunological mechanisms is likely.

The Ardystil syndrome represents, hitherto, the most convincing example of occupationally induced organizing pneumonia. This outbreak of severe respiratory disease occurred in 1992 in Spain and involved several workers from factories where textiles were air-sprayed with dyes. Most of the affected workers had worked in a factory named Ardystil, hence the name given to the disease. Six subjects died from the disease over the course of a few months (Moya 1994). A similar, though smaller, outbreak was also reported from Algeria (Ould Kadi 1994). The clinical features of the disease included cough, epistaxis, dyspnoea and chest pain, as well as crackles on auscultation. Radiology showed patchy infiltrates in two-thirds of patients and a micronodular pattern in one-third of the studied patients (Romero 1998). There was a restrictive functional impairment and rapid progression to irreversible respiratory failure, despite corticosteroid treatment, in several patients. The Ardystil syndrome seems to differ from cryptogenic organizing pneumonia with respect to its severity, with a rapidly fatal outcome in several patients and an evolution towards chronic pulmonary fibrosis in others.

Another recently described form of subacute toxic lung injury is "popcorn worker's lung" (Kreiss 2002, Akpinar-Elci 2004). This severe lung disease, characterized as bronchiolitis obliterans, occurred in subjects occupationally exposed to vapours of butter flavouring (containing diacetyl) in factories making microwave popcorn.

These outbreaks of bronchiolar disease make it conceivable that sporadic cases of organizing pneumonia or bronchiolitis obliterans are sometimes also caused by occupational or environmental exposures. It is, therefore, important to remain vigilant when such conditions are diagnosed and always think of the possibility of a toxic aetiology.

References

Akpinar-Elci M, Travis WD, Lynch DA, Kreiss K (2004) Bronchiolitis obliterans syndrome in popcorn production plant workers. Eur Respir J 24:298–302

Banauch GI, Alleyne D, Sanchez R, Olender K, Cohen HW, Weiden M et al (2003) Persistent hyperreactivity and reactive airways dysfunction in World Trade Center firefighters. Am J Respir Crit Care Med 168:54–62

Bismuth CH, Hall AH (1995) Paraquat poisoning. Mechanisms, prevention, treatment. Marcel Dekker, New York Basel Hong Kong

Blanc P, Boushey HA (1993) The lung in metal fume fever. Semin Respir Med 14:212–225

Blanc PD, Golden JA (1992) Unusual occupationally related disorders of the lung: case reports and a literature review. Occup Med 7:403–422

Brooks SM, Weiss MA, Bernstein IL (1985) Reactive airways dysfunction syndrome (RADS). Persistent asthma syndrome after high level irritant exposures. Chest 88:376–384

Burkhart KK, Britt A, Petrini G, O'Donnell S, Donovan JW (1996) Pulmonary toxicity following exposure to an aerosolized leather protector. Clin Toxicol 34:21–24

Cordasco EM, Stone FD (1973) Pulmonary edema of environmental origin. Chest 6497:182–185

Cordier J-F (2000) Organising pneumonia. Thorax 55:318–328

Das R, Blanc PD (1993) Chlorine gas exposure and the lung: a review. Toxicol Indust Health 9:439–455

Dhara R, Dhara VR (1995) Bhopal – A case study of international disaster. Int J Occup Environ Health 1:58–69

Douglas WW, Colby TV (1994) Fume-related bronchiolitis obliterans. In: Epler GR (ed). Diseases of the bronchioles. Raven Press, New York pp 187–213

Douglas WW, Hepper NGG, Colby TV (1989) Silo filler's disease. Mayo Clin Proc 64:291–304

Kreiss K, Gomaa A, Kullman G, Fedan K, Simoes EJ, Enright PL (2002) Clinical bronchiolitis obliterans in workers at a microwave-popcorn plant. N Engl J Med 347:330–338

Loke JS (2000) Thermal lung injury and acute smoke inhalation. In: Fishman AP (ed) Pulmonary diseases and disorders (Vol. 1), 3rd edn. Mc Graw-Hill, New York pp 989–1000

Moya C, Anto JM, Newman Taylor AJ (1994) Collaborative Group for the Study of Toxicity in Textile Aerographic Factories. Outbreak of organising pneumonia in textile printing sprayers. Lancet 344:498–502

Nemery B (1990) Metal toxicity in the respiratory tract. Eur Respir J 3:202–219

Nemery B (1996) Late consequences of accidental exposure to inhaled irritants: RADS and the Bhopal disaster. Eur Respir J 9:1973–1976

Nemery B (2002) Toxic pneumonitis. In: Hendrick DJ, Burge PS, Beckett W, Churg A (eds) Occupational disorders of the lung. Recognition, management, and prevention. WB Saunders–Harcourt Publishers, London, pp 201–219

Nemery B (2003) Reactive fallout of World Trade Center dust. Am J Respir Crit Care Med 168:2–3

Olson KR, Shusterman DJ (1993) Mixing incompatibilities and toxic exposures. Occup Med 8:549–560

Ould Kadi F, Mohammed-Brahim B, Fyad A, Lellou S, Nemery B (1994) Outbreak of pulmonary disease in textile dye sprayers in Algeria. Lancet 344:962–963

Rask-Andersen A (1996) Inhalation fever. In: Harber P, Schenker MB, Balmes JR (eds) Occupational and environmental respiratory disease, 1st edn. Mosby, St. Louis, pp 243–258

Rask-Andersen A, Pratt DS (1992) Inhalation fever: a proposed unifying term for febrile reactions to inhalation of noxious substances. Br J Ind Med 49:40

Reiffenstein RJ, Hulbert WC, Roth SH (1992) Toxicology of hydrogen sulfide. Annu Rev Pharmacol Toxicol 32:109–134

Reisz GR, Gammon RS (1986) Toxic pneumonitis from mixing household cleaners. Chest 89:49–52

Romero S, Hernández L, Gil J, Aranda I, Martín C, Sanchez-Payá J (1998) Organizing pneumonia in textile printing workers: a clinical description. Eur Respir J 11:265–271

Schwartz DA (1987) Acute inhalation injury. Occup Med 2:297–318

Shusterman DJ (1993) Polymer fume fever and other fluorocarbon pyrolysis-related syndromes. Occup Med 8:519–531

Tsao TCY, Juang YC, Lan RS, Shieh WB, Lee CH (1990) Respiratory failure of acute organophosphate and carbamate poisoning. Chest 98:631–636

Wesselius LJ (1997) Pulmonary disorders associated with use of illicit drugs. Clin Pulm Med 4:71–75

Willems JL (1989) Clinical management of mustard gas casualties. Ann Med Milit Belg 3[Suppl]:1–61

3 Diagnostic Techniques

Zelena A. Aziz, David M. Hansell, Vinicius C. S. Antao, John E. Parker, Sherwood Burge, Pascal Dumortier, Gabriel Reboux, Nadine Magy and Jean-Charles Dalphin

3.1 Occupational and Environmental Lung Disease: The Role of Imaging

Zelena A. Aziz and David M. Hansell

CONTENTS

3.1.1 Introduction 77
3.1.2 The Chest Radiograph 77
3.1.2.1 The ILO Classification 78
3.1.3 Computed Tomography 79
3.1.4 The Utility of the Chest Radiograph and CT 81
3.1.4.1 Establishing the Diagnosis 81
3.1.4.2 Quantification of Disease Severity 84
3.1.4.3 Prediction of Prognosis 84
3.1.4.4 Population Screening 84
3.1.4.5 Lung Cancer Screening of Asbestos-Exposed High-Risk Individuals 85
3.1.4.6 The Identification of Co-Existing or Alternative Diseases 85
3.1.5 Thin-Section CT Classification of Pneumoconiosis 87
3.1.6 Magnetic Resonance Imaging 87
3.1.7 Radionuclide Imaging 87
References 89

3.1.1 Introduction

Imaging contributes to the evaluation of occupational and environmental lung disease on many levels: in diagnosis (Lynch 1995), for the quantification of disease extent (Gamsu et al. 1995), as part of the evidence in medicolegal claims (Schachtman and Rhodes 1992), to screen high-risk individuals for lung cancer (Miller et al. 2004), and for identifying other (non-exposure-related) potential causes of pulmonary disability (Gaensler et al. 1991).

What follows is a discussion of the role of different imaging techniques in the evaluation of occupational and environmental lung disease, using asbestos-induced pleuroparenchymal disease as a model. The strengths and weaknesses of each technique will be discussed with particular emphasis given to the main workhorses of lung imaging – chest radiography and computed tomography (CT). The imaging features of specific diseases will not be discussed as they are dealt with in detail in other chapters.

Z. A. Aziz, MD; D. M. Hansell, MD, FRCP, FRCR
Department of Radiology, Royal Brompton Hospital, Sydney Street, London, SW3 6NP, UK

3.1.2 The Chest Radiograph

Chest radiography is the most commonly used diagnostic radiographic procedure in the imaging of lung disease. Most chest radiographs are still acquired with conventional film-screen radiography systems, which provide good image quality and high spatial resolution at low cost (Garmer et al. 2000). However, typical disadvantages of film-screen radiography techniques are a limited exposure range, a high retake rate and the inflexibility of image display and film management (Rong et al. 2000). As computer technology and storage capacities have developed during recent years, the considerable advantages of picture archiving and communication systems (PACS) have become increasingly evident. The implementation of PACS requires digital acquisition of images. Digital radiography systems offer instant image display, a wide dynamic range, and a linear signal response (Rong et al. 2000). Initially, storage phosphor plates were used in digital chest radiography; more recently, full-field digital amorphous silicon flat-panel X-ray detector radiography systems based on caesium iodide and amorphous silicon have become commercially available. These systems have excellent image quality (Floyd et al. 2001; Fink et al. 2002) and allow a significant reduction in effective dose compared with film-screen radiography (Bacher et al. 2003). With PACS, interpretation of images from a PC monitor is the norm. Workstation interpretation coupled with the availability of filmless standards on a disc would encourage and facilitate the use of standardised images, such as the International Labour Organization (ILO) classification scheme.

3.1.2.1 The ILO Classification

The ILO International Classification of Radiographs for the Pneumoconioses is a system used internationally for the recording of chest radiographic abnormalities related to the inhalation of dusts. Its intent was to improve workers' health surveillance by facilitating international comparisons of pneumoconiosis statistics and research reports (International Labour Office 1980). Thus, in contrast to most tests, it was designed primarily for population epidemiology rather than for individual diagnoses. The classification involves the identification of small opacities (p, q and r for rounded or nodular opacities; s, t and u for irregular opacities), large opacities (≥10 mm), graded as A, B and C based on the combined dimensions of all large opacities present, and pleural abnormalities, categorised according to the maximum width and length of chest wall involved. Profusion of the small opacities is classified into four categories (0–3) in comparison with standard films, category 0 indicating that there is no excess of small opacities above normal. The use of two profusion categories is useful when appearances lie between those of the standard films. Thus, 1/0 indicates that appearances most closely resemble category 1 but that the reader has also considered category 0. The latest edition (revised 2000) of the ILO classification includes digitised copies of most (20) of the 22 standard radiographs with 2 new standard radiographs for pleural abnormalities and u/u size small opacities.

A basic problem with the ILO classification system is that it attempts to integrate two concepts that by definition are at odds with each other: standardisation and interpretation (Henry 2002). A system that sets out to record chest radiographic findings produced by the inhalation of dusts for the purpose of detection and measurement is an apparently straightforward concept; however, controversy is inevitable when that goal is combined with a process that invites the subjective explanation of the radiographic findings to make them understandable. This blending of clinical interpretation with classification is a potential cause of reader variability, and studies have demonstrated that the attitude or perspective of the reader can have a significant impact on reader variability (Hilt et al. 1992).

In the absence of a histopathological "gold standard", the level of interobserver variability allows some inferences concerning the diagnostic value of a test to be drawn. Additionally, a classification system that may be factored into societal decisions concerning compensation, fitness for work and environmental policies will necessarily receive additional scrutiny when observers disagree. Problems of interobserver consistency have long been recognised in the context of pneumoconiosis chest radiography (Fletcher and Oldham 1949), and the criticism of the ILO classification is, in part, due to the fact that interobserver variation continues to be a substantial problem despite incremental improvements in the ILO classification system itself. In a review of interobserver studies, it has been shown that selected experts exhibited a twofold or greater range for the prevalence of abnormal profusions (Ducatman 1991). Factors contributing to interobserver variability include the experience of the reader, overall film quality and film reading in the presence of background small opacities that are unrelated to dust exposure. Several studies have demonstrated the presence of small opacities on chest radiographs in individuals who have no dust exposure, these opacities being attributed to smoking (Fig. 3.1.1.), age, gender and geography (Epstein et al. 1984; Dick et al. 1992; Barnhart et al. 2004; Zitting et al. 1996). Another factor is the "middling tendency", a bias by less proficient observers towards the central (more certain) minor category within each major category (Hessel 1985). Experts tend to express uncertainty by using the 1/0 minor category for their category 1 films; less experienced observers are more likely to use category 1/1.

The ILO classification was not intended to set, or imply, a level at which compensation is payable; yet, the system is frequently applied for this purpose (Ducatman 1991). In most cases of asbestos litigation, radiology is the dispositive evidence for or against the claim (Schachtman and Rhodes 1992), with a profusion level of 1/0 generally taken as "positive" evidence in the adjudication of compensation claims. A recent study by Gitlin et al. (2004) contains data that is disquieting and raises fundamental questions about the interpretations of chest radiographs made by attorney-hired B-reader radiologists. Of chest radiographs interpreted as ≥0/1 by *B* readers retained by plaintiffs' attorneys, 492 were reinterpreted by six other B-reader radiologists who had no knowledge of how the initial radiologists had interpreted the radiographs or even that the radiographs had been entered as evidence in asbestos-related litigation. The attorney-hired radiologists reported 96% of the cases as positive for asbestosis (≥1/0) compared with only 4.5% by the other six consulting B-reader radiologists; an aston-

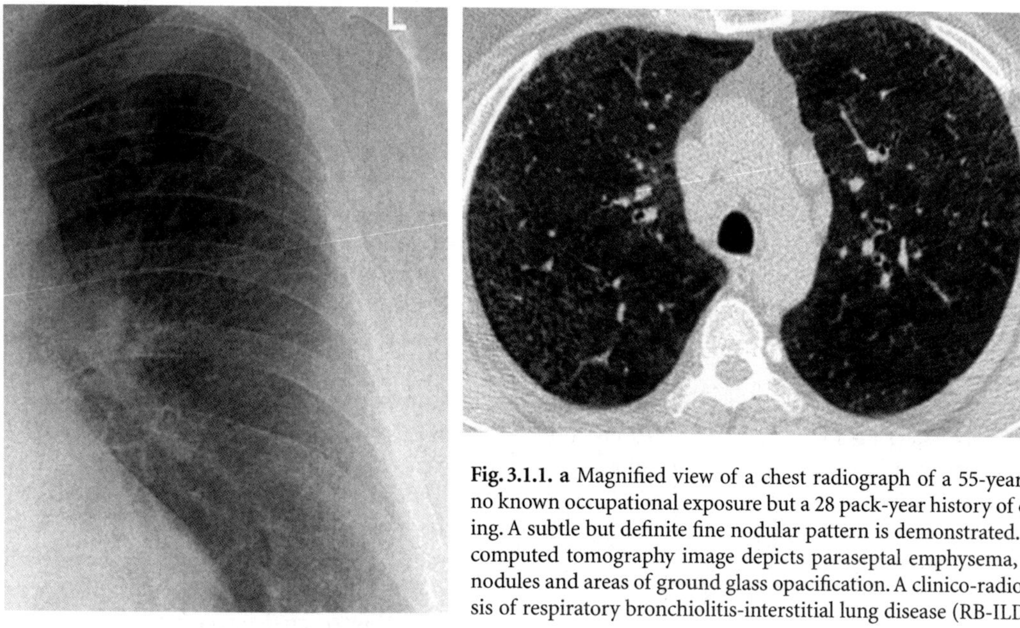

Fig. 3.1.1. **a** Magnified view of a chest radiograph of a 55-year-old male with no known occupational exposure but a 28 pack-year history of cigarette smoking. A subtle but definite fine nodular pattern is demonstrated. **b** Thin-section computed tomography image depicts paraseptal emphysema, poorly defined nodules and areas of ground glass opacification. A clinico-radiological diagnosis of respiratory bronchiolitis-interstitial lung disease (RB-ILD) was made

ishing discrepancy, far too great to be attributed to interobserver variability (Gitlin et al. 2004).

Despite its limitations, the ILO classification remains a beneficial shorthand, whose meaning is understood widely and used advantageously in population studies. As an epidemiological tool, the ILO classification provides the best recognised way, at present, of recording systematically abnormalities seen on a chest radiograph. The problems of misuse and variability that are associated with it can be regarded as reflecting problems with the "speakers" and not with the "language" (Ducatman 1991).

3.1.3 Computed Tomography

Multidetector CT (MDCT) represents the latest and possibly the most important breakthrough in CT technology. First introduced in 1992, the fundamental difference between MDCT and its predecessors lies in the design of the detector array. The strategy of replacing a single detector row by 4-, 16- or even 64- detector rows enables simultaneous acquisition of data from different slice locations during a single rotation of the X-ray source. The advantages of MDCT include rapid scanning (up to eight times faster than conventional single-slice helical CT), longer anatomic coverage, improved spatial resolution in the z-axis and the generation of "isotropic" (identical resolution of a structure in all dimensions) data. The ability to acquire volumetric data rapidly means that the entire thorax can be imaged with a high-resolution technique (16×1-mm collimation) in less than 10 s (Prokop 2003). The raw data can be reconstructed to provide thin sections (1.25 mm) and 5-mm sections; thus, MDCT offers the convenience of a single scan in patients who potentially have combined focal and diffuse lung disease (which would require two different examinations on an older CT machine). In the context of patients with occupational lung disease, MDCT enables the evaluation of asbestosis whilst also providing the opportunity to screen for lung cancer.

The combination of multidetector CT and low-dose techniques has stimulated interest in the use of CT as a first-line imaging modality for the diagnosis of asbestos-related lung disease. A recent study compared contiguous 5-mm-thick sections acquired with a low-dose MDCT protocol (4×2.5-mm collimation) with conventional thin-section CT in the evaluation of asbestos-related pleuropulmonary disease (Remy-Jardin et al. 2004). No differences were observed between the two protocols for the detection of pleural and asbestos-related parenchymal abnormalities, although the presence of honeycombing (n=1) was only visualised on the thin-section CT images (recorded as ground-glass opacity on the low-dose images). Not surprisingly, lung nodules were depicted with a higher frequency on the low-dose contiguous 5-mm-thick sections (Remy-Jardin et al. 2004). The estimated effective dose for the low-dose MDCT-acquired images was 1.9 mSv compared with

3.4 mSv (conventional thin-section CT). The authors did not use 4×1-mm collimation, as this would have led to a 20% increase in effective radiation dose. However, with 64-detector scanners, system performance is such that satisfactory 1.25-mm sections can be obtained with an effective dose as low as 1 mSv. For high-contrast structures such as the lung, the use of ultra-low-dose applications can entail a dose as low as 0.4 mSv comparable with a conventional posterior anterior and lateral chest radiograph using a modern screen-film system (Prokop 2003).

Conventional thin-section CT is still used routinely to evaluate interstitial lung disease. A typical protocol simply consists of thin (1–2 mm) collimation sections at 10-mm intervals from lung apices to the costophrenic angles with the patient breath-holding at full inspiration, in a supine position. For the evaluation of lung parenchyma, the majority of thoracic radiologists use a window level of –600 Hounsfield Units (HU) and a window width of 1500 HU (Stern et al. 1995).

In situations relating specifically to interstitial lung disease (as is often the case in occupational lung disease), a standard thin-section CT (interspaced thin sections) will suffice, the only caveat being the need to acquire prone images when evaluating individuals with suspected (and by definition limited) asbestosis. Prone thin-section CT images reliably differentiate the subtle gravity-induced increase in attenuation seen in the posterobasal segments on supine sections from that due to interstitial lung disease, which remains fixed on prone sections. This technique is crucial in the evaluation of asbestosis in which parenchymal abnormalities are most frequently seen in the caudal parts of the posterobasal segments (Fig. 3.1.2.) (Aberle et al. 1988a).

A further procedure that may improve diagnostic yield is the acquisition of end-expiratory images. Areas of air-trapping caused by small airways disease are seen as regional inhomogeneity on thin-section CT. End-expiratory images can accentuate this mosaic attenuation pattern (Fig. 3.1.3.). Non-smoking asbestos-exposed individuals have an element of small airways disease, which may contribute to their functional deficit (Kilburn and Warshaw 1994). Constrictive obliterative bronchiolitis is also associated with a wide variety of other occupational and environmental exposures: fly ash produced by the incineration of coal and oil (Boswell and McCunney 1995), amorphous and synthetic silicates (Spain et al. 1995) and butter flavouring in popcorn production (Akpinar-Elci et al. 2004). Although the diagnosis of obliterative bronchiolitis may be suggested by clinical features, the demonstration of air-trapping on CT may permit detection of small airways obstruction in exposed individuals with clinically suspected disease even when lung function tests are normal.

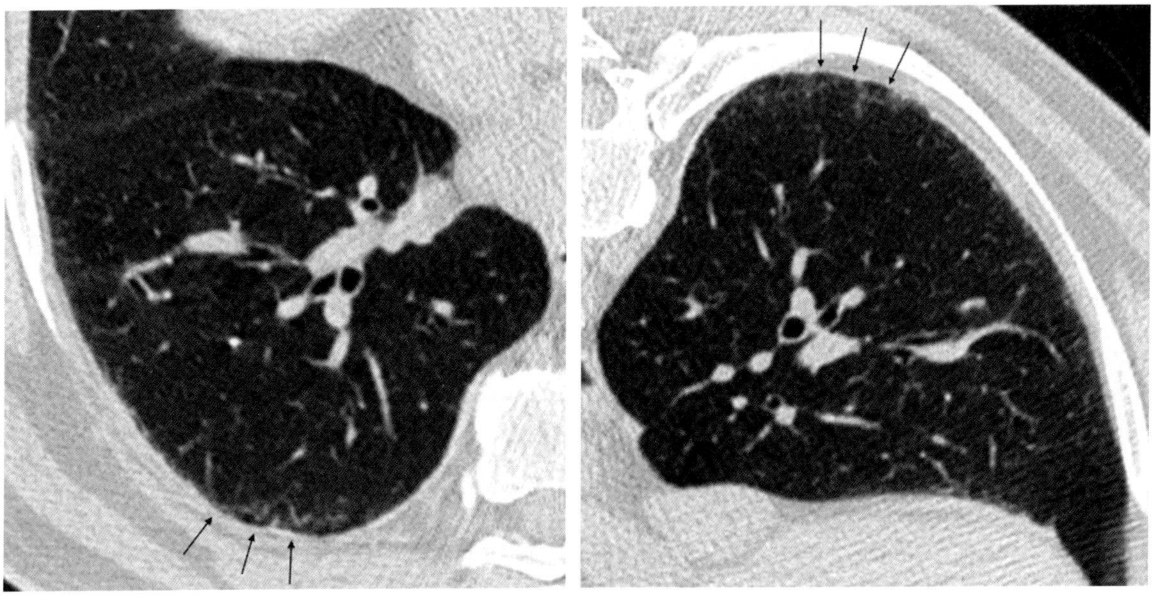

a b

Fig. 3.1.2a,b. Thin-section computed tomography images obtained supine **a** and prone **b** in a 73-year-old worker exposed to asbestos. A fine reticular pattern (*arrows*) and increased ground glass attenuation are seen on the supine image, predominantly in the dependent areas. These features persist on the prone images and are in keeping with early asbestosis a 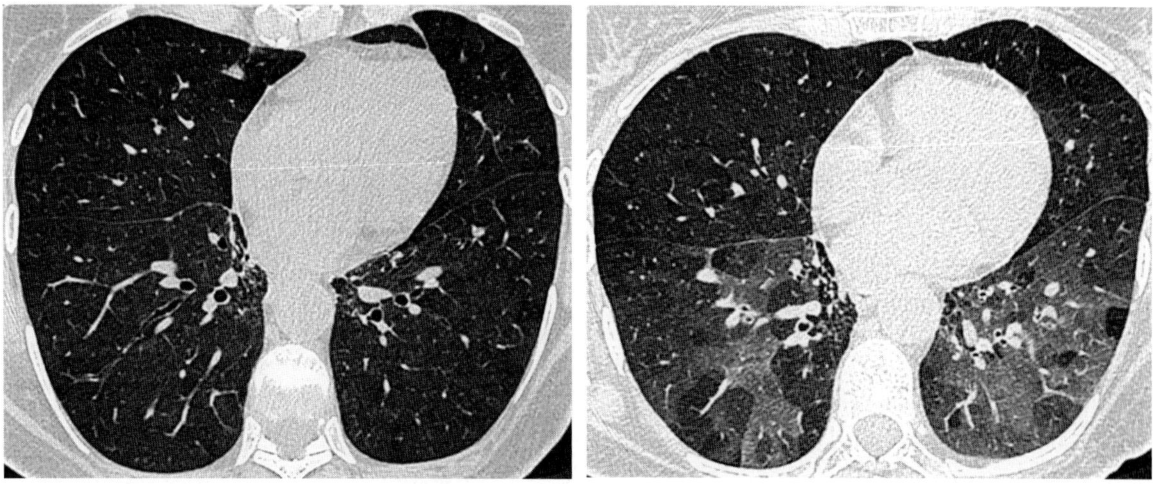 b

Fig. 3.1.3a,b. Thin-section computed tomography images obtained on inspiration (**a**) and expiration (**b**) in a 52-year-old farm worker. There is a suggestion of a mosaic attenuation pattern on the inspiratory image, but the appearances are far more striking on the expiratory image, with focal areas of air-trapping

3.1.4 The Utility of the Chest Radiograph and CT

The contribution of chest radiography and CT to the evaluation of subjects with suspected environmental or occupational lung disease can be divided into five key areas: as an aid to diagnosis, for the quantification of disease severity, in the prediction of prognosis, as a screening tool and for the identification of co-existing or alternative diseases as a cause of respiratory disability. What follows is a focused discussion of the usefulness of chest radiography and CT when applied to these specific areas using asbestos-induced disease as an example, although many of the considerations are equally applicable to the other occupational lung diseases. Asbestos-induced lung disease was an obvious example to use due to the more extensive literature on this subject compared with the other occupational lung diseases.

3.1.4.1 Establishing the Diagnosis

The diagnosis of asbestosis has significant implications for the patient in terms of prognosis, work ability and the possibility of receiving legal compensation. Both the chest radiograph and thin-section CT can confirm previous exposure (the identification of pleural plaques) and demonstrate interstitial changes compatible with asbestosis. Ultimately, however, the diagnosis of asbestosis is largely inferential. The recent American Thoracic Society document states that the diagnosis of asbestosis is dependent on demonstrating a compatible structural lesion, evidence of exposure and the exclusion of other plausible conditions. With regards to the chest radiograph, a distinction is made between category 0/1, considered "negative" for asbestosis, and 1/0, considered "positive" for asbestosis (American Thoracic Society Documents 2004). This is a shift from the 1986 guidelines, in which a grading of 1/1 was required for the diagnosis of asbestosis (American Thoracic Society 1986). The problem with defining diagnostic criteria based on the ILO classification (a use it was not intended for) is made apparent by several studies, which have shown that a profusion reading of 1/0 can be found in non-asbestos-exposed factory workers and in middle-aged smokers (Dick et al. 1992; Weiss 1991; Meyer et al. 1997).

Chest radiographs are limited with respect to sensitivity and specificity in the detection of mild or early asbestosis (Fig. 3.1.4.). Among individuals with asbestosis confirmed by histopathological findings, 15–20% had no radiographic evidence of parenchymal fibrosis (Kipen et al. 1987), similar to the proportion of other interstitial lung diseases that present with normal chest films (Epler et al. 1978). More recent studies have shown that between 5% (Paris et al. 2004) and 30% (Lee et al. 2003) of subjects with documented asbestos exposure and pulmonary

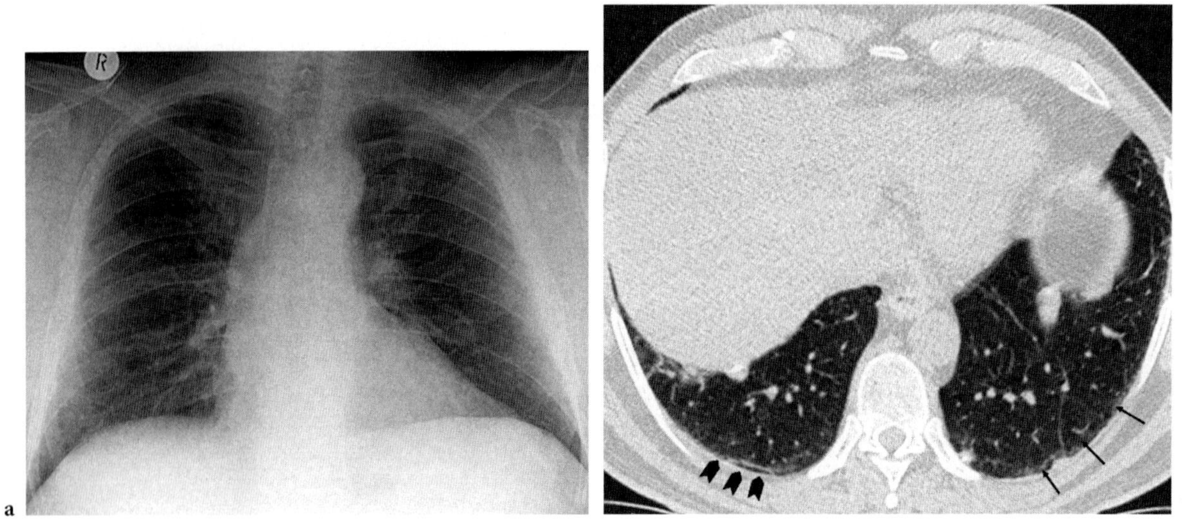

Fig. 3.1.4a,b. Chest radiograph (a) and thin-section computed tomography (b) of a 69-year-old male with asbestos exposure. The chest radiograph demonstrates pleural thickening within the left hemithorax, but there is no suggestion of interstitial lung disease. Changes compatible with early asbestosis are seen on the thin-section computed tomography image: subpleural line (*solid arrows*) and a fine reticular pattern (*line arrows*)

fibrosis on thin-section CT had no evidence of interstitial lung disease on chest X-ray (profusion 0/0 or 0/1). The chest radiograph may also be mildly abnormal in individuals who have never been exposed to asbestos. In an analysis of several studies performed in the United States and Europe, the number of radiographs that were read as being positive for asbestosis (ILO grade ≥1/0) among individuals who had not been exposed to asbestos varied from 0.21% to 11.7% (Meyer et al. 1997). A meta-analysis of the published data yielded a population prevalence of 5.3%; thus, with qualified readers, the specificity of the chest radiograph is at best 90–95%. Based on a literature analysis, Ross estimated the positive predictive value of the chest radiograph in asbestos-exposed individuals as approximately 40% and suggested that the chest radiograph was inadequate as the only clinical tool in the diagnosis of asbestosis (Ross 2003).

Several studies have demonstrated the superior sensitivity of thin-section CT over the chest radiograph for the identification of early fibrosis in asbestos-exposed individuals (Staples et al. 1989; Gamsu 1989; Akira et al. 1991). However, sensitivity is not 100%, and a histopathological diagnosis of asbestosis can be present in patients with normal or near-normal thin-section CTs (Gamsu et al. 1995). Nevertheless, the use of CT in the diagnosis of asbestosis has inevitably lead to "diagnostic dilution", a concept coined by Harber and Smitherman to illustrate the changing definition of asbestosis as a result of identifying early disease (Harber and Smitherman 1991). The value of identifying subtle disease was demonstrated in a study by Oksa et al. They demonstrated that early changes indicative of fibrosis (subpleural curvilinear lines, pleural-based nodular irregularities, parenchymal bands and septal lines) visualised only on thin-section CT (ILO<1/0) were functionally significant (Oksa et al. 1994) and suggested that asbestos-exposed workers with an ILO classification of <1/0 and functional impairment should proceed to thin-section CT.

The specificity of CT is difficult to tease out; in many studies, the presence or absence of disease is inevitably based on symptoms, exposure history and physiology rather than on a histological diagnosis. Bergin et al. found that a significant proportion of patients being investigated for a variety of indications had thin-section CT single features described in asbestosis (Bergin et al. 1994). A study by Aberle et al., which used certain thin-section CT features (subpleural density, subpleural curvilinear densities, thickened septal lines and parenchymal bands) to establish probability scores for asbestosis, found that 36% of subjects who did not satisfy the criteria for clinical asbestosis were judged to have a high probability of asbestosis (Aberle et al. 1988a). This emphasises, as with the other interstitial lung diseases, the importance of integrating clinical and radiographic information before a diagnosis is reached. Establishing the clinical "prior" or "pre-test" probability", a concept used in medical decision making, could be usefully applied to the diagnosis of asbestosis (JONES 1991). In the presence of a high pre-test probability (adequate exposure, an appropriate latency and the exclusion of confounders for the presence of pulmonary fibrosis), demonstration of the constellation of thin-section CT features described in asbestosis should enable the diagnosis to be reached with a degree of certainty.

Pleural plaques are frequently documented on chest radiographs, but CT is more sensitive for their detection. Only 50–80% of cases of documented pleural thickening (demonstrated by autopsy, conventional CT or thin-section CT) are detected using chest radiography (OKSA et al. 1994; ABERLE et al. 1988b; SCHWARTZ et al. 1993; FRIEDMAN et al. 1988). In the study by OKSA et al., the most common sites of pleural plaques missed on the chest radiograph were in the paravertebral and posterior regions of the costal pleural, areas that are poorly visualised on routine radiographs (Fig. 3.1.5.) (OKSA et al. 1994). Additionally, the distinction between mild pleural disease and extrapleural fat is difficult on a plain chest radiograph (Fig. 3.1.6.) (HARKIN et al.

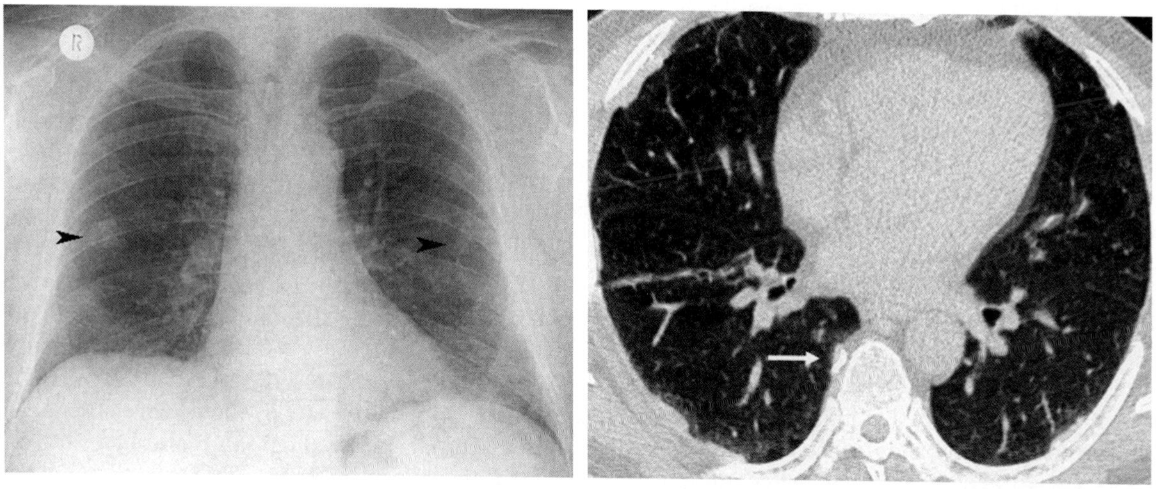

a b

Fig. 3.1.5a,b. There are abnormal opacities, possibly pleural in origin (*arrowheads*), demonstrated bilaterally on the chest radiograph (**a**) of a 52-year-old male with asbestos exposure. The thin-section computed tomography (**b**) shows several well-circumscribed pleural plaques, one located in the right paravertebral region (*arrow*) not visualised on the chest radiograph

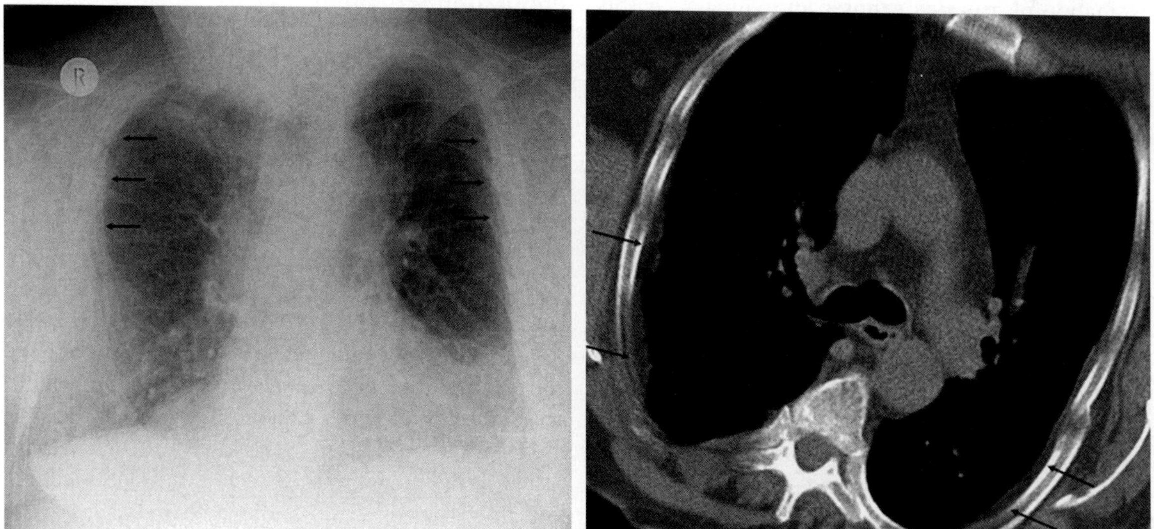

a b

Fig. 3.1.6a,b. Bilateral pleural thickening (*arrows*) documented on a chest radiograph (**a**) which on computed tomography (**b**) was found to represent extrapleural fat (*arrows*)

1996; LEE et al. 2001). Although oblique views can enhance detection of pleural abnormalities in cases where thin-section CT is unavailable, they may also fail to distinguish plaques from extrapleural fat (AMEILLE et al. 1993).

3.1.4.2 Quantification of Disease Severity

The radiological evaluation of workers exposed to asbestos has the potential to allow the quantification of parenchymal and/or pleural involvement. Traditionally, quantification of disease has relied on the measurement of the intensity (profusion score) and extent of disease (number of zones involved) on the basis of the ILO classification. Studies have shown that the profusion score on the chest radiograph predicts, to some extent, the degree of functional impairment (HARKIN et al. 1996; ROSENSTOCK et al. 1988; OKSA et al. 1998; MILLER et al. 1996). Additionally, ILO profusion scores and the extent of disease (number of zones involved) have been shown to independently predict arterial oxygen desaturation during exercise (LEE et al. 2003). JARAD et al. modified the ILO radiographic scoring system for CT to take into account the functional consequences of a combination of interstitial fibrosis, emphysema and diffuse pleural thickening (JARAD et al. 1992). There was better interobserver agreement for all features using the thin-section CT system compared with chest radiography. Gamsu et al. developed a combined semiquantitative and qualitative scoring system for the thin-section CT evaluation of asbestos-exposed individuals. In this classification, a combination of an extent and severity index and a cumulative score, which adds the different types of interstitial abnormalities, was used. The semiquantitative grade of asbestosis on thin-section CT correlated significantly with the severity of fibrosis measured histopathologically (GAMSU et al. 1995). More recently, SETTE et al. explored the relationship between interstitial abnormalities at thin-section CT and pulmonary gas exchange impairment at rest and during moderate exercise in workers exposed to asbestosis (SETTE et al. 2004). Using a system of quantifying parenchymal abnormalities based on that of Gamsu and co-workers, they demonstrated that the extent of disease on CT predicted the probability of pulmonary gas exchange impairment at rest and during exercise.

Pleural disease can also be quantified on CT. VAN CLEEMPUT et al. established that surface area occupied by pleural plaques on thin-section CT did not correlate with lung function parameters or with cumulative asbestos exposure (VAN CLEEMPUT et al. 2001). Similarly, the presence and number of pleural plaques did not improve model accuracy for gas exchange impairment prediction in a study by SETTE et al. (2004). This is in contrast to the extent of diffuse pleural thickening, which is strongly related to functional deficit (SCHWARTZ et al. 1993; JARAD et al. 1992; COPLEY 2000).

3.1.4.3 Prediction of Prognosis

Imaging may also contribute to predicting the natural history of disease. COOKSON et al. conducted a long-term comprehensive follow-up study of a group of heavily exposed miners from Western Australia. They found that the sojourn time in radiographic category 0 (ILO classification) predicted progression; that is, the likelihood of progressing from category 1 to category 2 was much higher if it took relatively little time to progress to category 1 (COOKSON et al. 1986). BOURGKARD et al. found that the presence and extent of micronodules on CT at baseline predicted radiographic worsening and the evolution to frank pneumoconiosis at 4 years in a cohort of coal miners with an initial chest radiograph classified as 0/1 or 1/0 (suspected pneumoconiosis) (BOURGKARD et al. 1998).

3.1.4.4 Population Screening

Despite its limitations, the chest radiograph remains the most widely used imaging tool in surveillance programs and in screening individuals with suspected pneumoconiosis (INTERNATIONAL LABOUR OFFICE 1980). It has survived in this role because it is widely available, can be performed at the workplace and is inexpensive; important considerations in population or work-force screening. CT could be promoted by offering low-cost, low-dose CT (LYNCH 2002), but at present there is insufficient evidence concerning which individuals would benefit from CT screening (PARIS et al. 2004). It is probable that the use of CT will increase, particularly in light of the recent development of thin-section CT classification systems (HERING et al. 2004); whether it will eventually replace the standard radiographic ILO classification will depend primarily on availability and on its yet untested applicability as an epidemiological tool.

3.1.4.5
Lung Cancer Screening of Asbestos-Exposed High-Risk Individuals

Interest has been expressed in the screening of high-risk asbestos-exposed subjects for lung cancer (International Expert Meeting 2000). Experts have estimated that the relative risk for lung cancer is roughly doubled for cohorts exposed to asbestos fibers at a cumulative exposure of 25 fiber-years or with an equivalent occupational history, at which asbestosis may or may not be present or detectable (Consensus Report 1997) (Fig. 3.1.7.). Clearly cost, availability and dose are factors when considering the implementation of screening using CT; however, a recent study performed in the US using a low-dose protocol and mobile scanners demonstrated that the screening of a large occupationally defined population (nuclear fuel workers) was at least feasible (Miller et al. 2004). The overall lung cancer rate was 0.7% (20/3598), lower than from other well-publicised North American series of at-risk individuals (cigarette smokers) (Swensen et al. 2002; Henschke et al. 1999), a probable reason being the inclusion of younger subjects with less of a smoking burden. Using CT, Tiitola et al. found a detection rate of lung cancer of 0.8% in Finnish construction workers with 10 years or more (mean 26 years) of asbestos exposure. However, the screening detected 111 of 602 patients with non-calcified nodules greater than 0.5 cm. Of these, 5 lung cancers were subsequently confirmed; thus, 106 cases represented false positives (Tiitola et al. 2002). Due to the sheer number of positive findings, patient selection is crucial in the establishment of screening programs for high-risk asbestos-exposed workers. Criteria suggested include subjects over 50 years of age, greater than 20 pack-years of smoking and greater than 25 fiber-years of asbestos exposure with an appropriate latency from first exposure (International Expert Meeting 2000).

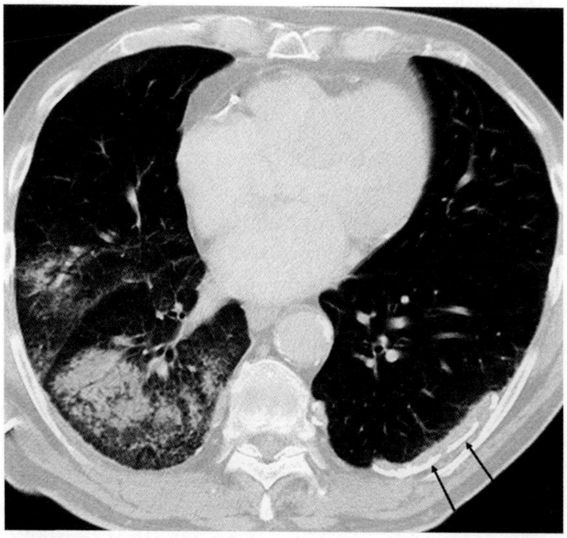

Fig. 3.1.7. Computed tomography image of a 67-year-old male with asbestos exposure and a 20 pack-year smoking history. There is extensive ground glass opacification in the right lower lobe and right middle lobe. Histology of this area demonstrated adenocarcinoma. No interstitial changes were demonstrated on the other sections. Pleural plaques (*arrows*) are evident on the left

At present, American Thoracic Society guidelines do not recommend the regular surveillance of subjects with a history of asbestos exposure for lung cancer or mesothelioma (American Thoracic Society Documents 2004).

3.1.4.6
The Identification of Co-Existing or Alternative Diseases

In individuals with coal workers' pneumoconiosis and silicosis, the development of chronic airflow obstruction is related to inorganic dust inhalation, although age and smoking are contributing factors (Begin et al. 1995; Coggon and Newman 2004; Ruckley et al. 1984; Kinsella et al. 1990). The association between emphysema and asbestos exposure is more contentious. Nevertheless, multiple morphological abnormalities often co-exist in the same patient. One of the main advantages of CT compared with the chest radiograph in evaluating individuals with occupational lung disease is the more accurate demonstration of coexisting pathology as CT enables the quantification of both the extent of emphysema and the extent of interstitial fibrosis (Fig. 3.1.8.). Whilst chest radiography is quite specific in moderate to severe emphysema, its use in mild disease is limited because of insensitivity, and it is even less reliable when coexisting chronic interstitial disease is present (Thurlbeck and Simon 1978). Thin-section CT is more sensitive than either chest radiography or pulmonary function testing for the detection of mild disease (Klein et al. 1992; Gurney et al. 1992); furthermore, techniques for the quantification of emphysema (both subjective and objective) have been established (Bankier et al. 2002). Separating the two pathologies (interstitial fibrosis and emphysema) is important as the level of pulmonary impairment is primarily dependent on the degree of

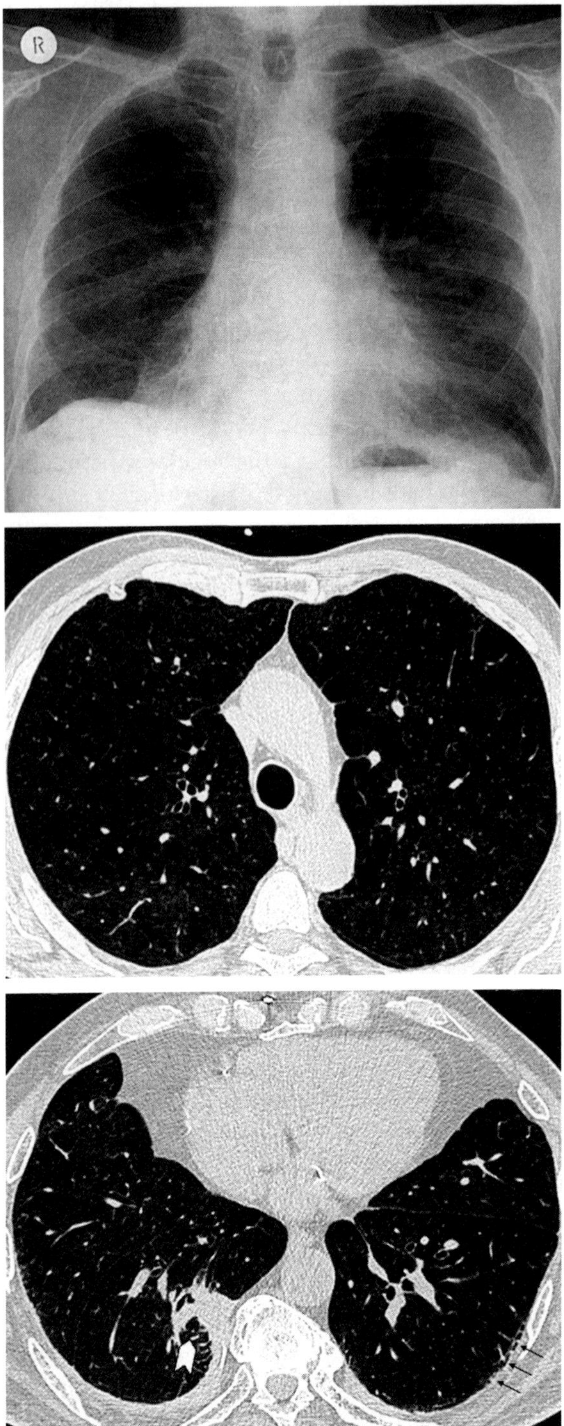

Fig. 3.1.8a-c. Thin-section computed tomography images from the upper (**b**) and lower (**c**) lobes of a 67-year-old male smoker with asbestos exposure demonstrate centrilobular emphysema in the upper lobes and thickened septal lines in the subpleural region on the left (*arrows*). The extent of emphysema and interstitial change is not readily apparent on the chest radiograph (**a**). An area of rounded atelectasis with a typical comet's tail appearance is seen within the right lower lobe (*arrowhead*)

emphysema rather than the degree of silicosis (Kinsella et al. 1990), even in never-smokers (Bergin et al. 1986). The ability to demonstrate emphysema is equally useful in patients exposed to asbestos. Here, quantification of emphysema and interstitial abnormalities enables the determination of disability (reflected by abnormalities in pulmonary function tests) attributable to asbestos-related disease versus emphysema (Copley 2000). This is particularly relevant in medicolegal disputes, when it may be important to establish what proportion of disability is a result of compensatable interstitial fibrosis and how much is due to non-compensatable emphysema.

One of the problems in interpreting the presence of interstitial fibrosis, whether on chest radiography or thin-section CT, is the fact that asbestos-exposed individuals are as likely as the rest of the population to develop other causes of fibrosis. It had previously been assumed that with a history of asbestos-exposure fulfilling dose–response and latency requirements and with findings typical of interstitial fibrosis, a clinical diagnosis of asbestosis was unequivocal. Gaensler's study in 1991 demonstrated the problems of an inferential diagnosis. In this study, 9 of 176 (5.2%) of individuals with clinical features compatible with asbestosis did not have asbestos bodies on pathological examination of lung biopsy specimens. Pathological diagnoses in this group ranged from idiopathic pulmonary fibrosis to organising pneumonia. Distinguishing asbestosis from idiopathic pulmonary fibrosis is probably most important, as asbestosis is associated with a much slower rate of progression and, hence, better prognosis. Discrimination between the two with thin-section CT is by no means straightforward. It has been suggested that subpleural dot-like or branching opacities are significantly more common in patients with asbestosis; whereas, honeycombing, traction bronchiectasis with areas of confluent fibrosis and a mosaic perfusion pattern resulting from air-trapping are more common in patients with idiopathic pulmonary fibrosis (IFP) (Akira et al. 2003). Additionally, pleural disease may be a useful discriminator; in Akira's study, pleural disease was found in 83% (66/80) of patients with asbestosis but only in 4% (3/80) of subjects with IPF (Akira et al. 2003). Copley et al. found no statistically significant differences in the coarseness of fibrosis between individuals with asbestosis and a cohort of individuals with biopsy-proven usual interstitial pneumonitis, although the CT findings of asbestosis were strikingly different to NSIP – the quality of fibrosis was coarser, there was a lower proportion of ground glass opacification and a higher likelihood of a basal and subpleural distribution (Copley et al. 2003).

3.1.5 Thin-Section CT Classification of Pneumoconiosis

At an international meeting in 2000, it was agreed that an international classification scheme should be established for the CT evaluation of subjects with occupational lung disease (International Expert Meeting 2000). This system would be comparable to the 1980 ILO Classification of Radiographs, the intention being to standardise documentation of CT findings in occupationally and environmentally related lung and pleural changes and to facilitate international comparisons of results. An thin-section CT classification has recently been published, which was originally devised in Germany (Hering et al. 2004) but subsequently developed and tested in Belgium, Finland, France, Japan, the USA and the United Kingdom. The CT classification is essentially analogous to the ILO classification in that it is descriptive and requires comparison with standard/reference films; the presence of rounded/irregular opacities, inhomogeneous attenuation, ground-glass opacification, honeycombing, emphysema and pleural disease are recorded in a standardised manner (Hering et al. 2004). It is too early to gauge whether this classification will be widely accepted and adopted.

3.1.6 Magnetic Resonance Imaging

Conventional magnetic resonance imaging (MRI) of the lung parenchyma is hampered by two very fundamental problems: first, ^{1}H spin density, as the "MR imaging agent" is prohibitively low within the $N_2/O_2/CO_2/H_2O$ environment in airways and alveoli, essentially because of the high air content of the lungs. Second, the vast number of gas–tissue interfaces creates magnetic-filed inhomogeneities, which impair image quality. Although still largely a research tool, the introduction of hyperpolarised noble gas imaging using either ^{3}He or ^{129}Xe has enabled the evaluation structure–function relationships in lung disease (Eberle et al. 2001). Diffusion-sensitive MRI techniques allow mapping of the "apparent diffusion coefficient" (ADC) of ^{3}He within lung spaces, where ADC is physically related to local bronchoalveolar dimensions (Hanisch et al. 2000). ADC values are increased in fibrosis and emphysema and show good agreement with predicted lung function (Kauczor 2003); however, these sophisticated techniques are not widely available at present. In the context of occupational lung disease, one potential use of MRI lies in the evaluation of pleural disease. In a study that compared MRI and CT in the differentiation of benign from malignant pleural disease, a combination of morphological features (mediastinal pleural involvement, circumferential pleural thickening, nodularity, irregularity of pleural contour and infiltration of chest wall and/or diaphragm) and signal intensity features (hyperintensity on T2-weighted images, hyperintensity on contrast-enhanced T1-weighted images) resulted in a sensitivity of 100% and a specificity of 93% (Hierholzer et al. 2000). Using the same discriminatory morphological features, CT had a sensitivity of 93% and a specificity of 87% for malignancy. Of note, however, is that the presence of pleural calcification on CT (a feature that cannot be identified on MRI) was suggestive of a benign cause with a specificity of 96%. Interobserver agreement has also been demonstrated to be higher for MRI in assessing pleural thickening, pleural effusion and extrapleural fat when compared with CT in asbestos-exposed individuals (Weber et al. 2004). It has been suggested that MRI should be more widely used in the evaluation of malignant mesothelioma (Knuuttila et al. 1998). CT is limited in its ability to depict the plate-like growth of malignant pleural mesothelioma. In a comparative study, MRI showed tumour spread into the interlobar fissures, invasion of the diaphragm and infiltration of bony structures better than CT (Knuuttila et al. 1998). Consequently, MRI may be used when evaluating tumour resectability and in research protocols when an accurate evaluation of disease extent is essential.

3.1.7 Radionuclide Imaging

Radionuclide imaging is not used routinely in the evaluation of occupational or environmental lung disease. Historically, the gallium-67 (Ga-67) lung scan has been reported to be positive in asbestosis (Begin et al. 1983) and silicosis (Siemsen et al. 1978). More recently, the Ga-67 scan was reported to be abnormal in subjects with coal workers' pneumoconiosis, with the Ga-67 uptake index correlating significantly with total dust exposure (Kanner et al. 1985). However, the Ga-67 scan provided no information that was not already available from a careful exposure history and chest radiography.

Another nuclear medicine technique, fluorine-18 fluorodeoxyglucose positron emission tomography (FDG-PET), has emerged as an important clinical tool and has an established role in the imaging of lung cancer (Coleman 1999). The principle of the technique involves imaging the distribution of injected FDG, an analogue of glucose that accumulates in most tumours in a greater amount than it does in normal tissue. PET is based on the simultaneous detection of the two annihilation photons produced when a positron is emitted from a radioisotope. Each coincidence is recorded, and the final raw data sample is a number for each detector pair, indicating the number of coincidences measured for that pair. The raw data represent projections of the distribution of radiotracer in the body, which are subsequently reconstructed into cross-sectional images.

A means of estimating the likelihood of a benign or malignant lesion is by use of the standardised uptake value (SUV) – a semiquantitative index of glucose metabolism in a particular anatomic location. In a preliminary study on the average SUV of pulmonary lesions (Patz et al. 1993), investigators found that at a cut-off value of 2.5, the specificity and sensitivity of PET for a benign lesion was 100% and 89%, respectively. Although the use of PET has not been widely investigated in subjects with occupational lung disease, one of the potential uses of PET lies in the differentiation between progressive massive fibrosis (PMF) from lung cancer (Fig. 3.1.9.)

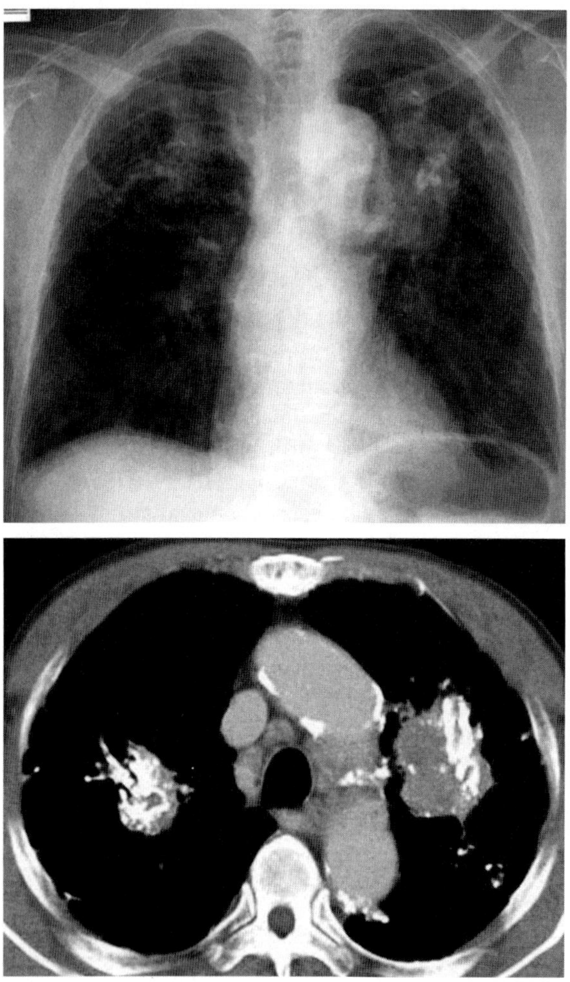

a

b

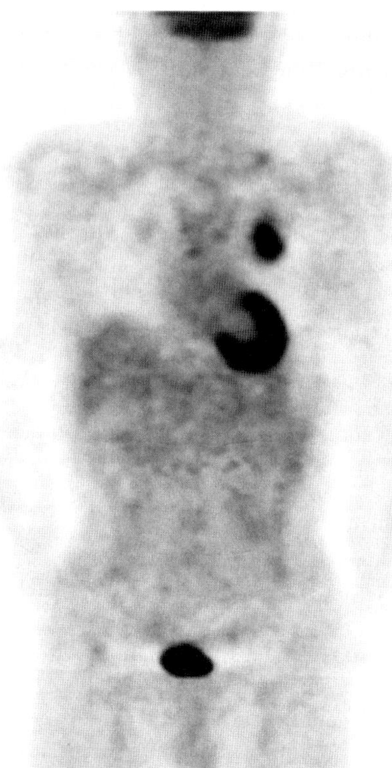

c

Fig. 3.1.9a-c. a Chest radiograph of a 79-year-old man who had been a tunnel worker for 15 years and had been diagnosed with silicosis and progressive massive fibrosis (PMF) 26 years previously. The chest radiograph demonstrates bilateral areas of confluent fibrosis. **b** These mass-like opacities are seen on computed tomography as having an irregular contour with areas of calcification, and appearances are consistent with PMF in pneumoconiosis. Note that the medial part of the mass in the left upper lobe is not calcified. **c** Coronal image of the fluorine-18 fluorodeoxyglucose (FDG) positron emission tomography scan shows marked uptake in the medial aspect of the PMF in the left upper lobe but no significant uptake within the conglomerate mass in the right upper lobe. Increased uptake of FDG is also observed in the left supraclavicular region, suggestive of a metastatic lymph node. Bronchial washings in this patient revealed adenocarcinoma. Images for Figure 3.1.9 are courtesy of Dr. Shuji Bandoh, Japan and have been published in Bandoh et al. (2003)

(Bandoh et al. 2003) – a difficult distinction to make particularly if the cancer develops within an area of PMF. Although pneumoconiotic lesions may show variable degrees of FDG uptake (Alavi et al. 2002), Bandoh et al. have reported significantly increased FDG uptake in a patient with PMF who developed adenocarcinoma (Bandoh et al. 2003). Further work is necessary, but preliminary studies demonstrate that PET may be able to contribute to the evaluation of subjects with occupational lung disease in a specific problem-solving capacity.

References

Aberle DR, Gamsu G, Ray CS, Feuerstein IM (1988a) Asbestos-related pleural and parenchymal fibrosis: detection with high resolution CT. Radiology 166:729-734

Aberle DR, Gamsu G, Ray CS (1988b) High-resolution CT of benign asbestos-related diseases: clinical and radiographic correlation. AJR 151:883-891

Akira M, Yokoyama K, Yamamoto S, Higashihara T, Morinaga K, Kita N, Morimoto S, Ikezoe J, Kozuka T (1991) Early asbestosis: evaluation with high-resolution CT. Radiology 178:409-416

Akira M, Yamamoto Y, Inoue Y, Sakatani M (2003) High-resolution CT of asbestosis and idiopathic pulmonary fibrosis. AJR Am J Roentgenol 181:163-169

Akpinar-Elci M, Travis WD, Lynch DA, Kreiss K (2004) Bronchiolitis obliterans syndrome in popcorn production plant workers. Eur Respir J 24:298-302

Alavi A, Gupta N, Alberini JL, Hickeson M, Adam LE, Bhargava P, Zhuang H (2002) Positron emission tomography imaging in nonmalignant thoracic disorders. Semin Nucl Med 32:293-321

Ameille J, Brochard P, Brechot JM, Pascano T, Cherin A, Raix A, Fredy M, Bignon J (1993) Pleural thickening: a comparison of oblique chest radiographs and high-resolution computed tomography in subjects exposed to low levels of asbestos pollution. Int Arch Occup Environ Health 64:545-548

American Thoracic Society Documents (2004) Diagnosis and initial management of nonmalignant diseases related to asbestos. Am J Respir Crit Care Med 170:691-715

American Thoracic Society (1986) The diagnosis of non malignant diseases related to asbestos. Am Rev Respir Dis 134:363-368

Bacher K, Smeets P, Bonnarens K, DeHauwere A, Verstraete K, Thierens H (2003) Dose reduction in patients undergoing chest imaging: digital amorphous silicon flat-panel detector radiography versus conventional film-screen radiography and phosphor-based computed radiography. AJR Am J Roentgenol 181:923-929

Bandoh S, Fujita J, Yamamoto Y, Nishiyama Y, Ueda Y, Tojo Y, Ishii T, Kubo A, Ishida T (2003) A case of lung cancer associated with pneumoconiosis diagnosed by fluorine-18 fluorodeoxyglucose positron emission tomography. Ann Nucl Med 17:597-600

Bankier AA, Madani A, Gevenois PA (2002) CT quantification of pulmonary emphysema: assessment of lung structure and function. Crit Rev Comput Tomogr 43:399-417

Barnhart S, Thornquist M, Omenn GS, Goodman G, Feigl P, Rosenstock L (2004) The degree of roentgenographic parenchymal opacities attributable to smoking among asbestos-exposed subjects. Am Rev Respir Dis 141:1102-1106

Begin R, Cantin A, Drapeau G, Lamoureux G, Boctor M, Masse S, Rola-Pleszczynski M (1983) Pulmonary uptake of gallium-67 in asbestos-exposed humans and sheep. Am Rev Respir Dis 127:623-630

Begin R, Filion RB, Ostiguy G (1995) Emphysema in silica- and asbestos-exposed workers seeking compensation. A CT scan study. Chest 108:647-655

Bergin CJ, Muller NL, Vedal S, Chan-Yeung M (1986) CT in silicosis: correlation with plain films and pulmonary function tests. AJR Am J Roentgenol 146:477-483

Bergin CJ, Castellino RA, Blank N, Moses L (1994) Specificity of high-resolution CT findings in pulmonary asbestosis: do patients scanned for other indications have similar findings? AJR 163:551-555

Boswell RT, McCunney RJ (1995) Bronchiolitis obliterans from exposure to incinerator fly ash. J Occup Environ Med 37:850-855

Bourgkard E, Bernadac P, Chau N, Bertrand J-P, Teculescu D, Pham QT (1998) Can the evolution to pneumoconiosis be suspected in coal miners. Am J Respir Crit Care Med 158:504-509

Coggon D, Newman TA (2004) Coal mining and chronic obstructive pulmonary disease: a review of the evidence. Thorax 53:398-407

Coleman E (1999) PET in lung cancer. J Nucl Med 40:814-820

Consensus report (1997) Asbestos, asbestosis and cancer: the Helsinki criteria for diagnosis and attribution. Scand J Work Environ Health 23:311-316

Cookson W, de Klerk N, Musk AW, Glancy JJ, Armstrong B, Hobbs M1986;. The natural history of asbestosis in former crocidolite workers of Wittenoom Gorge. Am Rev Respir Dis 133:994-998

Copley S (2000) Computed tomographic-functional relationships in asbestos-induced pleural and parenchymal disease. University of London

Copley S, Wells A, Sivakumaran P, Rubens MB, Lee YC, Desai SR, MacDonald SL, Thompson RI, Colby TV, Nicholson AG, Du Bois RM, Hansell DM, Musk AW (2003) Asbestosis and idiopathic pulmonary fibrosis: comparison of thin-section CT features. Radiology 229:731-736

Dick JA, Morgan WK, Muir DF, Reger RB, Sargent N (1992) The significance of irregular opacities on the chest roentgenogram. Chest 102:251-260

Ducatman AM (1991) Variability in interpretation of radiographs for asbestosis abnormalities: problems and solutions. Ann NY Acad Sci 643:108-120

Eberle B, Markstaller K, Schreiber WG, Kauczor HU (2001) Hyperpolarised gases in magnetic resonance: a new tool for functional imaging of the lung. Swiss Med Wkly 131(35/36):503-509

Epler GR, McLoud TC, Gaensler EA, Mikus JP, Carrington CB (1978; Normal chest roentgenograms in chronic diffuse infiltrative lung disease. N Engl J Med 298:935-939

Epstein DM, Miller WT, Bresnitz EA, Levine MS, Gefter WB (1984) Application of ILO classification to a population without industrial exposure: findings to be differentiated from pneumoconiosis. AJR 142:53-58

Fink C, Hallscheidt PJ, Noeldge G, Kampschulte A, Radeleff B, Hosch WP, Kaufmann GW, Hansmann J (2002) Clinical comparative study with a large-area amorphous silicon flat-panel detector: image quality and visibility of anatomic structures on chest radiography. AJR Am J Roentgenol 178:481-486

Fletcher CM, Oldham PD (1949) Problem of consistent radiological diagnoses in coal miners' pneumoconiosis. Br J Ind Med 6:168-183

Floyd CEJ, Warp RJ, Dobbins JT, Chotas HG, Baydush AH, Vargas-Voracek R, Ravin CE (2001) Imaging characteristics of an amorphous silicon flat-panel detector for digital chest radiography. Radiology 218:683-688

Friedman AC, Fiel SB, Fisher MS, Radecki PD, Lev-Toaff AS, Caroline DF (1988) Asbestos-related pleural disease and asbestosis: a comparison of CT and chest radiography. AJR 150:269-275

Gaensler EA, Jederlinic PJ, Churg A (1991) Idiopathic pulmonary fibrosis in asbestos-exposed workers. Am Rev Respir Dis 144:689-696

Gamsu G (1989) High-resolution CT in the diagnosis of asbestos-related pleuroparenchymal disease. Am J Ind Med 16:115-117

Gamsu G, Salmon CJ, Warnock ML, Blanc PD (1995) CT quantification of interstitial fibrosis in patients with asbestosis: a comparison of two methods. AJR 164(1):63-68

Garmer M, Hennigs SP, Jager HJ, Schrick F, van de LT, Jacobs A, Hanusch A, Christmann A, Mathias K (2000) Digital radiography versus conventional radiography in chest imaging: diagnostic performance of a large-area silicon flat-panel detector in a clinical CT-controlled study. AJR Am J Roentgenol 174(1):75-80

Gitlin JN, Cook LL, Linton OW, Garrett-Mayer E (2004) Comparison of "B" readers' interpretations of chest radiographs for asbestos related changes. Acad Radiol 11:843-856

Gurney JW, Jones KK, Robbins RA, Gossman GL, Nelson KJ, Daughton D, Spurzem JR, Rennard SI (1992) Regional distribution of emphysema: correlation of high-resolution CT with pulmonary function tests in unselected smokers. Radiology 183:457-463

Hanisch G, Schreiber W, Diergarten T, Markstaller K, Eberle B, Kauczor HU (2000) Investigation of intrapulmonary diffusion by 3He MRI. Eur Radiol 10 [Suppl 1]:S345

Harber P, Smitherman J (1991) Asbestosis: diagnostic dilution. J Occ Med 33:786-793

Harkin TJ, McGuinness G, Goldring R, Parker JE, Crane MD, Naidich DP (1996) Differentiation of the ILO boundary chest roentgenograph (0/1 to 1/0) in asbestosis by high-resolution computed tomography scan, alveolitis, and respiratory impairment. J Occup Environ Med 38:46-52

Henry DA (2002) International Labour Office classification system in the age of imaging: relevant or redundant. J Thorac Imaging 17:179-188

Henschke CI, McCauley DI, Yankelevitz DF, Naidich DP, McGuinness G, Miettinen OS, Libby DM, Pasmantier MW, Koizumi J, Altorki NK, Smith JP (1999) Early Lung Cancer Action Project: overall design and findings from baseline screening. Lancet 354:99-105

Hering KG, Tuengerthal S, Kraus T (2004) Standardized CT/HRCT-classification of the German Federal Republic for work and environmental related thoracic diseases. Radiologe 44:500-511

Hessel PA (1985) The middling tendency in reading chest films for pneumoconiosis: an important source of bias and variability. Am J Ind Med 8:43-48

Hierholzer J, Luo L, Bittner RC, Stroszcynski C, Schroder R-J, Schoenfeld N, Dorow P, Loddenkemper R, Grassot A (2000) MRI and CT in the differential diagnosis of pleural disease. Chest 118:604-609

Hilt B, Borgerson A, Lien JT, Langard S (1992) Chest radiographs in subjects with asbestos-related abnormalities: comparison between ILO categorizations and clinical reading. Am J Ind Med 21:862-868

International expert meeting on new advances in the radiology and screening of asbestos-related diseases (2000) Scand J Work Environ Health 26:449-454

International Labour Office (1980) Guidelines for the use of the ILO international classification of radiographs of the pneumoconioses, rev edn. International Labour Office, Geneva

Jarad NA, Wilkinson P, Pearson MC, Rudd RM (1992) A new high resolution computed tomography scoring system for pulmonary fibrosis, pleural disease, and emphysema in patients with asbestos related disease. Br J Ind Med 49:73-84

Jones RN (1991) The diagnosis of asbestosis. Am Rev Respir Dis 144:477-478

Kanner RE, Barkman HW Jr, Rom WN, Taylor AT Jr (1985) Gallium-67 Citrate Imaging in Underground Coal Miners. Am J Ind Med 8:49-55

Kauczor H (2003) Hyperpolarized helium-3 gas magnetic resonance imaging of the lung. Top Magn Reson Imaging 14:223-230

Kilburn KH, Warshaw RH (1994) Airways obstruction from asbestos exposure. Effects of asbestosis and smoking. Chest 106:1061-1070

Kinsella M, Muller N, Vedal S, Staples C, Abboud RT, Chan-Yeung M (1990) Emphysema in silicosis. A comparison of smokers with nonsmokers using pulmonary function testing and computed tomography. Am Rev Respir Dis 141:1497-1500

Kipen HM, Lilis R, Suzuki Y, Valciukas JA, Selikoff IJ (1987) Pulmonary fibrosis in asbestos insulation workers with lung cancer: a radiological and histopathological evaluation. Br J Ind Med 44:96-100

Klein JS, Gamsu G, Webb WR, Golden JA, Muller NL (1992) High-resolution CT diagnosis of emphysema in symptomatic patients with normal chest radiographs and isolated low diffusing capacity. Radiology 182:817-821

Knuuttila A, Halme M, Kivisaari A, Salo J, Mattson K (1998) The clinical importance of magnetic resonance imaging versus computed tomography in malignant pleural mesothelioma. Lung Cancer 22:215-225

Lee YC, Runnion CK, Pang SC, de Klerk NH, Musk AW (2001) Increased body mass index is related to apparent circumscribed pleural thickening on plain chest radiographs. Am J Ind Med 39:112-116

Lee YC, Singh B, Pang SC, de Klerk NH, Hillman DR, Musk AW (2003) Radiographic (ILO) readings predict arterial oxygen desaturation during exercise in subjects with asbestosis. Occup Environ Med 60:201-206

Lynch DA (1995) CT for asbestosis: value and limitations (comment). AJR 1:69-71

Lynch DA (2002) Imaging of occupational lung disease: time to enter the 21st century. J Thorac Imaging 17:177-178

Meyer JD, Islam SS, Ducatman AM, McCunney RJ (1997) Prevalence of small lung opacities in populations unexposed to dusts. A literature analysis. Chest 111:404-410

Miller A, Lilis R, Godbold J, Wu X (1996) Relation of spirometic function to radiographic interstitial fibrosis in two large workforces exposed to asbestos: an evaluation of the ILO profusion score. Occup Environ Med 53:808-812

Miller A, Markowitz S, Manowitz A, Miller JA (2004) Lung cancer screening using low-dose high-resolution CT scanning in a high-risk workforce. Chest 125:152S-153S

Oksa P, Suoranta H, Koskinen H, Zitting A, Nordman H (1994) High-resolution computed tomography in the early detection of asbestosis. Int Arch Occup Environ Health 65:299-304

Oksa P, Huuskonen MS, Jarvisalo J, Klockars M, Zitting A, Suoranta H, Tossavainen A, Vattulainen K, Laippala P (1998) Follow-up of asbestosis patients and predictors for radiographic progression. Int Arch Occup Environ Health 71:465-471

Paris C, Benichou J, Raffaelli C, Genevois A, Fournier L, Menard G, Broessel N, Ameille J, Brochard P, Gillon JC, Gislard A, Letourneux M (2004) Factors associated with early-stage pulmonary fibrosis as determined by high-resolution computed tomography among persons occupationally exposed to asbestos. Scand J Work Environ Health 30:206-214

Patz EF, Lowe VJ, Hoffman JM, Paine SS, Burrowes P, Coleman RE, Goodman PC (1993) Focal pulmonary abnormalities: evaluation with F-18 fluorodeoxyglucose PET scanning. Radiology 188:487-490

Prokop M (2003) General principles of MDCT. Eur J Radiol 45:S4-S10

Remy-Jardin M, Sobaszek A, Duhamel A, Mastora I, Zanetti C, Remy J (2004; Asbestos-related pleuropulmonary diseases: evaluation with low-dose four-detector row spiral CT. Radiology 233:182-190

Rong XJ, Shaw CC, Liu X, Lemacks MR, Thompson SK (2000) Comparison of an amorphous silicon/cesium iodide flat-panel digital chest radiography system with screen/film and computed radiography systems - a contrast-detail phantom study. Med Phys 28:2328-2335

Rosenstock L, Barnhart S, Heyer NJ, Pierson DJ, Hudson LD (1988) The relation among pulmonary function chest roentgenographic abnormalities and smoking status in an asbestos-exposed cohort. Am Rev Respir Dis 138:272-277

Ross RM (2003) The clinical diagnosis of asbestosis in this century requires more than a chest radiograph. Chest 124:1120-1128

Ruckley VA, Gauld SJ, Chapman JS, Davis JM, Douglas AN, Fernie J, Jacobsen M, Lamb D (1984) Emphysema and dust exposure in a group of coal workers. Am Rev Respir Dis 129:528-532

Schachtman NA, Rhodes CJ (1992) Medico-legal issues in occupational lung disease litigation. Semin Roentgenol 27:140-143

Schwartz DA, Galvin JR, Yagla SJ, Speakman SB, Merchant JA, Hunninghake GW (1993) Restrictive lung function and asbestos-induced pleural fibrosis. A quantitative approach. J Clin Invest 91:2685-2692

Sette A, Neder JA, Nery LE, Kavakama J, Rodrigues RT, Terra-Filho M, Guimares S, Muller N (2004) Thin-section CT abnormalities and pulmonary gas exchange impairment in workers exposed to asbestos. Radiology 232:66-74

Siemsen JK, Grebe SF, Waxman AD (1978) The use of gallium-67 in pulmonary disorders. Semin Nucl Med 128:1084-1089

Spain BA, Cummings O, Garcia JG (1995) Bronchiolitis obliternas in an animal feed worker. Am J Ind Med 28:437-443

Staples CA, Gamsu G, Ray CS, Webb WR (1989) High resolution computed tomography and lung function in asbestos-exposed workers with normal chest radiographs. Am Rev Respir Dis 139:1502-1508

Stern EJ, Frank MS, Godwin JD (1995) Chest computed tomography display preferences. Survey of thoracic radiologists. Invest Radiol 30:517-521

Swensen SJ, Jett JR, Sloan JA, Midthun DE, Hartman TE, Sykes AM, Aughenbaugh GL, Zink FE, Hillman SL, Noetzel GR, Marks RS, Clayton AC, Pairolero PC (2002) Screening for lung cancer with low-dose spiral computed tomography. Am J Respir Crit Care Med 165:508-513

Thurlbeck WM, Simon G (1978) Radiographic appearance of the chest in emphysema. AJR Am J Roentgenol 130:429-440

Tiitola M, Kivisaari L, Huuskonen MS, Mattson K, Koskinen H, Lehtola A, Zitting A, Vehmas T (2002) Computed tomography screening for lung cancer in asbestos-exposed workers. Lung Cancer 35:17-22

Van Cleemput J, de Raeve H, Verschakelen JA, Rombouts J, Lacquet LM, Nemery B (2001) Surface of localized pleural plaques quantitated by computed tomography scanning: no relation with cumulative asbestos exposure and no effect on lung function. Am J Respir Crit Care Med 163:705-710

Weber MA, Bock M, Plathow C, Wasser K, Fink C, Zuna I, Schmahl A, Berger I, Kauczor HU, Schoenberg SO (2004) Asbestos-related pleural disease: value of dedicated magnetic resonance imaging techniques. Invest Radiol 39:554-564

Weiss W (1991) Cigarette smoking and small irregular opacities. Br J Ind Med 48:841-844

Zitting AJ, Karjalainen A, Impivaara O, Kuusela T, Maki J, Tossavainen A, Jarvisalo J (1996) Radiographic small lung opacities and pleural abnormalities in relation to smoking, urbanization status, and occupational asbestos exposure in Finland. J Occup Environ Med 38:602-609

3.2 ILO Classification

Vinicius C. S. Antao and John E. Parker

CONTENTS

3.2.1 Introduction 93
3.2.2 The 2000 Revision 93
3.2.2.1 Parenchymal Abnormalities 94
3.2.2.2 Pleural Abnormalities 94
3.2.2.3 Symbols and Comments 94
3.2.2.4 The Quad Set 95
3.2.3 Proficiency in the Use of the ILO Classification 95
3.2.4 Correlation with Other Tests 95
3.2.5 Assessment of Disease Progression 96
3.2.6 Limitations of the Classification 96
3.2.6.1 Reader Variability 96
3.2.6.2 Insensitivity of Radiographs to Pneumoconiosis 96
3.2.6.3 Lack of Specificity to Pneumoconiotic Lesions 97
3.2.6.4 Importance of Film Quality 97
3.2.6.5 Additional Limitations of the Classification 97
3.2.7 Other Classifications 97
3.2.8 Future Trends in Digital Radiography and Computed Imaging 97
References 98

3.2.1 Introduction

The International Labour Office (ILO) International Classification of Radiographs of Pneumoconioses is an instrument intended to "standardize classification methods and facilitate international comparisons of data on pneumoconiosis, epidemiological investigations and research reports" (ILO 2002). The scope and purpose of the Classification are clearly stated in its guidelines: to describe and systematically record radiographic abnormalities seen on postero-anterior chest radiographs due to inhaled dust diseases. It is not designed to define pathological entities, and it does not take into account working capacity or compensation for disability (Jacobsen 1991). The initial version of the Classification was issued in 1930, with subsequent revisions published in 1950, 1958, 1968, 1971, 1980, and 2000. The first editions were focused on silicosis. In 1958, a single category was included to cover all types and profusions of linear markings. In the 1960s, the International Union Against Cancer (UICC) evolved a parallel system for linear (now called irregular) opacities, mainly spurred by asbestos exposure. In 1968, the UICC and ILO systems were merged for all dust-induced pneumoconioses, with the ILO embracing the UICC ideas (Henry 2002; ILO 2002; Shipley 1992).

3.2.2 The 2000 Revision

The 2000 revision of the Classification comprises a set of 22 standard radiographs (Complete Set) and the text guidelines for its use (ILO 2002). For this issue, 20 of the radiographs are made from digitized copies of the full-size standards distributed with the 1980 version of the Classification. A further composite film shows three different profusions of u/u size opacities plus an example of subcategory 0/0. A new film is provided to exemplify pleural abnormalities. It is recommended that standard reading sheets be used to record the classification. Because technical quality of the radiograph is essential to the interpretation, the reader must record a judgment regarding quality, using the following categories: (1) good; (2) acceptable, with minor defects; (3) acceptable, with considerable defects; and (4) unacceptable for classification purposes. Comments must be made about technical defects, if quality is not grade 1 (ILO 2002). The reporting system combines semi-quantitative and descriptive portions. The reader is required to record characteristics of the parenchyma or pleura

V. C. S. Antao, MD, PhD
Division of Respiratory Disease Studies -National Institute for Occupational Safety and Health, CDC, 1095 Willowdale Rd - MS 2800, Morgantown, WV 26505, USA
J. E. Parker, MD
Professor and Chief, Pulmonary and Critical Care Medicine, West Virginia University, HSC 4075A-9166, Morgantown, WV 26506-9166, USA

that are consistent with pneumoconiosis, as well as to note, under symbols and comments, other findings that are more likely to be due to other disease processes (Shipley 1992).

3.2.2.1 Parenchymal Abnormalities

There were no significant changes from the 1980 version of the Classification in the way parenchymal changes are reported. *Small opacities* are defined as parenchymal opacities less than 10 mm in size. They are described according to their shape (rounded or irregular), size, profusion level, and location. Rounded opacities are labeled *p*, *q*, *r*, according to their size (*p*, <1.5 mm; *q*, 1.5–3 mm; and *r*, 3–10 mm). Irregular opacities are identified by the letters *s*, *t*, and *u*, and categorized according to their width (*s*, <1.5 mm; *t*, 1.5–3 mm; and *u*, 3–10 mm). Two letters are used to record shape and size, and both rounded and irregular opacities may be described in the same film. For example, if the reader considers that virtually all lesions are irregular, with a width up to 1.5 mm, the film is coded *s/s*. A classification *r/s* would mean that the predominant type of opacity is rounded, 3–10 mm (*r*), but there are also a significant number of irregular opacities, up to 1.5 mm (*s*). The concentration of small opacities in affected zones of the lung is referred to as profusion. The profusion level is derived from comparisons with the standard films, which depict four categories: *0*, *1*, *2*, and *3*, for the increasing profusion. *Category 0* indicates the absence of small opacities or that there are fewer opacities than *category 1*. The classification includes 12 subcategories (Table 3.2.1). The first number denotes the category that the film resembles the most. If the appearance of the film closely matches the standard, the number is repeated (i.e., 2/2), but if another category is seriously considered (e.g., category 3), that is recorded as the second number, and the final classification should be 2/3. For the location of affected zones, the radiograph is divided into six zones: upper, middle, and lower on each side. *Large opacities* are defined as opacities having the longest dimension exceeding 10 mm. They are coded as *A* (longest dimension between 10 mm and 50 mm); *B* (greater than 50 mm but less than the area of the right upper zone); and *C* (greater than the area of the right upper zone). If there is more than one large opacity, the sum of the greatest dimensions of the large opacities is used for the categorization (ILO 2002).

Table 3.2.1. International Classification of Radiographs of Pneumoconioses: categories and subcategories for profusion of small opacities

Categories	0			1			2			3		
Subcategories	0/-	0/0	0/1	1/0	1/1	1/2	2/1	2/2	2/3	3/2	3/3	3/+

3.2.2.2 Pleural Abnormalities

Pleural abnormalities described by the Classification include *pleural plaques* (localized pleural thickening), *costophrenic angle obliteration*, and *diffuse pleural thickening*. *Pleural plaques* are classified on each hemithorax, according to their location (chest wall – in profile or face on, diaphragm, or other site), presence of calcification, and combined extent (*1*=up to 1/4; *2*=1/4 to 1/2; and *3*=more than 1/2 of lateral chest wall). For the 2000 version of the Classification, the recording of width is optional, and a minimum width of 3 mm is required for an in-profile plaque to be considered as present. If recorded, the width is categorized as *a* (3–5 mm); *b* (5–10 mm); or *c* (>10 mm). It is no longer necessary to measure the extent of calcification in this new version. *Costophrenic angle obliteration* is registered as either present or absent, for each hemithorax, and the lower limit for its classification is defined by comparison with the standard radiograph illustrating subcategory 1/1 t/t. *Diffuse pleural thickening* is recorded only if costophrenic angle obliteration is present. It is classified in the same manner as pleural plaques (ILO 2002).

3.2.2.3 Symbols and Comments

Important features seen on the radiograph that have not been registered previously are coded with the use of symbols. It is important to note that some of the symbols imply interpretations, rather than just descriptions, but are not definite diagnoses of specific findings. The 2000 Classification provides 29 symbols, an addition of 7 from the 1980 version. The new symbols are: *aa* (atherosclerotic aorta); *at* (significant apical pleural thickening); *cg* (calcified non-pneumoconiotic nodules (granulomas) or nodes); *me* (mesothelioma); *pa* (plate atelectasis); *pb* (parenchymal bands); and *ra* (rounded atelectasis). If the symbol *od* (other disease or significant abnormality) is used or other relevant information is necessary, the reader should provide further clarification in the comments section (ILO 2002).

3.2.2.4
The Quad Set

One of the main innovations of the 2000 version of the Classification was the introduction of a set of 14 standard radiographs that are compatible with the Complete Set. The Quad Set includes 9 of the original films (category 0/0 example 1; category 0/0 example 2; category 1/1 q/q; category 1/1 t/t; category 2/2 q/q; category 2/2 t/t; category 3/3 q/q; category 3/3 t/t; and the composite that shows pleural abnormalities). Of the films, 5 are composites of quadrant sections from the other radiographs in the Complete Set (4 of them show categories 1/1, 2/2, and 3/3 of small opacities p/p, r/r, s/s, and u/u, and 1 demonstrates large opacities A, B, and C). Prior to the issuance of the Quad, a reading trial was prepared by the ILO's Occupational Safety and Health Branch and by the Division of Respiratory Disease Studies of the United States National Institute for Occupational Safety and Health (NIOSH), with the collaboration of the Task Force on Pneumoconioses of the American College of Radiology (Jacobsen et al. 1998; NIOSH 1999). Chest radiographs (n=120) were evaluated in two rounds by 39 readers from 12 countries. The first reading was done with either the Complete or the Quad Set, which were switched for the subsequent round. In a third round, with the participation of 37 readers, each group of 60 radiographs was read with either set of standards. This trial showed that some readers, while using the Quad, recognized large opacities less frequently than when they used the Complete Set. A tendency to record higher profusion levels when using the Quad was also noted. Nevertheless, neither between- nor within-reader variability was influenced significantly by which set was used in the trial.

3.2.3
Proficiency in the Use of the ILO Classification

In the United States, NIOSH conducts a program aimed to train and certify physicians in the use of the ILO Classification. The NIOSH *B* Reader Program was developed to comply with U.S. Federal regulations that provide specifications for the interpretation and classification of radiographs. The creation of this program was also stimulated by the findings of large interreader variability in the classifications during the first years of NIOSH's Coal Workers' X-Ray Surveillance Program (Attfield and Wagner 1992). The first examinations began in 1974, but the program only went into full operation in 1978. The program certifies two categories of readers. The *A* readers are considered those who have applied for certification after attending a 2-day course on the Classification or have submitted to NIOSH six sample chest radiographs that are regarded as properly classified by a panel of *B* readers. A *B* reader is a physician who has been approved in one of the certification examinations administered monthly by NIOSH in Morgantown, West Virginia. *B* readers are certified for a period of 4 years and may apply for recertification during the last year before expiration of the certification. The certification examination requires classification of 125 radiographs, and the recertification is based on the classification of 50 films (Wagner et al. 1992). More than 1500 *B* readers have been certified up to December 2004. Currently, there are 438 *B* readers, of whom 26 are from foreign countries.

3.2.4
Correlation with Other Tests

The semi-quantitative approach of the Classification permits its comparison with several techniques, to assess its validity and also as a method to evaluate exposure-response relationships. Vallyathan et al. (1996) demonstrated good agreement between the ILO Classification and pathological abnormalities observed on whole-lung preparations from autopsied lungs of coal miners. Both micronodules and macronodules were strong predictors of both category ≥0/1 and ≥2/1. Nevertheless, the study showed that chest radiographs were insensitive for identifying coal workers' pneumoconiosis (CWP) macules. The impact of pneumoconioses on lung function has also been evaluated by correlations with parenchymal and pleural abnormalities seen on chest radiographs. Cowie (1998) showed that annual loss of forced expiratory volume in 1 s (FEV_1) was directly correlated with categories of small opacity profusion in gold miners. The presence of large opacities was also associated with significant impairment of lung function in silicotic patients (Henry 2002). Miller et al. (1996) showed that the forced vital capacity (FVC) was inversely correlated with ILO profusion scores among insulators and sheet metal workers exposed to asbestos. This study also provided evidence that both small opacity profusion and respiratory impairment were associated with different degrees of exposure to asbestos. Asbestos-related pleural abnormalities, such as diffuse pleural thickening, pleural plaques, and costophrenic angle obliteration, were related to decreased FVC as well (Cotes and King 1988). Several studies have addressed the relationship between chest radiographs and conventional computed tomography (CT) or high-resolution computed tomography (HRCT) in the evaluation of pneumoconioses. CT/HRCT was usually found to be more sensitive and specific in detecting both parenchymal lesions in silicosis, CWP, and asbestosis, as well as pleural abnormalities in asbestos-exposed individuals. Reader agreement is also consistently higher for CT/HRCT than for chest radiograph interpretations. (Bergin et al. 1986; Bégin et al. 1991, 1993; Huuskonen et al. 2001).

3.2.5 Assessment of Disease Progression

A number of approaches have been used to assess disease progression with the ILO Classification, all of them subject to biases (Wagner et al. 1993). In the *independent method*, films from the same patient are read apart from each other. According to Liddell and Morgan (1978), the order of readings may be immediate (as soon as they become available), serial (all first films in one occasion, all second films in another occasion, etc.), ranked (all films in a sequence of increasing radiographic change), or in randomized sequence. The *side-by-side method* may be carried out preserving the temporal order in which the films were taken, or this order may be concealed. Excessive variability has been associated with the *independent* method, whereas possible bias from knowing the temporal order may occur with *side-by-side* readings (Wagner et al. 1993). Usually, the side-by-side method is preferred (Amandus et al. 1973; de Klerk et al. 1990), although McMillan et al. (1982) states that whenever an estimate of prevalence is necessary, independent randomized readings should be used. Although the ILO Classification guidelines do not contemplate the assessment of serial radiographs, several studies have used progression of disease on sequential films as a health outcome. An example is the study of Oksa et al. (1998), which identified radiographic progression of asbestosis as an independent risk factor for lung cancer.

3.2.6 Limitations of the Classification

3.2.6.1 Reader Variability

One of the most important problems in the application of the ILO Classification is reader variability. Regardless of whether the readings are being conducted for epidemiological, clinical, or legal purposes, between- and within-reader variability creates significant problems for study comparisons and may undermine study validity (Wagner et al. 1993). The implications of reader variability for public health were observed by Parker et al. (1989), when initial readings of 566 radiographs showed a prevalence of 30% of pleural abnormalities in Minnesota. After being reviewed by a panel of three experts from NIOSH, only 4% of the films were considered abnormal. Nevertheless, Impivaara et al. (1998) found that the variability rarely exceeded one profusion subcategory in a large population sample in Finland. Poor film quality, lack of experience with the classification, and lack of familiarity with radiographic manifestations of pneumoconiosis have been implicated as causes of excessive variation (Felson et al. 1973). However, Copland et al. (1981) showed that individuals with no medical training were able to use the classification and achieved levels of variability comparable to experienced readers. Participation in quality-assurance panels and reliable feedback to readers are crucial and have been proposed as measures to reduce variability (Ducatman 1991). In Canada, a reading panel already provides this type of service (Muir et al. 1993). To address reader variability, it is also recommended that a minimum of two, but if possible more readers are employed in epidemiological studies (ILO 2002).

3.2.6.2 Insensitivity of Radiographs to Pneumoconiosis

Although not a problem of the Classification *per se*, radiographs are known to have inherent limitations in the assessment of early lesions of pneumoconiosis, regardless of film quality or reader expertise (Shipley 1992; Wagner et al. 1993). The threshold of visibility of very small pathological changes depends on the number of pneumoconiotic lesions per unit of lung volume, as well as the degree of summation of these changes. It has been reported that 10–20% of films of asbestos-exposed individuals may be classified as normal even in the presence of fibrotic lesions confirmed by histopathological examination (ROCKOFF and SCHWARTZ 1988).

3.2.6.3 Lack of Specificity to Pneumoconiotic Lesions

"Small opacities" seen on the chest radiograph may result from causes other than dust exposure and, thus, have a potential to create inaccuracies in the classification of pneumoconiosis. Cigarette smoking is recognized to cause an increase in the profusion of small opacities in asbestos-exposed workers (SHIPLEY 1992). Non-dust-related diseases, such as sarcoidosis, tuberculosis, and interstitial pneumonitis may also cause nodular or irregular lesions on the radiograph very similar to those of pneumoconioses. EPSTEIN et al. (1984) found that 11% of 200 symptomatic hospitalized patients with no recognized dust exposure or other medical etiology that could cause "small opacities" had a radiograph classified with a profusion of 1/0 or greater. In asymptomatic individuals, it is uncommon to find "small opacities." CASTELLAN et al. (1985) found only three radiographs with profusion greater than 1/0 in a cohort of 1,422 non-dust exposed workers.

3.2.6.4 Importance of Film Quality

Technical quality may seriously influence the classification of pneumoconiosis. A tendency to assign lower small opacity profusions to radiographs that are overexposed – or too "dark" or too "black" – has been reported. However, higher small opacity profusions are likely to be assigned in underexposed films (ROCKOFF and SCWARTZ 1988).

3.2.6.5 Additional Limitations of the Classification

The ILO classification system is designed primarily for the description of chronic radiographic abnormalities. It is not as powerful a tool in describing changes seen in acute silicosis, specifically those of the alveolar filling processes. The classification is also not, in and of itself, a great tool for differentiating chronic infectious changes, such as lung injury from tuberculosis, from those of pneumoconiosis. It may be particularly difficult when abnormalities from both tuberculosis and silicosis are present on a chest radiograph. This challenging task frequently requires skilled clinical expertise and culture material or consultation with treating physicians (WHITE et al. 2001; WHITE and DAVIES 2002). In addition, occupational dust exposure gives rise to various diseases, such as chronic airflow limitation, that are not detectable using chest radiographs.

3.2.7 Other Classifications

Instead of the ILO Classification, China and Japan have developed and often use their own systems. The Chinese Diagnostic Standard of Silicotic Radiographs has been used since 1963. Although 'suspect pneumoconiosis' categories and large opacities showed good agreement with the ILO Classification in a reading trial of 576 radiographs, recommendations were made to improve the Chinese scheme, such as the inclusion of subcategories for profusion, the subdivision of large opacities into three categories, and the adoption of standard films (HUANG and HONG 1984). The 1982 Japanese Classification of Radiographs of Pneumoconiosis utilizes their unique 23 standard films, which include mid-category films and so-called limit films. They also adopt a 12-point scale similar to the ILO Classification (KUSAKA and MORIMOTO 1992).

3.2.8 Future Trends in Digital Radiography and Computed Imaging

The increasing pace of change toward digital imaging around the world, and especially in developed nations, poses a challenge for the septuagenarian Classification. Theoretically, many advantages would arise from this technology, such as electronic transmission of images, significant reduction of storage space, and enhancement of image quality through manipulation of contrast, brightness, and other settings. Despite the substantial literature on digital imaging, only few studies have addressed this issue in the context of pneumoconioses. Digitized images acquired with laser scanners and conventional chest radiographs were examined in workers exposed to silica (KUNDEL et al. 1987) and coal-mine dust (MANNINO et al. 1993). Both studies showed very similar results on the interpretation of pneumoconiosis and on reader variability when the two techniques were compared. SCHAEFER et al. (1990) used digital storage phosphor radiography for the screening of pleural disease in asbestos-exposed workers and concluded that the method performed at least as well as conventional radiographs. KATSURAGAWA et al. (1990) employed a computer-aided system to obtain texture measures of the ILO standard radiographs. They observed that the measures corresponded closely to the profusion categories, and that this method could help radiologists to classify pneumoconiosis. In addition to the role of digital radiography and the ILO classification, the precise place for computed tomography, both CT and HRCT, is also awaiting delineation for the recognition, evaluation, and prevention of dust diseases. Substantial work has already been accomplished, including a computer-assisted system for the classification of radiographs and computed tomography of pneumoconiosis developed by German investigators (KRAUS et al. 1997). Also, outstanding work by Japanese scientists and others (SUGANUMA et al. 2001) continues to refine methods analogous to the ILO system for these advanced chest imaging techniques to supplement traditional chest radiography. Nevertheless, the current lack of widely adopted international descriptive classification schemes, both standard films and guidelines for the interpretation of digital radiographs, as well as CT and HRCT, demands that further studies be developed to enhance the utility of the ILO Classification system.

References

Amandus HE, Reger RB, Pendergrass EP et al (1973) The pneumoconioses: methods of measuring progression. Chest 63:736-743

Attfield MD, Wagner GR (1992) A report on a workshop on the National Institute for Occupational Safety and Health B reader certification program. J Occup Med 34:875-878

Bégin R, Ostiguy G, Fillion R et al (1991) Computed tomography scan in the early detection of silicosis. Am Rev Respir Dis 144:697-705

Bégin R, Ostiguy G, Filion R et al (1993) Computed tomography in the early detection of asbestosis. Br J Ind Med 50:689-698

Bergin CJ, Muller NL, Vedal S et al (1986) CT in silicosis: correlation with plain films and pulmonary function tests. AJR Am J Roentgenol 146:477-483

Castellan RM, Sanderson WT, Petersen MR (1985) Prevalence of radiographic appearance of pneumoconiosis in an unexposed blue collar population. Am Rev Respir Dis 131:684-686

Copland L, Burns J, Jacobsen M (1981) Classification of chest radiographs for epidemiological purposes by people not experienced in the radiology of pneumoconiosis. Br J Ind Med 38:254-261

Cotes JE, King B (1988) Relationship of lung function to radiographic reading (ILO) in patients with asbestos related lung disease. Thorax 43:777-783

Cowie RL (1998) The influence of silicosis on deteriorating lung function in gold miners. Chest 113:340-343

De Klerk NH, Musk AW, James A et al (1990) Comparison of chest radiograph reading methods for assessing progress of pneumoconiosis over 10 years in Wittenoom crocidolite workers. Br J Ind Med 47:127-131

Ducatman AM (1991) Variability in interpretation of radiographs for asbestosis abnormalities: problems and solutions. Ann NY Acad Sci 643:108-120

Epstein DM, Miller WT, Bresnitz EA et al (1984) Application of ILO classification to a population without industrial exposure: findings to be differentiated from pneumoconiosis. AJR Am J Roentgenol 142:53-58

Felson B, Morgan WK, Bristol LJ et al (1973) Observations on the results of multiple readings of chest films in coal miners' pneumoconiosis. Radiology 109:19-23

Henry DA (2002) International Labor Office Classification System in the age of imaging: relevant or redundant. J Thorac Imaging 17:179-188

Huang JQ, Hong YZ (1984) A comparison of Chinese diagnostic standards of silicotic radiographs and the ILO International Classification of Radiographs of Pneumoconioses. Ann Occup Hyg 28:13-18

Huuskonen O, Kivisaari L, Zitting A et al (2001) High-resolution computed tomography classification of lung fibrosis for patients with asbestos-related disease. Scand J Work Environ Health 27:106-112

Impivaara O, Zitting AJ, Kuusela T et al (1998) Observer variation in classifying chest radiographs for small lung opacities and pleural abnormalities in a population sample. Am J Ind Med 34:261-265

International Labour Office (ILO) (2002) Guidelines for the use of the ILO International Classification of Radiographs of Pneumoconioses, rev edn 2000. Occupational safety and health series, no 22 (rev). International Labour Office, Geneva

Jacobsen M (1991) The international labour office classification: use and misuse. Ann NY Acad Sci 643:100-107

Jacobsen M, Miller WE, Parker JE (1998) New composite ('quadrant') standard films for classifying radiographs of pneumoconioses. Ind Health 36:380-383

Katsuragawa S, Doi K, MacMahon H et al (1990) Quantitative computer-aided analysis of lung texture in chest radiographs. Radiographics 10:257-269

Kraus T, Raithel HJ, Lehnert G (1997) Computer-assisted classification system for chest X-ray and computed tomography findings in occupational lung disease. Int Arch Occup Environ Health 69:482-486

Kundel HL, Mezrich JL, Brickman I et al (1987) Digital chest imaging: comparison of two film image digitizers with a classification task. Radiology 165:747-752

Kusaka Y, Morimoto K (1992) A pilot study to evaluate Japanese standard radiographs of pneumoconioses (1982) according to the ILO 1980 International Classification of Radiographs of Pneumoconioses. Ann Occup Hyg 36:425-431

Liddell FD, Morgan WK (1978) Methods of assessing serial films of the pneumoconioses: a review. J Soc Occup Med 28:6-15

Mannino DM, Kennedy RD, Hodous TK (1993) Pneumoconiosis: comparison of digitized and conventional radiographs. Radiology 187:791-796

McMillan GH, Rossiter CE, Deacon R (1982) Comparison of independent randomised reading of radiographs with direct progression scoring for assessing change in asbestos-related pulmonary and pleural lesions. Br J Ind Med 39:60-61

Miller A, Lilis R, Godbold J et al (1996) Relation of spirometric function to radiographic interstitial fibrosis in two large workforces exposed to asbestos: an evaluation of the ILO profusion score. Occup Environ Med 53:808-812

Muir DC, Julian JA, Roos JO et al (1993) Classification of radiographs for pneumoconiosis: the Canadian Pneumoconiosis Reading Panel. Am J Ind Med 24:139-147

NIOSH (1999) Hazard evaluation and technical assistance report: a trial of additional composite standard radiographs for use with the ILO international classification of radiographs of pneumoconioses. National Institute for Occupational Safety and Health, Division of Respiratory Disease Studies, Morgantown, WV. US Department of Health and Human Services, Public Health Service, Centers for Disease Control and Prevention, National Institute for Occupational Safety and Health, NIOSH HETA Report No. 99-0340-2659, NTIS No. PB99-153-769. Available online at http://www.cdc.gov/niosh/hhe/reports/pdfs/1990-0340-2659.pdf

Oksa P, Klockars M, Karjalainen A et al (1998) Progression of asbestosis predicts lung cancer. Chest 113:1517-1521

Parker DL, Bender AP, Hankinson S et al (1989) Public health implications of the variability in the interpretation of 'B' readings for pleural changes. J Occup Med 31:775-780

Rockoff SD, Schwartz A (1988) Roentgenographic underestimation of early asbestosis by International Labor Organization classification. Analysis of data and probabilities. Chest 93:1088-1091

Schaefer CM, Greene R, Oliver LC et al (1990) Screening for asbestos-related pleural disease with digital storage phosphor radiography. Invest Radiol 25:645-650

Shipley RT (1992) The 1980 ILO classification of radiographs of pneumoconioses. Radiol Clin North Am 30:1135-1145

Suganuma N, Kusaka Y, Hosoda Y et al (2001) The Japanese classification of computed tomography for pneumoconioses with standard films: comparison with the ILO international classification of radiographs for pneumoconioses. J Occup Health 43:24-31

Vallyathan V, Brower PS, Green FH et al (1996) Radiographic and pathologic correlation of coal workers' pneumoconiosis. Am J Respir Crit Care Med 154:741-748

Wagner GR, Attfield MD, Kennedy RD et al (1992) The NIOSH B reader certification program. An update report. J Occup Med 34:879-884

Wagner GR, Attfield MD, Parker JE (1993) Chest radiography in dust-exposed miners: promise and problems, potential and imperfections. Occup Med 8:127-141

White NW, Davies A (2002) Chest radiography in the diagnosis of pneumoconiosis (letter). Int J Tuberc Lung Dis 6:273

White NW, Steen TW, Trapido AS et al (2001) Occupational lung diseases among former goldminers in two labour sending areas. S Afr Med J 91:599-604

3.3 Lung Function for Radiology

Sherwood Burge

CONTENTS

3.3.1 Introduction 101
3.3.2 Lung Volumes 101
3.3.3 Divisions of the Total Lung Capacity 102
3.3.4 Workers with Small Lungs 102
3.3.5 Measurement of the Transfer Factor (DLCO) and Transfer Coefficient (KCO) 103
3.3.6 Workers with Large Lungs 105
3.3.6.1 Measures of Forced Expiration and Inspiration 106
3.3.6.2 Asthma 109
3.3.7 Specific Bronchial Provocation Testing 112
3.3.7.1 What is Normal Lung Function? 112
3.3.7.2 Monitoring of Disease Progress 112
References 113

3.3.1 Introduction

This chapter will try and approach lung function as related to occupational disease from a radiological perspective. This puts some of the more complex tests before the simpler and more readily available ones to try and improve understanding. Many physiological texts are difficult to read for the non-specialist, because of the large range of symbols and abbreviations. I have tried to use as few as possible.

There are three main determinants of lung function: volume, time and pressure. Intrathoracic pressure measurement generally requires an oesophageal manometer, which is rarely used in routine testing. The rate of change of volume with time is flow. Volumes can be measured by integrating flow from a flow-measuring device, such as a pneumotachometer, or by measuring volumes directly with a spirometer (flow then being calculated as the rate of change of volume by time). Each method has its own problems, and they are not necessarily comparable.

S. Burge, MD
Department of Thoracic Medicine, Birmingham Heartlands Hospital, Bordesley Green East, Birmingham, B9 5SS, UK

3.3.2 Lung Volumes

The total lung capacity is the volume of air within the lungs at full inspiration. It is commonly estimated from the chest X-ray or computed tomography (CT) scan and can be formerly calculated radiographically, provided that care is taken to acquire the images truly at full inspiration (Clausen 1997). Taking a truly full inspiration is uncomfortable and takes longer than is often allowed in conventional radiological practice. It is also reduced in the supine position. Radiologically derived total lung capacity includes the air within the lungs, the intrapulmonary interstitial tissue and the intrapulmonary blood volume.

Lung function laboratories can measure total lung capacity by body plethysmography or inert gas dilution. The standard body plethysmograph is a sealed cabinet of constant volume. The subject sits inside, breathing through a mouthpiece that measures volume and pressure at the mouth. As the subject breathes in and out, the volume changes. As the cabinet is of fixed volume, the pressure of the air within the cabinet changes slightly. During the manoeuvre, a shutter obstructs the movement of air during an attempt at inspiration and expiration. The changes in pressure within the mouthpiece and the cabinet are measured; as the volume within the plethysmograph is constant, the volume of gas compressed within the subject can be calculated (by Boyles law, where pressure x volume is a constant). This method measures compressible gas volume. It would include air in non-communicating bullae, pneumothorax spaces, the oesophagus and some air within the stomach. It excludes the blood and interstitial volumes included radiographically. The measurement is accurate in those with low and normal lung volumes but can overestimate volume in those with significant airflow obstruction, as the mouth pressure measured may not be the same as the intra-alveolar pressure.

Gas dilution lung volumes are usually measured with helium. The subject is connected to a closed circuit system where the carbon dioxide is absorbed and oxygen replenished. Helium is normally neither secreted nor absorbed. The test continues until the expired helium concentration plateaus, as the inspired helium is diluted by the air within the lung at the time of connection. In normal subjects, this takes a few minutes, but in patients with significant emphysema, equilibrium may not be achieved for 10–20 min. Stopping before a steady state is reached is common in patients with severe emphysema. The Helium dilution lung volume measures air accessible to the mouth, excluding gas within the gastrointestinal tract, pneumothorax spaces or in non-communicating bullae, and, in a normal adult, is approximately 500 ml less than the volume measured by body plethysmography. The helium lung volume can also be measured with a single breath hold, where it is called the alveolar volume. This is a routine part of the gas-transfer measurement, where a 10-s breath hold is used. The lung volume accessible to helium in this time excludes poorly ventilated areas but is a measure of the volume of air that can be accessed by the subject during normal activities. The difference between the alveolar volume and the total lung capacity is a measure of trapped air, seen radiologically as the darker component of the mosaic pattern seen in patients with small airways disease.

3.3.3 Divisions of the Total Lung Capacity

After a full expiration, there is air left within the lungs; this is the residual volume and cannot be measured directly. It is calculated by measuring the total lung capacity and subtracting the vital capacity. The vital capacity (or forced vital capacity if the subject is asked to breathe out as hard and fast as possible) is measured directly by asking the subject to inhale until no more air can be inhaled and then breathe out until flow ceases.

The total lung capacity is reduced when the lungs are small, as in asbestosis, when the lungs are restricted by pleural effusion or thickening, or when the chest wall restricts lung expansion, as in obesity. It can also result from diaphragm palsy or compression by abdominal contents, such as in pregnancy or with ascites. The total lung capacity is increased when there is obstruction to airflow during exhalation, particularly in emphysema, where the obstruction is due to collapsing airways, and more severe asthma, where it is due to bronchial inflammation and narrowing.

3.3.4 Workers with Small Lungs

Figure 3.3.1 shows the total lung capacity, which is the sum of the vital capacity and the residual volume, expressed as a percentage of the expected normal value, for two workers with small lungs.

Worker 1 is an 82-year-old man who was a stoker in the engine room of an aircraft carrier between 1942 and 1947. He then became a school caretaker between 1947 and 1987, where he had to look after the boilers, which were initially coke fired and later converted to burn oil. He developed left-sided chest pain and breathlessness. Examination showed late inspiratory crackles at both bases and reduced movement and dull percussion on the left.

Worker 2 is a 55-year-old man who, for the past 11 years, serviced fork-lift trucks in a factory manufacturing car engines with incidental exposure to aerosols of metal-working fluid. He had been breathless for 6 months and lost 4 kg in weight but had improved considerably when off sick in the 3 months prior to being seen. Examination showed late inspiratory crackles at both lung bases.

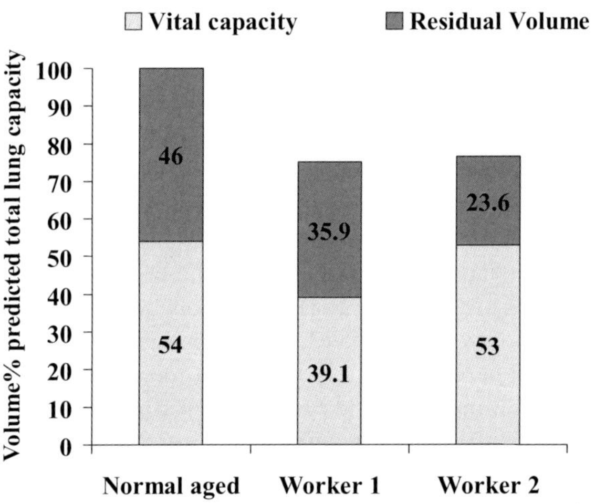

Fig. 3.3.1. Vital capacity and residual volume expressed as percentage of predicted total lung capacity. Worker 1 has a proportional reduction in vital capacity and residual volume. This could be due to external lung restriction or to intrinsic fibrotic lung disease. His alveolar volume (from a 10-s helium dilution breath hold) was 3.18 l, and his plethysmographic volume was 4.43 l, a 1.25 l difference (normal difference <500 ml). This would suggest some additional gas trapping. Worker 2 has a similarly reduced total lung capacity, but a greater proportion is due to a reduction in residual volume. His steady-state plethysmographic total lung capacity and alveolar volumes were 5.27 l and 5.46 l, respectively, compatible with small airways being less collapsible than normal

Finding the cause for a low total lung capacity is probably best done by reviewing the radiology, where it should be possible to differentiate between normal lungs whose volume is reduced externally and lungs with loss of volume usually caused by fibrosis or resection. In practice, it is often difficult to separate these from plain radiographs. To the physiologist, the separation is best made by measuring diffusing capacity (gas transfer).

3.3.5 Measurement of the Transfer Factor (DLCO) and Transfer Coefficient (KCO)

These tests measure the transfer of carbon monoxide (the CO in the abbreviations) from alveolar air to the pulmonary capillary. The afferent pulmonary capillary is assumed to have no carbon monoxide dissolved in the plasma, and the rate of transfer is assumed not to be rate limited by saturation of the plasma, as carbon monoxide is removed very rapidly and bound to haemoglobin. This means that the test can be carried out without measuring the carbon monoxide concentration in the pulmonary veins, something that would be required if the transfer of oxygen was being measured. The knowledge of the concentration of carbon monoxide in the alveolus is, however, necessary. Since any inhaled carbon monoxide will be diluted by the residual air in the lung at the start of inhalation, this dilution factor must also be measured. The standard test involves adding helium to the inspired air. The difference between the inspired and expired helium concentration can be used to calculate a dilution factor for the alveolar carbon monoxide concentration. It also measures the alveolar volume (the 10-s helium dilution lung volume mentioned above). The transfer factor (DLCO) is dependent on the alveolar volume, the capillary blood volume, a membrane factor, ventilation/perfusion matching and the haemoglobin concentration. The transfer coefficient (KCO) is the transfer factor (DLCO) divided by the alveolar volume. It, therefore, gives a value per unit of lung volume and is useful for differentiating between normal lungs whose volume is decreased by external factors and lungs that are, themselves, diseased. The main causes of a reduced transfer coefficient are lung fibrosis and emphysema (where the alveoli are destroyed). If the lungs are compressed externally, for instance by pleural disease or obesity, the transfer coefficient is often raised, as the same amount of blood has to pass through less lung volume, relatively increasing the pulmonary capillary volume.

The measurements for gas transfer for workers 1 and 2 are shown in Figure 3.3.2 and their radiology in Figure 3.3.3 and Figure 3.3.4.

Worker 1 has a low total lung capacity because of loss of volume of the left lung and left-sided pleural thickening and effusion (Fig. 3.3.3). His occupational history suggests significant asbestos exposure, starting in the navy 62 years prior to presentation and likely to have continued while caring for the boilers. Many boiler operators had their mess rooms in the boiler houses, as it was a warm place, and often had to clean up after pipe fitters and insulators had repaired pipe work insulated

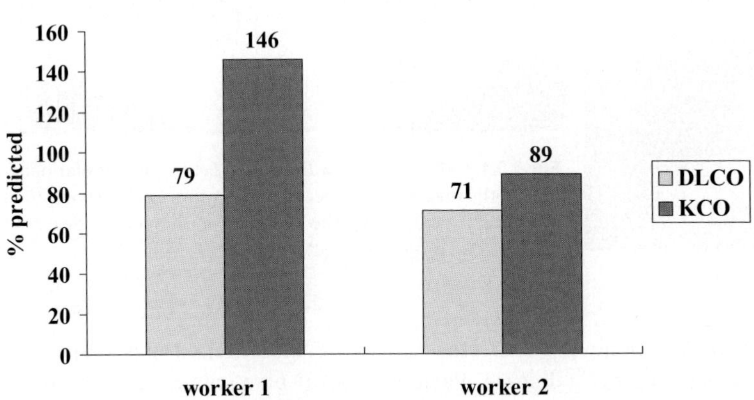

Fig. 3.3.2. Transfer factor (DLCO) and the transfer co-efficient (KCO, corrected for lung volume) for the workers in Fig. 3.3.1. Worker 1 has a reduced transfer factor (DLCO); when corrected for lung volume, the value is above predicted, suggesting that the available lung was not diseased. As the same cardiac output is going through less alveolar volume, the pulmonary capillary volume is high in relation to the alveolar volume, and the transfer co-efficient (KCO), therefore, increased over predicted values. The high transfer co-efficient makes it unlikely that there is any functionally important interstitial lung disease. Worker 2 has a low normal transfer coefficient (KCO), suggesting that the low lung volumes are likely to be due to the lungs themselves

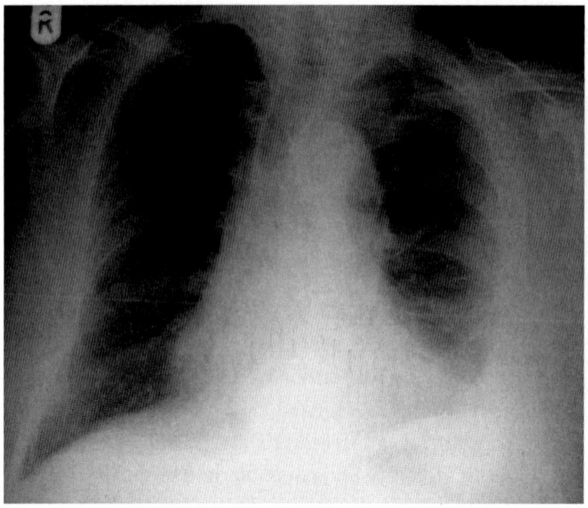
a

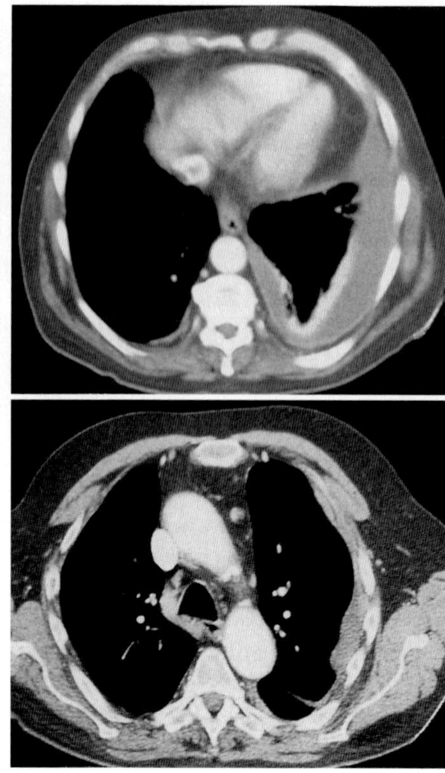
b

Fig. 3.3.3. a The chest X-ray of worker 1. There is a left-sided pleural effusion, loss of volume of the left lung and some cardiomegaly. The right lung appears normal in volume. **b** Two thin-section computed tomography images from worker 1. There is lower zone pleural thickening and effusion with parenchymal bands extending into the lung. The cut at the aortic arch shows that the pleural thickening does not involve the mediastinal pleura, a feature making mesothelioma less likely

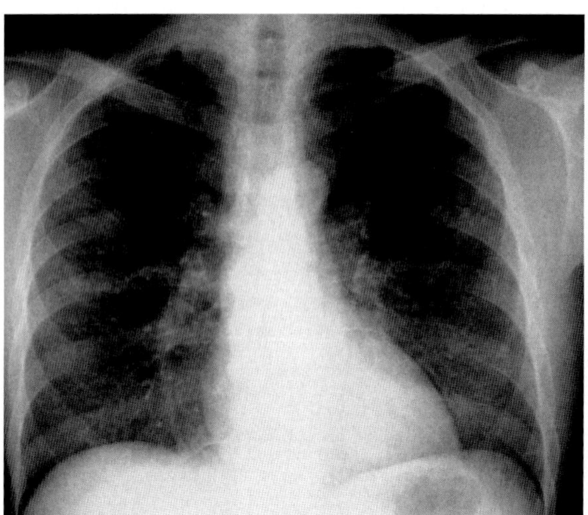
a

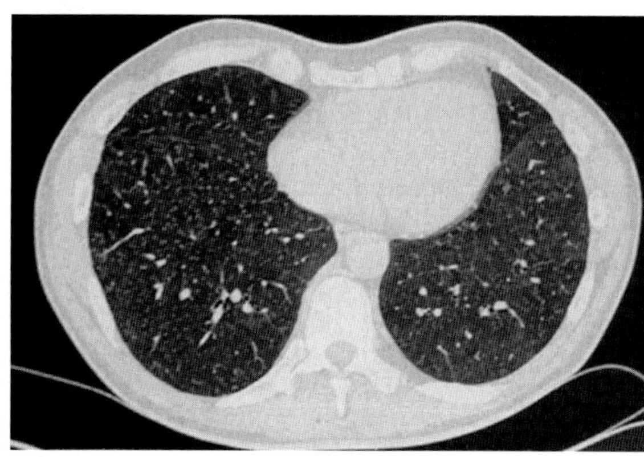
b

Fig. 3.3.4. a The chest X-ray in worker 2 showing nodular opacities in the middle and lower zones. **b** A thin-section computed tomography cut above the diaphragm showing widespread nodules and a mosaic effect

with asbestos lagging. Caring for school boilers alone (at least in the UK) has provided sufficient asbestos exposure for the development of asbestos-related pleural disease. Exposures at sea were often much higher, particularly during wartime, where many sailors lived on ships while they were being relagged, with considerable exposures in areas away from the lagging work, which would not have been sealed off.

Asbestos can cause four main types of pleural disease. Parietal pleural plaques produce the most recognisable radiological abnormality. They are not thought to cause impairment of lung function and are benign but are nearly always due to asbestos exposure. Visceral pleural thickening is commonly seen on CT scans when not obvious on plain chest X-rays. It stops the lung expanding on full inspiration and causes breathlessness, particularly on exertion, when the normal response is to increase tidal volume. The total lung capacity is usually reduced with a low transfer factor (DLCO) and a high transfer co-efficient (KCO), as in worker 1. Similar physiology is seen with a pleural mesothelioma or benign asbestos-related pleural effusion.

Asbestosis should be reserved for interstitial fibrosis due to asbestos exposure. It causes a loss of lung volume and a reduced transfer factor and transfer co-efficient. In its classical form, the spirometry is restrictive without airflow obstruction. In practice, nearly all have some airflow obstruction as well. This is most easily explained by smoking, as there is an association between smoking and working in very dusty occupations (the healthy worker and healthy smoker effects). However, only a minority of smokers develop airflow obstruction; an alternative explanation is that asbestos exposure is a cause of occupational chronic obstructive pulmonary disease (COPD) (Copes et al. 1985). Epidemiological studies have shown an interaction between smoking and working in dusty occupations on accelerated volume expired after 1 s (FEV_1) decline (and hence COPD), smokers showing a relatively larger effect than non-smokers.

The CT images confirm pleural thickening and effusion as the cause of the low total lung capacity. The sparing of the mediastinal pleura makes mesothelioma less likely, but it is often seen with secondary pleural malignancy. The parenchymal bands are not extensions of the pleura along the fissures (as seen in mesothelioma) and are a classical feature of benign asbestos-related visceral pleural thickening. This is thought to be preceded by pleural effusions in a number of instances. Thoracoscopic biopsies showed benign fibrous tissue, making benign asbestos-related pleural disease the most likely diagnosis. A benign biopsy does not, however, exclude mesothelioma, and careful follow-up is indicated.

Extrinsic allergic alveolitis (hypersensitivity pneumonitis in North America) and interstitial pulmonary fibrosis are the other main causes of small lungs with reduced gas transfer. Worker 2 had developed an allergic alveolitis from the aerosols from metalworking fluids. Many such workers also have some element of airflow obstruction, as pathologically the bronchioles are usually involved in the inflammatory response and are the probable cause of the mosaic pattern. The other main occupational causes of extrinsic allergic alveolitis would include: fungal antigens from mouldy grain and hay in farmers; mouldy wood in saw-mill workers and avian proteins in bird handlers. There are many other causes (Cormier et al. 2002). Exposure to hard metal dusts causes giant cell interstitial pneumonia, which has an acute and chronic fibrotic form, with similar physiology but distinct pathology. The cause is cobalt, which acts as a binder in the hard metal. The cobalt can dissolve in metalworking fluids when hard metal-tipped cutting tools are used, providing another possible source. Similar physiology is seen in patients with interstitial pulmonary fibrosis. These diseases are usually thought of as cryptogenic; however, there are occupational exposures associated with them, particularly in metal-working (including metal-working fluid exposure), farming and woodwork (Cormier et al. 2002). In some, the lung volumes are well preserved, and the main impairment is in gas transfer; in others, the disease is predominantly fibrotic with loss of lung volume. Physiological monitoring should include both measurements of gas transfer and spirometry.

3.3.6 Workers with Large Lungs

Figure 3.3.5 shows the total lung capacity, which is the sum of the vital capacity and the residual volume, expressed as a percentage of the expected normal value for two workers with large lungs.

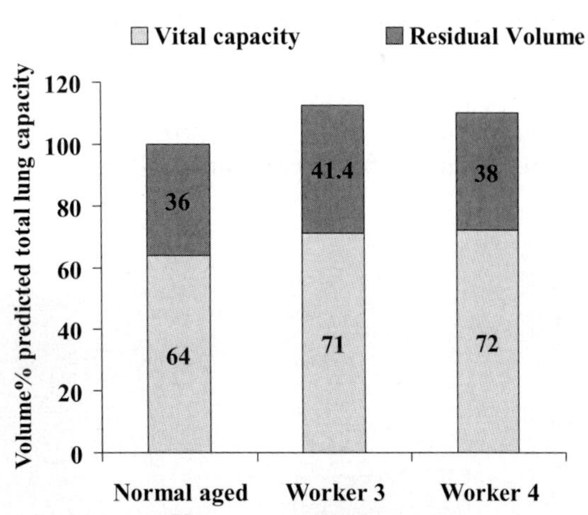

Fig. 3.3.5. Vital capacity and residual volume expressed as percentage of predicted total lung capacity. Worker 3 has a large residual volume and a preserved vital capacity, suggesting that any airflow collapse was insufficient to limit expiration. His alveolar volume (from a 10-s helium dilution breath hold) was 7.62 l and his plethysmographic volume 8.57 l, a 0.95-l difference showing some increased air-trapping. Worker 4 shows similar results with an alveolar volume (from a 10-s helium dilution breath hold) of 5.98 l and a plethysmographic volume 6.93 l, also a 0.95-l difference showing some increased air-trapping

Worker 3 is a 50-year-old male who spent 8 years heating iron and steel in a drop forge, then 3 years turning brass on a lathe with metal-working fluids before 7 years melting and casting an alloy of zinc and cadmium for use as sacrificial anodes for the feet of sea-based oil rigs. He then spent 16 years as a window fitter before having to give it up due to breathlessness at the age of 49 years. He was a lifelong non-smoker with a normal alpha-1 antitrypsin genotype. Examination showed scars from metal burns but no wheeze or crackles in the lungs.

Worker 4 is a 58-year-old male who had worked for 34 years digging and blasting tunnels, mostly for water and sewage, through many different strata, including sandstone, clay and granite, sometimes under pressure (caisson work), for which he had to have regular medicals. He was referred following an abnormal chest X-ray from one of these medicals. He was breathless on strenuous exertion and had a daily cough with clear sputum. He stopped smoking at the age of 43 years, variously recorded as 10–30 per day. Examination revealed vibration white finger and a cement burn on his forearm.

The measurements for gas transfer for workers 3 and 4 are shown in Figure 3.3.6 and their radiology is shown in Figure 3.3.7 and Figure 3.3.8.

3.3.6.1 Measures of Forced Expiration and Inspiration

The timed measurement of the volume of expired air after a full inspiration is the most reproducible lung-function measure, is widely available and is usually the most appropriate test for following the course of lung diseases. After a maximum inhalation, the subject blows out as hard and as fast as possible until flow ceases. The volume exhaled is the forced vital capacity (FVC). The test is more difficult to perform in patients with severe airflow obstruction, where the time taken to achieve no flow (the forced expiratory time) may fairly often exceed 20 s. The volume expired after specific time intervals gives a measure of airflow obstruction, the FEV_1 is the most commonly used. The ratio of FEV_1 to FVC forms the basis of separating obstructive (Fig. 3.3.9a) from restrictive (Fig. 3.3.9b) respiratory disease. Reductions of the forced vital capacity cannot be used alone to define restrictive lung diseases, as it goes down in obstructive disease as well but not as much as the FEV_1. In the presence of airflow obstruction, any additional restrictive disease should be defined from reductions in the total lung capacity (which is usually increased with airflow obstruction).

A reduced FEV_1/FVC ratio is the most common lung function abnormality. The usual causes are asthma, where the obstruction is due to inflammation and smooth muscle constriction in the large and small airways, to emphysema, where the problem is collapse of the airways that lack support in expiration, and obstructive bronchitis, where the main problem is small airway fibrosis and inflammation. COPD is an umbrella term to encompass emphysema and obstructive bronchitis, which usually coexist. Other less common causes include bronchiectasis, obstruction by extrinsic compression, tumour or foreign body. In clinical practice, the most difficult distinction is between asthma and COPD. By definition, asthma

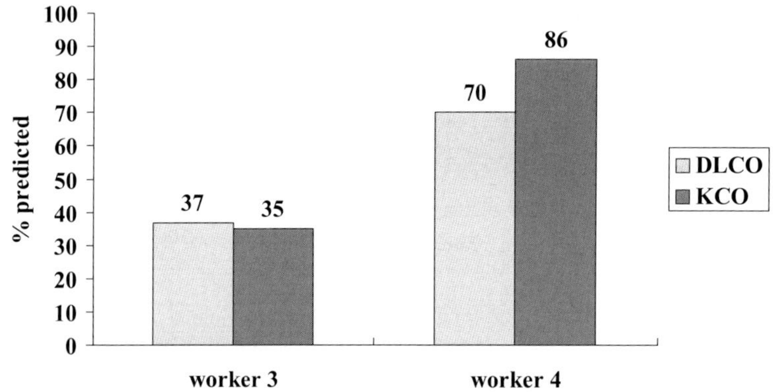

Fig. 3.3.6. Shows the transfer factor (DLCO) and the transfer co-efficient (KCO, corrected for lung volume) for the workers in Figure 3.3.5. Both have proportional reductions in transfer factor (DLCO) and coefficient (KCO). Worker 3 has severely reduced values. Provided that a very low haemoglobin has been excluded as a cause, measurements this low with large lungs is nearly always due to emphysema. The values for worker 4 are at the lower limit of normality and can be seen in more severe asthma, as well as chronic obstructive pulmonary disease with a more obstructive bronchiolitis element. Bronchiectasis and Langerhans cell granulomatosis would be other possibilities

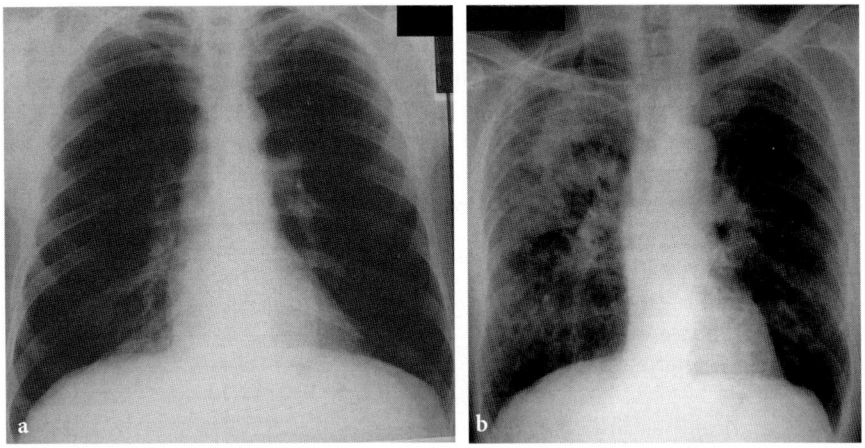

Fig. 3.3.7a,b. Chest X-ray of worker 3 (a) and 4 (b). Worker 3 has large lungs, somewhat enlarged pulmonary ateries and loss of peripheral vascular shadows. Worker 4 has large conglomerate lesions in the right upper and mid zones, with some bacjground nodulation best seen in the left lower zones. The lungs are over expanded.

a 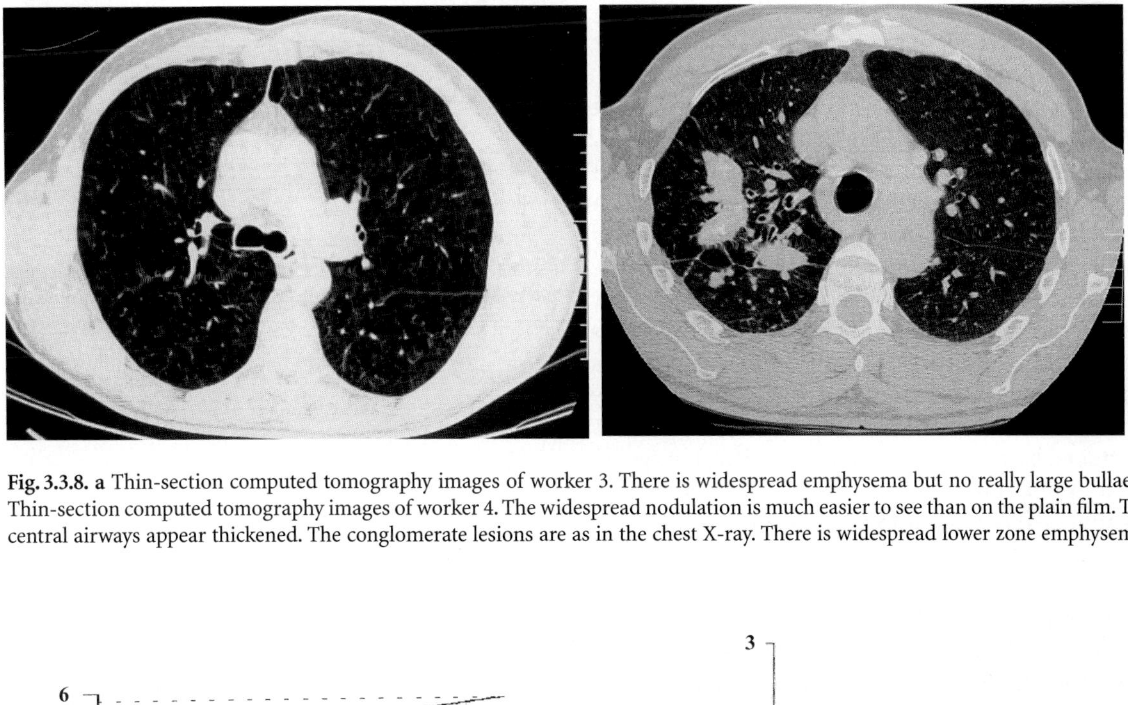 b

Fig. 3.3.8. a Thin-section computed tomography images of worker 3. There is widespread emphysema but no really large bullae. b Thin-section computed tomography images of worker 4. The widespread nodulation is much easier to see than on the plain film. The central airways appear thickened. The conglomerate lesions are as in the chest X-ray. There is widespread lower zone emphysema

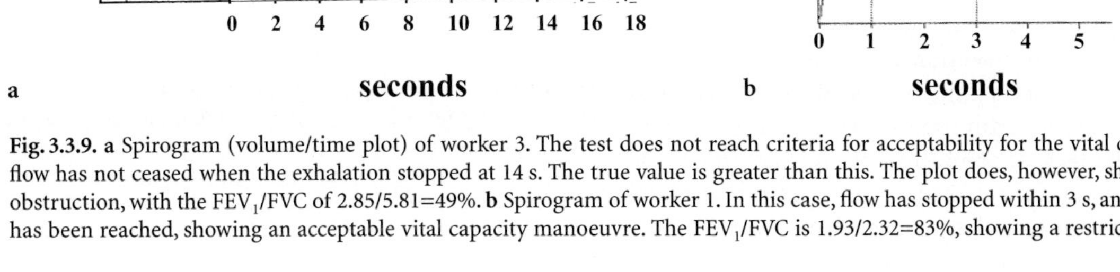

Fig. 3.3.9. a Spirogram (volume/time plot) of worker 3. The test does not reach criteria for acceptability for the vital capacity, as flow has not ceased when the exhalation stopped at 14 s. The true value is greater than this. The plot does, however, show airflow obstruction, with the FEV_1/FVC of 2.85/5.81=49%. b Spirogram of worker 1. In this case, flow has stopped within 3 s, and a plateau has been reached, showing an acceptable vital capacity manoeuvre. The FEV_1/FVC is 1.93/2.32=83%, showing a restrictive defect

is a reversible disease and COPD irreversible; tests of bronchodilator response, however, show a large overlap between the two conditions. Bad asthma can be temporarily irreversible (common in acute severe asthma), and responses up to 410 ml may be seen in patients with classical COPD (Calverley et al. 2003). Plotting flow against expired volume can often help distinguish the pressure-dependent airway collapse of emphysema from the airway inflammation of asthma and obstructive bronchitis. In addition, making measurements during forced inhalation shows no flow limitation in emphysema but a continuing limitation in both asthma and obstructive bronchitis.

The flow/volume loop plots exhalation (positive flow) upwards on the y-axis and inspiratory flow (negative flow) downwards. Volume is on the x-axis in liters (there is no time component in this plot, so the FEV_1 cannot be read from it). The time component is much faster at the beginning of exhalation, the peak usually being reached in less than 0.04 s. The maximum flow on a forced manoeuvre is the peak expiratory flow. Flow volume loops usually record flow in liters per second as here, whereas peak flow meters record in liters per minute. A normal expiratory limb has a near linear rise to peak expiratory flow and then a nearly straight line until vital capacity is reached. A reduction of flow below a straight line usually implies small airways obstruction. The normal inspiratory limb encloses about the same area on the plot as the expiratory limb but is semicircular. The inspiratory limb is flattened by reduced-compliance (stiffer) lungs, as seen in pulmonary fibrosis, by diaphragm muscle weakness and upper airways obstruction.

The two loops in Figure 3.3.10 both show some sagging of the expiratory limb implying small airways obstruction. The upper loop shows a large inspiratory limb, showing that the airflow obstruction is not due to fibrosed or inflamed small airways but due to pressure-dependent collapse. The negative intrathoracic pressure on inspiration reverses the obstruction. The lower trace shows some reduction of flow on inspiration, in keeping with reduced lung or chest wall compliance.

Worker 3 has large lungs, airflow obstruction, which reverses on inspiration, and a very low gas transfer. These are the features of emphysema, confirmed by thin-section CT. Emphysema due to occupational causes is not well established, the most specific cause is cadmium exposure (Davison et al. 1988). The lack of smoking, the normal alpha-one antitrypsin and the cadmium fume exposure make cadmium the most likely cause of his disease. In my experience, cadmium-induced emphysema is often centriacinar. This results in less disruption of alveolar attachments and, hence, less pressure-dependent airways collapse than panacinar emphysema. A flow–volume loop of a patient with panacinar emphysema showing more classical pressure-dependent airways collapse is shown in Figure 3.3.11.

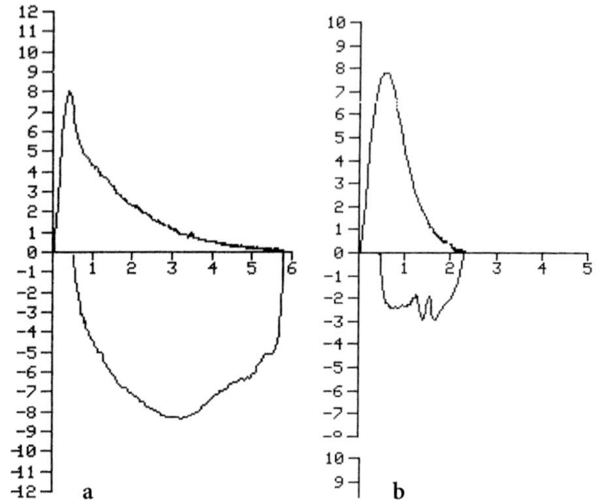

Fig. 3.3.10a,b The flow volume loops from worker 3 (**a**) and worker 1 (**b**) from the same manoeuvre as the volume/time plots in Figure 3.3.7

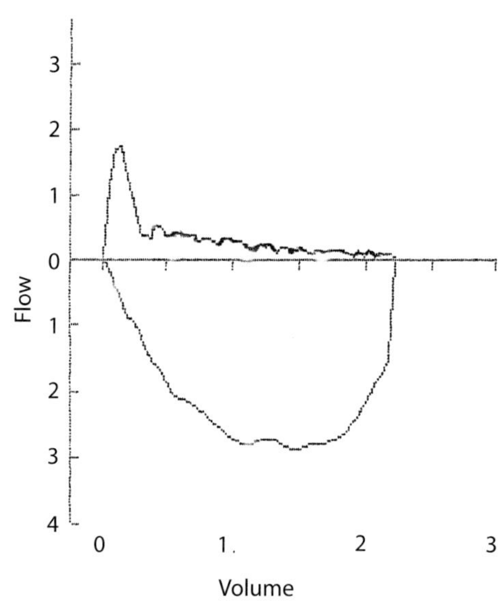

Fig. 3.3.11. Pressure-dependent airways collapse in a patient with smoking-related emphysema. The flow cuts off abruptly after peak flow. The volume contained in the expiratory limb is far less than during inspiration, where the negative intrathoracic pressure keeps the airways open. (Flow in liters/second, expiration upwards, inspiration downwards, volume in liters)

Worker 4 had obstructive spirometry with an FEV_1/FVC ratio of 2.83/4.66=61% (predicted 3.17/3.98=77%). The chest X-ray shows preservation of lung volumes despite nodular and conglomerate lesions classical of silica or coal pneumoconiosis. Tunnelling through silicious rocks is one of the commoner causes of silicosis, others being pottery work, quarry work, mining of metals in silicious rocks (particularly gold and tin), stone masonry and slate work. Silicosis and coal miners pneumoconiosis are often classified as restrictive lung diseases, and it is said that there is no physiological impairment without progressive massive fibrosis. Clinically, they present with a disease resembling COPD with large lungs and airflow obstruction, as shown by the physiology, and the airflow obstruction is not related to the presence or absence of radiologically visible nodules.

Early studies showed that lung function in miners with uncomplicated pneumoconiosis was similar to miners without pneumoconiosis (IRWIG and ROCKS 1978). This was interpreted as implying that silica or coal exposure had no effect on lung function in the absence of progressive massive fibrosis. Community studies have often identified increased risks in workers exposed to silica (foundry, quarry, tunnelling, stonemasons, etc.) (XU et al. 1992; HEEDERIK et al. 1989; HUMERFELT et al. 1993; KRZYZANOWSKI et al. 1986). Silica is one of the few exposures where there are good longitudinal workplace studies, mainly from the South African gold mines. A reasonable number of air measurements have been made, from which cumulative personal exposures can be estimated. These studies confirm the lack of effect of radiological uncomplicated pneumoconiosis (categories 1–3) on lung function but show that increasing silica exposure is associated with reducing levels of FEV_1 and FVC; i.e. the effect on lung function is acting independently of the effect of the nodular shadows on the chest X-ray. Similar effects occur with coal dust exposure.

South African gold miners are exposed to mine dust with 30% free silica. Studies have shown reductions in FEV_1 in workers with and without silicosis, with the major effects seen in smokers. After controlling for radiological silicosis, the excess annual loss of FEV_1 attributed to mining in Black African miners was 8 ml; that due to smoking 20 cigarettes a day was 6.9 ml/year (COWIE and MABENA 1991; HNIZDO 1992). The relationship between death from COPD, silica exposure and smoking has suggested that the effect of silica is predominantly in smokers, with 5% of the increased mortality due to dust alone, 34% due to smoking and 59% due to the interaction of smoking and dust (HNIZDO 1990). Similar to smoking, exposure in early adult life appeared to have more effect than later exposure. Attributing COPD to silica or coal exposure in an individual is difficult, as the epidemiology shows that smokers are at the most risk of silica or coal exposure, smokers obviously having an increased risk due to smoking alone.

For the same levels of exposure, coal has much less effect than silica. There is little evidence that coal dust per se is particularly toxic; its adverse effects are likely to be due to the dust burden retained in the lungs. The evidence favours an additive effect with smoking on FEV_1 decline. It is often argued that the average loss of FEV_1 is small in relation to that likely to cause significant disability. It depends on whether all of the exposed population decline at a rate close to the mean or whether there is wide variation, as in the effect of cigarette smoking. The evidence is tending to favour a large clinically significant effect in a few individuals. This has been calculated on the basis of 35 years exposure to the mean level of exposure per 1000 workers. For coal miners, a lifetime exposure of 122.5 gh/m^3 would result in 80 of 1000 having a 20% loss attributed to dust and 12 of 1000 a 35% loss. The comparable attributable risk for smokers is 66 of 1000 and 23 of 1000 respectively. The highest group cumulative dust exposure for the South African gold miners was only 21.3 gh/m^3, a tenth of the highest exposure group of British coal miners. Despite this, the attributable risk for an FEV_1 <80% was 4.9 for silica exposed gold miners versus 1.5 for coal miners (OXMAN et al. 1993).

There is some evidence that coal-dust exposure causes centrilobular emphysema, based on post-mortem lung sections, there being a relationship between emphysema score and lung-dust burden (COCKCROFT et al. 1982). The relationship is easier to demonstrate when dust-related fibrosis is present (RUCKLEY et al. 1984). The relationship between emphysema score and lung-dust burden is stronger in non-smokers than smokers (LEIGH et al. 1994).

3.3.6.2 Asthma

Asthma is the other common cause of airflow obstruction. Occupational asthma is separated from other causes of asthma by the periodicity of airflow obstruction in relation to occupational exposure. A worker with occupational asthma not only reacts to the occupational agents but to all the other non-specific provokers of non-occupational asthma. The main non-specific provokers are cold (or sometimes hot) air, fog, exercise, vehicle exhaust fumes, tobacco smoke, perfumes, menstruation and particularly upper respiratory infections. In addition, asthmatics have an increased diurnal variation in airway calibre, with the nadir around waking and the peak 4–12 h later. This means that for the average day-shift worker who wakes shortly before starting work, the spontaneous variation results in improving lung function over the working shift. Conversely, for an afternoon shift worker who sleeps shortly after the end of the shift, the spontaneous variation is for increasing airflow obstruction over the shift. In addition, the reactions to work exposure may occur within the first hour of exposure, or may be delayed for several hours. Many are at their worst in the evening and night after work rather than at work. Asking a worker for rest day improvement is, therefore, a more sensitive screening question than asking for work-shift deterioration. In addition, many with more severe occupational asthma get progressively worse with each day's exposure and may take several days to recover when away from exposure. The best method for the initial validation of occupational asthma is with 2-hourly measurements of peak expiratory flow over 3–4 weeks at work (Burge et al. 1999). Periods of recording should be selected where the worker is having periods at and away from work; consecutive periods of a least three workdays improve sensitivity. Treatment should be kept constant during the record, as the aim is to record the effects of exposure rather than monitor asthma control (the other principal use of serial peak expiratory flow records). Analysis of the records can be subjective but is improved by plotting the daily maximum, mean and minimum reading, with "days" starting with the first reading at work and continuing to the last reading before work on the next day. Records analysed with the Oasys plotter achieve a sensitivity of 70% and a specificity of 94% when compared with specific bronchial provocation testing (Burge et al. 1999).

Worker 5 is a lady who has worked as a radiographic assistant for the past 5 years. Her job is to assist patients in and out of X-ray and magnetic resonance imaging (MRI) suites and to help with dressing and undressing. She also has to clean the film processors weekly, add chemicals as necessary and clear film jams when they occur. She developed a sore throat, hoarse voice, rhinitis, cough, sputum, wheeze and chest tightness 3 years after starting this work. She started waking breathless during the night. She had several periods off work when she improved but deteriorated again within a few days of returning to work. She improved on days away from work and also noticed that she was better when working in a private hospital MRI suite without film processors on Saturdays, when she was not required in her regular job. She was also worse in hot environments, which was a problem in her regular job after installation of a second MRI machine, with room temperatures sometimes over 30°C. She was also worse in cold environments, in fog, with respiratory infections and some perfumes. She did not notice problems when wearing latex gloves and did not assist with invasive procedures. When seen on a day away from work, she had completely normal lung function (>100% predicted, with no response to bronchodilator). She kept a record of 2-hourly peak expiratory flow for 4 weeks (Fig. 3.3.12).

Fig. 3.3.12. a A peak flow plot of the radiographic assistant showing occupation asthma. She has kept approximately 2-hourly measurements for 4 weeks. The *top panel* shows daily diurnal variation as a percentage of the whole record mean. The *middle panel* shows the computer-generated score for each work-rest-work complex and rest-work-rest complex at the top. Below this are three lines; the uppermost is the best peak flow of the day, the middle bar is the mean and the lower line the minimum value. Days at work have a hatched background, days away from work a clear background. The *lower panel* shows the day and date, the number of readings taken each day, the hours worked and a comments line. On Saturdays, she works in a different hospital MRI department without radiographic films. The peak flow falls during the work week and is better on days away from work. She is also better in the second hospital MRI suite. Oasys gives scores from 1 (no evidence of occupational asthma) to 4 (definite occupational asthma) for each complex and gives an overall weighted score. The whole record score is 2.45, a score over 2.5 has a specificity of 94% and a sensitivity of 70% for occupational asthma. When the record is re-scored excluding the days in the second hospital, the score rises to 3.5. She kept a further record after redeployment shown in (**b**). **b** Second Oasys peak flow plot of worker 5 after redeployment as a lifting and handling trainer. The mean peak flow has increased, the diurnal variation reduced and the work effect gone showing successful relocation. She had specific bronchial provocation testing to X-ray film developer and fixer, as well as cleaning agents. None were convincingly positive. Despite this, the diagnosis of occupational asthma is secure and the place where it occurred identified

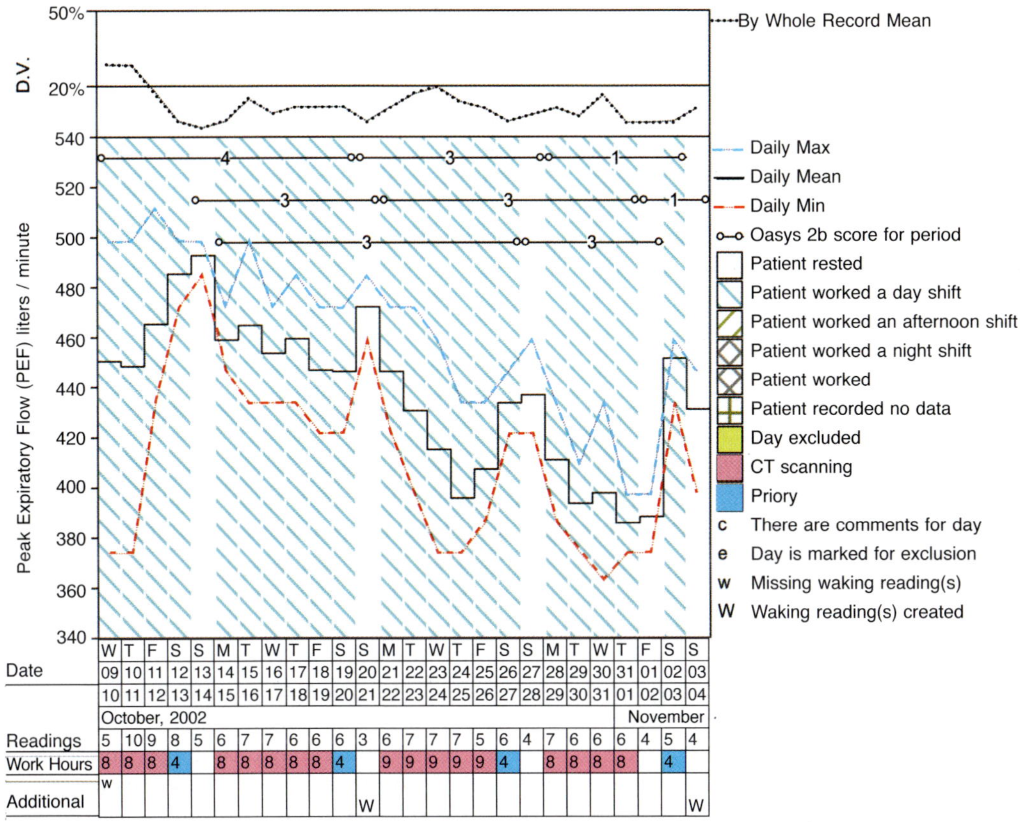
By Whole Record Mean
D.V.
50%
20%
Peak Expiratory Flow (PEF) liters / minute
Daily Max
Daily Mean
Daily Min
Oasys 2b score for period
Patient rested
Patient worked a day shift
Patient worked an afternoon shift
Patient worked a night shift
Patient worked
Patient recorded no data
Day excluded
CT scanning
Priory
c There are comments for day
e Day is marked for exclusion
w Missing waking reading(s)
W Waking reading(s) created
Date
October, 2002
November
Readings
Work Hours
Additional

a

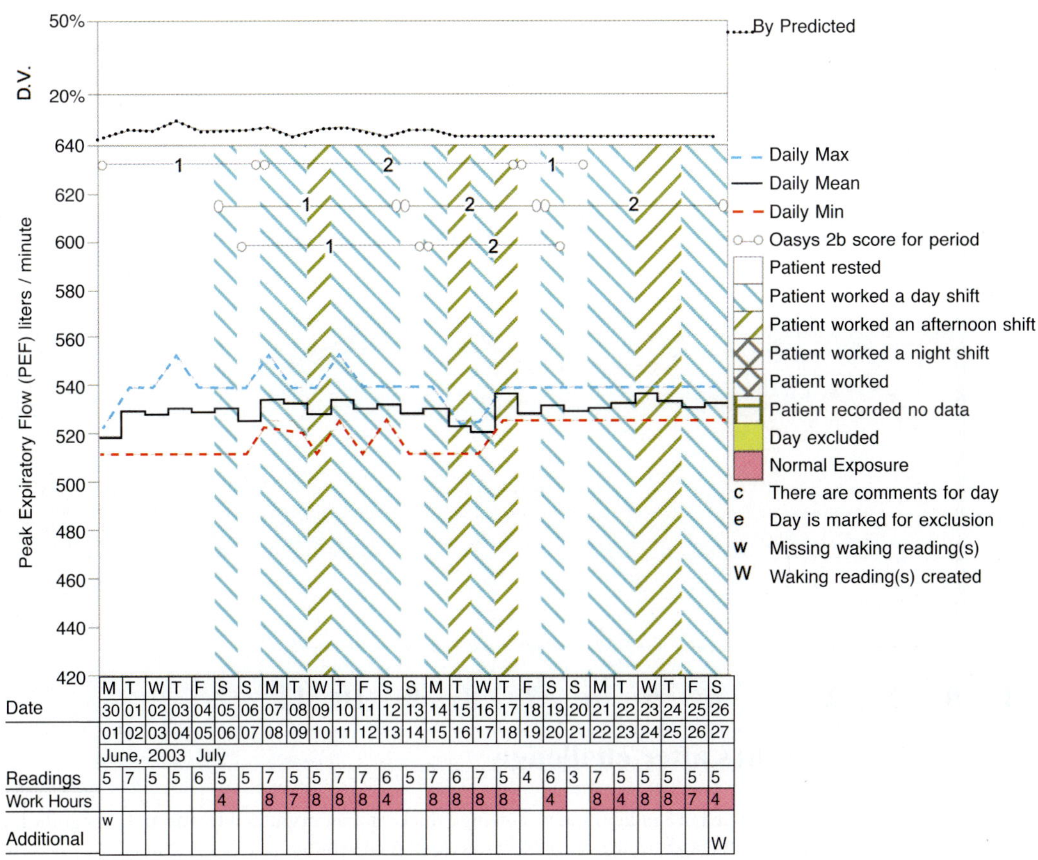
By Predicted
D.V.
50%
20%
Peak Expiratory Flow (PEF) liters / minute
Daily Max
Daily Mean
Daily Min
Oasys 2b score for period
Patient rested
Patient worked a day shift
Patient worked an afternoon shift
Patient worked a night shift
Patient worked
Patient recorded no data
Day excluded
Normal Exposure
c There are comments for day
e Day is marked for exclusion
w Missing waking reading(s)
W Waking reading(s) created
Date
June, 2003 July
Readings
Work Hours
Additional

b

3.3.7 Specific Bronchial Provocation Testing

The gold standard test for occupational asthma is the specific bronchial provocation test. These are time consuming and best done as hospital inpatients, where confounding factors can be better controlled. Reactions may be immediate or delayed for several hours. Control exposures on separate days are needed to make sure that any increase in airflow obstruction is due to the agent tested that day, rather than to a carryover from previous exposures or treatment withdrawal. An example of a radiographer is shown in Figure 3.3.13. Her role included adding chemicals to the daylight processors and work in a theatre darkroom, where peak flow records showed most problems. The challenge tests show a dual immediate and late reaction to glutaraldehyde with no reaction to similar concentrations of formaldehyde, making glutaraldehyde the most likely cause of her asthma. The role of glutaraldehyde in darkroom asthma has been debated (Ide 1993; Gannon et al. 1995), and most developers no longer contain glutaraldehyde. Sterilising agents, including glutaraldehyde, are often present in X-ray departments outside X-ray chemistry, for instance, for endoscope sterilisation. Operating theatres are a common source of sterilising agents, and it is at least possible that her sensitisation resulted from exposure there. She was relocated to areas without wet processing with success.

3.3.7.1 What is Normal Lung Function?

The large differences between measures of lung function in healthy individuals has hampered their general use. Lung volumes are related to height, age, sex and race.

Lungs grow from birth and continue growing after maximum height is achieved to a maximum at the age of about 25 years in a healthy non-smoker. There is then a plateau, followed by a decline from at least the age of 35 years, perhaps accelerating in old age. Women have smaller lungs than men of the same height. Predicted values related to standing height also differ by race, Black African races being about 15% less than Caucasian Europeans, Oriental races being intermediate. Normal values have been constructed from pooled results using different populations of normal people, using differing measurement devices but rarely including a full range of ages. All are approximations to the true predicted value for an individual, and the confidence intervals are wide, particularly for measurements of flow at low lung volumes. In Europe, the summary equations developed by the European Community for

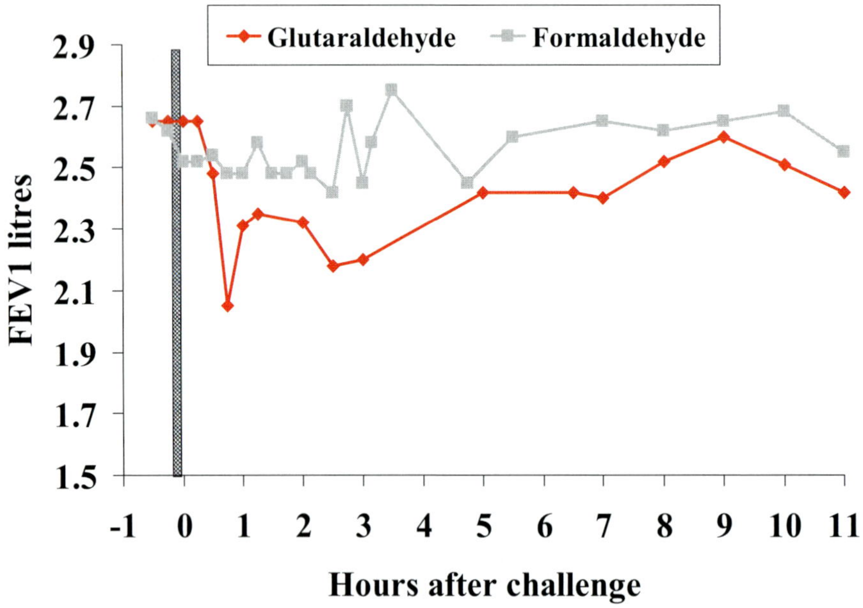

Fig. 3.3.13. Specific bronchial provocation testing in a radiographer showing a dual reaction to glutaraldehyde and no significant reaction to formaldehyde, confirming glutaraldehyde as the cause of her occupational asthma

Coal and Steel are generally used (Quanjer et al. 1993).

3.3.7.2 Monitoring of Disease Progress

Thus far, the examples of lung function have been used to aid diagnosis. A more important use is to follow the progress of disease, where the values that are "normal" for a particular worker can be established and changes monitored (Fig. 3.3.14). FEV_1 is the most appropriate measure for most airway diseases, the FVC and transfer factor (DLCO) for interstitial disease. Transfer factor is important where emphysema is predominantly centriacinar, when pressure-dependent airway collapse and airflow obstruction may be trivial.

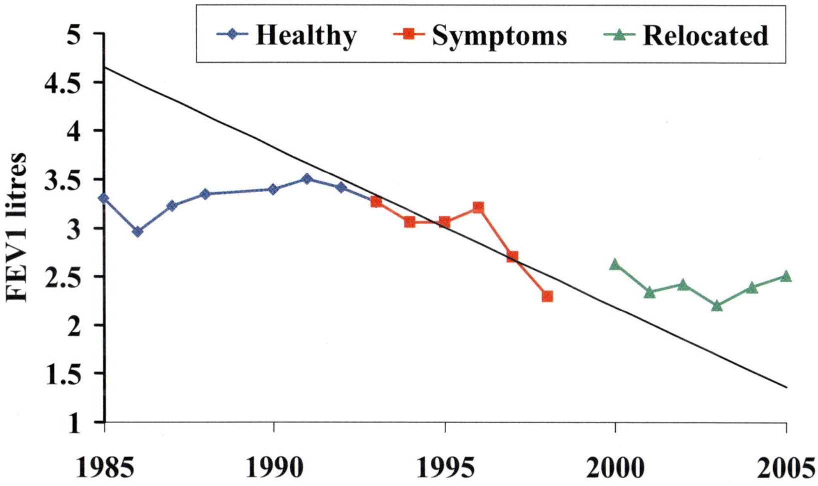

Fig. 3.3.14 The annual measurement of FEV_1 in a worker who sprayed vitamins onto cereals from 1981. He developed symptoms of occupational asthma in 1993 and was relocated completely away from exposure in 1998. During the symptomatic period with some thiamine exposure, his FEV_1 declined about 200 ml/year (normal 30 ml/year). Removal from exposure resulted in a modest improvement, with subsequent normalisation of FEV_1 decline (the black line is a best fit regression line through the measurements made while exposed with symptomatic occupational asthma)

References

Burge PS, Pantin CFA, Newton DT, Gannon PFG, Bright P, Belcher J, McCoach J, Baldwin DR, Burge CBSG (1999) Development of an expert system for the interpretation of serial peak expiratory flow measurements in the diagnosis of occupational asthma. Occup Environ Med 5:758-764

Calverley PMA, Burge PS, Spencer S, Anderson JA, Jones PW, on behalf of the Isolde study group (2003) Bronchodilator reversibility testing in chronic obstructive pulmonary disease. Thorax 58:659-664

Clausen J (1997) Measurement of absolute lung volumes by imaging techniques. Eur Respir J 10:2427-2431

Cockcroft A, Seal RM, Wagner JC, Lyons JP, Ryder R, Andersson N (1982) Post-mortem study of emphysema in coal workers and non-coal workers. Lancet 2:600-603

Copes R, Thomas D, Becklake MR (1985) Temporal patterns of exposure and non-malignant pulmonary abnormality in Quebec Chrysotile workers. Arch Environ Health 40:80-87

Cormier Y, Hendrick DJ, Burge PS, Beckett WS, Churg A (eds) (2002) Occupational disorders of the lung. Saunders, London, pp 229-239 (Hypersensitivity pneumonitis, vol 14)

Cowie RL, Mabena SK (1991) Silicosis, chronic airflow limitation, and chronic bronchitis in South African gold miners. Am Rev Respir Dis 143:80-84

Davison AG, Fayers PM, Newman Taylor AJ, Venables KM, Darbyshire J, Pickering CAC, Chettle DR, Franklin D, Guthrie CJ, Scott MC et al (1988) Cadmium fume inhalation and emphysema. Lancet 1:663-667

Gannon PFG, Bright P, Campbell M, O'Hickey SP, Burge PS (1995) Occupational asthma due to glutaraldehyde and formaldehyde in endoscopy and X-ray departments. Thorax 50:156-159

Heederik D, Pouwels H, Kromhout H, Kromhout D (1989) Chronic non-specific lung disease and occupational exposures estimated by means of a job exposure matrix: the Zutphen Study. Int J Epidemiol 18:382-389

Hnizdo E (1990) Combined effect of silica dust and tobacco smoking on mortality from chronic obstructive lung disease in gold miners. Br J Ind Med 47:656-664

Hnizdo E (1992) Loss of lung function associated with exposure to silica dust and with smoking and its relation to disability and mortality in South African gold miners. Br J Ind Med 49:472-479

Humerfelt S, Gulsvik A, Skjaerven R, Nilssen S, Kvale G, Sulheim O, Ramm E, Eilertsen E, Humerfelt SB (1993) Decline in FEV1 and airflow limitation related to occupational exposures in men in an urban community. Eur Respir J 6:1095-1103

Ide CW (1993) Developments in the darkroom: a cross-sectional study of sickness absence, work-related symptoms and environmental monitoring of darkroom technicians in a hospital in Glasgow. Occup Med 43:27-31

Irwig LM, Rocks P (1978) Lung function and respiratory symptoms in silicotic and nonsilicotic gold miners. Am Rev Respir Dis 117:429-435

Krzyzanowski M, Jedrychowski W, Wysocki M (1986) Factors associated with the change in ventilatory function and the development of chronic obstructive pulmonary disease in a 13-year follow-up of the Cracow Study. Risk of chronic obstructive pulmonary disease. Am Rev Respir Dis 134:1011-1019

Leigh J, Driscoll TR, Cole BD, Beck RW, Hull BP, Yang J (1994) Quantitative relation between emphysema and lung mineral content in coal workers. Occup Environ Med 51:400-407

Oxman AD, Muir DC, Shannon HS, Stock SR, Hnizdo E, Lange HJ (1993) Occupational dust exposure and chronic obstructive pulmonary disease. A systematic overview of the evidence. Am Rev Respir Dis 148:38-48

Quanjer PH, Tammeling GJ, Cotes JE, Pedersen OF, Peslin R, Yernault JC (1993) Lung volumes and forced ventilatory flows. Report Working Party Standardization of Lung Function Tests, European Community for Steel and Coal. Official Statement of the European Respiratory Society. Eur Respir J [Suppl] 16:5-40

Ruckley VA, Fernie JM, Chapman JS, Collings P, Davis JM, Douglas AN, Lamb D, Seaton A (1984) Comparison of radiographic appearances with associated pathology and lung dust content in a group of coalworkers. Br J Ind Med 41:459-467

Xu X, Christiani DC, Dockery DW, Wang L (1992) Exposure-response relationships between occupational exposures and chronic respiratory illness: a community-based study. Am Rev Respir Dis 146:413-418

3.4 Mineralogical Analysis of Lung Samples

Pascal Dumortier

CONTENTS

3.4.1 Introduction 115
3.4.2 Properties and Fate of Inhaled Particles 115
3.4.3 Role and Usefulness of Mineralogical Analysis of Lung Samples 117
3.4.4 Technical Aspects 118
3.4.4.1 Sampling 118
3.4.4.2 Sample Preparation 120
3.4.4.3 Analytical Techniques 120
3.4.5 Limitations of Mineralogical Analysis 124
3.4.6 Interpretation of Results 126
3.4.7 Conclusions 127
References 127

3.4.1 Introduction

The difficulties and uncertainties associated with the assessment of occupational or environmental dust exposures from occupational histories, job exposure matrixes or calculations from specific exposure databases have led clinicians, pathologists and epidemiologists to investigate the capacities associated with the mineralogical analysis of lung samples.

A number of specialised sampling and analytical techniques relying on instruments and methods commonly used in the determination of minerals have been developed to obtain relevant data about the concentrations and properties of particles retained in the lungs. Microscopic techniques are preferred, as the objects to be examined are generally in the micron or sub-micron size range. The first reports about the presence of inhaled mineral particles in histological sections of lung tissue date from the beginning of the 20th century (Marchand 1906; Watkins-Pitchford and Moir 1916; Cooke 1929; Gloyne 1929). Over time, analytical techniques became more and more accurate. Particularly, the usefulness of electron microscopy to characterise inhaled asbestos fibers was soon understood since a first publication about the subject (Kühn 1941) appeared approximately 10 years after the development of this instrument (Knoll and Ruska 1932). The most important progresses took place in the beginning of the 1970s, with the development of energy-dispersive X-ray spectrometers, which, when fitted on an electron microscope, allow the determination of the chemical composition of particles with diameters below 0.1 µm within seconds.

Meanwhile, less invasive sampling methods than open lung biopsies were introduced, such as bronchoalveolar lavage, transbronchial or thoracoscopic biopsies, facilitating the exploration of occupational and environmental lung diseases caused by mineral particles or fibers.

After considerations about the health-related properties of inhaled particles and their fate in the lung, this chapter will examine the role and usefulness of mineralogical analysis studies, the sampling and analytical techniques, the methodological limitations and the interpretation of the results.

3.4.2 Properties and Fate of Inhaled Particles

While breathing, airborne particles from occupational or environmental sources are continuously inhaled. To initiate pulmonary lesions, particles must be deposited and, to some extent, retained in the respiratory tract. According to deposition studies and modelling, particles with an aerodynamic diameter below 10 µm can reach the alveolar region of the lung. The deposited fraction varies as a function of diameter and typically ranges from approximately 10% to 60% for 0.1-µm and 5-µm particles, respectively (Parkes 1994). Modifications of breathing parameters (e.g. mouth versus nose breathing, respiratory rate at rest or during effort) influence

P. Dumortier, PhD
Chest Department – Laboratory of Mineralogy, Hôpital Erasme, Route de Lennik, 808, 1070 Brussels, Belgium

the deposited fraction and the location where the particles settle in the respiratory tract (Martonen and Katz 1993). For mineral fibers, the main determinant of penetration in the airways is the fiber diameter, regardless of its length. Asbestos or other mineral fibers with the same density are considered to be respirable for humans when they have physical diameters less than 3–3.5 µm (Timbrell 1965; NRCC 1982).

Once particles or fibers are deposited in the lungs, interaction may occur with alveolar fluids and cells. Kinetic studies show that inhaled dust phagocytosis by alveolar macrophages is a rapid phenomenon, occurring within hours or days after deposition. Differences in phagocytosis rate, however, occur according to the toxic properties of the particles (Le Bouffant et al. 1979; Brody et al. 1981). Lung clearance mechanisms will act to eliminate deposited particles by means of the mucociliary escalator or transport through lymphatics and storage in lymph nodes. Clearance rates may be affected by cigarette smoking, drugs and environmental pollutants (Lippmann et al. 1980). The inhibitory effects of cigarette smoking on pulmonary clearance mechanisms (McFadden et al. 1986) and its enhancement of asbestos penetration of respiratory epithelium (Churg et al. 1990a) have been proposed to explain why smoking appears to facilitate the development of lung fibrosis (asbestosis) (Tron et al. 1987). In cases of severe dust exposure, particle overload of the lung defence mechanisms results in an impairment of the alveolar macrophage-mediated lung clearance (Oberdorster 1995). Depending on their chemical composition, particles may also be completely or partially dissolved (e.g. sulphates, nitrates, cobalt) (Brain et al. 1994; Lison et al. 1994) or some man-made vitreous fibers (Hesterberg et al. 1998). Particles and fibers can also be transported from the deposition zones (respiratory bronchioles, alveoli) to the parietal pleura (Sebastien et al. 1980; Dodson et al. 1990; Boutin et al. 1996) and other extra-pulmonary target organs (Dodson et al. 2000). The mechanisms and pathways of the pleural dissemination of fibers and particles are still a matter of research (Mitchev et al. 2002). Finally, the fraction of the inhaled particles that is not translocated and cleared remains trapped for very long time in the alveolar macrophages or in the interstitial lung tissue, which acts as a sequestration compartment.

Lung or pleural lesions may result from numerous types of inorganic particles, including asbestos, erionite and refractory ceramic fibers, non-fibrous silicates (crystalline silica, talc mica, kaolinite, feldspar, montmorillonite), a variety of metals (iron, barium, tin, antimony, silver), rare earths (cerium, lanthanum), cobalt and hard metals (beryllium, aluminium, Cr-Co-Mo dental alloys) and silicon carbide (Parkes 1994).

Development, progression and severity of these lung and pleural diseases may vary widely according to particle-burden-related parameters. Shape and dimensions, which condition penetration and deposition, are important determinants of particle toxicity. Non-fibrous counterparts of asbestos minerals do not share the same toxic activity (Janssen et al. 1994). Short fibers are also less potent than long ones (Davis et al. 1986; Brown et al. 1990). Experimental studies by intrapleural and intraperitoneal instillation have demonstrated that the most carcinogenic fibers for the mesothelium are the longest and thinnest ones (lengths over 5–8 µm and diameters less than 0.25 µm) (Pott 1980; Stanton et al. 1981). Fiber size relevant for the induction of lung cancer may even be longer than for mesothelioma (Lippmann 1994).

Particle physicochemical structure and surface properties have also an influence on particle toxicity. The toxicity of particles of similar chemical composition may be affected by their crystalline structure. In this respect, quartz and cristobalite (two varieties of crystalline silica) are more fibrogenic than amorphous silica (Anonymous 1997). The production of oxygen radicals at the surface of particles could be an important step in fibrogenesis and carcinogenesis (Pezerat et al. 1989). Freshly ground quartz appears to be more active than aged quartz (Fubini et al. 2001). For asbestos fibers, the surface-oxidising properties depend largely on the nature of the fibers (Pezerat et al. 1989).

Biopersistence is another factor conditioning the health effects of inhaled particles. Particles resistant to the pulmonary clearance mechanisms, and which are not subject to physical breakdown or chemical dissolution are more likely to exert their bioactive effects and are thus potentially more fibrogenic and carcinogenic (Bignon et al. 1994). Studies involving measurements of asbestos fibers in lung tissue or bronchoalveolar lavage fluid from humans or experimental animals have demonstrated that the long-term retention is far greater for amphibole asbestos than for chrysotile (McDonald et al. 1989; Sebastien 1991). Epidemiological data consistently indicate that the incidence of malignant mesothelioma and excess of lung cancer are much higher in the cohorts exposed to amphiboles or mixtures (amphiboles/chrysotile) than to chrysotile alone

(McDonald and McDonald 1991; Hodgson and Darnton 2000).

The dose of particles or fibers retained in the lungs after deposition and clearance is a primary determinant of disease induction. Asbestosis or silicosis (lung fibrosis) are usually associated with high concentrations of asbestos fibers or silica particles in lung tissue resulting from heavy and/or prolonged exposures (Churg 1998b; Gibbs and Wagner 1998). Other diseases such as mesothelioma can be associated with short or low-dose exposures, as well as with low concentrations of fibers in lung tissue (Wagner et al. 1988; Roggli et al. 1992), despite the fact that a dose relationship has been demonstrated (Becklake and Case 1994).

Other factors suspected to play a role in lung and pleural disease development include individual factors (SV40, genetic, immunological) (Powers and Carbone 2002; Pfau et al. 2005) and exposure type (continuous versus intermittent, peaks of exposures) (Becklake 1991).

3.4.3 Role and Usefulness of Mineralogical Analysis of Lung Samples

The purpose of the mineralogical analysis of lung samples (lung tissue, bronchoalveolar lavage fluid, sputum) is to evaluate the particle burden retained in the lungs at the time of sampling. The measured particle levels integrate both phenomena of particle deposition and clearance.

The largest and most systematic body of data accumulated with mineralogical analysis deals with the presence of asbestos fibers and asbestos bodies (AB). Data about the non-fibrous particle burdens in the lungs is comparatively scarce and often concern case reports or small cohorts exposed to silica, various silicates or metallic compounds. Consequently, many considerations about theoretical and practical aspects of mineralogical analysis are derived from asbestos-related studies (Sébastien 1982; Roggli et al. 1992; Gibbs and Pooley 1996; Churg and Green 1998; De Vuyst et al. 1998; Pairon and Dumortier 1999).

Mineralogical analysis can be performed for individual cases or for groups of subjects, and results are useful for pathologists (Abraham et al. 1991; Dodson et al. 1991; Roggli et al. 1992; Gibbs and Pooley 1996; Dodson et al. 1997; Churg and Green 1998), clinicians (chest physicians) (De Vuyst et al. 1986a; De Vuyst et al. 1986b; De Vuyst et al. 1987a; De Vuyst et al. 1987b; De Vuyst et al. 1987c; Schwartz et al. 1991), epidemiologists (McDonald et al. 1989; McDonald et al. 1997; McDonald et al. 2001), compensation boards (Thimpont and De Vuyst 1998) and occupational health physicians (Paris et al. 2002) and are possibly produced in court trials (Motley and Patrick 1992).

Individual case studies mostly concern the assessment or clarification of exposures and the confirmation of the aetiological relationship between a specific mineral and a disease.

When compared with the collective or indirect character of airborne dust measurements or of occupational inquiry, mineralogical analysis provides an individual estimate of past exposure. It allows disclosing exposures not identified in occupational interview or after investigation of workplace conditions by occupational hygiene engineers. In a number of instances, exposure data are missing, not reliable, difficult to interpret quantitatively or not easily accessible as a consequence of the closure of a factory or workshop. The possible bias resulting from over- or under-scoring of exposure intensity when self estimated by patients is obviated. Indirect, occult and forgotten exposures can be highlighted.

Mineralogical analysis is particularly useful in assessing cases with short or remote exposures, since substantial amounts of fibers can be retrieved in lung tissue or bronchoalveolar lavage fluid (BALF) up to 50 years after short but intense exposures (De Vuyst et al. 1997; Wright et al. 2002).

According to local geology, non-industrially used tremolite-actinolite asbestos fibers are naturally present in the soils and eventually used for domestic applications in some areas of the world. Migrants originating from these countries may undergo further exposure to industrial asbestos in the host country. In this context, clarification of the fiber type(s) involved using electron microscopy analysis is helpful to asses the contribution of environmental/domestic and occupational exposures (Dumortier et al. 2001c).

Mineralogical analysis is also a useful adjunct to orient diagnosis in establishing the aetiology of a disease by confirming or excluding the presence and amount of a specific element or particle in lungs (Churg and Green 1998). In clinical practice, this may influence the treatment or result in a procedure of withdrawal from the risk. Typical examples are the differential diagnosis between idiopathic pulmonary fibrosis and asbestosis or between sarcoidosis and metal-induced granulomatosis (De Vuyst et al. 1987c; McDonald et al. 1997; Churg and Green 1998).

Mineralogical analysis may also be used to assess the contribution of asbestos to lung cancer development. The question whether a relevant asbestos exposure or asbestosis is responsible for asbestos-associated lung cancer remains open. Nevertheless, a series of exposure criteria were proposed for attribution of lung cancer cases to asbestos in the absence of asbestosis (Anonymous 1997). They correspond to exposures assumed to be associated with a doubling of the risk of developing lung cancer. In this context, association of lung cancer with asbestos exposure is plausible if lung burdens are over 5000 asbestos bodies, 5 million fibers (all sizes) or 2 million fibers longer than 5 microns per gram dry lung tissue, or more than 5 asbestos bodies per millilitre BALF.

In addition to individual cases, lung retention may be studied in cohorts of subjects for research purposes. Typical applications include comparison of retention among groups of subjects with different kinds of exposures (Gibbs et al. 1990; McDonald et al. 1997; Dumortier et al. 1998), clarification of exposure in terms of fiber or particle type and intensity (Jones et al. 1980; Wagner et al. 1986; Dumortier et al. 1998), clarification of usage of different materials at a facility (Jones et al. 1980), assessment of biopersistence (Pairon et al. 1994a; Churg and DePaoli 1988; Dumortier et al. 2001a), identification or confirmation of possible risks resulting from exposure to new materials (Dumortier et al. 2001a), correlation of burden and physical dimensions with severity of disease (Churg and Wiggs 1989; Churg et al. 1990b; Churg et al. 1989), clarification of fiber types causing disease (McDonald et al. 2001), validation of occupational hygiene assessment methods such as job-exposure matrix (Fischer et al. 2002) and identification of people with high exposures and, consequently, at highest risk of developing disease if a surveillance strategy is foreseen (Paris et al. 2002).

3.4.4 Technical Aspects

Technical aspects of fiber analysis were extensively reviewed by a workgroup of the European Respiratory Society and may be extended to mineralogical analysis of non-fibrous particles (De Vuyst et al. 1998). Relevant data are sought about the mineral(s) present (identification), their amount(s) (quantification), their size, composition and crystalline structure (characterisation) and about their association with lesions (importance as aetiological agent).

There are a number of methods described in the literature to perform mineralogical analysis on lung samples. They range from the basic examination of histological sections using light microscopy to very sophisticated electron microscopic analysis of individual particles isolated from the biological matrix.

3.4.4.1 Sampling

Sampling is a first critical step in particle or fiber analysis. The kind of sample available will determine the preparation and analytical methods. For an accurate quantification, the sample must be as representative as possible of the whole lung. If the question only concerns the types of fiber or particle present, small or unusual samples may be used.

Lung tissue analysis is considered as the "gold standard" for mineralogical analysis (De Vuyst et al. 1998). Fibers and particles are not uniformly distributed in the lung. There are marked variations from site to site. The largest distances over which such variations occur are not well defined. Fiber content of adjacent pieces of peripheral lung may differ in by a factor of 5–10 (Churg and Wood 1983; Morgan and Holmes 1983; Morgan and Holmes 1984). This effect appears to get worse as the pieces get smaller. The accumulation of non-fibrous carbonaceous and mineral dust in the lungs is significantly affected by the lung anatomy. In the large airways, particle deposits concentrate at the carinas (Churg and Brauer 2000). Respiratory bronchioles also accumulate particularly high particle loads, with the greatest retention in centres of lung acini (Pinkerton et al. 2000). Accordingly, small thoracoscopic samples and transbronchial biopsies are not reliable for quantification. The "ideal" lung tissue sample consists of a pool of three pieces of non-tumoral lung tissue having at least a volume of 1–2 cm^3, respectively, from the apex of the upper lobe and the apex and base of the lower lobe (Gibbs and Pooley 1996; De Vuyst et al. 1998). They must include subpleural tissue. The absence of tumoral tissue or pleural thickening must be controlled histologically on adjacent blocks. This procedure limits the variability of the results obtained when repeated analyses are performed in individual cases (Gibbs and Pooley 1996). Isolated samples obtained from lobectomy or from video-assisted thoracoscopy and paraffin blocks (see limitations) are "acceptable" if they represent a sufficient volume of lung tissue (GIBBS and POOLEY 1996; CHURG and GREEN 1998; DE VUYST et al. 1998). In addition to necropsy cases, invasive procedures to collect large specimens of lung tissue should only be considered when resection or thoracoscopic examination is justified for diagnostic or therapeutic reasons.

Other tissues should not be accepted for quantification. Samples with pleural thickening, pleural plaque and tumour tissue contain few particles and will result in false-negative counts. The particle content of lymph nodes may be influenced by their anatomical location. The parietal pleura is a very heterogeneous phase. Anatomical structures resorbing pleural fluid from the pleural space may trap and concentrate particles and fibers in localised areas called "black spots" because of their pigmentation (BOUTIN et al. 1996; MITCHEV et al. 2002). All these samples are "not suitable" for routine purposes, but may be used for research purposes, e.g. when studying the migration of fibers in the human body.

Due to the restrictions associated with lung tissue sampling, techniques to analyse the particle burden of BALF and sputum samples were developed by different teams (BIGNON et al. 1973; DE VUYST et al. 1982; SÉBASTIEN 1982; JOHNSON et al. 1986; DE VUYST et al. 1987b; DUMORTIER et al. 1989; DUMORTIER et al. 1990; DODSON et al. 1991; SCHWARTZ et al. 1991; MCDONALD et al. 1992; TUOMI et al. 1992; SCANSETTI et al. 1993; TESCHLER et al. 1993; VILKMAN et al. 1993; KARJALAINEN et al. 1994a; PAIRON et al. 1994a; PAIRON et al. 1994b; ROGGLI et al. 1994; FALCHI et al. 1996a; FALCHI et al. 1996b; TESCHLER et al. 1996; SULOTTO et al. 1997; DUMORTIER et al. 1998; FIREMAN et al. 1999; SARTORELLI et al. 2001; PARIS et al. 2002).

Bronchoalveolar lavage allows recovery of cells, biological fluids, mineral particles and infectious organisms present in the peripheral airways (WALLAERT et al. 1992). BALF is sampled through the broncho-fibroscope during the course of an endoscopic examination under local anaesthesia. This examination is simple, moderately invasive and without danger if contra-indications are respected and can eventually be repeated to follow the evolution of a disease (WALLAERT et al. 1992; REYNOLDS 2000). The area explored by BALF represents approximately 2.75% of the total lung volume (DAVIS et al. 1982). Comparatively, the fragments used for mineralogical analysis of lung parenchyma usually have a volume of 0.5–2 cm^3. This corresponds to less than 0.05% of the total lung volume (SEBASTIEN et al. 1988). The amounts of particles and fibers recovered using BAL are sufficient to carry out electron microscopy examinations (JOHNSON et al. 1986; GELLERT et al. 1986; DUMORTIER et al. 1989; DUMORTIER et al. 1990; GRIFFITH et al. 1993a; TESCHLER et al. 1993; PAIRON et al. 1994; ROGGLI et al. 1994; TESCHLER et al. 1994; FALCHI et al. 1996a; DUMORTIER et al. 1998; DUMORTIER et al. 2001a; DUMORTIER et al. 2001b; SARTORELLI et al. 2001). A non-trivial exposure to biopersistent particles can still be detected using BALF mineralogical analysis after several decades. Theoretically, particle clearance from the bronchial compartment and the alveoli tends to reduce the concentrations of particles used as markers of exposure. However, the long-term incidence of this phenomenon on concentrations measured in BALF must not be exaggerated. Indeed, its influence on the non-fibrous particle concentrations in BALF of subjects who ceased exposure for more than 1 year appears to be minimal (PAIRON et al. 1994b). However, there is no significant difference in the concentrations of asbestos bodies and tremolite fibers in BALF between Turks having emigrated from outside areas with environmental/domestic exposures since approximately 20 years prior to the sampling and those still exposed at the time of sampling (DUMORTIER et al. 2001c). Moreover, the good correlation between asbestos bodies counting on repeated BAL samples (DE VUYST et al. 1987b; SCHWARTZ et al. 1991) and the concordance of the results obtained on the successive fractions of a BAL (SÉBASTIEN 1982) indicate that the BAL procedure does not significantly affect the stock of asbestos bodies in the sampled area (SEBASTIEN et al. 1988). Several specific limitations must be taken into account when using BALF samples to analyse the inhaled particle load retained in the lungs. First, BAL only explores airway spaces and does not provide access to the particles retained in the lung interstitium. Second, there is no specific marker allowing estimation of the efficiency of the lavage procedure. In particular, there is currently no way to measure the level of dilution of the recovered elements (cells, secretions or particles) in the recovered fluid (WARD et al. 1997; HASLAM and BAUGHMAN 1999; REYNOLDS 2000). Third, the recovery of instilled fluid may be poor in patients presenting with severe chronic obstructive pulmonary disease, a tumour compressing the underlying lung tissue or in patients having a poor compliance to the endoscopic examination (DE VUYST et al. 1987b).

Sputum collection is a simple, costless and non-invasive method compared with lung tissue and BAL sampling. It was demonstrated that sputum analysis for asbestos bodies is an insensitive method for assessing the lung asbestos burden, much less sensitive than BALF analysis (Teschler et al. 1996). A sputum sample negative for AB does not exclude the possibility of a high lung burden. Nonetheless, AB in sputum is a highly specific marker for past asbestos exposure usually associated with significant fiber burden in the lungs. There is a high variation of the results obtained on sequential sputum samples, and the best performance is obtained by analysing a pool of daily samples collected on at least three different days (Teschler et al. 1996; Paris et al. 2002) or by analysing induced sputum samples (Fireman et al. 1999). Mineralogical analysis of sputum samples must be combined with a cytological examination to confirm the pulmonary origin of the sample by the demonstration of macrophages (Teschler et al. 1996; Fireman et al. 1999; Paris et al. 2002). The non-invasive nature of sputum collection may be interesting in occupational medicine to detect individuals with significant lung retention in a population (Sebastien et al. 1984; McDonald et al. 1992; Paris et al. 2002).

3.4.4.2 Sample Preparation

Mineralogical analysis can be performed in situ on routine histological sections prepared for light or scanning electron microscopy (Funahashi et al. 1984; Abraham et al. 1991) and on ultra-thin sections prepared for transmission electron microscopy (De Vuyst et al. 1987c). The main advantage is to preserve the geographical correlation between particles and surrounding tissue, cells or lesions. In situ analysis has, however, several disadvantages. It is inappropriate to quantify the lung dust burden, since the particles are heterogeneously distributed in the lungs, and the particle burden associated with a specific lesion is not representative the whole lung burden. The presence of tissue also tends to mask particles. In addition, particles or fibers may be cut or broken during the preparation of the sections, thus preventing accurate sizing. Finally, concerning transmission electron microscopy examinations, ultra-thin sections are approximately 100 nm in thickness and less than 1 mm wide. The very small volume of tissue examined may contain very few particles, while the lung burden can be very large. Moreover, the use of Os, U and Pb salts for fixation and contrast enhancement of sections may generate spurious signal interfering with the chemical analysis of the particles of interest.

Destruction of the biological material by *digesting* or *ashing* the sample allows one to isolate the particles or fibers and to concentrate them on membrane filters suitable for examination using light or electron microscopy. The pore size of the filters must be small enough to retain the particles of interest. Digestion by potassium hydroxide, sodium hypochlorite or formamide or low temperature ashing are most commonly used (De Vuyst et al. 1998). Concentrations are calculated knowing the number of particles of interest on a known surface of the filter, the total surface of the filter and the amount of lung tissue or BALF processed. The ability to process large quantities of biological material obviates the inconvenience resulting from the heterogeneous distribution of particles in the lung and allows the production of a mean estimate of the whole lung burden. Digestion or ashing preparations should be as conservative as possible for particle or fiber concentrations, chemistry or size distributions to provide the most accurate information on the sample content. Drying the tissue before low-temperature ashing and the uncontrolled use of ultrasonication to disperse the residue may break fibers and aggregates, resulting in higher counts and smaller sizes (De Vuyst et al. 1998). Particles or fibers may be lost during repeated centrifugation (Johnson et al. 1984). Ashing can introduce pronounced physical or structural alteration of the dusts (Gibbs and Pooley 1996) and destroys carbonaceous compounds that may be relevant, such as coal or soot particles. For lung tissue analysis, many laboratories express results as number of particles or fibers per gram dry lung tissue. The dry to wet weight ratio varies from 5% to 20% and should be measured for each sample. The use of a mean conversion factor of ten for the wet/dry ratio should be avoided (De Vuyst et al. 1998).

3.4.4.3 Analytical Techniques

Basic analytical techniques such as light microscopy examination of histological slides (Fig. 3.4.1a,b) are easily accessible, quick, inexpensive and provide a very rough estimate of the particulate burden, which may be sufficient for the pathological or clinical work-up of a case. More specialised particle-by-particle determination using analytical electron microscopy (Fig. 3.4.1c) can provide extremely precise quantitative data about particle concentrations, types and sizes. As a general rule, these procedures can only be performed routinely in a small number of dedicated laboratories and are expensive and time consuming.

a b c

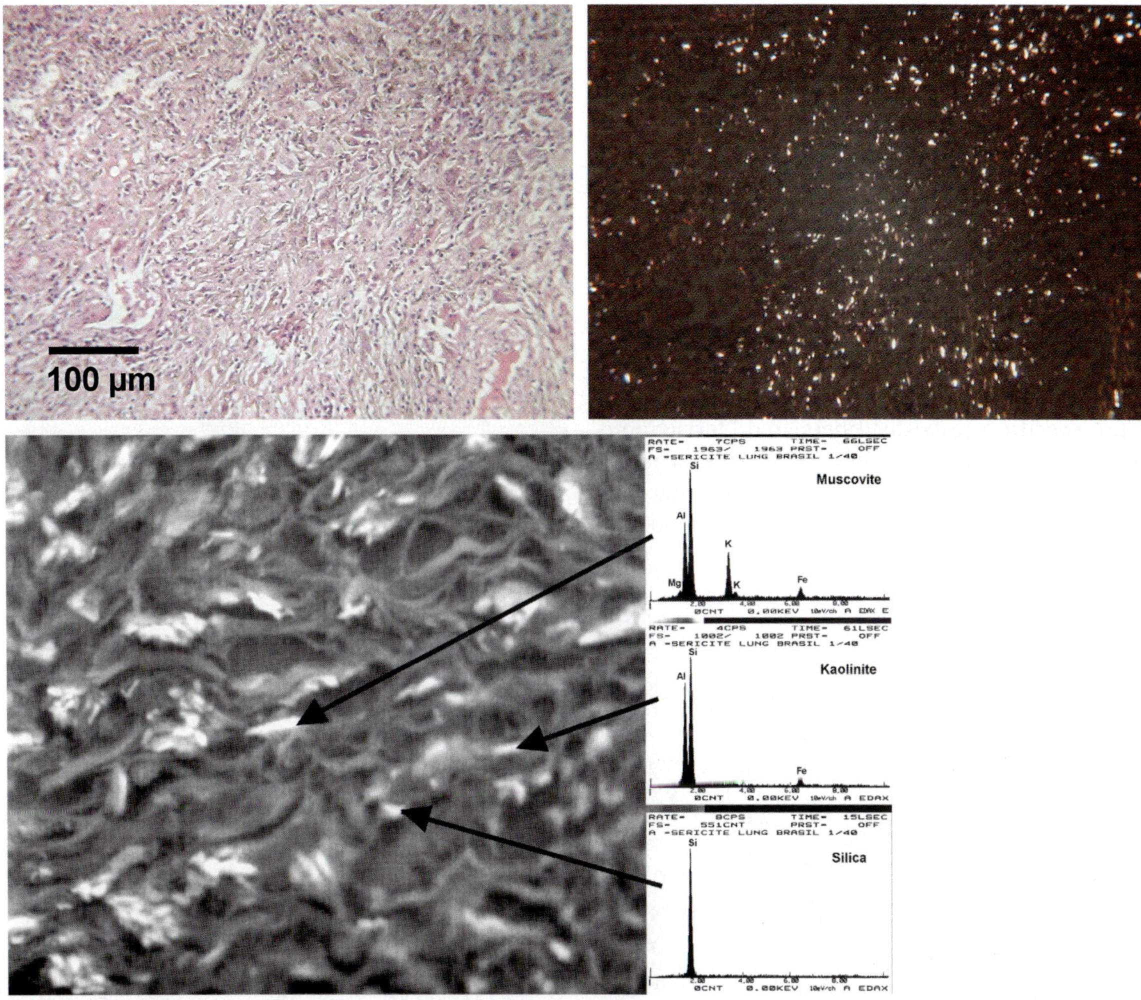

Fig. 3.4.1a–c. Histological section of lung tissue from a case with "sericite pneumoconiosis" (ALGRANTI et al. 2005) in natural (**a**) and polarised light microscopy (**b**). In situ particle analysis on corresponding section examined in back-scattered electrons mode using scanning electron microscopy (**c**). Chemical analysis of the particles by energy-dispersive X-ray spectrometry reveals the presence of silica, muscovite and kaolinite

Although suffering from a number of inherent limitations, *light microscopy* is a useful method for a first-line identification and quantification of the particulate burden in lungs and can be used routinely to examine large numbers of samples. Optical properties of the particles, including colour (Fig. 3.4.2), transparency, refractive index, birefringence and pleochroism, are helpful to roughly resolve the particle types. However, birefringence is difficult to assess for small particles or thin fibers, especially if they polarise weakly, as do silica or asbestos fibers. Morphology may eventually give an indication about their mode of formation. In this regard, a spherical shape is usually typical of a high temperature processes of formation, as in the case of flyash (GOLDEN et al. 1982) or welding fumes (Fig. 3.4.3).

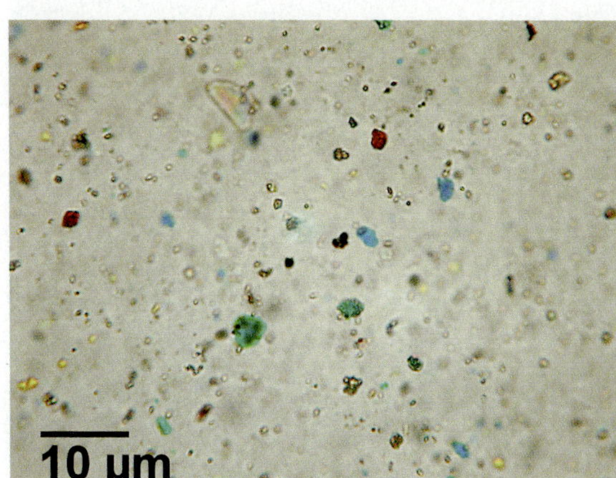

Fig. 3.4.2. Pigments in the bronchoalveolar lavage fluid of a paint maker

Resolution of light microscopy is limited to approximately 0.2 μm. Consequently, it can only detect large particles or fibers and asbestos bodies. The use of phase contrast (Fig. 3.4.4) enhances the capacity to visualise thin transparent fibers, which would otherwise be difficult or impossible to detect. It is recommended for asbestos fibers and bodies counting. AB (Fig. 3.4.5) are asbestos fibers too long to be completely phagocytised by macrophages, which become coated with an iron-rich protein layer deposited at the cell-fiber interface. AB mostly form on fibers longer than 10 μm (Churg and Warnock 1981; Morgan and Holmes 1985). This reaction is not specific to asbestos fibers, and "ferruginous bodies" may occur on a wide variety of materials, including sheet silicates (Fig. 3.4.6), diatomaceous earth, coal particles (Fig. 3.4.7), metal compounds

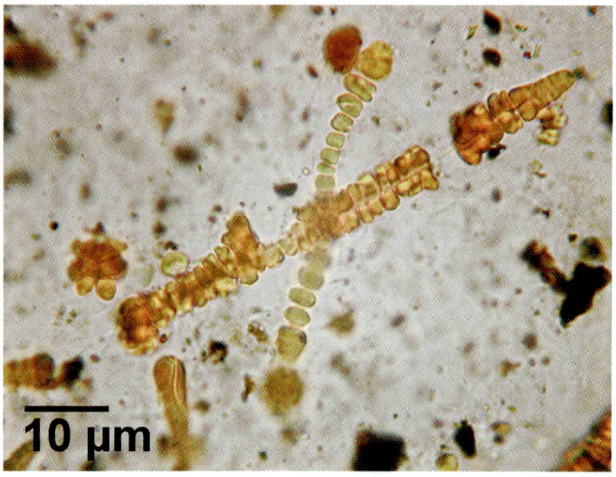

Fig. 3.4.5. Asbestos bodies in light microscopy

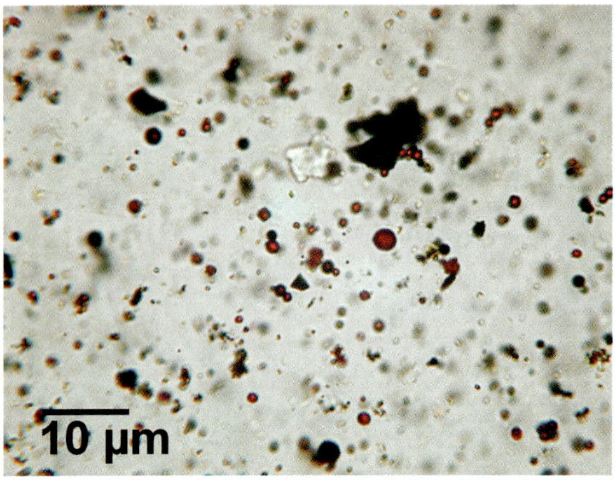

Fig. 3.4.3. Spherical iron oxide particles in the bronchoalveolar lavage fluid of a welder

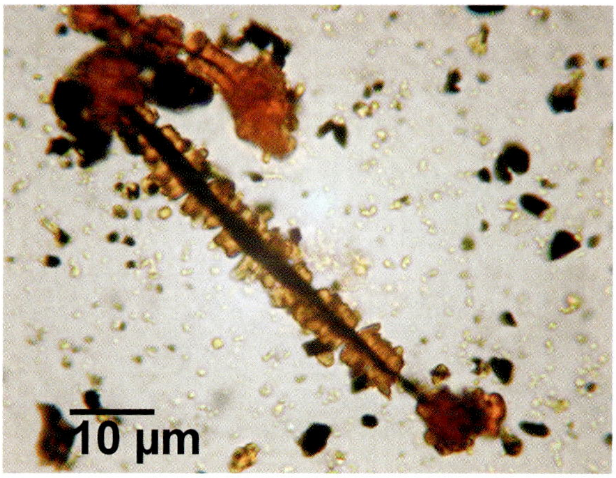

Fig. 3.4.6. Ferruginous body on an elongated coal particle

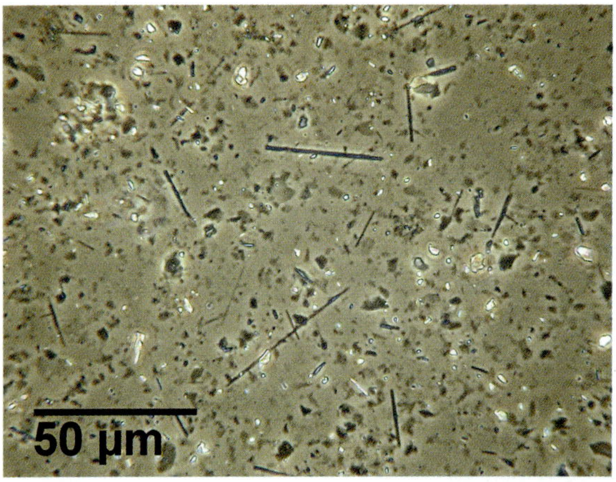

Fig. 3.4.4. Enhancement of thin uncovered asbestos fiber detection using phase-contrast light microscopy. Lung tissue of a Turk with environmental/domestic exposure to tremolite

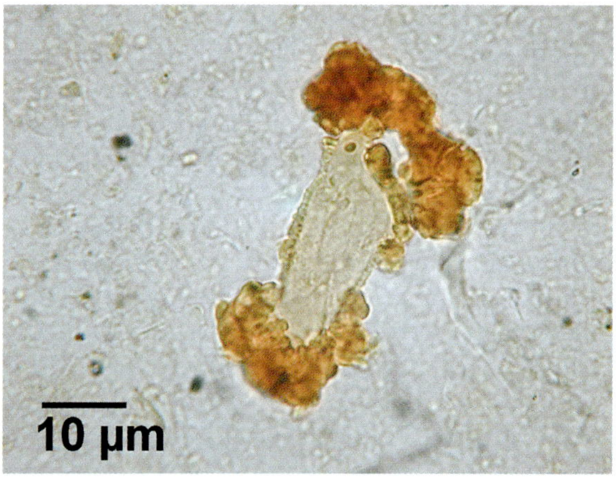

Fig. 3.4.7. Ferruginous body in the bronchoalveolar lavage fluid of a talc crusher

and silicon carbide (Churg et al. 1979; De Vuyst et al. 1986b; De Vuyst et al. 1987a; Dufresne et al. 1995). In light microscopy, the central core of a "typical" AB is a thin, straight, transparent and colourless fiber. The fiber is covered by a regularly segmented or continuous golden yellow to red brown coating. Some branched or curved forms can be observed (Churg et al. 1979; Churg and Warnock 1981; De Vuyst et al. 1987b). The validity of this definition is supported by numerous electron microscopy analyses, which have demonstrated that 95–98% of the core fibers of structures corresponding to this definition are indeed asbestos fibers (Churg and Warnock 1981; Dumortier et al. 1990). Most AB are built on amphibole asbestos fibers, and the AB burden correlates with the amphibole content of the lung (Warnock and Isenberg 1986; Karjalainen et al. 1996). AB on chrysotile have been observed in subjects recently exposed to this type of fiber, despite its shorter biopersistence (Dumortier et al. 1990). Typical AB can usually be discriminated from other ferruginous bodies, since the latter have brown to black cores or broad transparent to yellow cores, usually with an irregular coating (Churg et al. 1979). The only exceptions are ferruginous bodies on erionite and refractory ceramic fibers, which mimic AB, but their occurrence is limited to very particular exposures (Dumortier et al. 2001a; Dumortier et al. 2001b). AB and fiber counting using light microscopy allows the detection of low concentrations, down to 0.1 AB or fiber per millilitre BALF or 10 AB or fibers per gram dry lung tissue. Since it not possible to perform a precise typing of the fibers, uncovered fiber concentrations reported from light microscopy counts may include variable proportions of non-asbestos fibers.

Electron microscopy provides much better resolution than light microscopy. Moreover, interactions between incident electrons and matter generate different "signals" that can be analysed to obtain a very precise characterisation of the particles examined. According to the mode of formation of the images, there are basically two types of electron microscopes that should be distinguished: in a transmission electron microscope (TEM), the image of an electron beam passing through a thin sample is projected on a fluorescent screen (Fig. 3.4.8), and, in a scanning electron microscope (SEM), electrons re-emitted from a sample scanned by a small electron beam are amplified and imaged on a monitor. TEM is pre-

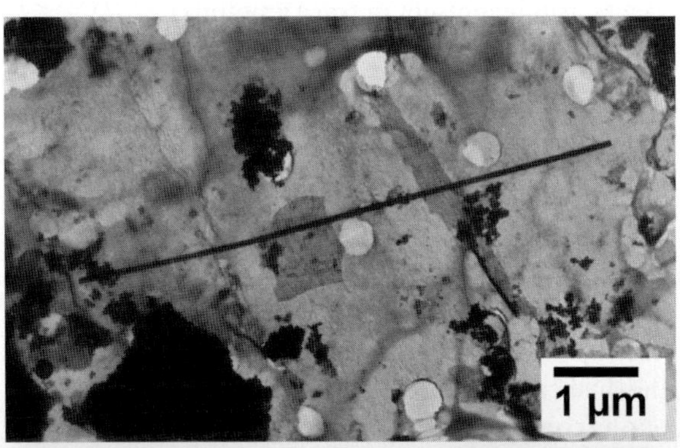

a

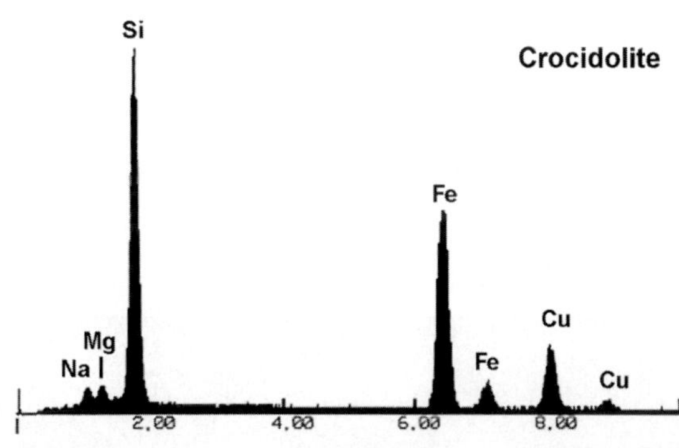

b

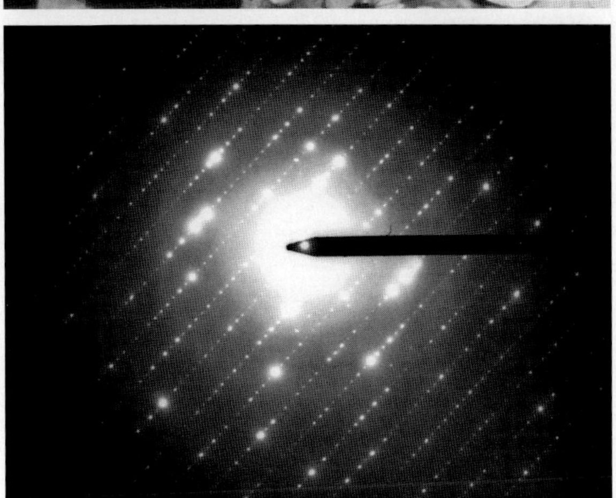
c

Fig. 3.4.8a–c. Transmission electron microscopy of a crocidolite asbestos fiber recovered from the lung tissue of an asbestos cement worker (**a**) with chemical composition spectrum (**b**) and selected area electron diffraction pattern (**c**). Copper peaks in the chemical spectrum are instrumental background ferred for asbestos-fiber counting, because it has a better resolution than SEM. It allows visualising of the thinnest chrysotile fibrils, measuring down to 0.01 μm. An analytical electron microscope is either a TEM or SEM fitted with an energy-dispersive X-ray spectrometer, allowing determination of the chemical composition of the particles or structures examined. It analyses the energy of the X-rays generated by the interactions between the incident electrons and the atoms constituting the particle analysed. Additionally, in TEM it is possible to obtain information on the crystalline structure of the particles by performing selected-area electron diffraction. This can help in the identification of structurally different compounds having the same chemical composition, such as talc and anthophyllite (Churg and Green 1998) or in distinguishing between crystalline and amorphous silica.

Two modes of imaging are available in SEM. Secondary electrons show the aspect of the surface of the particles (Fig. 3.4.9). Back-scattered electrons reflect the mean atomic number of the constituents of the particles or sample, brighter areas corresponding to the presence of heavier atoms. This is especially useful in finding out particles when performing in situ analysis on histological sections (Fig. 3.4.1c) or in cases where rare particles of heavy metal compounds should be specifically searched among numerous lighter compounds, such as silicates particles. In SEM, it is also possible to perform mapping of chemical elements to resolve complex structures, such as aggregates or altered particles (Fig. 3.4.10).

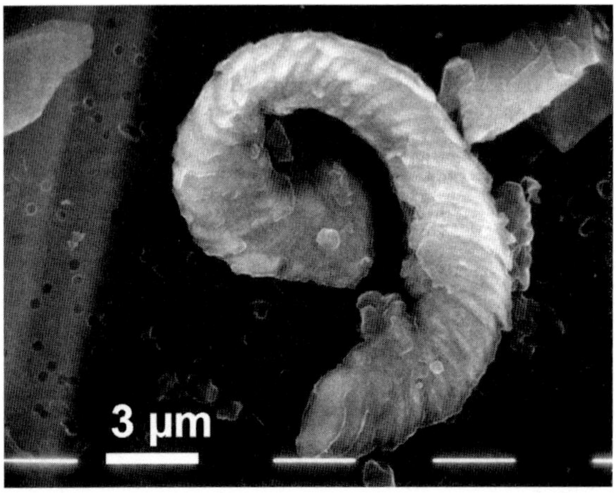

Fig. 3.4.9. Secondary electrons scanning electron microscopy of a chromium-cobalt-molybdenum shaving collected after digestion of lung tissue of a dental technician. Machining streaks reflect a mechanical formation process during grinding of dental prostheses

Due to the high magnification used in electron microscopy and the time required for detailed particle by particle analysis, only small surfaces of the sample can be examined and small numbers of particles analysed. Consequently, electron microscopy analyses have relatively poor analytical sensitivities, generally in the range of 10,000–50,000 fibers per gram dry lung tissue.

Miscellaneous techniques: in addition to light and analytical electron microscopy, a number of spectroscopic techniques have been used to analyse the bulk chemistry of lung tissue or BALF samples. Inductively coupled plasma atomic emission spectrometry (Gibbs and Pooley 1996), atomic absorption spectrometry (Fortoul et al. 1996; Harlyk et al. 1997; Tsuchiyama et al. 1997; Fortoul et al. 2002), X-ray fluorescence (Maier et al. 1987), particle induced X-ray emission (Corhay et al. 1995) or neutron activation analysis (Rizzato et al. 1992; Ishikawa et al. 1994; Saiki et al. 1999) allow the simultaneous determination of a large number of major and trace elements. These techniques can reach analytical sensitivities in the range of ppm or ppb. They are useful for disclosing elevations in concentrations of chemical elements with low atomic numbers ($n<11$) not detected by most analytical electron microscopy, such as beryllium, or in elements usually present in trace amounts.

X-ray diffraction (XRD) can identify crystalline components in digested lung dusts (Policard and Collet 1952; Gibbs et al. 1992; Gibbs and Pooley 1994; Algranti et al. 2005). It enables making the distinction between polymorphs of compounds having the same chemical composition but different crystalline habitus, such as quartz and cristobalite, two forms of crystalline silica. XRD is distinctly limited in sensitivity, and only major constituents of the dust can be detected. It does not assess the amorphous components such as coal or pumice, a kind of volcanic ash having a glass structure and associated with liparitosis (Mazziotti et al. 2004). With suitable standards, quantification of the major phases is possible (Gibbs and Pooley 1996, Dufresne et al. 1998a; Dufresne et al. 1998b).

3.4.5 Limitations of Mineralogical Analysis

In addition to limitations related to sampling, preparation and analytical methods described earlier, there are several limitations inherent to mineralogical analysis.

a
b
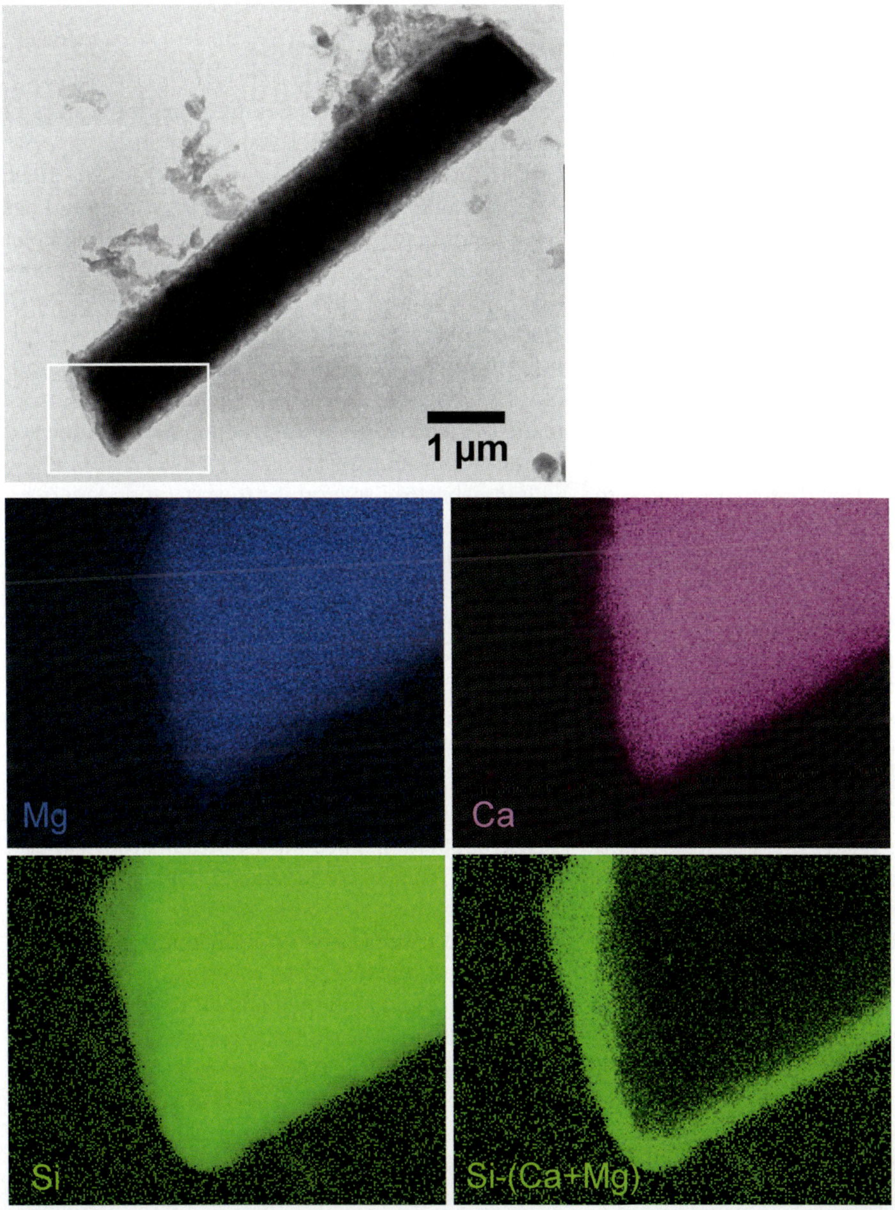

Fig. 3.4.10a,b. Transmission electron microscopy of an alkaline earth silicate fiber from bronchoalveolar lavage fluid of a worker producing high temperature insulation ropes (**a**). Chemical mapping reveal differential leaching of magnesium and calcium from the outer layer of the fiber (**b**).

Mineralogical analysis only provides a reflection of the particle burden retained in the sample at the time of sampling, and the effect of clearance should not be neglected. This may be especially relevant in cases with very old exposures or exposures to particles or elements having low biopersistence in the lung, such as chrysotile asbestos, cobalt or some man-made vitreous fibers.

Chrysotile fibers have a much faster clearance than amphiboles, and evaluation of exposures to this variety of asbestos (De Vuyst 1994) by analysing lung tissue (De Vuyst et al. 1998; Rees et al. 2001), BALF or sputum (Paris et al. 2002) samples is difficult. This restriction does not apply to recent exposures for which asbestos bodies on chrysotile fibers have been detected in BALF (Dumortier et al. 1990).

Hard-metal workers are exposed to dusts of cemented tungsten carbide containing 5–10% of cobalt. However, due to the solubility of metallic cobalt in the lung environment (Lison et al. 1994), particle analysis of lung tissue or BALF of hard metal workers show only trace amounts of cobalt (Dumortier et al. 1989).

Man-made glass or rock-wool fibers are widely used in insulation as substitutes for asbestos. In animal experiments, these fibers have relatively low biological persistence in lungs (Hesterberg et al. 1996). Accordingly, they are rarely found when performing mineralogical analysis of human lungs (McDonald et al. 1990; Dumortier et al. 2001a).

There are no standardised procedures for sample preparation and analysis. Technical differences, especially for electron microscopy counting, lead to a significant variability of results obtained by different laboratories. During an inter-laboratory trial by seven experienced laboratories to compare methods of counting asbestos fibers in lung tissue, all were able to rank samples according to concentrations, but there were marked differences in the absolute values obtained. Hence, participating laboratories appear to produce internally consistent results, but there is difficulty in comparing directly results from one laboratory to the next (Gylseth et al. 1985). The use of certified reference samples to standardise analytical procedures enables reducing these differences (Tossavainen et al. 2001). Much less variation is expected when comparing results of AB counts using light microscopy (Gylseth et al. 1985; De Vuyst et al. 1998). For non-fibrous particles, differences between analytical procedures are even more complex to assess than for asbestos fibers, and there is currently no inter-laboratory comparison about their burden in lung samples. Thus, each laboratory should obtain its own reference values from local control cases representing the general population of the study area (De Vuyst et al. 1998), and care must be taken when comparing results from laboratory to laboratory.

Interpretative errors can occur as a result of sample contamination. Possible contamination of paraffin blocks by asbestos fibers has been reported by some laboratories (Lee et al. 1995; Dodson et al. 1998). Therefore, asbestos fiber counts based on paraffin blocks should be interpreted with caution. Moreover, in a recent report, electron microscopy mineral analysis of lung tissue identified an unusual contamination by large amounts of fibrous sepiolite, a clay present in absorbent granules inadvertently used to provide the sample (Attanoos et al. 2003).

Finally, the influence of smoking on the particle load of lung tissue and BALF should be considered. It is a discussed issue (Lippmann et al. 1980). Some studies failed to demonstrate a significant effect on retention of fibers (Mollo et al. 1983; Corhay et al. 1990; Schwartz et al. 1991; Griffith et al. 1993b; Karjalainen et al. 1994a; Karjalainen et al. 1994b) or particles (Griffith et al. 1993b; Pairon et al. 1994a), while others tend to demonstrate a higher retention among smokers (Albin et al. 1994; Falchi et al. 1996a).

3.4.6 Interpretation of Results

Several papers report rules to interpret results of mineralogical analysis (Gibbs and Pooley 1994; Churg and Green 1998; De Vuyst et al. 1998; Pairon and Dumortier 1999). Each individual has some amount of particles and fibers in his lungs. Not all dust in lungs is of occupational origin. Greater amounts are expected in those living in polluted environments. For reliable interpretation of quantitative results, it is crucial that standardised methodologies have been used and that comparisons can be made to an adequate reference population analysed by the same laboratory.

For asbestos, several European and American laboratories consider that concentrations exceeding the following values are indicative of nontrivial exposure to asbestos: 1 AB per millilitre in BALF, 1000 AB per gram dry lung tissue, 1 10^6 amphibole fibers longer than 1 micron per gram dry lung tissue and 0.1 10^6 amphibole fibers longer than 5 microns per gram dry lung tissue. These levels are seldom exceeded in lifetime white-collar workers.

A result above reference level indicates an elevated retention of fibers compared with the unexposed reference population. Such positive results confirm past exposures, usually occupational. When compared against work histories, there are large overlaps in the fiber or AB counts between individuals classified as exposed and unexposed to asbestos. However, concentrations found in individuals with high cumulative exposures largely exceed the above-mentioned values.

A positive result is a proof of exposure but not of disease nor even an absolute proof of a causal relationship between exposure and disease. Mineralogical analysis is only one factor in the attribution of a disease to a particular exposure. Determining whether an element or mineral is responsible for a disease process depends on appropriate clinical, radiological and pathological findings (Churg and Green 1998).

A negative result does not exclude a low level or cleared exposure and cannot overrule a clear exposure history, especially when exposure to chrysotile is concerned. Significant past exposure to chrysotile can be associated with low concentration of fibers in lung (Churg 1988a; Pooley and Wagner 1988).

Quantifying asbestos bodies in lung tissue or BALF using light microscopy provides some crude estimate of the lung burden of amphibole asbestos (Teschler et al. 1994; Karjalainen et al. 1996), especially long ones, but it is a poor indicator of the lung burden of chrysotile asbestos fibers (Churg and Green 1998).

Several studies have investigated the correlation between AB concentrations in BAL fluid and in lung parenchyma (De Vuyst et al. 1988; Sebastien et al. 1988; Teschler et al. 1994; Karjalainen et al. 1996). The regression equations predicting the underlying parenchymal concentration from the concentration in BALF were very similar (Karjalainen et al. 1996). A concentration of greater than 1 AB per millilitre of BALF was associated with a high probability of having more than 1000 AB per gram dry lung (Pairon and Dumortier 1999).

Interpretation of the results of mineral fiber levels in particular cases will vary according to the disease considered. It is important to realise that there are different dose–response relationships between lung parenchyma and pleura in response to asbestos exposure, and there is a gradient of fiber levels for the various asbestos-related diseases. The highest pulmonary AB and fiber levels are found in asbestosis (De Vuyst et al. 1987b; Becklake and Case 1994). A fiber burden within the normal range of the unexposed reference population together with an absence of obvious history of asbestos exposure is a strong argument against asbestosis.

Lower levels may occur in mesothelioma and in pleural plaques. In a significant number of cases, retention is very low (De Vuyst et al. 1987b; Becklake and Case 1994; Orlowski et al. 1994; Pairon et al. 1994b), corresponding to low cumulated exposure. AB or fiber concentrations may even be in the range observed in the reference population. It must be stressed that BAL and lung tissue analyses are markers of alveolar and parenchymal retention of fibers but do not reflect directly the accumulation of fibers in the parietal pleura, where these lesions occur (Boutin et al. 1996). As mesothelioma and pleural plaques are most specifically related to asbestos exposure, it appears useless to perform mineralogical analysis only to assess their aetiology.

The finding of high fiber concentrations in lung tissue or BALF of lung cancer patients, much higher than in the reference population, is an argument for an aetiological attribution to asbestos exposure (see above). In surgically treated lung cancers, systematic counting of AB in specimens of resected lung tissue can be used to detect cases possibly related to asbestos that require careful evaluation of the occupational history or the lung fiber content using EM analysis.

Most of the above rules can be extended to interpret findings in cases with exposure to non-fibrous particles, provided consistent analytical methods are used, and reference levels for the general population are available, which is currently a rare situation.

3.4.7 Conclusions

Mineralogical analysis allows a detailed systematic study of the inhaled particles or fibers retained in human lungs. It is a powerful tool that complements the other methods used to investigate occupational or environmental exposures and related diseases. There are, however, a number of different methods available, and it is important to be aware of the technical factors and intrinsic limitations that could influence the results. The choice of the method will depend on the question to solve, the sample type and amount and the available analytical tools. The more sophisticated techniques, such as electron microscopy, are only used in a number of specialised laboratories. Currently, each laboratory should have its own reference values obtained from local control populations.

Threshold limit values for hazardous minerals were reduced, and the use of asbestos was banned in many Western countries during the two last decades. However, uncontrolled exposures can still occur in some trades, and more permissive hygiene standards may exist in other parts of the world. Thus, health consequences of occupational exposures to airborne particles or fibers are still expected in the future, since long latencies may be associated with the development of pneumoconiosis and asbestos-related diseases, especially in cases with low cumulative exposures. Moreover, atypical exposure circumstances, such as environmental exposures to asbestos-containing materials in buildings or exposures to soils naturally containing tremolite asbestos due to the local geology of some areas around the Mediterranean Sea or in California, are now a matter of concern. Mineralogical analysis of lung samples will remain useful to assess diseases possibly caused by these exposures. Mineralogical analysis is also helpful to point out new risks, and upcoming exposures to nanoparticles will likely become a challenging issue.

References

Abraham JL, Burnett BR, Hunt A (1991) Development and use of a pneumoconiosis database of human pulmonary inorganic particulate burden in over 400 lungs. Scanning Microsc 5:95–108

Albin M, Pooley FD, Stromberg U, Attewell R, Mitha R, Johansson L, Welinder H (1994) Retention patterns of asbestos fibers in lung tissue among asbestos cement workers. Occup Environ Med 51:205–211

Algranti E, Handar AM, Dumortier P, Mendonca EM, Rodrigues GL, Santos AM, Mauad T, Dolhnikoff M, De Vuyst P, Saldiva PH, Bussacos MA (2005) Pneumoconiosis after sericite inhalation. Occup Environ Med 62:e2

Anonymous (1997) Asbestos, asbestosis, and cancer: the Helsinki criteria for diagnosis and attribution. Scand J Work Environ Health 23:311–316

Attanoos RL, Griffiths DM, Gibbs AR (2003) Unusual contaminant fibers on mineral analysis. Histopathology 43:405–406

Becklake MR (1991) The epidemiology of asbestosis. In: Liddell D, Miller K (eds) Mineral fibers and health. CRC Press, Boca Raton, Florida, pp 103–119

Becklake MR, Case BW (1994) Fiber burden and asbestos-related lung disease: determinants of dose- response relationships. Am J Respir Crit Care Med 150:1488–1492

Bignon J, Depierre A, Bonnaud G, Goni J, Brouet G (1973) Mise en évidence de corps ferrugineux par microfiltration de l'expectoration. Corrélation avec le risque asbestosique. Nouv Presse Med (Paris) 2:1697–1700

Bignon J, Saracci R, Touray JC (1994) Introduction: INSERM-IARC-CNRS workshop on biopersistence of respirable synthetic fibers and minerals. Environ Health Perspect 102[Suppl 5]:3–5

Boutin C, Dumortier P, Rey F, Viallat JR, De Vuyst P (1996) Black spots concentrate oncogenic asbestos fibers in the parietal pleura. Thoracoscopic and mineralogic study. Am J Respir Crit Care Med 153:444–449

Brain JD, Godleski J, Kreyling W (1994) In vivo evaluation of chemical biopersistence of nonfibrous inorganic particles. Environ Health Perspect 102[Suppl 5]:119–125

Brody AR, Hill LH, Adkins B, O'Connor RW (1981) Chrysotile asbestos inhalation in rats: deposition pattern and reaction of alveolar epithelium and pulmonary macrophages. Am Rev Respir Dis 123:670–679

Brown RC, Hoskins JA, Miller K, Mossman BT (1990) Pathogenetic mechanisms of asbestos and other mineral fibers. Mol Aspects Med 11: 325–349

Churg A (1988a) Chrysotile, tremolite, and malignant mesothelioma in man. Chest 93:621–628

Churg A (1998b) Nonneoplastic diseases caused by asbestos. In: Churg A, Green FHY (eds) Pathology of occupational lung diseases, 2nd edn. Williams and Wilkins, Baltimore, pp 277–338

Churg A, Warnock ML (1981) Asbestos and other ferruginous bodies: their formation and clinical significance. Am J Pathol 102:447–456

Churg A, Wood P (1983) Observations on the distribution of asbestos fibers in human lungs. Environ Res 31:374–380

Churg A, DePaoli L (1988) Clearance of chrysotile asbestos from human lung. Exp Lung Res 14:567–574

Churg A, Wiggs B (1989) The distribution of amosite asbestos fibers in the lungs of workers with mesothelioma or carcinoma. Exp Lung Res 15:771–783

Churg A, Green FHY (1998) Analytic methods for identifying and quantifying mineral particles in lung tissue. In: Churg A, Green FHY (eds) Pathology of occupational lung diseases, 2nd edn. Williams and Wilkins, Baltimore, pp 45–55

Churg A, Brauer M (2000) Ambient atmospheric particles in the airways of human lungs. Ultrastruct Pathol 24:353–361

Churg A, Warnock ML, Green N (1979) Analysis of the cores of ferruginous (asbestos) bodies from the general population. II. True asbestos bodies and pseudoasbestos bodies. Lab Invest 40:31–38

Churg A, Wright JL, DePaoli L, Wiggs B (1989) Mineralogic correlates of fibrosis in chrysotile miners and millers. Am Rev Respir Dis 139:891—896

Churg A, Hobson J, Wright J (1990a) Effects of cigarette smoke dose and time after smoke exposure on uptake of asbestos fibers by rat tracheal epithelial cells. Am J Respir Cell Mol Biol 3:265–269

Churg A, Wright J, Wiggs B, Depaoli L (1990b) Mineralogic parameters related to amosite asbestos-induced fibrosis in humans. Am Rev Respir Dis 142:1331–1336

Cooke WE (1929) Asbestos dust and the curious bodies found in pulmonary asbestosis. BMJ 2:578–580

Corhay JL, Delavignette JP, Bury T, Saint-Remy P, Radermecker MF (1990) Occult exposure to asbestos in steel workers revealed by bronchoalveolar lavage. Arch Environ Health 45:278–282

Corhay JL, Bury T, Delavignette JP, Baharloo F, Radermecker M, Hereng P, Fransolet AM, Weber G, Roelandts I (1995) Nonfibrous mineralogical analysis of bronchoalveolar lavage fluid from blast-furnace workers. Arch Environ Health 50:312–319

Davis GS, Giancola MS, Costanza MC, Low RB (1982) Analyses of sequential bronchoalveolar lavage samples from healthy human volunteers. Am Rev Respir Dis 126:611–616

Davis JM, Addison J, Bolton RE, Donaldson K, Jones AD, Smith T (1986) The pathogenicity of long versus short fiber samples of amosite asbestos administered to rats by inhalation and intraperitoneal injection. Br J Exp Pathol 67:415–430

De Vuyst P (1994) Biopersistence of respirable synthetic fibers and minerals: point of view of the chest physician. Environ Health Perspect 102[Suppl 5]:7–9

De Vuyst P, Jedwab J, Dumortier P, Vandermoten G, Vande Weyer R, Yernault JC (1982) Asbestos bodies in bronchoalveolar lavage. Am Rev Respir Dis 126:972–976

De Vuyst P, Dumortier P, Rickaert F, Van de Weyer R, Lenclud C, Yernault JC (1986a) Occupational lung fibrosis in an aluminium polisher. Eur J Respir Dis 68:131–140

De Vuyst P, Vande Weyer R, De Coster A, Marchandise FX, Dumortier P, Ketelbant P, Jedwab J, Yernault JC (1986b) Dental technician's pneumoconiosis. A report of two cases. Am Rev Respir Dis 133:316–320

De Vuyst P, Dumortier P, Leophonte P, Weyer RV, Yernault JC (1987a) Mineralogical analysis of bronchoalveolar lavage in talc pneumoconiosis. Eur J Respir Dis 70:150–156

De Vuyst P, Dumortier P, Moulin E, Yourassowsky N, Yernault JC (1987b) Diagnostic value of asbestos bodies in bronchoalveolar lavage fluid. Am Rev Respir Dis 136:1219–1224

De Vuyst P, Dumortier P, Schandene L, Estenne M, Verhest A, Yernault JC (1987c) Sarcoidlike lung granulomatosis induced by aluminum dusts. Am Rev Respir Dis 135:493–497

De Vuyst P, Dumortier P, Moulin E, Yourassowsky N, Roomans P, de Francquen P, Yernault JC (1988) Asbestos bodies in bronchoalveolar lavage reflect lung asbestos body concentration. Eur Respir J 1:362–367

De Vuyst P, Dumortier P, Gevenois PA (1997) Analysis of asbestos bodies in BAL from subjects with particular exposures. Am J Ind Med 31:699–704

De Vuyst P, Karjalainen A, Dumortier P, Pairon JC, Monso E, Brochard P, Teschler H, Tossavainen A, Gibbs A (1998) Guidelines for mineral fiber analyses in biological samples: report of the ERS Working Group. European Respiratory Society. Eur Respir J 11:1416–1126

Dodson RF, Williams MG Jr, Corn CJ, Brollo A, Bianchi C (1990) Asbestos content of lung tissue, lymph nodes, and pleural plaques from former shipyard workers. Am Rev Respir Dis 142:843–847

Dodson RF, Garcia JG, O'Sullivan M, Corn C, Levin JL, Griffith DE, Kronenberg RS (1991) The usefulness of bronchoalveolar lavage in identifying past occupational exposure to asbestos: a light and electron microscopy study. Am J Ind Med 19:619–628

Dodson RF, O'Sullivan M, Corn CJ, McLarty JW, Hammar SP (1997) Analysis of asbestos fiber burden in lung tissue from mesothelioma patients. Ultrastruct Pathol 21:321–336

Dodson RF, Huang J, Williams MG, Bruce JR, Hammar SP (1998) Lack of asbestos contamination of paraffin. Arch Pathol Lab Med 122:1103–1106

Dodson RF, O'Sullivan MF, Huang J, Holiday DB, Hammar SP (2000) Asbestos in extrapulmonary sites: omentum and mesentery. Chest 117:486–493

Dufresne A, Loosereewanich P, Armstrong B, Infante-Rivard C, Perrault G, Dion C, Masse S, Begin R (1995) Pulmonary retention of ceramic fibers in silicon carbide (SiC) workers. Am Ind Hyg Assoc J 56:490–498

Dufresne A, Begin R, Dion C, Jagirdar J, Rom WN, Loosereewanich P, Muir DC, Ritchie AC, Perrault G (1998a) Angular and fibrous particles in lung in relation to silica-induced diseases. Int Arch Occup Environ Health 71:263–269

Dufresne A, Loosereewanich P, Begin R, Dion C, Ecobichon D, Muir DC, Ritchie AC, Perrault G (1998b) Tentative explanatory variable of lung dust concentration in gold miners exposed to crystalline silica. J Expo Anal Environ Epidemiol 8:375–398

Dumortier P, De Vuyst P, Yernault JC (1989) Non-fibrous inorganic particles in human bronchoalveolar lavage fluids. Scanning Microsc 3:1207–1218

Dumortier P, De Vuyst P, Strauss P, Yernault JC (1990) Asbestos bodies in bronchoalveolar lavage fluids of brake lining and asbestos cement workers. Br J Ind Med 47:91–98

Dumortier P, Coplu L, de Maertelaer V, Emri S, Baris I, De Vuyst P (1998) Assessment of environmental asbestos exposure in Turkey by bronchoalveolar lavage. Am J Respir Crit Care Med 158:1815–1824

Dumortier P, Broucke I, De Vuyst P (2001a) Pseudoasbestos bodies and fibers in bronchoalveolar lavage of refractory ceramic fiber users. Am J Respir Crit Care Med 164:499–503

Dumortier P, Coplu L, Broucke I, Emri S, Selcuk T, de Maertelaer V, De Vuyst P, Baris I (2001b) Erionite bodies and fibers in bronchoalveolar lavage fluid (BALF) of residents from Tuzkoy, Cappadocia, Turkey. Occup Environ Med 58:261–266

Dumortier P, Gocmen A, Laurent K, Manco A, De Vuyst P (2001c) The role of environmental and occupational exposures in Turkish immigrants with fiber-related disease. Eur Respir J 17:922–927

Falchi M, Biondo L, Conti C, Cipri A, Demarinis F, Gigli B, Paoletti L (1996a) Inorganic particles in bronchoalveolar lavage fluids from nonoccupationally exposed subjects. Arch Environ Health 51:157–161

Falchi M, Paoletti L, Mariotta S, Giosue S, Guidi L, Biondo L, Scavalli P, Bisetti A (1996b) Non-fibrous inorganic particles in bronchoalveolar lavage fluid of pottery workers. Occup Environ Med 53:762–766

Fireman E, Greif J, Schwarz Y, Man A, Ganor E, Ribak Y, Lerman Y (1999) Assessment of hazardous dust exposure by BAL and induced sputum. Chest 115:1720–1728

Fischer M, Gunther S, Muller KM (2002) Fiber-years, pulmonary asbestos burden and asbestosis. Int J Hyg Environ Health 205:245–248

Fortoul TI, Osorio LS, Tovar AT, Salazar D, Castilla ME, Olaiz-Fernandez G (1996) Metals in lung tissue from autopsy cases in Mexico City residents: comparison of cases from the 1950s and the 1980s. Environ Health Perspect 104:630–632

Fortoul TI, Quan-Torres A, Sanchez I, Lopez IE, Bizarro P, Mendoza ML, Osorio LS, Espejel-Maya G, Avila-Casado Mdel C, Avila-Costa MR, Colin-Barenque L, Villanueva DN, Olaiz-Fernandez G (2002) Vanadium in ambient air: concentrations in lung tissue from autopsies of Mexico City residents in the 1960s and 1990s. Arch Environ Health 57:446–449

Fubini B, Fenoglio I, Elias Z, Poirot O (2001) Variability of biological responses to silicas: effect of origin, crystallinity, and state of surface on generation of reactive oxygen species and morphological transformation of mammalian cells. J Environ Pathol Toxicol Oncol 20[Suppl 1]:95–108

Funahashi A, Schlueter DP, Pintar K, Siegesmund KA (1984) Value of in situ elemental microanalysis in the histologic diagnosis of silicosis. Chest 85:506–509

Gellert AR, Kitajewska JY, Uthayakumar S, Kirkham JB, Rudd RM (1986) Asbestos fibers in bronchoalveolar lavage fluid from asbestos workers: examination by electron microscopy. Br J Ind Med 43:170–176

Gibbs AE, Pooley FD, Griffiths DM, Mitha R, Craighead JE, Ruttner JR (1992) Talc pneumoconiosis: a pathologic and mineralogic study. Hum Pathol 23:1344–1354

Gibbs AR, Pooley FD (1994) Fuller's earth (montmorillonite) pneumoconiosis. Occup Environ Med 51:644–646

Gibbs AR, Pooley FD (1996) Analysis and interpretation of inorganic mineral particles in "lung" tissues. Thorax 51:327–334

Gibbs AR, Wagner JC (1998) Diseases due to silica. In: Churg A, Green FHY (eds) Pathology of occupational lung diseases, 2nd edn. Williams and Wilkins, Baltimore, pp 209–233

Gibbs AR, Griffiths DM, Pooley FD, Jones JS (1990) Comparison of fiber types and size distributions in lung tissues of paraoccupational and occupational cases of malignant mesothelioma. Br J Ind Med 47:621–626

Gloyne SR (1929) Presence of asbestos fibers in lungs of asbestos workers. Tubercle 10:404–407

Golden EB, Warnock ML, Hulett LD, Churg AM (1982) Fly ash lung: a new pneumoconiosis? Am Rev Respir Dis 125:108–112

Griffith DE, Garcia JG, Dodson RF, Levin JL, Kronenberg RS (1993a) Airflow obstruction in nonsmoking, asbestos- and mixed dust-exposed workers. Lung 171:213–224

Griffith DE, Garcia JG, Dodson RF, Levin JL, Kronenberg RS (1993b) Airflow obstruction in nonsmoking, asbestos- and mixed dust-exposed workers. Lung 171:213–224

Gylseth B, Churg A, Davis JM, Johnson N, Morgan A, Mowe G, Rogers A, Roggli V (1985) Analysis of asbestos fibers and asbestos bodies in tissue samples from human lung. An international interlaboratory trial. Scand J Work Environ Health 11:107–110

Harlyk C, Mccourt J, Bordin G, Rodriguez AR, van der Eeckhout A (1997) Determination of copper, zinc and iron in

broncho-alveolar lavages by atomic absorption spectroscopy. J Trace Elem Med Biol 11:137–142
Haslam PL, Baughman RP (1999) Guidelines for the measurement of acellular components and recommendations for standardization of bronchoalveolar lavage (BAL). Report of the European Respiratory Society Task Force. Introduction. Eur Respir Rev 9:25–27
Hesterberg TW, Miiller WC, Musselman RP, Kamstrup O, Hamilton RD, Thevenaz P (1996) Biopersistence of man-made vitreous fibers and crocidolite asbestos in the rat lung following inhalation. Fundam Appl Toxicol 29:269–279
Hesterberg TW, Hart GA, Chevalier J, Miiller WC, Hamilton RD, Bauer J, Thevenaz P (1998) The importance of fiber biopersistence and lung dose in determining the chronic inhalation effects of X607, RCF1, and chrysotile asbestos in rats. Toxicol Appl Pharmacol 153:68–82
Hodgson JT, Darnton A (2000) The quantitative risks of mesothelioma and lung cancer in relation to asbestos exposure. Ann Occup Hyg 44:565–601
Ishikawa Y, Nakagawa K, Satoh Y, Kitagawa T, Sugano H, Hirano T, Tsuchiya E (1994) "Hot spots" of chromium accumulation at bifurcations of chromate workers' bronchi. Cancer Res 54:2342–2346
Janssen YM, Marsh JP, Absher MP, Gabrielson E, Borm PJ, Driscoll K, Mossman BT (1994) Oxidant stress responses in human pleural mesothelial cells exposed to asbestos. Am J Respir Crit Care Med 149:795–802
Johnson NF, Lincoln JL, Wills HA (1984) Analysis of fibers recovered from lung tissue. Lung 162:37–47
Johnson NF, Haslam PL, Dewar A, Newman-Taylor AJ, Turner-Warwick M (1986) Identification of inorganic dust particles in bronchoalveolar lavage macrophages by energy dispersive x-ray microanalysis. Arch Environ Health 41:133–144
Jones JS, Smith PG, Pooley FD, Berry G, Sawle GW, Madeley RJ, Wignall BK, Aggarwal A (1980) The consequences of exposure to asbestos dust in a wartime gas-mask factory. IARC Sci Publ 30:637–653
Karjalainen A, Anttila S, Mantyla T, Taskinen E, Kyyronen P, Tukiainen P (1994a) Asbestos bodies in bronchoalveolar lavage fluid in relation to occupational history. Am J Ind Med 26:645–654
Karjalainen A, Vanhala E, Karhunen PJ, Lalu K, Penttila A, Tossavainen A (1994b) Asbestos exposure and pulmonary fiber concentrations of 300 Finnish urban men. Scand J Work Environ Health 20:34–41
Karjalainen A, Piipari R, Mantyla T, Monkkonen M, Nurminen M, Tukiainen P, Vanhala E, Anttila S (1996) Asbestos bodies in bronchoalveolar lavage in relation to asbestos bodies and asbestos fibers in lung parenchyma. Eur Respir J 9:1000–1005
Knoll M, Ruska E (1932) Das Electronenmikroskop. Z Physik 78:318–339
Kühn J (1941) Übermikroscopische Untersuchungen an Asbeststaub und Asbestlungen. Arch Gewerbepath Gewerbhyg 10:473–485
Le Bouffant L, Martin JC, Daniel H (1979) Facteurs influençant l'épuration et la migration des particules minérales inhalées. Nouv Presse Med 8:2083–2088
Lee RJ, Florida RG, Stewart IM (1995) Asbestos contamination in paraffin tissue blocks. Arch Pathol Lab Med 119:528–532
Lippmann M (1994) Deposition and retention of inhaled fibers: effects on incidence of lung cancer and mesothelioma. Occup Environ Med 51:793–798
Lippmann M, Yeates DB, Albert RE (1980) Deposition, retention, and clearance of inhaled particles. Br J Ind Med 37:337–362
Lison D, Buchet JP, Swennen B, Molders J, Lauwerys R (1994) Biological monitoring of workers exposed to cobalt metal, salt, oxides, and hard metal dust. Occup Environ Med 51:447–450
Maier EA, Dietemann-Molard A, Rastegar F, Heimburger R, Ruch C, Maier A, Roegel E, Leroy MJ (1987) Simultaneous determination of trace elements in lavage fluids from human bronchial alveoli by energy-dispersive x-ray fluorescence. 3. Routine analysis. Clin Chem 33:2234–2239
Marchand F (1906) Über eigentümlichte Pigmentkristalle in den Lungen. Verhandl d Deutsch path Gesellsch 10:223–228
Martonen TB, Katz IM (1993) Deposition patterns of aerosolized drugs within human lungs: effects of ventilatory parameters. Pharm Res 10:871–878
Mazziotti S, Gaeta M, Costa C, Ascenti G, Barbaro Martino L, Spatari G, Settineri N, Barbaro M (2004) Computed tomography features of liparitosis: a pneumoconiosis due to amorphous silica. Eur Respir J 23:208–213
McDonald AD, Case BW, Churg A, Dufresne A, Gibbs GW, Sebastien P, McDonald JC (1997) Mesothelioma in Quebec chrysotile miners and millers: epidemiology and aetiology. Ann Occup Hyg 41:707–719
McDonald JC, McDonald AD (1991) Epidemiology of mesothelioma. In: Liddell D, Miller K (eds) Mineral fibers and health. CRC Press, Boca Raton, pp 147–168
McDonald JC, Armstrong B, Case B, Doell D, McCaughey WT, McDonald AD, Sebastien P (1989) Mesothelioma and asbestos fiber type. Evidence from lung tissue analyses. Cancer 63:1544–1547
McDonald JC, Case BW, Enterline PE, Henderson V, McDonald AC, Plourde M, Sébastien P (1990) Lung dust analysis in the assessment of past exposure of man-made mineral fiber workers. Ann Occup Hyg 34:427–441
McDonald JC, Sebastien P, Case B, McDonald AD, Dufresne A (1992) Ferruginous body counts in sputum as an index of past exposure to mineral fibers. Ann Occup Hyg 36:271–282
McDonald JC, Armstrong BG, Edwards CW, Gibbs AR, Lloyd HM, Pooley FD, Ross DJ, Rudd RM (2001) Case-referent survey of young adults with mesothelioma: I. Lung fiber analyses. Ann Occup Hyg 45:513–518
McFadden D, Wright JL, Wiggs B, Churg A (1986) Smoking inhibits asbestos clearance. Am Rev Respir Dis 133:372–374
Mitchev K, Dumortier P, De Vuyst P (2002) 'Black Spots' and hyaline pleural plaques on the parietal pleura of 150 urban necropsy cases. Am J Surg Pathol 26:1198–1206
Mollo F, Andrion A, Bellis D, Pira E, Tallone MV (1983) Optical determination of coated and uncoated mineral fibers in lungs of subjects without professional exposure. Appl Pathol 1:276–282
Morgan A, Holmes A (1983) Distribution and characteristics of amphibole asbestos fibers, measured with the light microscope, in the left lung of an insulation worker. Br J Ind Med 40:45–50
Morgan A, Holmes A (1984) The distribution and characteristics of asbestos fibers in the lungs of Finnish anthophyllite mine-workers. Environ Res 33:62–75
Morgan A, Holmes A (1985) The enigmatic asbestos body: its formation and significance in asbestos- related disease. Environ Res 38:283–292

Motley RL, Patrick CWJ (1992) Medicolegal aspects of asbestos-related diseases: plaintiff's attorney's perspective. In: Roggli VL, Greenberg SD, Pratt PC (eds) Pathology of asbestos-associated diseases. Little, Brown and Company, Boston Toronto London, pp 347–364

NRCC (National Research Council of Canada (NRCC) Associate Committee on Scientific Criteria for Environmental Quality) (1982) Effects of inhaled particles on human health: influence of particle size and shape. Pulications NRCC/CNRC, Ottawa

Oberdorster G (1995) Lung particle overload: implications for occupational exposures to particles. Regul Toxicol Pharmacol 21:123–135

Orlowski E, Pairon JC, Ameille J, Janson X, Iwatsubo Y, Dufour G, Bignon J, Brochard P (1994) Pleural plaques, asbestos exposure, and asbestos bodies in bronchoalveolar lavage fluid. Am J Ind Med 26:349–358

Pairon JC, Dumortier P (1999) [Role of biometric analysis in the retrospective assessment of exposure to asbestos]. Rev Mal Respir 16:1219–1235

Pairon JC, Billon-Galland MA, Iwatsubo Y, Bernstein M, Gaudichet A, Bignon J, Brochard P (1994a) Biopersistence of nonfibrous mineral particles in the respiratory tracts of subjects following occupational exposure. Environ Health Perspect 102[Suppl 5]:269–275

Pairon JC, Orlowski E, Iwatsubo Y, Billon-Galland MA, Dufour G, Chamming's S, Archambault C, Bignon J, Brochard P (1994b) Pleural mesothelioma and exposure to asbestos: evaluation from work histories and analysis of asbestos bodies in bronchoalveolar lavage fluid or lung tissue in 131 patients. Occup Environ Med 51:244–249

Paris C, Galateau-Salle F, Creveuil C, Morello R, Raffaelli C, Gillon JC, Billon-Galland MA, Pairon JC, Chevreau L, Letourneux M (2002) Asbestos bodies in the sputum of asbestos workers: correlation with occupational exposure. Eur Respir J 20:1167–1173

Parkes RW (1994) Occupational lung disorders. 3rd edn. Butterworth-Heinemann Ltd., Oxford

Pezerat H, Zalma R, Guignard J, Jaurand MC (1989) Production of oxygen radicals by the reduction of oxygen arising from the surface activity of mineral fibers. IARC Sci Publ 90:100–111

Pfau JC, Sentissi JJ, Weller G, Putnam EA (2005) Assessment of autoimmune responses associated with asbestos exposure in Libby, Montana, USA. Environ Health Perspect 113:25–30

Pinkerton KE, Green FH, Saiki C, Vallyathan V, Plopper CG, Gopal V, Hung D, Bahne EB, Lin SS, Menache MG, Schenker MB (2000) Distribution of particulate matter and tissue remodeling in the human lung. Environ Health Perspect 108:1063–1069

Policard A, Collet A (1952) Deposition of siliceous dust in the lungs of the inhabitants of the Saharan regions. Arch Ind Hyg Occup Med 5:527–534

Pooley FD, Wagner JC (1988) The significance of the selective retention of mineral dusts. Ann Occup Hyg 32[Suppl 1]:187–194

Pott F (1980) Animal experiments on biological effects of mineral fibers. IARC Sci Publ 30:261–272

Powers A, Carbone M (2002) The role of environmental carcinogens, viruses and genetic predisposition in the pathogenesis of mesothelioma. Cancer Biol Ther 1:348–353

Rees D, Phillips JI, Garton E, Pooley FD (2001) Asbestos lung fiber concentrations in South African chrysotile mine workers. Ann Occup Hyg 45:473–477

Reynolds HY (2000) Use of bronchoalveolar lavage in humans–past necessity and future imperative. Lung 178:271–293

Rizzato G, Fraioli P, Sabbioni E, Pietra R, Barberis M (1992) Multi-element follow up in biological specimens of hard metal pneumoconiosis. Sarcoidosis 9:104–117

Roggli VL, Pratt PC, Brody AR (1992) Analysis of tissue mineral fiber content. In: Roggli VL, Greenberg SD, Pratt PC (eds) Pathology of asbestos-associated diseases. Little, Brown and Company, Boston Toronto London, pp 299–345

Roggli VL, Coin PG, MacIntyre NR, Bell DY (1994) Asbestos content of bronchoalveolar lavage fluid. A comparison of light and scanning electron microscopic analysis. Acta Cytol 38:502–510

Saiki M, Saldiva PH, Alice SH (1999) Evaluation of trace elements in lung samples from coal miners using neutron activation analysis. Biol Trace Elem Res 71–72:291–297

Sartorelli P, Scancarello G, Romeo R, Marciano G, Rottoli P, Arcangeli G, Palmi S (2001) Asbestos exposure assessment by mineralogical analysis of bronchoalveolar lavage fluid. J Occup Environ Med 43:872–881

Scansetti G, Pira E, Botta GC, Turbiglio M, Piolatto G (1993) Asbestos exposure in a steam–electric generating plant. Ann Occup Hyg 37:645–653

Schwartz DA, Galvin JR, Burmeister LF, Merchant RK, Dayton CS, Merchant JA, Hunninghake GW (1991) The clinical utility and reliability of asbestos bodies in bronchoalveolar fluid. Am Rev Respir Dis 144:684–688

Sébastien P (1982) Possibilités actuelles de la biométrologie des poussières sur échantillons de liquide de lavage bronchoalvéolaire. Ann Biol Clin (Paris) 40:279–293

Sébastien P (1991) Pulmonary deposition and clearannce of airborne mineral fibers. In: Liddell D, Miller K (eds) Mineral fibers and health. CRC Press, Boca Raton, pp 229–248

Sébastien P, Janson X, Gaudichet A, Hirsch A, Bignon J (1980) Asbestos retention in human respiratory tissues: comparative measurements in lung parenchyma and in parietal pleura. IARC Sci Publ 30:237–246

Sébastien P, Awad L, Bignon J, Petit G, Baris YI (1984) Ferruginous bodies in sputum as an indication of exposure to airborne mineral fibers in the mesothelioma villages of Cappadocia. Arch Environ Health 39:18–23

Sébastien P, Armstrong B, Monchaux G, Bignon J (1988) Asbestos bodies in bronchoalveolar lavage fluid and in lung parenchyma. Am Rev Respir Dis 137:75–78

Stanton MF, Layard M, Tegeris A, Miller E, May M, Morgan E, Smith A (1981) Relation of particle dimension to carcinogenicity in amphibole asbestoses and other fibrous minerals. J Natl Cancer Inst 67:965–975

Sulotto F, Capellaro E, Chiesa A, Villari S, Bontempi S, Scansetti G (1997) Relationship between asbestos bodies in sputum and the number of specimens. Scand J Work Environ Health 23:48–53

Teschler H, Konietzko N, Schoenfeld B, Ramin C, Schraps T, Costabel U (1993) Distribution of asbestos bodies in the human lung as determined by bronchoalveolar lavage. Am Rev Respir Dis 147:1211–1215

Teschler H, Friedrichs KH, Hoheisel GB, Wick G, Soltner U, Thompson AB, Konietzko N, Costabel U (1994) Asbestos fibers in bronchoalveolar lavage and lung tissue of former asbestos workers. Am J Respir Crit Care Med 149:641–645

Teschler H, Thompson AB, Dollenkamp R, Konietzko N, Costabel U (1996) Relevance of asbestos bodies in sputum. Eur Respir J 9:680–686

Thimpont J, De Vuyst P (1998) Occupational asbestos related diseases in Belgium. In: Peters GA, Peters BJ (eds) Sourcebook on asbestos diseases, vol 17. Lexis Law Publishing, Charlottesville, VA, pp 311–328

Timbrell V (1965) The inhalation of fibrous dusts. Ann NY Acad Sci 132:255–273

Tossavainen A, Dumortier P, Billon-Galland MA, Burdett G, Mitha R, Monso E, Rödelsperger K, Taikina-Aho O, Tuomi T, Vanhala E, Maier EA (2001) The certification of the contents of asbestos fibers in lung tissue (BCR-665 and BCR-666). European Commission, Office for Official Publications of the European Communities, Luxemburg

Tron V, Wright JL, Harrison N, Wiggs B, Churg A (1987) Cigarette smoke makes airway and early parenchymal asbestos-induced lung disease worse in the guinea pig. Am Rev Respir Dis 136:271–275

Tsuchiyama F, Hisanaga N, Shibata E, Aoki T, Takagi H, Ando T, Takeuchi Y (1997) Pulmonary metal distribution in urban dwellers. Int Arch Occup Environ Health 70:77–84

Tuomi T, Oksa P, Anttila S, Taikina-aho O, Taskinen E, Karjalainen A, Tukiainen P (1992) Fibers and asbestos bodies in bronchoalveolar lavage fluids of asbestos sprayers. Br J Ind Med 49:480–485

Vilkman S, Lahdensuo A, Mattila J, Tossavainen A, Tuomi T (1993) Asbestos exposure according to different exposure indices among Finnish lung cancer patients. Int Arch Occup Environ Health 65:269–274

Wagner JC, Pooley FD, Gibbs A, Lyons J, Sheers G, Moncrieff CB (1986) Inhalation of china stone and china clay dusts: relationship between the mineralogy of dust retained in the lungs and pathological changes. Thorax 41:190–196

Wagner JC, Newhouse ML, Corrin B, Rossister CER, Griffiths DM (1988) Correlation between fiber content of the lung and disease in east London asbestos factory workers. Br J Ind Med 45:305–308

Wallaert B, De Vuyst P, Israel-Biet D (1992) Le lavage broncho-alvéolaire. Des aspects techniques aux règles d'interpretation. Rev Mal Respir 9:39–56

Ward C, Fenwick J, Booth H, Walters EH (1997) Albumin is not suitable as a marker of bronchoalveolar lavage dilution in interstitial lung disease. Eur Respir J 10:2029–2033

Warnock ML, Isenberg W (1986) Asbestos burden and the pathology of lung cancer. Chest 89:20–26

Watkins-Pitchford W, Moir J (1916) On the nature of the doubly-refracting particles seen in microscopic sections of silicotic lungs. Rep S African Inst Med Res 1:000–000

Wright RS, Abraham JL, Harber P, Burnett BR, Morris P, West P (2002) Fatal asbestosis 50 years after brief high intensity exposure in a vermiculite expansion plant. Am J Respir Crit Care Med 165:1145–1149

3.5 Immunological Methods

Gabriel Reboux, Nadine Magy, and Jean-Charles Dalphin

CONTENTS

3.5.1 Immunological Diagnosis of Hypersensitivity Pneumonitis 133
3.5.1.1 Antigen 139
3.5.1.1.1 Antigen Type 139
3.5.1.1.2 Nature of Microbe Antigens 140
3.5.1.1.3 Nature of Avian Antigens 140
3.5.1.2 Choice of Micro-Organisms Involved in HP for Producing Antigens 141
3.5.1.3 Serological Methods 142
3.5.1.3.1 Methods Demonstrate Presence or Absence of Precipitins (Semi-Quantitative Method) 142
3.5.1.3.2 Methods Produce Results as a Level of Antibodies (Quantitative Methods) 144
3.5.1.3.3 Methods Revealing Bands from Several Immunoglobulins 144
3.5.1.4 Limits and Diagnostic Value of the Tests 145
3.5.1.4.1 Diagnostic Value of the Tests 145
3.5.1.4.2 Durability of Antibody Response 146
3.5.1.5 Technical Considerations and Choices 146
3.5.1.5.1 Fine or Crude Antigens? 146
3.5.1.5.2 Spore or Mycelium Antigens? 146
3.5.1.5.3 Accuracy of Techniques 146
3.5.1.5.4 Choice of Isotypes 147
3.5.1.6 Conclusion 147
3.5.2 Immunological Diagnosis of Berylliosis 148
3.5.2.1 General Considerations 148
3.5.2.2 Immunological Diagnosis 149
3.5.2.2.1 Development of Laboratory Methods and Current Status of the BeLPT 149
3.5.2.2.2 Genetic Testing and Future Directions 150
3.5.3 Immunological Diagnosis for Interstitial Lung Diseases Associated with Collagen-Vascular Disorders 151
3.5.3.1 Systemic Sclerosis 151
3.5.3.1.1 Definition (Gilliland 2001a) 151
3.5.3.1.2 Pathophysiology 151
3.5.3.1.3 Pulmonary Involvement 151
3.5.3.1.4 Immunological Diagnosis 151
3.5.3.1.5 Association Between SSc and Silica Dust 152
3.5.3.2 Rheumatoid Arthritis 152
3.5.3.2.1 Definition (Lipsky 2001) 152
3.5.3.2.2 Pathophysiology 152
3.5.3.2.3 Pulmonary Involvement 152
3.5.3.2.4 Immunological Diagnosis (Schumacher et al. 2003) 152
3.5.3.2.5 Association Between Rheumatoid Arthritis and Silicosis 152
3.5.3.3 Mixed Connective Tissue Disease 152
3.5.3.3.1 Definition (Sharp 1994) 152
3.5.3.3.2 Pathophysiology 152
3.5.3.3.3 Pulmonary Involvement 153
3.5.3.3.4 Immunological Diagnosis 153
3.5.3.4 Sjögren's Syndrome 153
3.5.3.4.1 Definition (Moutsopoulos 2001) 153
3.5.3.4.2 Pathophysiology 153
3.5.3.4.3 Pulmonary Involvement 153
3.5.3.4.4 Immunological Diagnosis 153
3.5.3.5 Churg and Strauss Syndrome 153
3.5.3.5.1 Definition (Fauci 2001) 153
3.5.3.5.2 Pathophysiology 154
3.5.3.5.3 Pulmonary Involvement 154
3.5.3.5.4 Immunological Diagnosis (Abril et al. 2003) 154
3.5.3.6 Other Auto-Immune Diseases 154
3.5.3.6.1 Polymyositis and Dermatopolymyositis (Dalakas 2001) 154
3.5.3.6.2 Systemic Lupus Erythematosus (Hahn 2001) 154
3.5.3.6.3 Relapsing Polychondritis (Gilliland 2001b) 154
3.6 Conclusion 154
References 155

Immunological methods for diagnosis of occupational and environmental infiltrative lung diseases mainly concern hypersensitivity pneumonitis and berylliosis. Collagen – vascular disorders, which frequently involve lungs, must also been considered as differential diagnoses. Therefore, useful immunological diagnostic tools in these three situations will be described.

3.5.1 Immunological Diagnosis of Hypersensitivity Pneumonitis

Diagnosis of hypersensitivity pneumonitis (HP), or extrinsic allergic alveolitis, has most often relied

G. Reboux, PhD
Department of Mycology and Parasitology, Hôpital Jean Minjoz, Boulevard Fleming, 25030 Besançon cedex, France
N. Magy, MD, PhD
Department of Internal Medicine, Hôpital Jean Minjoz, Boulevard Fleming, 25030 Besançon cedex, France
J.-C. Dalphin, MD
Professor, Department of Respiratory Disease, Hôpital Jean Minjoz, Boulevard Fleming, 25030 Besançon cedex, France

on an array of non-specific clinical symptoms and signs developed in an appropriate setting, with the demonstration of interstitial marking on chest X-rays, lymphocytic alveolitis on bronchoalveolar lavage (BAL), serum precipitins against offending antigens (Ag) and/or a granulomatous reaction on lung biopsies (American Thoracic Society 1998; Patel et al. 2001).

Farmer's lung disease (FLD) is the most common form of HP. The diagnostic value of serological tests in FLD is controversial (Burrel and Rylander 1981; Eduard 1995; Husman et al. 1987). For some authors, serology is a reliable diagnostic tool; whereas for others, it fails to discriminate FLD subjects from healthy exposed subjects and appears to be a mere indicator of exposure (American Thoracic Society 1998; Marx et al. 1978; Cormier et al. 2004). This discrepancy may be due to the choice of antigens and/or the serological techniques applied, to the methodology used, with variations in diagnostic criteria for cases or, more importantly, to the level of exposure for controls.

To compare studies in the same field is very difficult, notably because of the choice of serological techniques – the types of antigens used as well as their quality and origin (Salvaggio 1972; Kaukonen et al. 1994). Despite the same choice of techniques in a long-term retrospective study, the quality of each lot of antigens could not be guaranteed (Cormier et al. 2004; Rask-Andersen 1989; Table 3.5.1).

Bird breeder's lung (BBL), often called pigeon breeder's lung or pigeon fancier's lung, would appear to be the next most frequent form of HP, considerably more frequent wherever bird breeding is commonplace. The relatively good efficacy of serology (Toubas et al. 1995; Mc Sharry et al. 2002; Baldwin et al. 1998), the nature of the antigen involved in this disease and its high specificity with respect to each bird species puts this form of HP in a class of its own (Kokkarinen et al. 1993). A specific comment will be made about it further on in the text.

Other HPs are less frequent and are strongly correlated with specific environmental conditions. In cheese worker's lung, for example, it is difficult to compare workers from the Swiss cheese-making area (Gruyère or Mont d'Or) with workers who produce cheddar or mimolette cheese. Problems are also encountered with mushroom workers who are exposed to different fungal spores (shiitake, pleurotus) involved in mushroom worker's lung disease. However, many of the same moulds or actinomycetes are found in different forms of HP related to agriculture or the food industry (Table 3.5.2).

Table 3.5.1. Four decades of farmer's lung antibodies detection (1962–2004). Subjects: *FLD* farmer's lung disease certain, *FLDp* farmer's lung disease possible, *BFL* bird fancier lung, *HEF* healthy exposed farmer, *Ctrl* unexposed subject, *Pul* patients with pulmonary disease, *Asth* asthmatic patients, *NERC* non-exposed rural controls. Methods: *DD* double diffusion or Ouchterlony test, *IEP* immunoelectrophoresis, *ES* electrosyneresis, *BIDI* bi-dimensionnal electrophoresis, *ELIEDA* electrosyneresis revealed with Ig/peroxydase, *ELISA* enzyme linked immunosorbent assay, *ELIFA* enzyme linked immunosorbent filtration assay, *WB* western-blot. Antigens (Ag): *Mf Micropolyspora faeni* = *Saccharopolyspora rectivirgula*, *Tv Thermoactinomyces vulgaris*, *Tc Thermoactinomyces candidus*, *Ts Thermoactinomyces sacchari*; *Tt Thermoactinomyces talophilus*, *Sv Saccharomonospora viridis*, *St Streptomyces* « mesophilic », *Stt Streptomyces* « thermophilic », *Af Aspergillus fumigatus*, *Au Aspergillus umbrosus*, *Ea Eurotium amstelodami*, *Asp* other *Aspergillus*, *Rh Rhizopus*, *Mu Mucor*, *Ac Abisdia corymbifera*, *Pae Paecilomyces*, *Pen Penicillium*, *Cla Cladosporium*, *Hum Humicola grisea*, *Ws Wallemia sebi*, *Fus Fusarium* sp., *Rho Rhodotorula*, *Fun* other fungi, *HE* hay extract, *SE* silage extract

References	Subjects	Tests	Ag	Conclusions
Aiache et al. (1976) Pathol Biol	3 FLD, 7 BFL, 20 HEF	BIDI IEP	Mf HE	BIDI better than IEP and DD to distinguish FLD from healthy farmers
Aznar et al. (1988) J Clin Microbiol	10 FLD, 10 Ctrl	ES WB	Mf	28 Kd, 49 Kd bands IgA and IgM correlated with disease
Bamdad (1980) Clin Allergy	88 FLD, 80 HEF, 61 Ctrl	ELISA DD	Mf	ELISA is specific and sensitive and allows differentiation of FLD from HEF except for 10 from 80 HEF (false positive)
Brummund et al. (1988) J Allergy Clin Immunol	4 FLD, 3 HEF (same family)	ELISA, IgG, A, M, D, E, BIDI	Mf, Tv, Tc, Sv, Af	High level of all Ig for all FLD with exposure up to 1 year. Serological technique distinguishes FLD from HEF
Cormier et al. (1985) Thorax, Cormier et al. (1989) Thorax	888 HEF, 445 HEF	DD	Mf, Af, Tv	There were 8.4% positive precipitins. In 5 years, 34 remain positive, 14 became negative. A single precipitin-positive farmer correlated with the disease. Of the farmers, 28 initially negative became positive. In all, 13.9% subjects changed precipitin status. Authors concluded a fluctuation of precipitin over time

References	Subjects	Tests	Ag	Conclusions
Cormier et al. (2004) Eur Respir J	27 HEF	?	?	Precipitin only correlated with decrease in forced expiratory volume. No long-term consequences
Dalphin et al. (1994) Allergy	35 FLD, 140 FLDp, 376 Pul, 100 HEF, 20 Ctrl	DD, IEP	HE, Mf	DD unable to distinguish the different groups. Conversely, IEP can distinguish the four groups. Number of arcs correlates with level of exposure
Erkinjuntti-Pekkanen et al. (1999) Allergy	87 FLD, 81 HEF	ELISA IgG	Au, Pen, Ac, Af, Hum, Mf, Tv, Rho	Clearest differences between groups obtained, in order of effectiveness: Absidia, Mf, Tv and Rh. glutinis
Fasani et al. (1987) Ann All	58 FLDp	ELISA IgG,M DD/ IEP/BIDI isofocusing electrophoresis	Mf	ELISA has a good specificity and sensitivity. ELISA level in correlation with DD results. Cut-off obtained in reference to DD threshold
Gangwar et al. (1991) Antonie Van Leeuwenhoek	112 HEF	ELISA	Mf, Sv, Ts, Tv, Tt	With Mf, 25% positive; 3% with Sv, 1.5% with T. talophilus: discrepancy with microbiological results (Sv 56%, Tv and T. Talophilus 5% Mf 5%)
Gari et al. (1982) Mycopath, Gari et al. (1984) Sem Hop Paris, Gari et al. (1986) Clin Allergy	10 FLD, 17 FLD, 60 HEF, 185Ctrl, 24FLD, 1376 Ctrl	IEP, ES	Mf, HE	Electrosyneresis: greater efficacy than IEP. Chymotrypsic arc is inconstant in FLD. Level of precipitins not correlated to the severity of disease. More IgG present using HES. When serology shows presence of chymotrypsic arc + IgG + other Ig, FLD is more likely
Gariepy et al. (1989) Am Rev Respir Dis	33 HEF	DD	Mf, Tv, Af	For this 7-year survey, numerous variations between positive and negative precipitin status was seen in the HEF group. Only one subject developed the disease. Author concludes that precipitins and lymphocytes in BAL have no diagnostic value
Gruchow et al. (1981) Am Rev Respir Dis	1400 HEF	DD	Mf, Tv, Af, Sv, Tc, Ts, HE	Of HEF, 10% have precipitins; not all FLD patients are positive. Rainfall, crop type and tobacco composition decrease the level of precipitins. Conversely, precipitin levels enhanced by size of farm, number of cattle and hay volume
Gump et al. (1979) Respiration	258 FLD, 125 Pul_1, 27 Pul_2, 115 $Ctrl_1$, 76 $Ctrl_2$	DD, IF	Mf, Tv	Of HEF, 5.4% are positive to Mf, 1.2% to Tv. Of patients with fibrosis, 5.6% are positive to Mf, 14.4% to Tv. DD is more effective than immunofluorescence
Homma et al. (1986) Respiration	442 HEF, 94 Ctrl	ES	Mf, Tv	Precipitin level reflects number of hours of daily farm work and volume of hay used
Huizinga and Berrens (1985) Clin Allergy	18 FLD, 19 HEF, 29 Ctrl	ELISA IgG,A,M, Rast IgE, DD	Mf	No difference IgM or IgE level found between FLD and HEF. Author concludes necessity to use IgG and IgA against Mf for FLD serology
Husman et al. (1987) Eur J Resp	2440 HEF	DD	Mf, Tv, Af, Au	Demonstrated that 18% of FLD, 8% of HEF and 10% of bronchitis patients have precipitins to one of four Ag tested. Tv is the antigen most correlated to FLD, however, Aspergillus umbrosus is the Ag most present in farms
Iranitalab et al. (1989) Allergy	25 FLD, 31 FLDp, 14 HEF, 13 Ctrl	WB	Mf	FLD gave 12-, 25- and, 60-Kd bands in IgG, IgM, IgA, sometimes 15–62 Kd bands but HEF have similar results. HEF react more variably to 11-, 25- and 60-Kd Ag. No correlation found between disease and all Ig tested
Katila et al.(1978) Clin Allergy	22 FLD, 26 FLDp, 325 HEF, 80 Ctrl	DD	Mf, Tv, Af	DD is a less sensitive method. Finnish farmers reacts poorly with Mf. Author asks why urban controls react massively against Tv Ag and where this sensitivity to Tv comes from

References	Subjects	Tests	Ag	Conclusions
Katila et al. (1986a) Clin Allergy (1986b) Am J Ind Med	325 HEF, 107 Ctrl	DD	Mf, Tv, Af, Au	In 6-year follow-up, level fluctuation represented 25%. Level for Mf Ag and Au Ag higher in HEF than in NERC. Ag level similar for HEF and NERC. Level of Tv HEF much lower than for NERC group
Katila and Mäntyjärvi (1987) Eur J Respir	292 HEF	DD	Mf, Tv, Af	Higher level of precipitins found (1) in older subjects (2) in women with respect to related to feeding time in the stable
Kaukonen et al. (1993) Clin Exp Allergy	57 FLD, 10 HEF, 10 Ctrl	ELISA, WB	Au	High specificity of IgG manane and mamoprotein fraction of *A. umbrosus*. Cross-reaction due to presence of polysaccharoside in fungal wall
Kaukonen et al. (1994) Clin Exp Immunol	12 FLD, 12 HEF, 5 Ctrl	ELISA	Au	Higher level IgG antibodies for FLD than controls. Levels maintained 1 year with slight decrease or increase if re-exposure
Kumar et al. (1993) Int Arch Allergy	7 FLD, 8 HEF	WB, ELISA, DD	Mf	FLD gave numerous IgG bands (28, 35, 60, 65 Kd and four components above100 Kd with a monoclonal Ag
Kurup et al. (1984) Mol Immunol	?	WB	Mf	16-, 29-, 51-Kd fractions are correlated with FLD
Kurup et al. (1987a) Diag Clin Immunol	?	WB	Mf	45-, 55-, 60-Kd are correlated with FLD, treatment management possible in relation to antibody study
Kurup et al. (1997b) Mycopathologia	69 FLD, 28 Ctrl	ELISA (biotine-avidine)	Mf, Tc, Tv, Sv, Af, Pen, Au	US FLD patients reacted more than Finnish patients with MF. Finnish patients reacted more with Tv. FLD patients from four countries reacted with Tc. Authors give an exposure value to the Tc levels but not a diagnostic value alone
Kusaka et al. (1989) Am Rev Respir Dis	92 HEF	ES (agar)	Mf	A 6-year follow-up demonstrates some fluctuation of antibody levels (18.5% positive in 1979 and 19.6% in 1984). Tobacco consumption decreases levels of antibodies. Oldest farmers and long-term exposure farmers are negative with Mf Ag, except farmers with FLD. Cellular immunity evolve in same way. No correlation with the duration of hay feeding
Lappaleinen et al. (1998) Ann Allergy Asthma Immunol	24 FLD, 19 Asth, 20 HEF, IgG+, 20 HEF, IgG-,16 Ctrl	ELIFA, ELISA	Ac, Af, Au, Hum Mf Rh Tv Ws 2Fus	Increase of IgG in FLD and chronic bronchitis patients and in some HEF with 10^4 ufc/m3 or higher concentration of microorganisms in hay. Half-life of IgG antibodies, few weeks. Cross-reaction between species. IgG considered as exposure marker
Larsson et al. (1988) Int Arch Allergy Appl Immunol	10 HEF, 25 Ctrl	DD, ELISA	Pen, Cla, Af Botrytis, Pullularia, Pae	Positive correlation between level of antibodies from Paecilomyces, Af and Penicillium Ag and the number of lymphocytes
Marcer et al. (1983) Clin Allergy	36 FLD, 39 Pul, 113 Asth, 131 HEF	Cutaneous tests (10Ag), DD, ES, IEP	Mf, Tv, Af Acremonium, Cryptostroma, Pullularia, Trichoderma	Precipitins always present in the acute phase. FLD positive with Mf 22%, Tv 2%

References	Subjects	Tests	Ag	Conclusions
MARX et al. (1978) J Allergy Clin Immunol	40 HEF precipitin +	ELISA	Mf, Tv, Tc, Ts, Sv, Af, 3 Asp	Precipitins present in 38% of FLD, 12% of FLDp and 50% of HEF
MELINN and MCLAUGHLIN (1989) Ir J Med Sci	?	ELISA, ES	Mf	Precipitins present in 25% of FLD
MUNDT et al. (1996) J Allergy Clin Immunol	? FLD, ? Ctrl	WB, dot blot, Polyacrylic, BIDI	Mf	IgG2 correlated with FLD. HEF and blood donors give no IgG2 level but only IgG. IgG does not distinguish FLD from controls
OJANEN et al. (1980) Allergy	17 FLD, 18 HEF, 20 Ctrl	ELISA, DD	Mf, Tv, Af	FLD gave higher levels than HEF and Ctrl with the three Ag. Somatic antigens much better than metabolic antigens
OJANEN et al. (1982) Allergy	30 FLD	ELISA, DD	Af, Au	More specificity for Au Ag than Af. Cross-reactions between these two aspergillus Ag compounds are influenced by the quality of the Ag, which is influenced by culture conditions
OJANEN et al. (1987) Eur J Respir Dis	13 FLD	ELISA IgG, G3, G4	Au, Af, Tv, Mf	IgG3 and IgG4 present in FLD patients tested with TvAg. Only Mf found for Ag IgG3. For Au, IgG3 was present in 2/3 of cases and IgG4 in 1/2 of cases
OJANEN (1992)Br J Ind Med	24 FLD, 24 HES (spouses)	ELISA IgG,M,A,E	Au, Af, Tv, Mf	A serological interpretation was proposed: presence of IgA against Af Ag concomitant with presence of IgG against Tv Ag may be correlated with the disease
PEPYS et al. (1962) Thorax	FLD, Pul, HEF Ctrl, rabit sera	DD	11 HE, Af, Muc, Cla, Hum	Moist hay, Mucor species and A. fumigatus are incriminated on the basis of precipitin response. Actinomycetes was initially remote as FLD cause on the basis of its low responsiveness (18%)
PEPYS et al. (1963) Lancet	?	DD, IEP	Muc, Af, Cla, HE, Mf, Tv	Mf and Tv produced FL Ag, which can induce FLD
PEPYS and JENKINS (1965) Thorax	205 FLD, 532 Ctrl, (asthma, sarcoidosis)	DD, IEP	Muc, Af, Mf, Tv	Of FLD patients, 89% are positive against Mf Ag, 50% for other FLD exposed on plants other than hay. Further, 18% of HEF were positive, 15% of asthma patients and 21% of patients with other pulmonary diseases
PEPYS (1969) Monographie	?	BIDI, Rocket	Af, 3Asp, Fun	Cross-reactivity was found with five fungal Ag (from 19% to 35% of common antigenic compounds)
PEPYS (1994) ACI News	10 FLD1, 61 FLD2, 50 HES, 250 Pul1, 654 Pul2, 205 FLD3	DD, IEP	2 HE, Af, Cla, Pen, Muc, Hum, Mf	All FLD patients have precipitins to one of eight Ag used to test. Per Ag responsiveness varies from 6% to 52% of the 61 FLD tested. For the second group of FLD patients tested (n=205) serological responsiveness went from 87% to 91% positiveness, but 49% of this group were not in an acute phase of the disease. Cross-reaction present. IEP less sensitive than DD but also specific
RASK-ANDERSEN (1989) Uppsala J Med Sci	21 FLD 17 FLDp, Retrospective study on 20 years (n=6267)	DD	Mf tv af Alt, Bot, Cla, Pae Muc Pen, Rh, Pul	Of FLD patients, 68% have precipitins against 4 Ag for 11 tested on average. In descending order, the most reactive Ag are: Rh, Pae, Mucor, Mf and Af. Tv in one case only
RAUTALAHTI et al. (1990) Ann Allergy	91 HEF, 90 Ctrl	ELISA IgG	Mf, Tv, Af, Au	IgG level is higher in December using HEF than Ctrl. Specific IgG against A. umbrosus Ag decreases in April (year with a good crop season)

References	Subjects	Tests	Ag	Conclusions
Reboux (2001a) Am J Respir Crit Care Med	15 FLD, 15 HEF, 30 Ctrl	Es, DD, ELISA, WB	Ac, Ea, Ws, Mf	ES and DD are more effective with the offending antigen to distinguish patients from controls. No evidence to obtain effectiveness cut-off for ELISA IgG. Impossible to obtain specific bands correlated to the disease with WB. IgA do not seem related to the disease
Reboux et al. (2001b) Am J Respir Crit Care Med	11 FLD, 11 HEF, 22 Ctrl	ES, DD	Ac, Ea, Ws, Af, Asp, St, Stt, Mf HE, SE	Most effective to distinguish patients from HEF and controls in descending order are Ac Ag, Ec Ag and to a lesser degree Ws Ag. Other Ag do not distinguish patients from controls. Thresholds are different for each antigen. Specificity with Ac Ag by ES is 100% and 80% sensitivity
Recco et al. (1978) Bull SFMM	402 Pul	DD, IEP	7 HE, Mf, Tv, Sv	Of patients with pulmonary disease, 12% have precipitins. Of these, half were FLD patients, and half were HEF with pulmonary problems
Roberts et al. (1976) J Allergy Clin Immunol	1045 HEF	DD	Mf, Tv, Sv, Asp	Of farmers, 8.9% have precipitins, including 68% against Mf Ag, 7.5% against Tv Ag and 17% against both. Age has no influence, but exposure to grain silo increases the level of IgG in those with chronic bronchitis
Roussel et al. (2004) OEM	5 FLD, 5 HEF	ES	Ac, Ea, Ws	Precipitins were sought in FLD patients and HEF at the beginning and end of winter. Levels fluctuated for both groups but remained above the threshold required for FLD diagnosis for the FLD group
Scribner et al. (1980) Clin Allergy	443 FLDp, 339 BFL, 944 other HP, 1072 Ctrl	DD	Mf, Tv, Af, pigeon serum	High level of precipitins against Mf Ag and Tv Ag present in industrial environment. Farmers: 8% positive precipitins against Af Ag, 13% against Mf Ag and 6% against Tv Ag. Controls were positive in only 3% of one of the tested antigens
Solal-Céligny et al. (1982) Am Rev Respir Dis	7 FLD, 10 HEF(Mf+), 10 HEF(Mf–)	?	Mf, Af, Tv	Very good correlation between presence of precipitins and high level of lymphocytes in BAL for cases in acute phase of the disease. All FLD were not positive with the three Ag tested, but may have been with other Ag
Stokes et al. (1981) Clin Allergy	33 FLD, 33 HEF, 33 Ctrl	IgG, G1, 2, 3, 4 dosages	Mf	All farmers produced IgG and IgG1, but FLD produced more IgG3
Terho et al. (1987) Eur J Respir Dis	54 FLD	DD	Mf, Tv, Af, Au	100% sensitivity for FLD. Of farmers, 8.6% are positive. A. umbrosus and T. vulgaris are the most present Ag
Treuhaft et al. (1979) Am Rev Respir Dis	12 FLD, 16 HEF, (Mf+)	BIDI	Mf	The authors found 36 peaks for FLD, with 3 specific for the disease, and 10 peaks related to other exposure
Vohlonen (1987) Eur J Respir Dis	2530 HEF	DD	Mf, Tv, Af, Au	Of farmers, 11% were positive at one of the 4 Ag tested -- 7% against Au, 2% against Af, 2.5% against Mf
Wardrop et al. (1977) Br J Ind Med	11 FLD, 14 HEF1, 13 HEF2	DD, IEP	Mf and 59 Ag	The authors used 60 Ag. Response against HES induced doubt as to the usefulness of this test for FLD diagnosis. FLD related more to more in relation to Mf
Wenzel et al. (1974) Am Rev Respir Dis	1122 FLDp	?	Mf, Tv, Sv, Ts	Of FLDp, 10% were positive. Half of these were sensitive against Mf Ag. Several cases of sensitivity against Mf and Sv were seen

Table 3.5.2. Some causes of hypersensitivity pneumonitis (adapted from Yi 2002). *MDI* diphenylmethane diisocyanate; *TDI* toluene diisocyanate, *TMA* trimetallic anhydride, *HP* hypersensitivity pneumonitis

Disease	Main source of antigen	(Probable) antigen
Vegetable products, Farmer's lung disease	Mouldy hay	Thermophilic actinomycetes, *Saccharopolyspora rectivirgula, Thermoactinomyces vulgaris*, Fungi
Bagassosis (bagasse)	Mouldy pressed sugar cane	Thermophilic actinomycetes, *Thermoactinomyces sacchari, T. vulgaris*
Mushroom workers' disease	Mouldy compost	Thermophilic actinomycetes ? Mushroom spores
Suberosis	Mouldy cork	*Penicillium* spp
Malt workers' lung	Contaminated barley	Aspergillus clavatus
Maple bark disease	Contaminated maple logs	Cryptostroma corticale
Sequoiosis	Contaminated wood dust	*Graphium* spp, *pullularia* spp
Wood pulp workers' disease	Contaminated wood pulp	*Alternaria* spp
Humidifier lung	Contaminated humidifiers, air conditioners, dehumidifiers	Thermophilic actinomycetes, Fungi, Amoebas
Cheese washers' disease	Cheese casings	*Penicillium* spp
Wood trimmers' disease	Contaminated wood trimmings	*Rhizopus* spp, *Mucor* spp, *Penicillium* spp
Cephalosporium HP	Contaminated basement (sewage)	Cephalosporium
Sauna takers's disease	Sauna water	*Pulluluria* spp
Detergent workers' disease	Detergent	*Bacillus subtilis*, enzymes
Paprika splitters' lung	Paprika dust	*Mucor stolonifer*
Japanese summer HP	Contaminated houses, walls	Trichosporon cutaneum
Familial HP	Contaminated wood dust in walls	Bacillus subtilis
Domestic HP	Contaminated organic materials	Fungi
Animal products		
Pigeon breeders' disease	Pigeon droppings	Altered pigeon serum (probably IgA)
Duck fever	Duck feathers	Duck proteins
Turkey handlers' disease	Turkey products	Turkey proteins
Laboratory workers' HP	Rat fur	Male rat urine
Pituitary snuff takers's disease	Pituitary powder	Bovine and porcine proteins
Mollusc shell HP	Mollusc shell	Mollusc proteins
Insect products		
Millers' lung	Wheat weevils	Sitophilus granarius
Cheese worker lung	Cheese	Acarus siro
Chemical products		
TDI HP	TDI	Altered proteins (albumin+others)
TMA HP	TMA	Altered proteins
MDI HP	MDI	Altered proteins
Epoxy resin lung	Heated epoxy resin	Phthalic anhydride
Pyrethrum HP	Insecticide spray	

Fungi are clearly involved in domestic-related HP. Moreover, it should be mentioned that these HPs, in which the role of bacterial antigens other than actinomycetes (*Klebsiella* or *Mycobacteria*) is probably underestimated, need to be investigated in future environmental studies.

3.5.1.1 Antigen

3.5.1.1.1 Antigen Type

The importance of antigens in the diagnosis of HP is frequently underestimated. The quality of the antigen preparation might have a significant effect on the specificity and sensitivity of diagnostic tests (Kim et al. 1979). Varying degrees of cross-reactivity have been shown among micro-organism species (Salvaggio 1991, 1997). Conversely, in numerous studies comparing microbiological environmental data to the immunological response for exposed workers, not all antigens react favourably (Dutkiewicz et al. 2001, 2002; Moran et al. 2002; Miyazaki et al. 2004; Flandes et al. 2004). In addition, an increasing number of potentially new antigen sources for which commercial extracts are not available are being identified (Lappalainen et al. 1998; Dalphin et al. 2000). There are few standardised antigen products available because of the difficulties inherent to manufacturing and standardising fungal and bacterial extracts (Ramasamy et al. 1987; Reese et al. 1989; Melinn and McLaughlin 1992; Horner et al. 1995; Mundt et al. 1996). In fact, only crude antigens for infrequent or new aetiologies are produced by diagnostic centres themselves and used for HP diagnosis (Esch 2004).

The three types of crude antigens are:

- Total crude extracts from crude sample materials (hay, corn, water from humidifiers, oil from metalworking, food products such as cheese and salami, glass fiber, dust mites, rat excrement, chemical products). For BBL, droppings and feathers are either produced by each centre or, for common antigens, purchased from a manufacturer (e.g. FSK Avian Immunodiffusion system, Microgen Bioproducts, Camberley, UK). Pure or diluted bird sera are also used for BBL diagnosis without transformation.
- Somatic antigens (also called "surface antigens" or "soluble antigens") from bacterial, actinomycetes or pure fungal culture. A crude antigen including the micro-organism itself is obtained by cultivation on solid media on Petri dishes (spores present) or on shacked liquid broth (mycelium predominant).
- Metabolic antigens from the broth of bacterial, actinomycetes or pure fungal culture without micro-organisms.

Somatic and metabolic extracts are formed by a patchwork of numerous individual antigens (approximately 60 for some yeasts or moulds). Ojanen and colleagues found that the somatic antigens of fungi gave more positive results than the metabolic antigens. The opposite was true for actinomycetes. These authors recommend using either a somatic antigen or a combination of somatic and metabolic antigens for routine enzyme-linked immunosorbent assay (ELISA) tests (Ojanen et al. 1980).

The development of recombinant antigens concerns allergy tests, and, to a lesser extent, HP diagnosis.

- As we know, only *Aspergillus* and *Saccharopolyspora* recombinant purified antigens have been used to diagnose HP (Kumar et al. 1993; Kaukonen et al. 1993) and allergic bronchopulmonary aspergillosis (ABPA) (Moss 2002). No particular fraction has been correlated with HP diseases; hence, the development of small antigen fractions does not appear useful to diagnose HP. Further investigation may well change this notion in the future.

3.5.1.1.2 Nature of Microbe Antigens

The nature of microbe antigen compounds is rarely given. Some enzymatic functions are characterised as protease, oxidase, catalase or chymotrypsinase in some species (*Aspergillus fumigatus* or *Alternaria*) (Roberts et al. 1976; Latge 1999). The biochemical nature of antigens is defined as either a glycoprotein or a polysaccharidic compound. Hence, in summer-type HP fever in Japan, a high-weight polysaccharidic compound, extracted from a *Trichosporon cutaneum* yeast, may be responsible for immunological response (Trentin et al. 1988). It is true that certain glycoproteic complex antigen compounds are partially or totally shared by numerous mould antigens. Up to now, their presence has always been assessed by rough precipitin, double immuno-diffusion (DD) or electrophoresis techniques: precipitin arcs indicate totally or partially immunological identity (either a continuous line between two arcs indicating total identity or the presence of a forked arc indicating partial identity). However, this compound is not characterised or matched with a protein control with a known molecular weight. Using the Western blot (WB) technique, Ag characteristics are often only summarised as a fraction with a molecular weight in kilodaltons and not compared together (Edwards 1972).

3.5.1.1.3 Nature of Avian Antigens

In pigeon droppings, numerous Ag have been found – essentially gamma globulins, which are very antigenic. Hydrolytic and esterolytic enzymes Ag properties have also been found; they may play an important role in the pathogenesis of the disease by increasing the inflammatory process on the alveoli wall. However, intestinal mucin seems to be the principal antigenic compound of BBL (Baldwin et al. 1998). This substance is a high-molecular-weight glycoprotein, only slightly biodegradable (Boyd et al. 1982) and assumed to be the best antigen for BBL serology (Todd et al. 1993).

3.5.1.2 Choice of Micro-Organisms Involved in HP for Producing Antigens

Pepys opened Pandora's box four decades ago (Pepys 1994). Numerous microorganisms, if the length of their spore or bacteria is less than 4 μm, are able to induce HP. Their immunological capacity to induce disease and antibody reactions is probably widely shared by all micro-organism species. Some publications give cumulative lists of aetiological agents (Table 3.5.2) without taking long-term validity or the modification of environmental circumstances into account. Certain professional and personal settings or practices, such as round baling crops, air-conditioned dwellings, Jacuzzis and do-it-yourself wood joinery, are modifying exposure in terms of the level and kind of microorganisms involved in HP. This evolution implies the need for regular re-evaluation of those micro-organisms that may be useful for serology diagnosis.

In the past decade, new aetiologies of HP have been described in the field of agriculture. Although the relative humidity of hay or grain crops has been seen to decrease with better agricultural practice and education about biohazards, this change, paradoxically, does not imply a decrease in the frequency of the disease but the discovery of new species that require less humidity.

As the microbiological flora of mouldy hay varies widely from one country to another, the antigens for serological studies should be selected on the basis of specific local species (Kurup et al. 1987).

Despite recent reports describing "new" antigens in FLD [*Absidia corymbifera, Humicola grisea, Penicillium brevicompactum* and *Rhodotorula glutinis* (Erkinjutti-Pekkanen et al. 1999); *A. corymbifera, Eurotium amstelodami* and *Wallemia sebi* (Reboux et al. 2001a,b)], it is not always possible to perform environmental microbiological analyses prior to selecting the appropriate antigens to use in serological tests for each patient. What is needed in routine serology is a standard panel of Ag for each professional or domestic activity. The choices of today are not universal and should evolve to take into account human activity, professional practice and the geographic area where patients come from. Proposals from three centres – the National Jewish Medical & Research Centre (http://nationaljewish.org), the Occupational Health Centre Kuopio (Dr. M. Reiman) and the experience of our department (University Hospital of Besançon, Parasitology Mycology Laboratory, Besançon) are given in Table 3.5.3.

Table 3.5.3. Choice of screening panel antigens extracts involved in hypersensitivity pneumonitis (HP) for serology tests without specific microbiologic or activity information about patient environment. *Centre I NJMRC* National Jewish Medical & Research Center, *Centre II OHCK* Finnish Institute of Occupational Health (Kuopio), *Centre III UHB* University Hospital of Besançon, *Z* For HP screening in centre I

HP types	Farmer's lung			Food workers			Timber and wood workers			Bird breeder's lung			Domestic HP		
Centres	I	II	III	I	II	III	I	II	III	I	II	III	I	II	III
S. rectivirgula	x	x	x		x								x		
T. vulgaris	x	x	x										x		
Streptomyces (mesophilic)			x												
Streptomyces (thermophilic)			x						x						
Absidia corymbifera		x	x											x	
Mucor					x	x								x	
Eurotium		x	x												
Wallemia		x	x												
Rhodotorula		x				x			x					x	
Penicillium		x			x	x		x	x					x	
Aspergillus fumigatus	x	x	x		x	x		x	x					x	
Aspergillus polyvalent	x														
Candida	z			z			z			z			z		
Aureobasidium	x			z		x	z		x	z			x		
Other moulds					x			x	x					x	x
Mites					x	x									
Crop product: hay, grain, oats, soy...	x	x	x												
sawdust, dust								x	x						x
Chicken, rat, mouse serum	x														
Avian sera and droppings (pigeon)	z			z			z			x	x	x	z	x	
Exotic bird (Budgerigar, parrot, canary)										x	x	x			

Antigens from patient environment (total extracts and microorganism extracts): for all unusual situations for the three centres

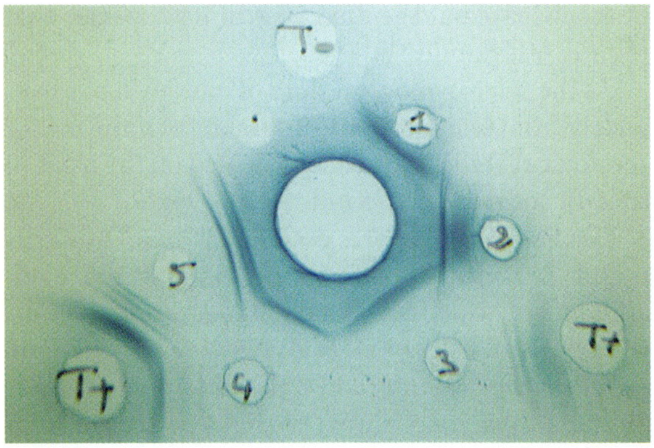

Fig. 3.5.1. Double diffusion plate. One to five wells filled with five different Bird antigens. *Central well* patient sera, *T-* negative control sera, *T+* positive control sera. (Photo G. Reboux)

3.5.1.3 Serological Methods

More than ten serological tests and numerous variants have been used to identify and quantify specific antibodies. DD, immunoelectrophoresis (IEP) and electrosyneresis (ES), with some variants and immunoenzymatic tests (ELISA), have been widely used to evaluate humoral immune response in patients with HP. WB has been used more recently to seek any specific antibody response correlated with the disease; no results have been obtained as yet. Some authors have given a highly complex formula with combined results coming from different antigens and different immunoglobulins (IgG, IgA) (Ojanen 1992). Bi-dimensional immunoelectrophoresis (BIDI) has been used to dissociate immunological response for any antigen in multiple signals (peaks). Efficacy was limited by the excessive quantity of serum needed to test one antigen (>1 ml). The efficacy and limits of each method will be commented on in section 3.5.1.4.

3.5.1.3.1 Methods Demonstrate Presence or Absence of Precipitins (Semi-Quantitative Method)

Serum precipitins are antibodies that form visible lines of precipitated glycoprotein when they encounter their specific antigen in an agarose gel or on an acetate cellulose sheet. The chemical nature of precipitins is still unknown. Precipitins are usually, but not exclusively, of the IgG or IgM antibody class and result from exposure of the patient's immune system to the antigen. The number of precipitin lines reflects the intensity of the immune response to one or more components present in a given antigen.

3.5.1.3.1.1 Ouchterlony Test or DD

Since the end of 1950s, the Ouchterlony method (Ouchterlony 1953) has been widely used with a large variety of antigen-antibody systems: bacteria, moulds, yeasts and other organic material with antigenic properties. The fact that the Ouchterlony method is of low cost and is easy to use and to reproduce explains the long-term use of this technique.

Procedure

On a glass plate, serum (300 µl) from each subject is placed in the large central well cut in 0.9% agar gel in a diethylmalonylurea sodium-buffered solution, pH=8.2. The smaller surrounding wells are filled with different antigens. After 48 h at room temperature, (time needed for passive diffusion between serum and antigens), the plate is washed with a 5% sodium citrate solution for 4 h to dissolve the C-reactive protein present in most sera, then with physiological water for 48 h to rinse the plate. The agar on the glass plate is covered with a filter sheet, desiccated under a fan (4 h) and then stained with amidoschwartz.

The number of arcs is counted for each antigen under a lighted magnifier.

3.5.1.3.1.2 ES [Countercurrent Immunoelectrophoresis or Immunoelectrodiffusion]

Two variants exist: one uses agar gel (Flaherty et al. 1974); the other uses a sheet of cellulose acetate and lasts 4 h (Gari et al. 1982) (Fig. 3.5.2).

Procedure

ES is performed with an ES apparatus on cellulose acetate sheet (Sartorius, Goettingen, Germany). After 10 min in a bath of buffered Tris glycine solution, 6 cellulose acetate sheets are immersed in a buffered Tris glycine solution, pH=8.8, and then soft-dried between 2 filter papers and placed in the electrophoresis vat filled with buffered Tris glycine solution, pH=8.8. Next, 15 µl of each serum are placed on three spots on the anode side, and a 15-µl line of antigen is placed on the cathode side. A 110-V current is applied for 2 h 15 min. After washing, the cellulose acetate sheets are stained with Coomassie blue.

3.5.1.3.1.3
Enzyme-linked Immunoelectrodiffusion Assay

Enzyme-linked immunoelectrodiffusion assay (ELIEDA) is a variant that combines ES and immunoblotting. This technique consists of revealing bands obtained using ES on an acetate cellulose membrane, with several anti-human globulins (IgG, IgM, IgA or IgE) (Aznar et al. 1988).

3.5.1.3.1.4
Immunoelectrophoresis

IEP is done in two phases (Williams and Grabar 1955). First, the antigen (15 µl) is separated on 1% agar plate using electrophoresis in an electrophoresis vat containing a diethylmalonylurea sodium-buffered solution, pH=8.75 (110 V for 2 h). The second phase consists of passive diffusion (48 h) between the serum (200 ml) placed in a trough cut into the gel along the zone where the antigens were separated using electrophoresis. After washing and staining, the arcs are enumerated. This process takes 5 days (Fig. 3.5.3).

The IEP test was considered by Pepys and generally by several other biologists as a less sensitive but more discriminating method than the DD test. This technique is widely used in routine diagnosis of several fungal diseases (aspergillosis, candidiasis) and often used in BBL diagnosis (Pepys 1994).

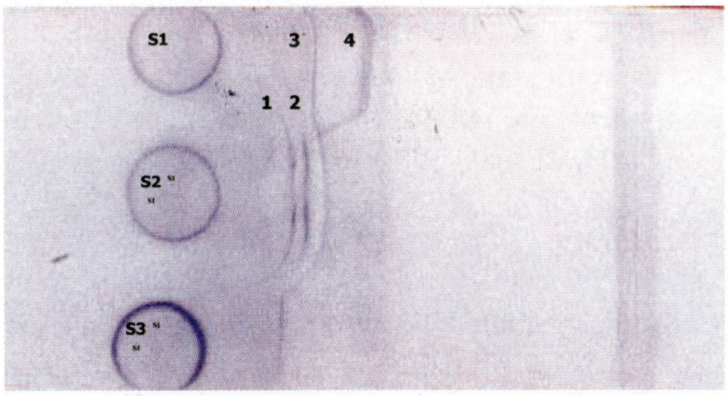

Fig. 3.5.2. Electrosyneresis on cellulose acetate. *Blue line* Ag line, *S1, S2, S3* three patients sera. *S1* 2 arcs; *S2* 3 arcs; *S3* 1 arc. Arc n°3 from S1 is composed of the same compound as arcs on S2 and S3 (*continuous line*). Arc n°4 has no common compound with those from S2. Note the sharp angle at the end of arc n°4. (Photo G. Reboux)

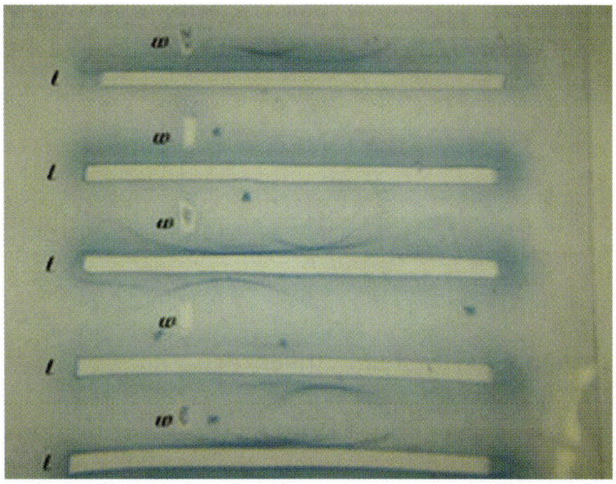

Fig. 3.5.3. Immunoelectrophoresis plate. [*W* five wells for different antigens (Ag); *T* five troughs for sera]. Electrophoresis phase deposits Ag from left to right. Second phase: sera diffuse from the trough towards the Ag line and form arcs. (Photo G. Reboux)

3.5.1.3.1.5
BIDI or Crossed Immunoelectrophoresis

Here, a double electrophoresis is performed: first, it is done as in the first phase of IEP, then a second time at 90° through an agar gel containing the subject's serum. Finally, after staining, many peaks are obtained for each sera (Axelsen 1973).

As each test needs up to 1 ml of serum, this serological test can be used with only immunised animals for the study of antigenic compounds involved in HP (Treuhaft et al. 1979; Pavesi et al. 1984; Brummund et al. 1988; Ylönen et al. 1989; Fig, 3.5.4).

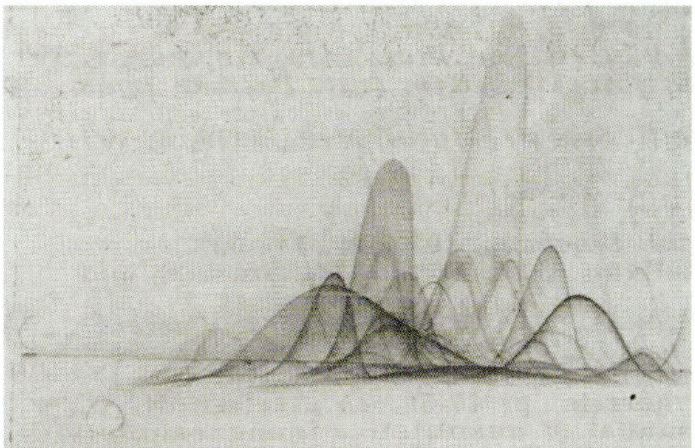

Fig. 3.5.4. Bi-dimensional electrophoresis. *Arrow 1* indicates the first direction of the electrophoresis; *arrow 2* indicates the second. (Photo G. Reboux)

For 1 arc obtained using DD, it is often possible to obtain 2 or 3 arcs by IEP, 3–12 arcs by ES and more than 20 peaks by BIDI.

3.5.1.3.2 Methods Produce Results as a Level of Antibodies (Quantitative Methods)

3.5.1.3.2.1 Enzyme-Linked Immunosorbent Assay

ELISA (Engwall and Perlman 1971) uses antibody systems able to release a chromogen substance. The "sandwich technique" is the most commonly used variant. The Ag is first coated on a solid surface - often, plastic wells of a microplate. The antibodies (Ab) present in the serum are then bound with the Ag. Finally, the Ab–Ag complex is both bound with an anti-human immunoglobulin conjugate able to bind with it and combined with an enzyme, which when it reacts with a chromogenic substrate, releases a coloured compound. The intensity of coloration, which is proportional to Ab concentration, is read by a spectrometer. Results are expressed as an optical density or with a reference to a pooled sera and expressed as arbitrary units (Fig. 3.5.5).

(an example of one procedure)

The wells of flat-bottom microtitre plates are coated with 200 µl of 1 µg/ml antigen solution in 50 mmol/l K_2HPO_4 buffer, pH 8.5 at 4°C for 72 h. Excess binding sites are blocked at 37°C for 1 h with 250 µl of 50 mmol/l NaH_2PO_4, containing 0.5% bovine serum albumin and 60 g/l of sorbitol. Next, 100-µl serum samples diluted 1:100 are added in duplicate to all wells (§1). The plates are incubated at 37°C for 1 h, shaken constantly, then washed four times with washing buffer (100 mmol/l Tris-HCl, pH 7.5, containing 0.25% Tween). Then, 100 µl of peroxidase-conjugated goat anti-human IgG diluted or IgA diluted 1:4000 are added to all wells, and the plates are incubated at 37°C for 1 h and shaken constantly (§2). The washing procedure is repeated and 100 µl of 3.3'.5.5' tetramethylbenzidine solution (TMB One-Step Substrate System, Dako, Carpinteria, California) (§2) is added to the wells at room temperature for 10 min. To stop the TMB reaction, 100 µl of an acid solution (a mixture of 1N HCl and 3N H_2SO_4) are added. Wells are read spectrophotometrically at 450 nm, and the results are expressed in optical density (od) (§3).

§1: A preliminary assay must be done to find which dilution of the serum gives the best decrease in optical density. A graph is made to record the best value for each lot of plates with each antigen.

§2: Several other globulins, conjugates (essentially peroxidase and alkaline phosphatase) and chromogen solutions can be used.

§3: Results can be also expressed as a percentage of a pooled reference sera.

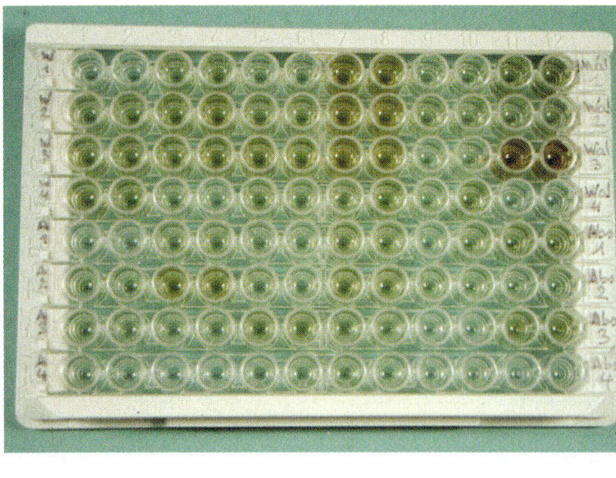

Fig. 3.5.5. ELISA microplate. Sera are distributed in duplicate in columns 1 and 2, then 3–4 from top to bottom. Notice the slightly different colours between the different duplicates. (Photo G. Reboux)

3.5.1.3.3 Methods Revealing Bands from Several Immunoglobulins

3.5.1.3.3.1 Western Blot

Antigens are separated by polyacrylamide gel electrophoresis, electroblotted onto a membrane and then incubated with serum samples from subjects. Antigen-antibody reactions are detected by treatment of the strips with antiserum to human IgG (or other globulin) and a specific stain. Molecular weights of the antigenic components are obtained with a pre-stained protein standard (Laemmli 1970) (Fig. 3.5.6).

Procedure:

The antigen diluted 1:5 in a sample buffer solution (Tris 0.5 M, pH 6.8, ethylenediaminetetraacetate 0.25 M, pH 7.5, beta-mercaptoethanol, 2% sodium dodecyl sulphate) is denatured for 3 min at 100°C and separated by electrosyneresis in a 10% polyacrylamide running gel at 110 V for 140 min on the Mini-Protean Electrophoresis Cell (Bio-Rad, Hercules, California). Blotting is performed on 0.45-µm pore-

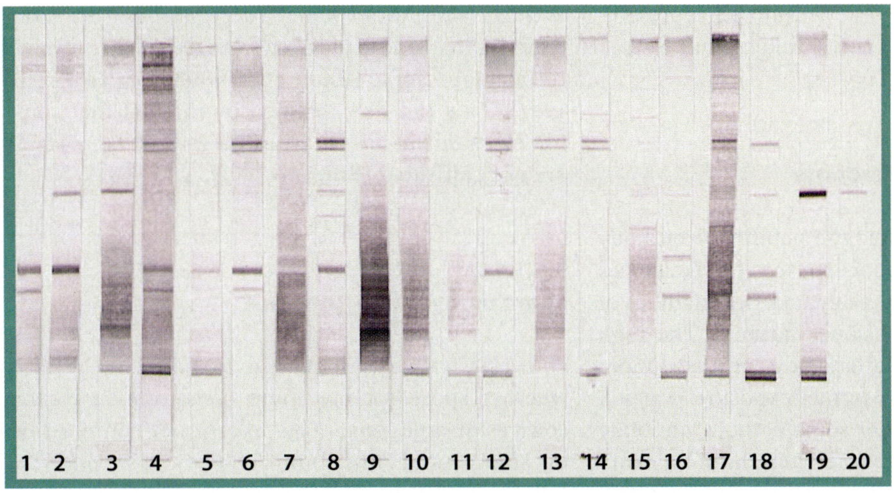

Fig. 3.5.6. Western blot with *Wallemia sebi* antigen revealed using IgG phosphatase alkaline conjugate (alternate of bands exposed with 10 farmer's lung disease sera – *uneven numbers* – and with 10 control sera – *even numbers*). (Photo G. Reboux)

size nitrocellulose transfer membrane (Schleicher & Schuell, Dassel, Germany) with Trans-blot semi-dry (Bio-Rad) at 10 V for 35 min. The nitrocellulose sheets are then saturated for 30 min using mechanical agitation in Tris buffered saline (10mM Tris/HCl, pH 8.1, 50 mM NaCl with 0.05%), Tween 20 and 5% non-fat milk (TBSTm). Each serum is diluted 1:200 in TBSTm. After four 5-min washings with TBSTm, the nitrocellulose sheets are incubated at room temperature for 1 h, with mechanical agitation and goat anti-human IgG (or another globulin) phosphatase alkaline conjugates diluted, respectively 1:1000, 1:500 in TBSTm (Sigma, Steinheim, Germany). After this cycle of washing with TBST, bands are visualised with 0.15 mM nitroblue tetrazolium plus 0.15 mM 5-bromo-4-chloro-3-indolyl phosphate (Combo Gibco Life Technology, Little Chalfont, England) in phosphate buffer, pH 9.5 (100 mM Tris 100 mM NaCl, 5 mM $MgCl_2$) for 30 min. The reaction is stopped by distilled water washes.

The number of bands is counted for each antigen, and the position is assessed with reference to the pre-stained protein standard.

3.5.1.4 Limits and Diagnostic Value of the Tests

3.5.1.4.1 Diagnostic Value of the Tests

The effectiveness of tests is less often evaluated in routine conditions than in specific studies, where trained operators and the standardisation of antigens provide optimum conditions.

Serological tests can be useful to study different aspects of HP, such as helping to establish a differential diagnosis (ABPA, organic dust toxicity syndrome or other lung involvement), assessing antigen exposure, or helping to identify new aetiologies.

A recent study with a cohort of 400 patients (116 with HP, 284 control subjects) re-evaluated precipitins as a diagnostic tool for HP (Lacasse et al. 2003). Six significant predictors were identified: exposure to a known offending antigen and positive precipitating to the offending antigen ranked first and second, respectively, ahead of recurrent episodes of symptoms, inspiratory crackles on physical examination, symptoms occurring 4–8 h after exposure and weight loss. It follows that the diagnosis of HP can often be reached or rejected with confidence, especially in areas of high or low prevalence, respectively, without BAL or biopsy. However, the importance of the role of serological tests changes according to the type of HP. Results obtained with precipitins in BBL are considered to have more value than those in other HP, due to the omnipresence of antigens in the environment. This may be one of the reasons for the difference and the negative assessment of the role of precipitins in HP diagnosis. Some authors are reticent as to the role of precipitins in farmer's lung diagnosis. A recent 20-year retrospective follow-up study of 27 farmers is a case in point (Cormier et al. 2004). The same cohort, initially used in two studies conducted 5 years apart (Cormier et al. 1985; Cormier and Belanger 1989) showed only 9.2% of the cohort (n=445) to have inexplicable variations. In the 20-year follow-up study, the only difference was that, compared with the sero-negative farmers, farmers with positive precipitins had a statistically significant greater decrease in their forced expiratory volume in 1 s. The authors conclude that serum precipitins in asymptomatic, exposed dairy farmers have no clinically meaningful long-term consequences.

These two studies by the same team are representative of the limits and diagnostic value of this test.

3.5.1.4.2 Durability of Antibody Response

Some authors have evaluated the stability of antibody response at a few weeks from exposure (Spiegelberg 1974). Other authors have evaluated this stability at more than 5 years in pensioner farmers. The high level of antibodies in the latter study correlated more with the disease than with former exposure (Katila and Mäntyjärvi 1987). For some authors, antibody response is the result of only a few months of exposure (Eduard 1995; Homma et al. 1986; Kusaka et al. 1989). Kaukonen and colleagues used ELISA to measure the antigen-binding avidity of *A. umbrosus*-specific IgG antibodies in FLD, in healthy farmers and urban controls during a 1-year follow-up. During the first acute phase, FLD patients with long exposure (>25 years) exhibited a high avidity of *A. umbrosus*-specific IgG antibodies that remained high throughout the 1-year follow-up, although the titre did decrease (Kaukonen et al. 1994). We had similar results with the measurement of *A. corymbifera* precipitins using ES before and after the winter period with FLD and healthy farmers. FLD precipitins fluctuate: either they decrease slightly if the patient is asymptomatic or increase if the patient has had a relapse. In all FLD cases, the precipitin titre remained over the threshold; whereas, in controls, it remained under the threshold required to classify the patient as FLD (Roussel et al. 2004). In our experience, low fluctuation was detected between autumn and spring in serology from FLD and exposed control subjects and did not modify the ability of the test to distinguish FLD subjects from controls (Roussel 2004).

3.5.1.5 Technical Considerations and Choices

3.5.1.5.1 Fine or Crude Antigens?

Contrary to what has been described in ABPA, where IgE serological response to recombinant purified allergen from *A. fumigatus* showed better sensitivity and specificity than with the crude antigen (Knutsen et al. 2004), crude antigen and rough serological methods with precipitin antibodies gave better results than sophisticated antigens and methods for diagnosis of HP (Reboux et al. 2001a). In some cases, total crude extracts (humidifier water, fiberglass dust) are more effective than antigens taken from the culture of environmental sample (Baur et al. 1992; Nolard et al. 1994). This can be explained by the fact that some microorganisms or parasites present in the sample are not cultivated (Eduard 1997).

3.5.1.5.2 Spore or Mycelium Antigens?

One classic question related to fungi antigens is whether spores or mycelium constitute the better source of antigens. The allergenic composition of spores and mycelium is obviously different (Hoffman et al. 1981). For some subunits, spore extract are more active than those from mycelium (Hoffman et al. 1981; Rosen et al. 1999). For other subunits, located in the cytoplasm, antigens are found both in spores and in mycelium (Paris et al. 1990). The spiculose part of spores contains more antigen compounds than smooth part does (Kaukonen et al. 1993).

3.5.1.5.3 Accuracy of Techniques

Precipitin techniques have shown reproducibility to be 89% for double diffusion (n=108) and 78% for electrosyneresis (n=202), with results showing ± 1 arc considered to be the same (Reboux et al. 2001b).

The ELISA is considered by several authors to be a sensitive, specific and quantitative test, which is readily available and widely applicable to HP diagnosis. FLD commonly have significantly higher values in the ELISA than exposed but asymptomatic farmers. Bamdad concluded that ELISA (IgG) correlated better than DD with clinical diagnosis (Bamdad 1980). In this paper and in others, the difficulty lies in establishing the best cut-off to distinguish FLD patients from exposed asymptomatic farmer.

In a recent study concerning the diagnosis of pigeon breeder's disease, specific measurement to avian antigens using the ELISA method showed greater effectiveness (10–10,000 ng/ml) than classic precipitating methods. Significant differences were found between non-exposed controls and the asymptomatic fancier control group, but no significant differences were found between asymptomatic and symptomatic patients (Rodrigo et al. 2000). The greater technical effectiveness of this method is frequently misunderstood to be the higher sensitivity of the diagnostic tool. Another widely accepted opinion states the advantage of automatic lecture methods (Spectrometer), due to less operator influence. This is certainly true. However, the other phases of the process, which require producing each reaction in duplicate or, better yet, in triplicate are equally as meticulous and often more difficult to manipulate precipitin methods. An internal reference sera is absolutely necessary to obtain a useful reference value between the batches of microtitre plates or as an arbitrary unit, in absence of a standard. Therefore, a cut-off is not easy to give in routine practice.

For other sophisticated techniques, with numerous bands (WB) or peaks (BIDI), interpretation is difficult due to excessive number of signals without specific bands or peaks correlated with the disease.

3.5.1.5.4 Choice of Isotypes

Patients in the acute phase of farmer's lung often have antibodies of several Ig classes against several microbes, in contrast with controls, who have only IgG antibodies against one or two microbes. In the acute phase of HP, total IgG is elevated. IgG_1 levels determine the levels of total IgG found both in non-exposed individuals and in farmers. IgE concentrations are generally normal or low, with no diagnostic value (Kaukonen et al. 1997). Conversely, IgG bound with the causative agent are elevated in acute reactions (Patel et al. 2001). Mundt and colleagues demonstrated specific binding of FLD patients' IgG_2 to *S. rectivirgula* antigens but found no such antibodies in exposed, unaffected subjects. Thus, IgG_2 antibodies reacting with *S. rectivirgula* antigens are useful for serological diagnosis of patients with FLD (Mundt et al. 1996). Conversely, a study by Stoke and colleagues showed no difference between patient and exposed controls in level of IgG, IgG_1, IgG_2 and IgG_4 but only with IgG_3. They explain that FLD patients are separated from exposed population on the basis of their propensity to produce IgG_3 in response to certain types of antigens stimulus (Stokes et al. 1981).

IgA antibodies against fungus have been found in patients with FLD and healthy exposed farmers. Except for Ylönen and colleagues, who assess that the presence of IgA is correlated with the disease, or for Ojanen, who highlights the value of the presence of IgA from *A. fumigatus* in the diagnosis of FLD, no other authors have given a special value to the presence of IgA in FLD. Exposed controls often have either IgG or IgA antibodies (Ojanen 1992). Our experience demonstrates that the highest levels of IgA were found using ELISA in healthy exposed farmers (personal unpublished data).

In BBL serodiagnosis, Martinez-Cordero showed positive IgA anti-avian antibodies to be the most frequent abnormalities, with values above those of the reference groups. A relationship of IgM-positive tests, using avian-pooled serum as antigen for subjects with a recent history of avian antigen exposure, was found to be reliable in the acute stage of the disease (Martinez-Cordero et al. 2000). Baldwin et al. (1998) found positive differences in the composition of subclasses against mucin antigen with significantly higher IgG1 titres in the patients than in the controls. Similar results were found by Rodrigo in a group of patients with HP caused by inhalation of mollusc shell dust (Rodrigo et al. 2000).

3.5.1.6 Conclusion

The presence of seric precipitins is one of the diagnostic criteria for HP and is important in epidemiological studies and research on new aetiologies. However, the diagnostic value of precipitins remains controversial. The sensitivity of tests varies according to the study, from 18% to 91%. Although some studies show what is often a considerable number of false negative subjects, the number of false positives is more problematic in that they may lead authors to consider precipitins as markers of exposure rather than of disease. Therefore, the presence of precipitins in an exposed asymptomatic subject does not predict an increased risk of developing the disease. Differences of results in the literature are due to several factors, which stem, on one hand, from the variety of techniques and antigens used and, on the other, from the misunderstanding of the nature and precise meaning of precipitins in HP. Consequently, it is important to recall that:

- Aetiological agents are varied, and the realisation of serological tests with inappropriate antigens can lead to false negatives and to results that do not reflect clinical features. Antigens related to domestic forms of HP are little known. We have attempted to solve this difficulty by producing custom-made antigens that allow identification of the aetiological agents at the origin of HP. This practice consists of taking environmental samples (air and surfaces), analysing them using

classic methods of culture to determine the microorganisms with which the patient has been in contact and then producing somatic antigens, useful in serological tests, from pure cultures of microorganisms.
- Detection of precipitins uses different methods, depending on the study. Besides the intrinsic problems inherent with each technique (standardisation, reproducibility, repeatability), this variety makes comparison between studies difficult. Rough methods seem preferable to sophisticated uninterpretable methods with several unspecific signals.
- Methods of preparing antigens are not standardised. They may be metabolic antigens, somatic antigens, a mixture of both, total extracts or purified antigenic fractions. Culture medium (solid or liquid), length and temperature for incubation, growth stage of fungi, extract and purification method are also factors liable to vary antigen quality. The reactivity of each extract needs to be evaluated by WB with reference sera to be sure that the extract reveals the maximum number of antigen compounds.
- Clinical criteria for inclusion in a study are variable, as are the criteria for constituting control groups. Some authors have said that the test sensitivity of precipitins research borders on 100% in the acute stage of the disease. For all new antigens, an evaluation with a large healthy exposed group is necessary to provide a robust, well-founded interpretation.
- Some factors cause antibody level to vary: smoking decreases precipitin production; dairy size and weekly duration of exposure increases seric immunoglobulin rates. Immunoglobulin rates seem to fluctuate over the seasons or one's lifetime; although, these studies show variations for approximately 10% of subjects only.

Despite the aforementioned difficulties, precipitin research contributes to HP diagnosis by demonstrating exposure to antigens liable to provoke the disease. Recently, the diagnostic value of precipitins was re-evaluated in an international multi-centric study: 78% of patients with HP showed positive serology against 31% for control subjects. Presence of seric precipitins was one of the six significant predictors for diagnosis of HP.

3.5.2 Immunological Diagnosis of Berylliosis

Owing to its material properties – very light and very strong – beryllium is an important industrial metal. Generally alloyed with other metals such as copper, it is a key component of materials used in the aerospace and electronics industries. In addition, beryllium has a small neutron cross-section, which makes it useful in the production of nuclear weapons and in sealed neutron sources (Taylor et al. 2003). Unfortunately, beryllium is responsible for a severe lung disease, chronic beryllium disease (CBD) or berylliosis and, in addition, was listed in 1993 as a Class A human carcinogen by the International Agency for Research on Cancer (1993).

In this sub-chapter, we first present generalities concerning this disease: sources of exposure, frequency, bases for prevention and methods of diagnosis. Second, we will develop data on the beryllium lymphocyte-proliferation test (BeLPT), which is considered as a relevant immunological diagnostic test, given its high level for sensitivity and, to a lesser degree, for positive predictive value. Finally, a few data on genetic tests for individual susceptibility will be described.

3.5.2.1 General Considerations

Because of its properties, beryllium is now widely used in a variety of industrial applications, including inertial guidance systems, turbine rotor blades, laser tubes, rocket engine liners, springs, aircraft brakes and landing gear, ball bearings, injection and blow mould tooling, electrical contacts, automotive electronics, X-ray tubes windows, spark plugs, electrical components, ceramic applications, gears, aircraft engines, oil and gas industries, welding electrodes, computer electronics and golf clubs. It is extremely light, with a high modulus of elasticity (stiffness), a low thermal expansion coefficient, high thermal and electrical conductivities and a high melting point. Pure beryllium metal is used in the nuclear industry as a moderator to slow down neutrons, increasing the effectiveness of fission. More frequently, it is used as an oxide or an alloy with copper, aluminium, magnesium or nickel. The beryllium content and its attendant hazards may not be obvious to workers generating dust and fumes (Barna et al. 2003; Infante and Newman 2004).

Occupations with the highest risk involve processes that generate particles, especially metal production and machining. In general, the risk of disease is proportional to the intensity and duration of exposure to beryllium (Kreiss et al. 1993a, 1996, 1997). However, well-documented cases have occurred in susceptible individuals with brief and trivial exposures: people residing near beryllium processing plants or secretaries working in offices attached to factories (Barna et al. 2003). Beryllium particles may also be liberated into the air in unexpected settings or circumstances, such as after the collapse of the World Trade Center (Lioy et al. 2002).

CBD can be identified in both current and former beryllium workers with a well-established blood assay, the BeLPT. This test of T-lymphocyte activation identifies individuals with beryllium sensitisation. Individuals are generally sensitised to beryllium before CBD develops. The latency period for sensitisation and CBD is very variable. Although CBD can take more than 30 years to develop, beryllium sensitisation can occur within 2 months and CBD within 3 months of initial exposure (Kelleher et al. 2001).

Prevalence of sensitisation and CBD depend mainly on the level and duration of exposure. The 8-h time-weighted-averages permissible exposure limits (PELs) for beryllium are generally 1–2 μg/m² (Infante and Newman 2004). In plants complying with these PELs, the prevalence of CBD has ranged from 2% to 15%, depending on the jobs being surveyed (Infante and Newman 2004). However, CBD can occur in workers whose average beryllium exposure levels are 20–100 times lower than the current PELs (Kelleher et al. 2001; Kolanz 2001). There is growing evidence that particle size and chemical forms may be important factors that influence the risk of developing CBD (Kolanz 2001).

CBD is an irreversible disease that mainly involves the respiratory tract. Common manifestations include the insidious onset of exertional dyspnoea, non-productive cough, fatigue, arthralgias and chest pain (Infante and Newman 2004; Rossman 1996). Non-pulmonary organs, including the skin, liver, spleen, myocardium, kidneys, salivary glands and bones, may also be affected (Stoeckle et al. 1969). Lung function test may demonstrate restrictive, obstructive or mixed defect, usually with a decreased pulmonary diffusing capacity. Chest radiographs are often normal in early disease; with progression, diffuse infiltrates typically occur. In absence of medical treatment and in cases of continuing exposure, severe lung fibrosis is a common outcome. Radiographic and physiological abnormalities are similar to those in sarcoidosis. A positive BeLPT, although non-specific, is indicative of CBD in a patient who presents the previous clinical and paraclinical signs. A diagnosis of CBD requires a bronchoscopy with BAL and occasionally, transbronchial biopsy. BAL fluid typically reveals a lymphocytosis in individuals with both beryllium sensitisation and CBD. The percentage of BAL lymphocytes is higher in CBD patients than in sensitised patients. Lymphocytes are CD4-positive T-lymphocytes. The percentage of BAL lymphocytes may correlate with a severity of physiological and radiographic disease (Newman et al. 1994). Biopsy reveals evidence of non-necrotising granulomas and lymphocytic interstitial infiltration indistinguishable from those due to other granulomatous disorders, such as sarcoidosis. Prolonged treatment with corticosteroids is usually necessary for patients with significant symptoms or physiological abnormalities. Although response to therapy is generally excellent, patients can progress to end-stage lung disease.

3.5.2.2 Immunological Diagnosis

3.5.2.2.1 Development of Laboratory Methods and Current Status of the BeLPT

In the late 1960s, the advent of in vitro techniques for studying cellular immune responses led to the development of laboratory methods for detecting beryllium sensitivity (Deodhar and Barna 1991). In 1973, Deodhar and co-workers reported a correlation between the clinical status of CBD and in vitro responses to beryllium in a lymphocyte proliferation test (Deodhar et al. 1973). In 1982, the test was adapted to use tritiated thymidine uptake as an indicator of response (Williams and Williams 1982). In these developments, elevated responses to beryllium were observed in patients with clinically verified CBD. Slightly elevated responses were also observed in healthy beryllium-exposed subjects, suggesting sensitisation to the metal but also demonstrating the lack of specificity of the method. Later, it was suggested that the BeLPT using BAL fluid cells was more sensitive and specific than that with blood (Rossman et al. 1988). However, these findings have not been confirmed to date, and BAL BeLPT is not routinely used.

Kreiss and co-workers in 1989 and 1993 carried out two studies that suggested that the test might be helpful in preventing clinical CBD by allowing early diagnosis of subclinical disease (Kreiss et al. 1989, 1993b). However, more recent studies have not demonstrated this to be a consistent finding, and we continue to think that a positive test may be only a biological manifestation of exposure, which does not necessarily lead to a clinical or even histological disease.

A major concern encountered with the test, in addition to its lack of specificity, is a high-level of variability, which also contributes to the lack of specificity. Results from a larger industrial study reviewing the use of BeLPT as a surveillance tool, including 5483 records representing 3 080 samples from 1510 subjects, showed a single abnormal blood BeLPT to have a positive predictive value of only 39% and a first-time double abnormal test pf 49%, with very high intra- and inter-laboratory variability (Deubner et al. 2001).

In the U.S., laboratories performing the test formed a working group, the Committee to Accredit Beryllium Sensitivity Testing, to address technical issues (Barna et al. 2003).

The consensus BeLPT method uses challenge of peripheral blood mononuclear cells with three incremental doses of beryllium sulphate solution at two different culture periods, thus providing six different responses for analysis. Tritiated thymidine is added to cultures 1 day prior to harvest, and uptake of radio-labelled thymidine is measured as counts per minute with a beta counter. Final results are expressed as a stimulation index (SI), where the mean counts per minute of control (beryllium-free) cultures are divided into the mean counts per minute of each beryllium-exposed culture. The test is interpreted as abnormal if an SI of 3.0 or higher occurs in two of six beryllium-exposed cultures. An SI of 3.0 or higher in one of six cultures is considered borderline, and a SI of 3.0 or higher in zero of six cultures is considered negative. The least-absolute-values method of statistical analysis has been proposed as a means to improve identification of borderline and abnormal BeLPT results (Frome et al. 2003).

This new statistical-biological positive method reflects the clinical judgement that: (1) at least two SIs show a "positive" response to beryllium and (2) the maximum of the six SIs must exceed a cut-point that is determined from a reference data set of normal individuals whose blood has been tested by the same method in the same serum. This statistical method applied to the Y-12 National Security Complex in Oak Ridge, consisting of 1080 workers and 33 non-exposed control BeLPTs (all tested in the same serum), showed sensitivity to be 86% and specificity 97% (Frome et al. 2003).

To discriminate beryllium sensitisation (BeS) from CBD, some authors have questioned whether Be-stimulated neopterin production by peripheral blood cells in vitro might be useful in the diagnosis of CBD (Maier et al. 2003). CBD, BeS and Be-exposed workers without disease normal controls and sarcoidosis subjects were compared. CBD patients produced higher levels of neopterin in both unstimulated and Be-stimulated conditions than all other subjects. Using a neopterin concentration of 2.5 ng/ml as a cut-off, Be-stimulated neopterin had an 80% sensitivity and 100% specificity for CBD and was able to differentiate CBD from BeS. These results, nevertheless, have to be confirmed before this test could be used in workplace screening.

3.5.2.2.2 Genetic Testing and Future Directions

The human leukocyte antigen (HLA) complex is a series of genes located on chromosome 6 that are important in normal immune function. Susceptibility to CBD is modified by genetic variants of the HLA-DP sub-region. Evaluation of HLA-DPB1 sequence motifs in current and former beryllium workers implicated a glutamic acid residue at position 69 [HLA-DPB1(Glu69)] in CBD.

Studies have demonstrated an association of CBD with HLA-DPB1 (Glu69) alleles in up to 97% of subjects with CBD, but also 30–40% of controls. Two copies of the Glu69 gene may be a disease-specific genetic risk factor. The TNF-alpha-308 A variant is associated with beryllium-stimulated TNF-alpha production, which, in turn, is associated with more severe CBD. Whether the TNF-alpha-308 A is a genetic risk factor in CBD, sensitisation or more severe disease still needs to be determined. It is likely that sensitisation and CBD are multigenetic processes and that these genes interact with exposure to determine risk of a disease (Maier 2002; Maier et al. 2003). A close association of HLA-DR Arg 74 with beryllium sensitisation but not with CBD has also been noted (Saltini et al. 2001). Testing for carrier status in a pre-employment population is, however, problematic, not only because of ethical or financial issues but because the HLA-DPB1 (Glu69) is a haplotype, frequently found within the general population, that leads to a low positive predictive value of this test (Deodhar and Barna 1991).

3.5.3 Immunological Diagnosis for Interstitial Lung Diseases Associated with Collagen-Vascular Disorders

Interstitial lung diseases related to environmental factors have many immunological differential diagnoses. Actually, many auto-immune diseases present with pulmonary involvement and should be properly identified. The diagnosis of those auto-immune diseases is mostly clinical and immunological. The most frequent differential diagnoses and their clinical and immunological features are presented below.

3.5.3.1 Systemic Sclerosis

3.5.3.1.1 Definition (Gilliland 2001a)

Systemic sclerosis (SSc), also named scleroderma, is a systemic disease characterised by thickening of the skin due to an accumulation of connective tissue and by the involvement of various organs such as the lungs, gastrointestinal tract, heart and kidneys. The annual incidence has been estimated to be 19 cases per million population, and the reported prevalence of SSc is between 19 and 75 per 100,000 persons.

3.5.3.1.2 Pathophysiology

The main feature of SSc is overproduction and accumulation of collagen and some other extracellular matrix proteins in the skin and other organs. The fibrosis is usually preceded by vascular injury involving small arteries, arterioles and capillaries in the skin, lungs, gastrointestinal tract, kidneys and heart.

3.5.3.1.3 Pulmonary Involvement

Pulmonary involvement concerns at least two-thirds of patients with SSc. The most common symptom is exertional dyspnea associated with dry cough. The symptoms are not directly related to pulmonary fibrosis. Approximately 10% of SSc patients will develop pulmonary hypertension, which is a very severe complication related to obliteration of pulmonary arteries and arterioles. The mean duration of survival for SSc patients with pulmonary hypertension is approximately 2 years.

3.5.3.1.4 Immunological Diagnosis

In SSc patients, different autoantibodies could be detected, some of which are unspecific, while others are highly specific for SSc.

3.5.3.1.4.1 *Unspecific Autoantibodies* (Khalaley 1991)

In SSC, antinuclear antibodies detected using immunofluorescence are present in 95% of patients.

A rheumatoid factor (IgG anti-IgM), detected using the Waaler–Rose latex test and usually associated with rheumatoid arthritis, is present in 25% of patients.

High titres of anti-ribonucleoprotein (RNP), detected using an ELISA, are present in patients with features of mixed connective tissue disease.

3.5.3.1.4.2 *Specific Autoantibodies* (Dick et al. 2002)

Soluble antinuclear antibodies that have high specificity for SSc are:

- Anti-topoisomerase 1 (originally called anti-Scl-70 for scleroderma 70), anti-nucleolar and anti-centromere. Anti-topoisomerase (anti-Scl-70) recognises the nuclear enzyme DNA topoisomerase 1. These antibodies are detected in 20% of SSc patients and are associated with generalised skin involvement and interstitial pulmonary disease.
- Antinucleolar antibodies are relatively specific for SSc and are present in 20% of patients. Different anti-nucleolar antibodies has been identified in SSc patients: anti-RNA polymerase 1 found in patients with diffuse cutaneous SSc are associated with a high prevalence of renal and cardiac involvement, anti-PM-Scl (formerly anti-PM1) are found SSc patients with polymyositis and renal involvement. Anti-U3 nucleolar RNP are highly specific for SSc, more common in African-American patients and associated with skeletal muscle disease and pulmonary arterial hypertension.

- Anti-centromere antibodies react with antigen located in the kinetochore region of chromosomes and are strongly associated with CREST syndrome (i.e. calcinosis + Raynaud phenomenon + oesophageal hypomotility + skin abnormalities + telangiectasia). Those antibodies are only found in 10% of patients with diffuse disease.

3.5.3.1.5
Association Between SSc and Silica Dust

Coal and gold miners developed SSc more frequently than other workers. A relationship was established between pulmonary disease induced by silica and the development of SSc, and the association between silicosis and SSc is called the Erasmus syndrome.

3.5.3.2
Rheumatoid Arthritis

3.5.3.2.1
Definition (Lipsky 2001)

Rheumatoid arthritis (RA) is also a multi-system disease of unknown cause. The characteristic feature is a persistent inflammatory synovitis concerning peripheral joints with a symmetric distribution. The prevalence of RA is approximately 1% of the population.

3.5.3.2.2
Pathophysiology

Microvascular injury and an increase in the number of synovial-limited cells appear to be the earliest lesion in rheumatoid synovitis. Family studies indicate a genetic predisposition. There is a strong association between RA and the class II major histocompatibility complex gene product HLA-DR4 (and especially DR^1-0404).

3.5.3.2.3
Pulmonary Involvement

The pulmonary involvement in more common in men. Pulmonary manifestations include interstitial fibrosis, pleuropulmonary nodules (single or clusters), pneumonitis and arteritis. Rarely, pulmonary hypertension secondary to obliteration of the pulmonary vasculature occurs.

3.5.3.2.4
Immunological Diagnosis
(Schumacher et al. 2003)

Rheumatoid factors: autoantibodies reactive with the Fc portion of IgG are found in more than two-thirds of RA patients. The tests (latex and Waaler-Rose) detect IgM rheumatoid factors. Its presence is not specific to RA, it is found in 5% of healthy persons (and in 10–20% of persons over 65 years old). Patients with high titres of rheumatoid factors tend to have more severe and progressive disease with extra-articular manifestations.

A number of additional autoantibodies may be found in patients with RA, including antibodies to *filaggrin, citrulline, calpastatin, components of the spliceosome (RA-33)*. Some of these are useful in diagnosis because they may occur in the disease before a rheumatoid factor or may be associated with severe disease.

3.5.3.2.5
Association Between Rheumatoid Arthritis and Silicosis

When the rheumatoid pulmonary nodules appear in patients with pneumoconiosis, a diffuse nodular fibrotic process, called Caplan's syndrome, may develop.

3.5.3.3
Mixed Connective Tissue Disease

3.5.3.3.1
Definition (Sharp 1994)

Mixed connective tissue disease (MCTD) is an overlap syndrome characterised by a combination of clinical features similar to those of systemic lupus erythematosus, scleroderma, polymyositis, rheumatoid arthritis and unusually high titres of circulating antibody to RNP antigen.

3.5.3.3.2
Pathophysiology

Characteristic immune findings include immunoregulatory abnormalities (high titres of anti-RNP), a marked polyclonal hypergammaglobulinaemia indicating B-cell hyperactivity and circulating immune complexes during active disease with normal clearance by the reticuloendothelial system in most patients.

3.5.3.3.3 Pulmonary Involvement

Pulmonary involvement occurred in 85% of one series of MCTD patients and appeared latent until an advanced stage. Pulmonary hypertension is the most frequent serious complication in MCTD.

3.5.3.3.4 Immunological Diagnosis

Almost all patients have high titres of positive fluorescent *antinuclear antibodies* with a speckled pattern and very high titres of *anti-RNP*, a component of extractable nuclear antigen.

Anti-native DNA antibodies and *anti-ribonuclease resistant Sm* antibodies are usually uncommon in MCTD and are associated with a severe flare-up of lupus-like features.

Rheumatoid factor is found usually at very high titres in half the patients.

3.5.3.4 Sjögren's Syndrome

3.5.3.4.1 Definition (Moutsopoulos 2001)

Sjögren's syndrome is a slowly progressive chronic auto-immune disease characterised by lymphocytic infiltration of the exocrine glands enhancing xerostomia and dry eyes. One-third of patients present with extraglandular manifestations. The most severe complication is the development of malignant lymphoma.

3.5.3.4.2 Pathophysiology

There are two main autoimmune features: lymphocytic infiltration of exocrine glands and B-lymphocyte hyperreactivity illustrated by circulating autoantibodies. Immunogenetics studies have demonstrated that HLA B8, DR3 and DRw52 are prevalent in primary Sjögren's syndrome patients as compared with the normal control population.

3.5.3.4.3 Pulmonary Involvement

Pulmonary involvement in Sjögren's syndrome is frequent but rarely clinically relevant. Subclinical diffuse interstitial lung disease is the most common feature.

3.5.3.4.4 Immunological Diagnosis

The incidence of autoantibodies found in the sera of patients with Sjögren's syndrome is very high. Some of them are unspecific, and some are strongly correlated with Sjögren's syndrome.

3.5.3.4.4.1 Unspecific Autoantibodies

Rheumatoid factor is found in 80% of patients with Sjögren's syndrome. Almost all patients have high titres of positive fluorescent *antinuclear antibodies*.

3.5.3.4.4.2 More Specific Autoantibodies

Antibodies directed against extractable nuclear and cytoplasmic antigens (*Ro/SSA and La/SSB*) are found preferentially in Sjögren's syndrome patients. Anti-SSA is found in 60% of patients and anti-SSB in 50% of patients. Both antibodies are detected using an ELISA technique. The presence of anti-SSA and anti-SSB autoantibodies is associated with earlier disease onset, longer disease duration and salivary gland enlargement.

Autoantibodies to organ-specific antigens, such as salivary duct cells, thyroid gland cells and gastric mucosa, have also been described.

3.5.3.5 Churg and Strauss Syndrome

3.5.3.5.1 Definition (Fauci 2001)

Also named allergic angiitis and granulomatosis, the disease is characterised by granulomatous vasculitis of multiple organ systems, particularly the lung. Another feature of the disease is the presence of a strong association between asthma and peripheral eosinophilia.

3.5.3.5.2 Pathophysiology

The vasculitis is similar to that of classic polyarteritis nodosa. The characteristic histopathological features are granulomatous reactions, which are present in the tissues or even within the vessel walls. These are usually associated with infiltration of the tissues with eosinophils.

3.5.3.5.3 Pulmonary Involvement

The pulmonary findings clearly dominate the clinical picture of Churg and Strauss syndrome. Patients present with severe asthmatic attacks and pulmonary infiltrates.

3.5.3.5.4 Immunological Diagnosis

(Abril et al. 2003)

The only autoantibodies found to be related to Churg and Strauss syndrome are the *antineutrophil cytoplasmic antibodies (ANCA),* especially the perinuclear ANCA, also referred to as p-ANCA; they are directed against myeloperoxidase. High titres of those autoantibodies could be detected in one-half of patients with Churg and Strauss syndrome (Garini G).

Elevated serum IgE levels also characterise Churg and Strauss syndrome.

3.5.3.6 Other Auto-Immune Diseases

3.5.3.6.1 Polymyositis and Dermatopolymyositis

(Dalakas 2001)

Polymyositis and dermatopolymyositis are diseases in which the skeletal muscle is damaged by a non-suppurative inflammatory process dominated by infiltration. The aetiology of those disorders is presumed to be auto-immune. One-third of cases are associated with various mixed connective tissue disorders. Although interstitial lung disease is reported to occur in only 5–10% of patients, its presence is more common in the subgroup of patients with an *anti-Jo-1 antibody* that is directed to tRNA synthetase. Weakness of respiratory muscles contributing to aspiration pneumonitis is a common occurrence.

3.5.3.6.2 Systemic Lupus Erythematosus

(Hahn 2001)

Systemic lupus erythematosus (SLE) is a systemic auto-immune disease of unknown cause in which tissues and cells are damaged by pathogenic autoantibodies and immune complexes. Ninety per cent of cases are in women, usually of childbearing age. Pleurisy and pleural effusions are common manifestations of SLE. Interstitial pneumonitis leading to fibrosis occurs occasionally. Pulmonary hypertension is a serious, uncommon manifestation of SLE. Many autoantibodies could be detected in SLE patients; the most frequent are *antinuclear antibodies* (Keren) (90% of patients); the most specific antibodies are *anti-DNA* (70% of patients) and *anti-Sm* (30% of patients).

3.5.3.6.3 Relapsing Polychondritis

(Gilliland 2001b)

Relapsing polychondritis is an episodic and often progressive inflammatory disorder of unknown cause affecting predominately the cartilage of ears, nose tracheobronchial tree as well as the internal structure of the eyes and ears. It is most common between the ages of 40–60 years. Collapse of cartilage in bronchi leads to pneumonia and, when extensive, to respiratory insufficiency. *Anti-collagen type-II* antibodies may be found in patients with relapsing polychondritis but are not specific to the disease as well as are the *pANCA* autoantibodies.

3.6 Conclusion

In the presence of an interstitial lung disease assumed to be related to environmental factors, it is essential to carry out a differential diagnosis with an auto-immune disease with pulmonary involvement, because most of those diseases need an appropriated treatment, which can improve the pulmonary disease.

References

Abril A, Calamia KT, Cohen MD (2003) The Churg and Strauss syndrome (allergic ganulomatous angiitis): review and update. Semin Arthritis Rheum 33:106-114

Aiache JM, Jeanneret A, Molina C et al (1976) Applications de la technique d'immunoélectrophorèse bidimensionnelle aux pneumopathies d'hypersensibilité par inhalation d'antigènes organiques. Pathol Biol 24:525-529

American Thoracic Society, Medical Section of the American Lung Association (1998) Respiratory health hazards in agriculture. Am J Respir Crit Care Med 158:S1-S76

Axelsen NH (1973) Quantitative immunoelectrophoretic methods as tools for a polyvalent approach to standardization in the immunochemistry of *Candida albicans*. Infect Immun 7:949-960

Aznar C, Andre PM, Deunff J et al (1988) Investigation of human immune response to *Micropolyspora faeni* antigens by enzyme-linked immunoelectrodiffusion assay and immunoblotting. J Clin Microbiol 26:443-447

Baldwin CI, Stevens B, Connors S et al (1998) Pigeon fanciers' lung: the mucin antigen is present in pigeon droppings and pigeon bloom. Int Arch Allergy Immunol 117:187-193

Bamdad S (1980) Enzyme-linked immunosorbent assay (ELISA) for IgG antibodies in farmers' lung disease. Clin Allergy 10:161-171

Barna BP, Culver DA, Yen-Lieberman B et al (2003) Clinical application of beryllium lymphocyte proliferation testing. Clin Diagn Lab Immunol 990-994

Baur X, Richter G, Pethran A et al (1992) Increased prevalence of IgG-induced sensitization and hypersensitivity pneumonitis (humidifier lung) in nonsmokers exposed to aerosols of a contaminated air conditioner. Respiration 59:211 214

Boyd G, Mc Sharry CP, Banham SW et al (1982) A current view of pigeon fancier lung: a model for pulmonary extrinsic allergic alveolitis. Clin Allergy 12 [Suppl]:53-59

Brummund W, Kurup VP, Resnick A et al (1988) Immunologic response to *Faenia rectivirgula* (*Micropolyspora faeni*) in a dairy family. J Allergy Clin Immunol 82:190-195

Burrel P, Rylander R (1981) A critical review of the role of precipitins in hypersensitivity pneumonitis. Eur J Respir Dis 62:332-343

Cormier Y, Belanger J (1989) The fluctuant nature of precipitating antibodies in dairy farmers. Thorax 44:469-473

Cormier Y, Belanger J, Durant P et al (1985) Factors influencing the development of serum precipitins to farmer's lung antigen in Quebec dairy farmers. Thorax 40:138-142

Cormier Y, Letourneau L, Racine G (2004) Significance of precipitins and asymptomatic lymphocytic alveolitis: a 20-yr follow-up. Eur Respir J 23:523-525

Dalakas MC (2001) Polymyositis and dermatopolymyositis. In : Braunwald E, Fauci AS, Kasper DL, Hauser SL, Longo DL, Jameson JL (eds) Harrison principles of internal medicine, 15th edn. McGraw Hill, New York pp 2524-2529 (PM)

Dalphin JC, Toson B, Monnet E et al (1994) Farmer's lung precipitins in Doubs (a department of France): prevalence and diagnostic value. Allergy 49:744-750

Dalphin JC, Reboux G, Westeel V et al (2000) Importance de la démarche étiologique dans les pneumonies d'hypersensibilité, à propos d'un cas dû à un oreiller en plume d'oie. Rev Mal Resp 17:869-872

Deodhar SD, Barna BP (1991) Immune mechanisms in beryllium lung disease. Clev Clin J Med 58:157-160

Deodhar SD, Barna BP, van Ordstrand HS (1973) A study of the immunologic aspects of chronic berylliosis. Chest 63:309-313

Deubner DC, Goodman M, Iannuzzi J (2001) Variability, predictive value, and uses of the beryllium blood lymphocyte proliferation test (BLPT) : preliminary analyses of the ongoing workforce survey. Appl Occup Environ Hyg 16:521-526

Dick T, Mierau R, Bartz-Bazanella P et al (2002) Coexistence of antitopoiomerase I and anticentromere antibodies in patients with systemic sclerosis. Ann Rheum Dis 61:121-127

Dutkiewicz J, Skorska C, Dutkiewicz E et al (2001) Response of sawmill workers to work-related airborne allergens. Ann Agric Environ Med 8:81-90

Dutkiewicz J, Skorska C, Krysinska-Traczyk E et al (2002) Precipitin response of potato processing workers to work-related microbial allergens. Ann Agric Environ Med 9:237-242

Eduard W (1995) Immunoglobulin G antibodies against moulds and actinomyces as biomarkers of exposure in the work environment. Occup Hyg 1:247-260

Eduard W (1997) Exposure to non-infectious microorganisms and endotoxins in agriculture. Ann Agric Environ Med 4:179-186

Edwards JH (1972) The isolation of antigens associated with farmer's lung. Clin Exp Immunol 11:341-355

Engwall E and Perlman P (1971) Enzyme-linked immunosorbent assay (ELISA). Quantitative assay of immunoglobulin G. Immunochemistry 8:871-874

Erkinjuntti-Pekkanen R, Reiman M, Kokkarinen JI et al (1999) IgG antibodies, chronic bronchitis, and pulmonary function values in farmer's lung patients and matched controls. Allergy 54:1181-1187

Esch RE (2004) Manufacturing and standardizing fungal allergen products. J Allergy Clin Immunol 113:210-215

Fasani F, Bossi A, Caramia V (1987) Double diffusion and ELISA for the detection of IgG and IgM antibodies against *Micropolyspora faeni*. Ann Allergy 59:451-454

Fauci AS (2001) Churg and Strauss syndrome. In : Braunwald E, Fauci AS, Kasper DL, Hauser SL, Longo DL, Jameson JL (eds) Harrison principles of internal medicine, 15th edn. McGraw-Hill, New York, pp 1960-1961 (cHURG)

Flaherty DK, Barboriak J, Emanuel D et al (1974) Multilaboratory comparison of three immunodiffusion methods used for the detection of precipitating antibodies in hypersensitivity pneumonitis. J Lab Clin Microbiol 84:298-306

Flandes J, Heili S, Gomez Seco J et al (2004) Hypersensitivity pneumonitis caused by esparto dust in a young plaster worker: a case report and review of the literature. Respiration 71:421-423

Frome EL, Newman LS, Cragle DL et al (2003) Identification of an abnormal beryllium lymphocyte proliferation test. Toxicology 183:39-56

Gangwar M, Khan ZU, Gaur SN et al (1991) Occurrence and significance of precipitating antibodies against thermophilic actinomycetes in the sera of dairy herd workers, Nangali, Delhi. Anatomie Van Leeuwenhoek 59:167-175

Gari M, Smets P, Pinon JM et al (1982) Use of immuno-electrodiffusion on cellulose acetate for the research of the precipitating antibodies in the screening of patients suspected of farmer's lung disease. Mycopathologia 78:151-153

Gari M, Recco P, Pinon JM, Seguela JP (1984) Intérêt de la co-immunoélectrodiffusion sur acétate de cellulose dans le diagnostic du poumon de fermier pour la mise en évidence de systèmes précipitants remarquables. Sem Hop Paris 60:776-779

Gari M, Pinon JM, Poirriez J et al (1986) Enzyme-linked immunofiltration (ELIFA) for the detection of specific antibodies (IgG-IgM-IgA-IgE) in farmer's lung disease. Clin Allergy 16:553-562

Gariepy L, Cormier Y, Laviolette M et al (1989) Predictive value of bronchoalveolar lavage cells and serum precipitins in asymptomatic dairy farmers. Am Rev Respir Dis 140:1386-1389

Gilliland BC (2001a) Systemic sclerosis. In: Braunwald E, Fauci AS, Kasper DL, Hauser SL, Longo DL, Jameson JL (eds) Harrison principles of internal medicine, 15th edn. McGraw-Hill, New York, pp 1937-1946

Gilliland BC (2001b) Relapsing polychondritis. In: Braunwald E, Fauci AS, Kasper DL, Hauser SL, Longo DL, Jameson JL (eds) Harrison principles of internal medicine, 15th edn. McGraw-Hill, New York, pp 2005-2007

Gruchow HW, Hoffman RG, Marx JJ et al (1981) Precipitating antibodies of farmer's lung antigens in a Wisconsin farming population. Am Rev Respir Dis 124:411-415

Gump DW, Babbott FL, Holly C et al (1979) Farmer's lung disease in Vermont. Respiration 37:52-60

Hahn BH (2001) Systemic lupus erythematosus. In: Braunwald E, Fauci AS, Kasper DL, Hauser SL, Longo DL, Jameson JL (eds) Harrison principles of internal medicine, 15th edn. McGraw-Hill, New York, pp 1922-1928

Hoffman DR, Kozak PP Jr, Gillman S et al (1981) Isolation of spore specific allergens from *Alternaria*. Ann Allergy 46:310-316

Homma Y, Terai T, Matsuzaki M (1986) Incidence of serum-precipitating antibodies to farmer's lung antigens in Hokkaido. Respiration 49:300-306

Horner WE, Helbling A, Salvaggio JE et al (1995) Fungal allergens. Clin Microbiol Rev 8:161-179

Huizinga M, Berrens I (1985) Detection of class-specific antibodies against Micropolyspora faeni antigens in farmers'lung. Clin Allergy 15:139-145

Husman K, Vohlonen I, Terho EO et al (1987) Precipitins against microbes in mouldy hay in the sera of farmers with farmer's lung or chronic bronchitis and of healthy farmers. Eur J Respir Dis [Suppl] 152:122-127

Infante PF, Newman LS (2004) Beryllium exposure and chronic beryllium disease. Lancet 363:415-416

International Agency for Research on Cancer, World Health Organization (1993) IARC monographs on the evaluation of carcinogenic risks to humans: beryllium, cadmium, mercury and exposures in the glass manufacturing industry, vol 58. IARC, Lyon, pp 41-117

Iranitalab M, Jarolim E, Rumpold H et al (1989) Characterization of *Micropolyspora faeni* antigens by human antibodies and immunoblot analysis. Allergy 44:314-321

Katila ML, Mäntyjärvi RA (1978) The diagnostic value of antibodies to the traditional antigens of farmer's lung in Finland. Clin Allergy 8:581-587

Katila ML, Ojanen TH, Mäntyjärvi RA (1986a) A six-year follow-up of antibody levels against microbes present in the farming environment in a group of dairy farmers in Finland. Am J ind Med 10:307-309

Katila ML, Ojanen TH, Mäntyjärvi RA (1986b) Significance of IgG antibodies against environmental microbial antigens in a farming population. Clin Allergy 16:459-467

Katila ML, Mäntyjärvi RA (1987) Prognosis value of precipitins for working ability in dairy farmers. Eur J Respir Dis 152 [Suppl]:146-154

Kaukonen K, Savolainen J, Viander M et al (1993) Characterization of *Aspergillus umbrosus* carbohydrate antigens by biotinylated lectins and IgG response to mannan/mannoprotein antigens in patients with farmer's lung. Clin Exp Allergy 23:21-27

Kaukonen K, Savolainen J, Viander M et al (1994) Avidity of Aspergillus umbrosus IgG antibodies in farmer's lung disease. Clin Exp Immunol 95:162-165

Kaukonen K, Savolainen J, Nermes M, et al (1997) IgE antibody response against *Aspergillus umbrosus* in farmer's lung disease. Int Arch Allergy Immunol 112:313-316

Kelleher PC, Martyny JW, Mroz MM et al (2001) Beryllium particulate exposure and disease relations in a beryllium machining plant. J Occup Environ Med 43:238-249

Keren DF (2002) Antinuclear antibody testing. Clin Lab Med 22:447-474

Khalaleh MB (1991) Soluble immunologic products in scleroderma sera. Clin Immunol Pathol 58:139

Kim SJ, Chaparas SD, Buckley HR (1979) Characterisation of antigens from *Aspergillus fumigatus*. IV. Evaluation of commercial and experimental preparations and fractions in the detection of antibody in aspergillosis. Am Rev Respir Dis 120:1305-1311

Knutsen AP, Hutcheson PS, Slavin RG et al (2004) IgE antibody to *Aspergillus fumigatus* recombinant allergens in cystic fibrosis patients with allergic bronchopulmonary aspergillosis. Allergy 59:198-203

Kokkarinen JI, Tukiainen HO, Terho EO (1993) Recovery of pulmonary function in farmer's lung. A five-year follow-up study. Am Rev Respir Dis 147:793-796

Kolanz ME (2001) Introduction to beryllium: uses, regulatory history, and disease. Appl Occup Environ Hyg 16:559-567

Kreiss K, Newman LS, Mroz MM et al (1989) Screening blood test identifies subclinical beryllium disease. J Occup Med 31:603-608

Kreiss K, Mroz MM, B Zhen, et al (1993a) Epidemiology of berylllium sensitization and disease in nuclear workers. Am Rev Respir Dis 148:985-991

Kreiss K, Wasserman S, Mroz MM et al (1993b) Beryllium disease screening in the ceramics industry. J Occup Med 35:267-274

Kreiss K, Mroz MM, LS Newman et al (1996) Machining risk of beryllium disease and sensitization with median exposures below 2 micrograms/m3. Am J Ind Med 30:16-25

Kreiss K, Mroz MM, Zhen B et al (1997) Risks of beryllium disease related to work processes at a metal, alloy, and oxide production plant. Occup Environ Med 54:605-612

Kumar A, Elms N, Kurup VP (1993) Monoclonal antibodies against farmer's lung antigens having specific binding to IgG antibodies. Int Arch Allerg Immunol 102:67-71

Kurup VP, John KV, Ting EY et al (1984) Immunochemical studies of a purified antigen from *Micropolyspora faeni*. Mol Immunol 21:215-221

Kurup VP, Mäntyjärvi RA, Terho EO et al (1987a) Circulating IgG antibodies against fungal and actinomycetes antigens in the sera of farmer's lung patients from different countries. Mycopathologia 98:91-99

Kurup VP (1987b) Detection of the relevant farmer's lung antigens by using immunoblots of two-dimensional electrophoresis. Diagn Clin Immunol 5:25-29

Kusaka H, Homma Y, Ogasawara H et al (1989) Five-year follow-up of *Micropolyspora faeni* antibody in smoking and nonsmoking farmers. Am Rev Respir Dis 140:695-699

Lacasse Y, Selman M, Costabel U et al (2003) Clinical diagnosis of hypersensitivity pneumonitis. Am J Respir Crit Care Med 168:952-958

Laemmli UK (1970) Cleavage of structural proteins during the assembly of the head of bacteriophage T4. Nature 227:680-685

Lappalainen S, Pasanen AL, Reiman M et al (1998) Serum IgG antibodies against *Wallemia sebi* and *Fusarium* species in Finnish farmers. Ann Allergy Asthma Immunol 81:585-592

Larsson K, Malmberg P, Eklund A et al (1988) Exposure to microorganisms, airway inflammatory changes and immune reactions in asymptomatic dairy farmers. Int Arch Allergy Appl Immunol 87:127-133

Latge JP(1999) *Aspergillus fumigatus* and aspergillosis. Clin Microbiol Rev 12:310-350

Lioy PJ, Weisel CP, Millette JR et al (2002) Characterization of the dust/smoke aerosol that settled east of the World Trade Center (WTC) in lower Manhattan after the collapse of the WTC 11 September 2001. Environ Health Perspect 110:703-714

Lipsky PE (2001) Rheumatoid arthritis. In : Braunwald E, Fauci AS, Kasper DL, Hauser SL, Longo DL, Jameson JL (eds) Harrison principles of internal medicine, 15th edn. McGraw-Hill, New York, pp 1928-1937

Maier LA (2002) Genetic and exposure risks for chronic beryllium disease. Clin Chest Med 23:827-839

Maier LA, Kittle LA, Mroz MM et al (2003) Beryllium-stimulated neopterin as a diagnostic adjunct in chronic beryllium disease. Am J Ind Med 43:592-601

Marcer G, Simioni L, Saia B et al (1983) Study of immunological parameters in farmer's lung. Clin Allergy 13:443-449

Martinez-Cordero E, Aguilar Leon DE, Retana VN (2000) IgM antiavian antibodies in sera from patients with pigeon breeder's disease. J Clin Lab Anal 14:201-207

Marx JJ, Emanuel DA, Dovenbarger WV et al (1978) Farmer's lung disease among farmers with precipitating antibodies to the thermophilic actinomycetes: a clinical and immunologic study. J Allergy Clin Immunol 62:185-189

McSharry C, Anderson K, Bourke SJ et al (2002) Takes your breath away - the immunology of allergic alveolitis. Clin Exp Immunol 128:3-9

Melinn M, McLaughlin H (1989) Farmer's lung : a three year survey and comparison of ELISA and CIEP technique in antibody detection. Ir J Med Sci 15:173-174

Melinn M, McLaughlin H (1992) Comparison of methods of production of farmer's lung antigens. Int Arch Allergy Immunol 99:56-62

Miyazaki H, Gemma H, Uemura K, et al (2004) Hypersensitivity pneumonitis induced by *Aspergillus niger* – a case report. Nihon Kokyuki Gakkai Zasshi 42:676-681

Moran JV, Greenberger PA, Patterson R (2002) Long-term evaluation of hypersensitivity pneumonitis: a case study follow-up and literature review. Allergy Asthma Proc 23:265-270

Moss RB (2002) Allergic bronchopulmonary aspergillosis. Clin Rev Allergy Immunol 23:87-104

Moutsopoulos HM (2001) Sjögren's syndrome. In : Braunwald E, Fauci AS, Kasper DL, Hauser SL, Longo DL, Jameson JL (eds) Harrison principles of internal medicine, 15th edn. McGraw-Hill, New York, pp 1947-1949

Mundt C, Becker WM, Schlaak M (1996) Farmer's lung: patients' IgG2 antibodies specifically recognize *Saccharopolyspora rectivirgula* proteins and carbohydrate structures. J Allergy Clin Immunol 98:441-450

Newman LS, Bobka C, Schumacher B et al (1994) Compartmentalized immune response reflects clinical severity of beryllium disease. Am J Respir Crit Care Med 150:135-142

Nolard N, Symoens F, Beguin H (1994) Mycological surveys in dwellings and factories: application to diagnosis of extrinsic allergic alveolitis. In: Samson RA, Flannigan B, Flannigan ME et al (eds) Air quality monographs. Health implication in indoor environments. Elsevier, Amsterdam, pp 201-209

Ouchterlony O (1953) Antigen-antibody reactions in gels. Acta Pathol Microbiol Scand 32:231-240

Ojanen T (1992) Class specific antibodies in serodiagnosis of farmer's lung. Br J Ind Med 49:332-336

Ojanen TH, Katila ML, Mäntyjärvi RA (1980) The use of enzyme-linked immunosorbent assay (ELISA) in the diagnosis of farmer's lung. Allergy 35:537-542

Ojanen TH, Terho EO, Mäntyjärvi RA (1982) Comparison of *Aspergillus fumigatus* and *Aspergillus umbrosus* antigens in serological tests of farmer's lung. Allergy 37:297-301

Ojanen TH, Terho EO, Mantyjarvi RA (1987) IgG subclasses in farmer's lung, Eur J Respir Dis [Suppl] 154:145-150.

Paris S, Fitting C, Latge JP et al (1990) Comparison of conidial and mycelial allergens of *Alternaria alternata*. Arch Allergy Appl Immunol 92:1-8

Patel AM, Ryu JH, Reed CE (2001) Hypersensitivity pneumonitis: current concepts and future questions. J Allergy Clin Immunol 108:661-670

Pavesi F, Fasani F, Rancati E et al (1984) *Micropolyspora faeni* antigens of three commercial extracts. Mycopathologia 84:165-169

Pepys J, Riddell RW, Citron KM et al (1962) Precipitins against extracts of hay and moulds in the serum of patients with farmer's lung, aspergillosis, asthma and sarcoidosis. Thorax 17: 366-374

Pepys J, Jenkins PA, Festenstein GN et al (1963) Farmer's lung, thermophilic actinomycetes as a source of "farmer's lung hay" antigen. Lancet 41:607-611

Pepys J, Jenkins PA (1965) Precipitin (FLH) test farmer's lung. Thorax 20:21-35

Pepys J (1969) Hypersensitivity disease of the lung due to fungi and other organic dusts. Karger, Basel (Monographs in allergy, vol 4)

Pepys J (1994) Farmer's lung. A needle in a haystack and Pandora's box. ACI News 6:63-72

Ramasamy M, Khan ZU, Kurup VP (1987) A partially purified antigen from *Faenia rectivirgula* in the diagnosis of farmer's lung disease. Microbios 49:171-182

Rask-Andersen A (1989) Allergic alveolitis in Swedish farmers. Upsala J Med Sci 94:271-285

Rautalahti M, Terho EO, Ojanen T (1990) Changes in the titers of IgG antibodies against farmer's lung antigens in the sera of healthy dairy farmers. Ann Allergy 64:455-458

Reboux G, Piarroux R, Bardonnet K et al (2001a) Comparison of four serological techniques in immunological diagnosis of farmer's lung disease. Am J Respir Crit Care Med 163:A747 (abstract)

Reboux G, Piarroux R, Mauny F et al (2001b) Role of molds in farmer's lung disease in Eastern France. Am J Respir Crit Care Med 163:1534-1539

Recco P, Pourciel D, Borderies M et al (1978) Poumon de fermier, poumon des éleveurs d'oiseaux notre expérience en midi-pyrénées. Bull Soc Fr Mycol Méd 7:281-284

Reese G, Trompelt J, Becker WM et al (1989) Extrinsic allergic alveolitis: IgG subclass reactivities and monoclonal antibodies against *Micropolyspora faeni* and *Aspergillus fumigatus*. Immun Infekt 17:165-168

Roberts RC, Wenzel FJ, Emanuel DA (1976) Precipitating antibodies in a Midwest dairy farming population toward the antigens associated with farmer's lung disease. J Allergy Clin Immunol 57:518-524

Rodrigo MJ, Benavent MI, Cruz MJ et al (2000) Detection of specific antibodies to pigeon serum and bloom antigens by enzyme linked immunosorbent assay in pigeon breeder's disease. Occup Environ Med 57:159-164

Rosen S, Yu JH, Adams TH (1999) The *Aspergillus nidulans* sfaD gene encodes a G protein beta subunit that is required for normal growth and repression of sporulation. EMBO J 18:5592-5600

Rossman MD (1996) Chronic beryllium disease: diagnosis and management. Environ Health Perspect 104S:945-947

Rossman MD, Kern JA, Elias JA et al (1988) Proliferative response of bronchoalveolar lymphocytes to beryllium. Ann Intern Med 108:687-693

Roussel S (2004) Influence des pratiques agricoles sur la flore microbiologique des fourrages et sur le risque de maladie du poumon de fermier. Thesis, Besançon

Roussel S, Reboux G, Dalphin JC et al (2004) Microbiological evolution of hay and relapse in patients with farmer's lung. Occup Environ Med 61:e3

Saltini C, Richeldi L, Losi M et al (2001) Major histocompatibility locus genetic markers of beryllium sensitization and disease. Eur Respir J 18:1-8

Salvaggio JE (1972) Diagnostic significance of serum precipitins in hypersensitivity pneumonitis. Chest 62 242-252

Salvaggio JE (1991) Immune reactions in allergic alveolitis. Eur Respir J 4 [Suppl 13]:47s-59s

Salvaggio JE (1997) Extrinsic allergic alveolitis (hypersensitivity pneumonitis): past, present and future. Clin Exp Allergy 27 [Suppl 1]:18-25

Schumacher HR, Pessler F, Chen LX (2003) Diagnosing early rheumatoid arthritis (RA). What are the problems and opportunities? Clin Exp Rheumatol 21 [Suppl 31]:S15-S19

Scribner GH, Barboriak JJ, Fink JN (1980) Prevalence of precipitins in group at risk of developing hypersensitivity pneumonitis. Clin Allergy 10:91-95

Sharp GC (1994) Mixed connective tissue disease arthritis. In: Isselbacher KJ, Braunwald E, Wilson JD, Martin JB, Fauci AS, Kasper DL (eds) Harrison principles of internal medicine, 13th edn. McGraw-Hill, New York, pp 1660-1661

Solal-Céligny PH, Laviolette M, Hébert J et al (1982) Immune reactions in the lungs of asymptomatic dairy farmers. Am Rev Respir Dis 126:964-967

Spiegelberg HL (1974) Biological activities of immunoglobulins of different classes and subclasses. Adv Immunol 19:259-294

Stoeckle JD, Hardy HL, Weber AL (1969) Chronic beryllium disease. Long-term follow-up of sixty cases and selective review of the literature. Am J Med 46:545-561

Stokes TC, Turton CWG, Turner-Warwick M (1981) A study of immunoglobulin G subclasses in patients with farmer's lung. Clin Allergy 11:201-207

Taylor TP, Ding M, Ehler DS et al (2003) Beryllium in the environment: a review. J Environ Sci Health A Tox Hazard Subst Environ Eng 38:439-469

Terho EO, Husman K, Vohlonen I et al (1987) Serum precipitins against microbes in mouldy hay with respect to age, sex, atopy and smoking of farmers. Eur J Respir Dis 152 [Suppl]:115-121

Todd A, Coan R, Allen A (1993) Pigeon breeders' lung: IgG subclasses to pigeon intestinal mucin and IgA antigens. Clin Exp Immunol 92:494-499

Toubas D, Prevost A, Deschamps F et al (1995) Les alvéolites allergiques extrinsèques d'origine professionnelle. Presse Med 24:1391-1396

Trentin L, Marcer G, Chilosi M et al (1988) Longitudinal study of alveolitis in hypersensitivity pneumonitis patients: an immunologic evaluation. J Allergy Clin Immunol 82:577-585

Treuhaft MW, Roberts RC, Hackbarth C et al (1979) Characterization of precipitin response to *Micropolyspora faeni* in farmer's lung disease by quantitative immunoelectrophoresis. Am Rev Respir Dis 119:571-578

Vohlonen I, Husman K, Terho EO et al (1987) Prevalence of serum precipitins against microbes in mouldy hay, and of chronic bronchitis and farmer's lung with respect to farmer's occupational health hazards. Eur J Respir Dis 152 [Suppl]:139-145

Wardrop VE, Blyth W, Grant WB (1977) Farmer's lung in a group of Scottish dairy farms. Br J Ind Med 34:186-195

Wenzel F, Gray R, Roberts RC et al (1974) Serologic studies in farmer's lung. Am Rev Respir Dis 109:464-468

Williams CA Jr, Grabar PJ (1955) Immunoelectrophoretic studies on serum proteins. I. The antigens of human serum. Immunology 74:158-168

Williams WR, Williams WJ (1982) Development of beryllium lymphocyte transformation in chronic beryllium disease. Int Arch Allergy Appl Immunol 67:175-180

Yi ES (2002) Hypersensitivity pneumonitis. Crit Rev Clin Lab Sci 39:581-629

Ylönen JK, Ojanen TH, Jägerroos HJW et al (1989) Comparative immunochemical analysis of five *Thermoactinomyces* strains. Int Arch Allergy Appl Immunol 90:405-410

Part II:

Imaging

4 Lung Effects of Cigarette Smoking

SUJAL R. DESAI and DAVID M. HANSELL

CONTENTS

4.1 Introduction 161
4.2 Historical Concepts 161
4.3 Histopathological Considerations 162
4.3.1 Histopathological Overlap Among Smoking-Related Diseases 162
4.4 Emphysema 163
4.4.1 Plain Chest Radiography in Emphysema 163
4.4.2 CT in Emphysema 164
4.5 Langerhans' Cell Histiocytosis 164
4.5.1 Classification and Clinical Issues 164
4.5.2 Histopathological Features of Pulmonary LCH 165
4.5.3 Imaging of LCH 165
4.5.3.1 Chest Radiography 165
4.5.3.2 Computed Tomography 166
4.5.4 Radiological Differential Diagnosis 167
4.6 Respiratory Bronchiolitis, Respiratory Bronchiolitis-Associated Interstitial Lung Disease and Desquamative Interstitial Pneumonia 167
4.6.1 Histopathological and Clinical Issues 167
4.6.2 Imaging of RB, RBILD and DIP 168
4.6.2.1 Plain Chest Radiography 168
4.6.2.2 Computed Tomography 168
4.7 Radiological Differential Diagnosis 170
4.7.1 Natural History of Smoking-Related Interstitial Lung Diseases 170
4.8 Cigarette Smoking, Interstitial Fibrosis and Other Idiopathic Interstitial Pneumonias 171
4.8.1 Usual Interstitial Pneumonia 172
4.8.2 Non-Specific Interstitial Pneumonia 172
4.8.3 Other Idiopathic Interstitial Pneumonias and Diffuse Lung Disorders 173
4.9 Summary 173
References 173

S. R. DESAI, MD, MRCP, FRCR
Consultant Radiologist, Department of Radiology, King's College Hospital, Denmark Hill, London, SE5 9RS, UK
D. M. HANSELL, MD, FRCP, FRCR
Professor of Thoracic Imaging, National Heart and Lung Institute and Division of Investigative Science, Imperial College School of Medicine, London *and* Department of Radiology, Royal Brompton Hospital, Sydney Street, London, SW3 6NP, UK

4.1 Introduction

The concept that smoking has a deleterious effect on health is not new (BRITTON et al. 2000). The implications for health care are truly global, with bronchogenic carcinoma, chronic obstructive lung disease and ischaemic heart disease proportionately accounting for the greatest smoking-related morbidity (BRITTON et al. 2000; BARTECCHI et al. 1994; WHO CHRONICLES 1982). In recent years, there has been increasing awareness about the potential for smokers to develop pulmonary diseases other than lung cancer, chronic bronchitis and emphysema. Whilst briefly revisiting emphysema, this chapter will focus on the imaging of interstitial lung diseases related to smoking, particularly as demonstrated thin-section computed tomography (CT) abnormalities. The sometimes complex interrelationships among the smoking-related pulmonary disorders will be explored, and the more speculative association between pulmonary fibrosis and smoking will also be discussed.

4.2 Historical Concepts

The list of disorders that are known (or presumed) to be causally linked to cigarette smoking has grown steadily (Table 4.1). The association between smoking and lung cancer, chronic bronchitis and emphysema have long been established and are not contentious. However, smoking has been linked to other pulmonary disorders. In historical terms, the notion that smoking can lead to pulmonary fibrosis (a link that remains unproven) was first posited in 1969 (WEISS 1969). Within 5 years, Niewoehner and colleagues had demonstrated what are now taken to be the characteristic histopathological changes in the lungs of smokers: the study was the first to report the features of respiratory bronchiolitis at autopsy

Table 4.1. Lung disorders related to cigarette smoking

Definite association:
• Bronchogenic carcinoma
• Emphysema
• Chronic bronchitis
Probable association:
• Respiratory bronchiolitis
• Respiratory bronchiolitis-associated interstitial lung disease
• Langerhans' cell histiocytosis
• Desquamative interstitial pneumonitis
Possible association:
• Cryptogenic fibrosing alveolitis/Idiopathic pulmonary fibrosis
• Non-specific interstitial pneumonia pattern
• Eosinophilic pneumonia
• Pulmonary haemorrhage

in a small cohort of young smokers (Niewoehner et al. 1974). The entity of desquamative interstitial pneumonia (DIP), first described in 1965 (Liebow et al. 1965), has radiological features that overlap with respiratory bronchiolitis (RB) and respiratory-bronchiolitis-associated interstitial lung disease (RBILD) on histopathological examination. More importantly, clinical and epidemiological data suggest that DIP is almost invariably an idiosyncratic reaction to cigarette smoke (Gaensler et al. 1966; King et al. 2000; Travis et al. 2002; Moon et al. 1999), and the view that DIP is an "early" or cellular form of cryptogenic fibrosing alveolitis has been discredited (Fromm et al. 1980).

4.3 Histopathological Considerations

A common theme in the smoking-induced lung diseases is macrophage-related lung damage: there are variable abnormalities of macrophage function, accumulation or activation (Marten and Hansell 2005). Animal studies have shown that an excess of macrophages can accumulate within the alveoli even after a relatively short exposure to cigarette smoke (Frasca et al. 1983). In the related entities of RB, RBILD and DIP, the striking cellular abnormality is an excess of macrophages within the lungs. In this context, the recent observation on serial CT studies that the centrilobular nodules of RB (reflecting bronchiolocentric macrophage infiltration) may, in some patients, be replaced by the lesions of centrilobular emphysema is a tantalising one (Remy-Jardin et al. 2002). Indeed, a potential link between the excess of smoking-induced pulmonary macrophages and the venerable "elastase–antielastase" theory may be proposed, with macrophage recruitment by neutrophil elastase seemingly the key event in the development of emphysema (Janoff 1985; Shapiro et al. 2003; Hautamaki et al. 1997). In pulmonary Langerhans' cell histiocytosis (LCH), cigarette smoke is likely to be the initiating factor [possibly through the release of bombesin-like neuropeptides (Aguayo et al. 1989)] for the recruitment, proliferation and activation of so-called Langerhans' cells, which themselves are differentiated cells of the monocyte-macrophage system (Vassallo et al. 2000). However, unlike lung disorders that are linked to specific cells types, the pathogenesis of macrophage-driven diseases has not been fully elucidated.

4.3.1 Histopathological Overlap Among Smoking-Related Diseases

The evaluation of lung biopsy material in patients with suspected smoking-related lung disease is not an easy undertaking. One of the main problems is that a mixture of histopathological abnormalities is not uncommon [and often reflected in findings at thin-section CT (Fig. 4.1)]. Features of RB and

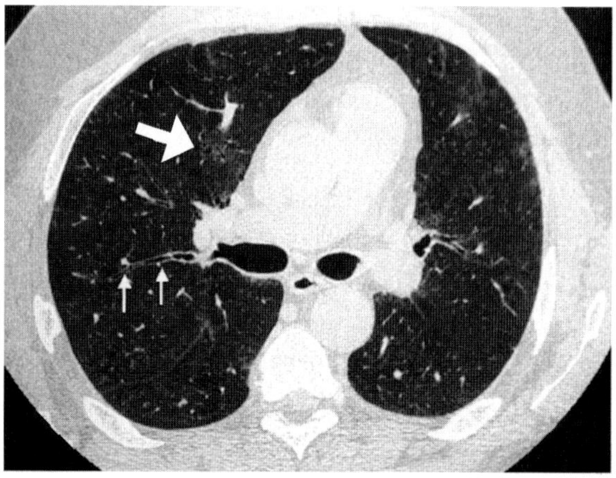

Fig. 4.1. Mixed thin-section computed tomography patterns in an adult smoker. There is generalised ground-glass opacification in both lungs (taken to represent a component of respiratory bronchiolitis). In addition, there are signs of fibrosis: a fine superimposed reticular pattern is seen, and there is evidence of traction bronchiectasis (*thin arrows*) in the right lung. There is also centrilobular emphysema, of limited extent, in the right lung (*thick arrow*)

DIP and emphysema are often noted in patients with pulmonary LCH (Colby and Lombard 1983; Travis et al. 1993; Vassallo et al. 2003); in some patients, the macrophage accumulation around the lesions of LCH is so florid that the distinction from DIP may be impossible (Colby and Carrington 1995). Even the apparently simple histological exercise of detecting emphysema is not entirely straightforward. Although there is little difficulty for the pathologist in confirming that there is the *de rigueur* alveolar wall destruction, the requirement that there must be no obvious fibrosis (Snider et al. 1985) is often more difficult to satisfy: in some patients with emphysema, there is biochemical (Cardoso et al. 1993; Lang et al. 1994) and radiological (Tonelli et al. 1997) evidence of fibrosis. To confuse matters further, there is the view that tobacco smoke may be the common denominator in the causation of not only emphysema but also pulmonary fibrosis (Weiss 1969; Niewoehner et al. 1982; Baumgartner et al. 1997). Proponents of the hypothesis usually quote the indirect evidence from animal studies (Frasca et al. 1983) and also observations about the prevalence of smoking (Turner-Warwick et al. 1980; Johnston et al. 1997), together with the frequent coexistence of emphysema on CT in patients with cryptogenic fibrosing alveolitis (Wiggins et al. 1990; Doherty et al. 1997; Wells et al. 1997).

4.4 Emphysema

The histopathological definition of emphysema (i.e. abnormal, permanent enlargement of the air spaces distal to the terminal bronchiole, accompanied by *destruction* of their walls but without obvious fibrosis) is cumbersome but emphasises the importance of identifying parenchymal destruction before a pathological diagnosis of emphysema can be made (Snider et al. 1985).

The main histopathological subtypes of emphysema are categorised according to the distribution of disease within the acinus (Thurlbeck 1995): in centrilobular (centriacinar) emphysema, there is abnormal dilatation of respiratory bronchioles but sparing of the more distal structures of the acinus (Thurlbeck et al. 1970; Thurlbeck 1995). This type of emphysema shows striking heterogeneity, so that adjacent lobules are variably affected. Paraseptal emphysema (characterised by enlargement of alveoli adjacent to connective tissue septa or the pleura) is typically seen at the periphery of the secondary lobule. Finally, in panlobular (otherwise known as panacinar) emphysema, there may be more selective involvement of the alveolar ducts, at least in the early stages, compared with other regions of the acinus; the changes are most pronounced in the lower zones (Thurlbeck et al. 1970; Thurlbeck and Simon 1978; Gishen et al. 1982). As the term implies, the histopathological hallmark of panacinar emphysema is the virtually uniform involvement of the whole acinus. Thus, perhaps not surprisingly, panlobular emphysema is most often associated with clinically significant disease.

4.4.1 Plain Chest Radiography in Emphysema

The plain radiograph is usually the first radiological test to be requested in patients with suspected obstructive airways disease. However, it must be stressed that only emphysema of moderate-to-marked severity can be depicted on plain radiographs (Thurlbeck and Simon 1978). The key radiographic abnormalities of emphysema were first identified by Kerley in 1936: hyperinflation and abnormalities of peripheral small vessels (a diminution in the number and calibre) were the key features. Laws and Heard evaluated radiographic features in patients with histopathologically-proven disease (Laws and Heard 1962). Not surprisingly, the plain radiograph was normal in patients with limited centrilobular emphysema. However, there was broad correlation between the extent of emphysema and the likelihood of there being abnormalities on the plain radiograph, a relationship validated in subsequent publications (Thurlbeck and Simon 1978; Burrows et al. 1966). With extensive disease, and particularly when there was panacinar emphysema, the radiograph was frequently abnormal. Unlike the sign of peripheral vascular attenuation, hyperinflation is a more robust indicator of emphysema on plain radiographs (Nicklaus et al. 1966; Katsura and Martin 1967). Flattening of the hemidiaphragm is a typical finding and is sometimes better appreciated on the lateral view (Nicklaus et al. 1966; Katsura and Martin 1967). A consequence of diaphragmatic flattening is the change in the configuration of the cardiac silhouette, leading to the characteristic "narrow" heart on frontal radiographs (Simon 1964).

4.4.2 CT in Emphysema

The ability of CT to detect emphysema was recognised nearly two decades ago (GODDARD et al. 1982; HAYHURST et al. 1984). The earliest observations, made using older CT machines (with thick collimation images), were that there was a reduction in *global* lung density in patients with emphysema (HAYHURST et al. 1984). However, the advent of faster CT imaging and specifically, thin-section CT facilitated the recognition of the more specific morphological features of centrilobular emphysema. The characteristic thin-section CT pattern is foci of decreased attenuation, usually without visible walls, that are distributed non-uniformly and interspersed with regions of apparently normal lung (FOSTER et al. 1986; AUSTIN et al. 1996). Because of the permeative nature of parenchymal destruction, the lungs have a "moth-eaten" appearance (Fig. 4.2). In more advanced disease, there is distortion of pulmonary vessels. It is often possible to see a high-density structure (the lobular arteriole) in the centre of the lesions of centrilobular emphysema and, whilst the intervening normal lung parenchyma can usually be identified, with more extensive disease, this may prove difficult. The lesions of centrilobular emphysema may appear to have well-defined walls, and the walls of such "cysts" are probably composed of retracted residual alveoli that have collapsed against lobular septa. Furthermore, there may also be a component of fibrosis within interlobular septa that contributes to the impression on an identifiable wall.

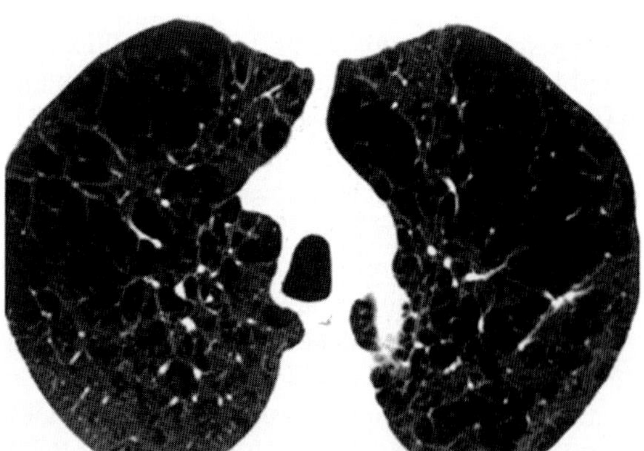

Fig. 4.2. Centrilobular emphysema on thin-section computed tomography. There is characteristic symmetrical and "permeative" lung destruction

In centrilobular emphysema, the brunt of disease is generally in the upper lobes, particularly in the early stages. However, with progression, the lesions of centrilobular can become confluent, and, in such cases, the distinction between centrilobular and panacinar emphysema on CT can become blurred (COPLEY et al., in press). Paraseptal emphysema frequently coexists with the changes of centrilobular emphysema. This type of emphysema may be seen giving rise to a "saw-tooth" type of appearance along mediastinal and pleural surfaces. In contrast to centrilobular disease, the lung destruction in panacinar emphysema is generally more uniform, and there are widespread areas of low density and vascular attenuation; it is notable that there is often little or no architectural disturbance as shown by the normal disposition of attenuated vessels.

4.5 Langerhans' Cell Histiocytosis

4.5.1 Classification and Clinical Issues

The terminology and classification of the histiocytic disorders has recently been revised and simplified (VASSALLO et al. 2000; FAVARA and FELLER 1997). LCH is a term that encompasses three historical clinical conditions, namely Hand-Schüller-Christian disease, Letterer-Siwe disease and eosinophilic granuloma; the term histiocytosis X was first used in 1953 to encompass all three disorders (LICHTENSTEIN 1953). Whilst the basic dichotomy between localised and systemic disease remains in the new classification, the older eponymous titles have been rejected (FAVARA and FELLER 1997), and all patients, regardless of the site(s) of disease, are deemed to have LCH.

The lungs may be involved in the systemic forms of LCH, but pulmonary disease most frequently occurs in isolation. Although the age distribution is wide, LCH usually affects young adults. Males outnumber females by about 4 to 1, and the great majority of adult patients are cigarette smokers (TRAVIS et al. 1993; FRIEDMAN et al. 1981; HOWARTH et al. 1999). Indeed, in contrast to systemic forms, the pulmonary disease is considered to be a reactive condition (YOUSEM et al. 2001). The symptoms reported by patients are non-specific and include cough and dyspnoea. As with other diffuse lung disease, patients with LCH are prone to develop pneumothoraces. Constitutional symptoms such as weight loss and fever may also occur, but some patients are surprisingly asymptomatic despite evidence of radiographic lung disease. Lung function tests usually show a restrictive defect physiological defect. Patients with pulmonary LCH have an increased but variable (1–25%) number of Langerhans' cells in bronchoalveolar lavage fluid compared with healthy non-smokers (fewer than 1%) and with normal smokers and patients with other interstitial lung diseases (up to 3%).

The pathogenesis of pulmonary LCH is not known. However, it is very likely that cigarette smoke is an important aetiological agent: over 90% of patients with pulmonary LCH give a history of smoking (Travis et al. 1993; Friedman et al. 1981; Howarth et al. 1999). Further support of a link between smoking and LCH comes from experimental data, which associate components of cigarette smoke with the development of pulmonary LCH (Casolaro et al. 1988; Youkeles et al. 1995; Zeid and Muller 1995). Aside from smoking, there is an interesting but unexplained association between LCH and certain malignancies (typically lung and haematological) (Howarth et al. 1999; Burns et al. 1983; Neumann and Frizzera 1986; Tomashefski et al. 1991; Vassallo et al. 2002). Malignant neoplasms in patients with pulmonary LCH may predate, follow or occur concurrently with the disease (Vassallo et al. 2002).

4.5.2 Histopathological Features of Pulmonary LCH

The unifying cytological feature, in the various forms of LCH, is the proliferation of and infiltration by CD1+ histiocytes (Langerhans' cells) (Favara and Feller 1997; Yousem et al. 2001). The earliest abnormality is an interstitial infiltrate, which tends to be centred on the small airways (Colby 1983; Colby and Carrington 1995). At high power, the cellular lesions of LCH can be seen to be comprised of aggregates of Langerhans' cells, containing a moderate amount of light eosinophilic cytoplasm devoid of pigment. The cells may be mitotically active and generally associated with variable numbers of eosinophils. Scanty numbers of neutrophils and lymphocytes may be present.

As the disease progresses, the infiltrate becomes appreciably nodular. There may be florid infiltration of the surrounding air spaces by pigmented macrophages (essentially a "DIP-type" reaction). Indeed, a component of respiratory bronchiolitis and/or DIP are a common (and sometimes florid) feature of the lungs in patients with proven LCH (Vassallo et al. 2003). Cavitation [which, in some cases, can be traced to a dilated airway lumen (Ambouchner et al. 1996)] is a characteristic feature of the nodules of LCH, and the cardinal histopathological lesion of LCH is a roughly symmetrical nodule with central scarring and a stellate outline (Colby 1983). Another characteristic is the temporal heterogeneity, so that "new" cellular lesions often coexist with "old" scarred nodules. There may be co-existent emphysema. In the end-stage, there is confluent scarring associated with widespread emphysema producing a peculiar form of honeycombing with overinflation of the lungs.

4.5.3 Imaging of LCH

4.5.3.1 Chest Radiography

In established pulmonary disease, the chest radiograph is usually abnormal. The most common abnormalities are a reticular pattern, micronodules (measuring up to 2 mm in diameter) and cysts (Lacronique et al. 1982). There is no obvious predilection for the central or peripheral lung. A useful diagnostic clue on chest radiographs (but not necessarily confined to cases of LCH) is that, despite the apparently extensive interstitial disease, lung volumes may be preserved or, in some patients, even increased (Lacronique et al. 1982) (Fig. 4.3). Indeed, hyperinflation becomes

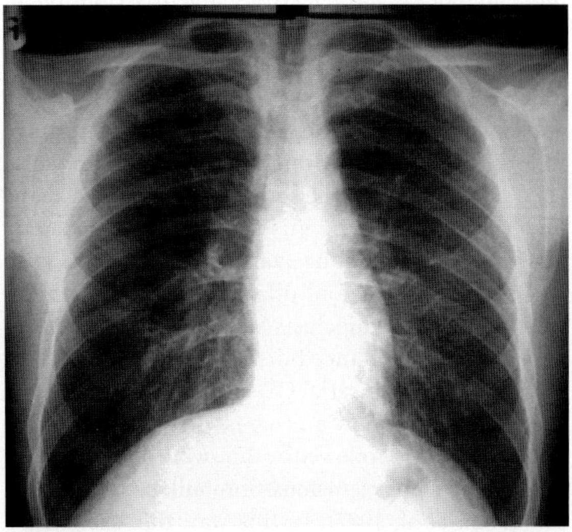

Fig. 4.3. Chest radiograph in a young smoker with Langerhans' cell histiocytosis. There is a diffuse reticulo-nodular pattern in both lungs but, despite the apparently extensive disease, lung volumes are increased

more evident with disease progression; given that the disease is so strikingly bronchiolocentric, it seems likely that small airways obstruction is responsible for the hyperinflation (Travis et al. 1993). A rare complication (which may also be explained by the bronchovascular microscopic distribution of LCH lesions) is severe pulmonary arterial hypertension (Fartoukh et al. 2000).

Pleural effusions, hilar lymph-node enlargement, endoluminal masses, pneumothorax and a solitary pulmonary nodule are less common manifestations of pulmonary LCH (Lacronique et al. 1982; Pomeranz and Proto 1986; O'Donnell et al. 1987; Fichtenbaum et al. 1990). The appearances on serial radiographs vary, but, in general, nodular opacities tend to regress (with or without treatment). In some patients, there may be almost complete radiographic resolution following the cessation of smoking (von Essen et al. 1990; Mogulkoc et al. 1999); whereas, in others, a period of disease stability can be followed (sometimes many years later) by florid relapse (Tazi et al. 1998) or a slow inexorable progression characterised by airflow obstruction and disproportionate pulmonary hypertension (Fartoukh et al. 2000). Disease recurrence has also been reported after lung transplantation (Etienne et al. 1998).

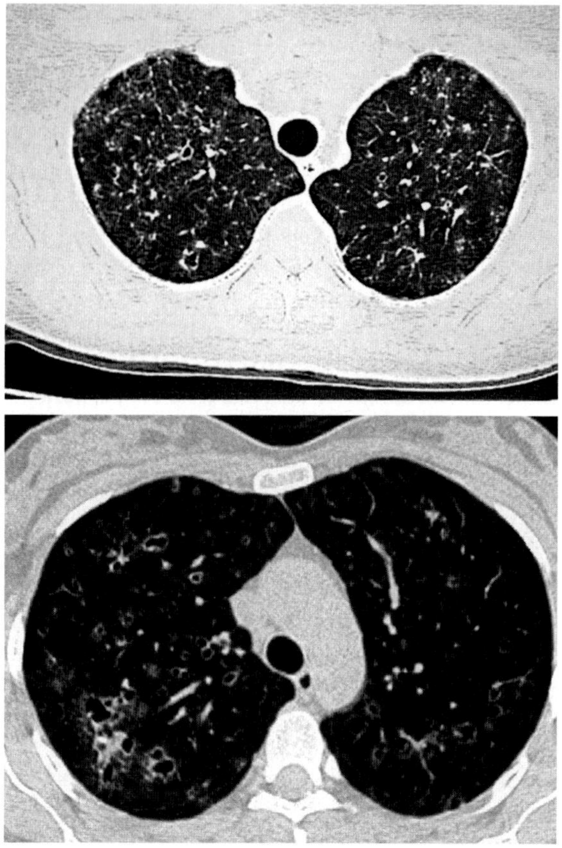

Fig. 4.4a,b. Two patients with Langerhans' cell histiocytosis (LCH). **a** Thin-section computed tomography through the upper zones demonstrates numerous small (1–2 mm diameter) nodules, an unusual pattern in LCH. There is evidence of cavitation in one or two of the larger nodules. **b** A more typical pattern demonstrating larger cavitating nodules. Many of the cavities have an unusual outline

4.5.3.2 Computed Tomography

Thin-section CT can show with great clarity the morphological characteristics and distribution of disease in LCH. Furthermore, on serial examinations, the natural history of the disease can also be followed. The classical and virtually pathognomonic appearances on CT comprise nodules, which range in size from a few millimetres to 2 cm in diameter (Fig. 4.4). Because of the sometimes elongated shape of cysts, some may be mistaken for bronchiectatic airways; whilst it is conceivable that some lesions do represent distorted and dilated airways, it is noteworthy that bronchiectasis is not a reported feature on CT, even in advanced disease.

Observations on serial CT studies indicate that the nodules of LCH show a progression through certain stages: cavitation, followed by thin-walled cystic lesions and finally emphysematous/fibrobullous destruction (Brauner et al. 1997). In this way, thin-section CT may predict "disease activity" in LCH, although one recent study has shown that there may be extensive microscopic cellular infiltration even in the presence of apparently end-stage cystic lung disease (Soler et al. 2000). The CT appearances, at any point in time, are governed by the stage of the disease in an individual patient: thus, in the early phase, nodules tend to predominate; whereas, at follow-up, cysts are seen more often (Brauner et al. 1997). In one series, both nodules and cysts were seen at CT in 13 of 18 (72%) patients; however, isolated cysts or nodules (22% and 6%, respectively) were also noted in a minority of cases (Brauner et al. 1989). The cysts of pulmonary LCH initially tend to be small (generally less than 1 cm in diameter) and have a variable wall thickness. A helpful diagnostic feature on CT is the sometimes strikingly bizarre outline of cysts, which is presumed to be because of the coalescence of adjacent cysts. The sparing of the costophrenic recesses and the tip of the middle lobe/lingula is also said to be a characteristic finding on CT (Moore et al. 1989). In some patients, CT will not demonstrate any of the recognised features of LCH, despite histopathological proof of the diagnosis (Moore et al. 1989); it seems possible that such cases represent "occult" pulmonary LCH (Pai and Tomashefski 2002).

Other thin-section CT abnormalities may coexist in patients with LCH: in a small proportion of patients, there is diffuse ground-glass opacification, which is likely to reflect a component of respiratory bronchiolitis and/or DIP (Vassallo et al. 2003). The coexistence of centrilobular and paraseptal emphysema, at a time when the LCH is largely nodular or showing early cavitation of the nodules, reflects the fact that almost all patients are cigarette smokers. Later in the evolution of the disease, the distinction between pre-existing smoking-related emphysema and end-stage LCH may be more difficult.

4.5.4 Radiological Differential Diagnosis

On individual CT images, the appearances of pulmonary LCH may be mistaken for those of bronchiectasis. However, review of adjacent sections will generally confirm the cystic nature of lesions in LCH. Another problem in diagnosis is the differentiation on CT between emphysema and LCH. True cysts, in contrast to the low attenuation lesions of centrilobular emphysema, generally have a definable wall (Austin et al. 1996); however, when the lesions of emphysema extend to the periphery of the secondary pulmonary lobule, the distinction can become difficult (Fig. 4.5). Multiple intrapulmonary cysts are also a feature in patients with lymphangioleiomyomatosis (LAM) (Rappaport et al. 1989; Sherrier et al. 1989; Aberle et al. 1990). In most instances, the radiological differentiation from LCH is relatively straightforward, since nodules are not a CT feature at any stage in patients with LAM. Finally, intrapulmonary cysts are also reported in patients with pulmonary lymphocytic infiltration (Desai et al. 1997; Johkoh et al. 1999b; Honda et al. 1999). In this context, because most cases of lymphocytic interstitial pneumonia occur on a background of other disorders [including Sjögren's syndrome, acquired immunodeficiency syndrome and Castleman's disease (Anderson and Talal 1971; Koss et al. 1986)], the distinction from Langerhans' cell histiocytosis is not usually difficult.

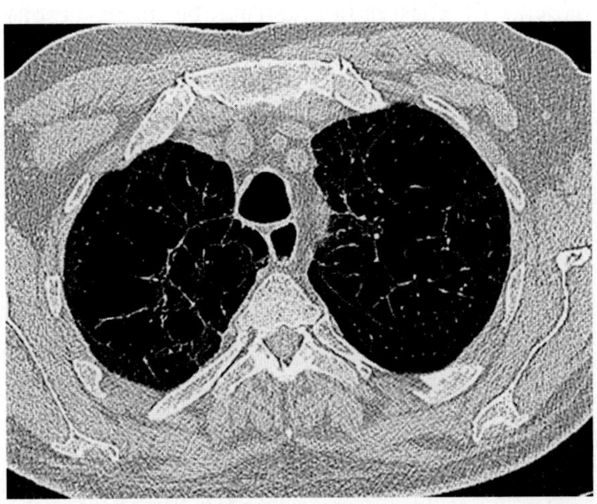

Fig. 4.5. Thin-section computed tomography through the upper zones in a patient with severe centrilobular emphysema. Many of the low attenuation lesions of emphysema appear to have a well-defined wall, and the appearances may be mistaken for those seen in "end-stage" Langerhans' cell histiocytosis

4.6 Respiratory Bronchiolitis, Respiratory Bronchiolitis-Associated Interstitial Lung Disease and Desquamative Interstitial Pneumonia

4.6.1 Histopathological and Clinical Issues

Because of overlapping histopathological appearances and the association with smoking, RB, RBILD and DIP will be considered together in the following sections (Carrington et al. 1978; Yousem et al. 1989). The entity of RB (sometimes called "smoker's bronchiolitis") is an incidental but invariable finding in the lungs of otherwise healthy smokers (Niewoehner et al. 1974; Fraig et al. 2002). Niewoehner and colleagues were the first to recognise the characteristic histopathological abnormality of RB in an autopsy study of 24 young subjects, 19 of whom had a documented smoking history (Niewoehner et al. 1974): there was mild chronic peribronchiolar inflammation (with characteristic pigmented macrophages), and fibrosis was noted in the walls of respiratory bronchioles and adjacent alveoli.

The changes of RB are, barring a few exceptions [namely, the cases of so-called "variant RB" in non-smokers (Fraig et al. 2002)], consistently associated with a history of smoking (Fraig et al. 2002) and, in the vast majority of cases, clinically silent. However, in 1987, Myers and colleagues reported the histopathological features in six heavy smokers who presented with the clinical features of an interstitial lung disease but who, on histopathological examination of open lung biopsy material, were shown to have changes identical to those previously reported in RB (Myers et al. 1987). The term "respiratory bronchiolitis-associated interstitial lung disease" was coined to distinguish the airway-centred nature of changes in RBILD from those seen in DIP (Yousem et al. 1989). Indeed, for the pathologist, the key features that distinguish RBILD from DIP are the distribution and extent of involvement: in the RBILD, macrophage accumulation and fibrosis is centred on the small airways, and there is limited extension into adjacent alveoli. In contrast, lung involvement in DIP is generally more diffuse. The alveoli are filled by cells, which were at first thought to be pneumocytes shed from the alveolar epithelium (Fromm et al. 1980; Corrin et al. 1985). Not surprisingly, despite the apparent simplicity of this distinction, there is an overlap in appearance between DIP and RBILD, making the exercise of histopathological differentiation sometimes difficult (Moon et al. 1999; Colby and Carrington 1995; Yousem et al. 1989). Current opinion dictates that the patterns of RBILD and DIP should be regarded as separate entities, since there are differences in the range of associated clinical disorders (Travis et al. 2002), with the DIP pattern seen in the context of reaction to certain dusts (Herbert et al. 1982), drugs (Hamadeh et al. 1992) and some inborn errors of metabolism (Amir and Ron 1999). Furthermore, it must be remembered that DIP is exceedingly rare: the largest CT series, comprising a mere 22 patients, was published only after culling the records, over an 8-year period, from five tertiary centres (Hartman et al. 1993).

Patients with RBILD generally present between the second and fifth decades, and there is an equal sex distribution (Moon et al. 1999; Yousem et al. 1989; Fraig et al. 2002; Myers et al. 1987; Park et al. 2002). The commonest presenting features are a gradual onset of dyspnoea and a prominent cough (King 1993). Much less frequent symptoms include chest pain, weight loss but very rarely fever and haemoptysis. DIP usually presents in the fourth to fifth decades and, as a "pure" entity, is rare (Carrington et al. 1978). Clubbing, fever, lethargy and weight loss are recognised symptoms, but most patients complain of shortness of breath and a dry cough.

4.6.2 Imaging of RB, RBILD and DIP

4.6.2.1 Plain Chest Radiography

To date, there is relatively little in the literature about the plain radiographic abnormalities in RBILD. It seems likely that previous descriptions, referring to the presence of low-profusion, small irregular opacities on chest radiographs, were reporting RB and RBILD; the exact relationship of the historical and vexing term "dirty lung" to the entities of RB and RBILD is not entirely clear (Carilli et al. 1973; Dick et al. 1992; Gückel and Hansell 1998). The chest radiograph is usually abnormal in patients with symptoms ascribable to RBILD. In two of the earliest reports (including Myers' original description), comprising a total of 24 patients, the majority (70%) had evidence of a fine diffuse or basal reticulonodular pattern (Yousem et al. 1989; Myers et al. 1987). There may be bibasal areas of atelectasis (Yousem et al. 1989; Myers et al. 1987; Holt et al. 1993). Unlike CT, ground-glass opacification is a surprisingly uncommon finding on plain radiography in patients with RBILD. In the Mayo Clinic study, there was no evidence of ground-glass opacification in any of 18 patients (Yousem et al. 1989), and ground-glass opacification was a dominant feature in only 3 of 10 patients in another series (Moon et al. 1999).

The plain film abnormalities in DIP are variable and non-specific. In the original report of DIP by Liebow and colleagues, ground-glass opacification in the lower zones was the dominant radiographic abnormality in the majority of patients (Liebow et al. 1965). However, in at least three subsequent series, a reticulo-nodular pattern was the most common abnormality on plain radiographs; ground-glass opacification was a less frequent finding in both of these studies (Carrington et al. 1978; Patchevsky et al. 1973; Feigen and Friedman 1980). In some patients, the chest radiograph may be normal despite histopathologically proven disease (Liebow et al. 1965; Carrington et al. 1978; Yousem et al. 1989).

4.6.2.2 Computed Tomography

In RB and RBILD, there are variable and overlapping CT features; the constellation of reported thin-section CT features (in approximate decreasing order of frequency) are summarised in Table 4.2 (Fig. 4.6). In a study that was clearly ahead of its time, Remy-Jardin and colleagues were the first to report the "early" morphological effects of smoking cigarettes (Remy-Jardin et al. 1993a). The authors compared HRCT features in 98 current smokers, 26 ex-smokers and 51 lifelong non-smokers with essentially normal lung function and showed that parenchymal micronodules (upper zone predominant and measuring

Table 4.2. A summary of thin-section computed tomography features in respiratory bronchiolitis/respiratory bronchiolitis-associated lung disease

- Poorly defined small centrilobular nodules
- Areas of ground glass opacity
- Bronchial wall thickening
- Areas of decreased attenuation reflecting small airways disease
- Emphysema (paraseptal and centrilobular) – limited
- Thickened interlobular septa
- Features of established interstitial fibrosis

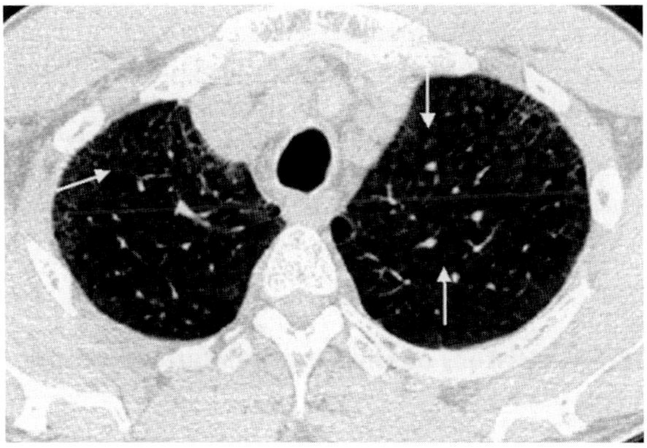

Fig. 4.6. Computed tomography through the upper lobes in respiratory bronchiolitis-associated interstitial lung disease. There is generalised ground-glass opacification and numerous ill-defined parenchymal micronodules (*arrows*). A fine peripheral reticular pattern and emphysema, both of limited extent, are noted

2–3 mm in diameter) were found in over one quarter of smokers but not in any of the non-smokers. Similar differences were observed for areas of ground-glass attenuation and emphysema [20% of smokers versus none of the non-smokers (for both comparisons)]. Parenchymal micronodules and ground-glass opacification were only seen in a minority (4% each) of ex-smokers. With the benefit of hindsight, it seems probable that Remy-Jardin et al. (1993a) were reporting the thin-section CT features of RB. In another paper from the same group, the authors showed that the main areas of ground-glass opacification corresponded to the accumulation of pigmented macrophages and mucus in the alveolar spaces, whereas the poorly defined parenchymal nodules (seen in their earlier study) were related to bronchiolectasis and peribronchiolar fibrosis (Remy-Jardin et al. 1993b).

A more recent study of 21 patients with pathologically proven RBILD demonstrated centrilobular nodules in 71% of cases, areas of ground glass opacity in two-thirds and patchy regions of decreased attenuation (most probably reflecting small airways obstruction) in over one-third (Park et al. 2002). Interestingly, in contrast to the study by Remy-Jardin and colleagues, the majority of patients had wall thickening of both proximal and distal airways (90% and 86%, respectively), presumably reflecting chronic bronchitis (Park et al. 2002).

Thickening of interlobular septa is seen in some patients with RBILD (Fig. 4.7); more obvious features of established interstitial fibrosis are unusual but evident in some patients with RBILD (Moon et al. 1999). A mosaic attenuation pattern, denoting the bronchiolitic element component of RBILD, is usually not a dominant feature but, when present, tends to be more conspicuous in the lower lobes (Park et al. 2002). In terms of differential diagnosis, it is worth noting that the combination of infiltrative and small airways disease on thin-section CT can also be encountered in subacute hypersensitivity pneumonitis, and this differential diagnosis is an important one for radiologists (see below). Emphysema is often present in patients with RBILD but usually of limited extent and confined to the lung apices.

Because there is widespread macrophage infiltration and consequent displacement of air from the alveoli, diffuse ground-glass opacification is the most frequent CT abnormality in DIP (Hartmann et al. 1993; Vedal et al. 1988; Heyneman et al. 1999). In the largest study to date, bilateral ground-

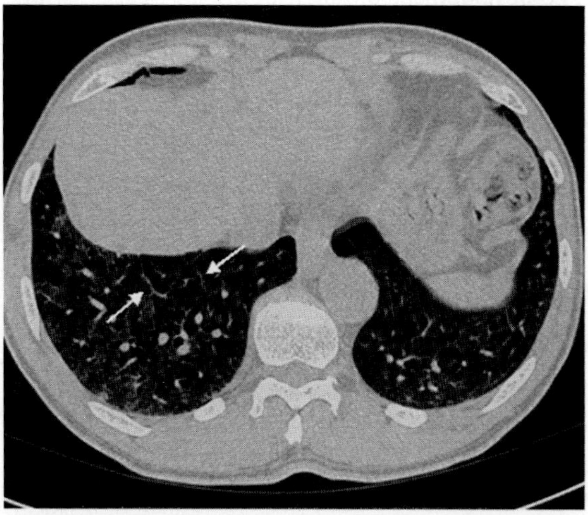

Fig. 4.7. Computed tomography through the lower zones in respiratory bronchiolitis-associated interstitial lung disease demonstrating smooth thickening of interlobular septa (*arrows*). There is also generalised ground-glass opacification and a fine reticular pattern in the subpleural lung

glass opacification was seen in all cases (Hartman et al. 1993). The mid and lower zones were affected in all patients. Although there was abnormality in the upper zones in the majority of patients, predominantly upper zone disease was seen in only three cases (Hartman et al. 1993), findings that were mirrored in a subsequent study (Heyneman et al. 1999). There was a predilection for the subpleural lung in 13 of 22 (59%) patients, but the distribution of ground-glass opacification was entirely random in nearly one quarter of cases. Other findings at CT include irregular lines together with signs of parenchymal distortion plus traction bronchiectasis (taken to denote underlying fibrosis), cystic spaces, emphysema and parenchymal nodules (Hartman et al. 1993). It is worth emphasising that the CT appearances of DIP are wholly non-specific. Thus, in one recent study, a confident diagnosis of DIP, made by experienced thoracic radiologists, was correct in only 59% of cases (Johkoh et al. 1999b).

The prognosis of patients with DIP is generally favourable (Carrington et al. 1978), and the CT appearances at follow-up have been evaluated in previous studies (Vedal et al. 1988; Hartman et al. 1996; Akira et al. 1997). In general, there is a tendency for regions of ground-glass opacification to regress with corticosteroid treatment. However, steroid-responsive disease is not invariable, and the extent of ground-glass opacification may be relatively "fixed" or even increase over time; in the absence of histopathological proof, it is difficult to be certain about the significance of persistent ground-glass opacification on CT. The development of small cystic air spaces (which may represent dilatation of bronchioles and alveolar ducts or indeed early emphysematous destruction), within regions of ground-glass opacification has also been reported on serial CT in DIP (Hartman et al. 1996; Akira et al. 1997).

4.7 Radiological Differential Diagnosis

Widespread ground-glass opacification on CT (a pattern seen with varying severity in patients with DIP and RBILD) is a non-specific sign that may be related to diseases in the air spaces and/or the interstitium (Colby and Swensen 1996; Collins and Stern 1997). Other and sometimes commoner causes of diffuse ground-glass opacification than DIP and RBILD include pulmonary oedema, infection (such as *Pneumocystis carinii* pneumonia) and pulmonary haemorrhage. Thus, for all patients with widespread ground-glass opacification and no ancillary features on CT, it is crucial to consider all available clinical and, if possible, histopathological data. Distinguishing between the CT appearances of RBILD and subacute hypersensitivity pneumonitis is sometimes challenging: diffuse ground-glass opacification, ill-defined centrilobular nodules and regions of low attenuation are the typical CT findings in subacute hypersensitivity pneumonitis (Silver et al. 1989; Hansell and Moskovic 1991; Remy-Jardin et al. 1993c). In practice, the differentiation between subacute hypersensitivity pneumonitis and the smoking-related disorders is aided by knowledge of the apparent protective effect of cigarette smoke in subacute hypersensitivity pneumonitis; thus, the patient's smoking history is particularly important in this situation (Hapke et al. 1968; Waren 1977).

4.7.1 Natural History of Smoking-Related Interstitial Lung Diseases

It must be appreciated that the signs of smoking-related damage on conventional chest radiographs represent relatively advanced lung disease. Theoretically, inferences about the development of smoking-related disease might be drawn from biopsy material taken from individual patients during the natural course of the disease. However, serial histopathological examinations, from a single patient, are rarely forthcoming. In this context, by providing highly detailed images, thin-section CT has been able to shed light both on the subtle, early morphological changes induced by cigarette smoking and, more importantly, their natural history.

Serial thin-section CT studies can provide valuable information about the development and progression of smoking-related changes in susceptible individuals. This is illustrated by considering the intriguing evolution, over time, of parenchymal changes seen in subjects who smoke. In the elegant study by Remy-Jardin et al. (2002), 111 otherwise healthy smokers were followed over an average of approximately 5.5 years. Compared with non-smokers, there was a significantly higher frequency of pulmonary abnormalities (comprising ill-defined parenchymal micronodules, areas of ground-glass opacification and emphysema) on initial CT studies in the groups of current and ex-smokers. Significant differences in CT abnormalities between the initial and follow-up studies were confined to the group of 57 persistent current smokers: the frequency of regions of ground-glass opacification and emphysema had increased at follow-up (Fig. 4.8). Whilst the progression of already established centrilobular emphysema in individuals who continue to smoke was hardly surprising, REMY-JARDIN also showed that that, in 7 of 19 subjects, there had been an increase in the profusion of ill-defined micronodules (likely to represent RB) since the first examination (REMY-JARDIN et al. 2002). Furthermore, the authors made the potentially important pathophysiological observation (admittedly in a relatively small number of subjects) that ill-defined micronodules on the initial study were replaced by emphysematous lesions at follow-up (Fig. 4.9).

In subjects who stop smoking, parenchymal abnormalities may regress. However, REMY-JARDIN et al. (2002) also made the salient observation (albeit in only one individual who quit smoking in the interval between the two thin-section CT studies) that the micronodular pattern may persist, presumably indicating residual inflammation, mirroring the known potential on histopathological examination for persisting changes reported in ex-smokers (FRAIG et al. 2002). Clearly, the subtle insights from the study of REMY-JARDIN et al. are not possible from the global and non-specific picture provided by pulmonary function tests. Furthermore, it seems likely that serial thin-section CT examinations will elucidate the highly variable progression of smoking-related pulmonary damage.

4.8 Cigarette Smoking, Interstitial Fibrosis and Other Idiopathic Interstitial Pneumonias

It must be stated at the outset that, whilst the debate about the relationships between tobacco smoke [including some of the more exotic cigarettes brands (MILLER et al. 1968)] and pulmonary fibrosis has been long running (WEISS 1969; AUERBACH et al. 1963), there is no direct evidence for a causal link. Early post-mortem studies demonstrated fibrosis within the alveolar septa of smokers (AUERBACH et al. 1963). Although the histopathological abnormalities could conceivably have been attributed to the effects of aging, the authors showed that all the changes were more frequent in subjects who had smoked (AUERBACH et al. 1963). More recently, it has been argued that smoking may be a risk factor for the development of pulmonary fibrosis (TURNER WARWICK et al. 1980; JOHNSTON et al. 1997). However, in general, the interpretation of clinical and epidemiological data about the relationships between smoking and interstitial fibrosis must be regarded with some cau-

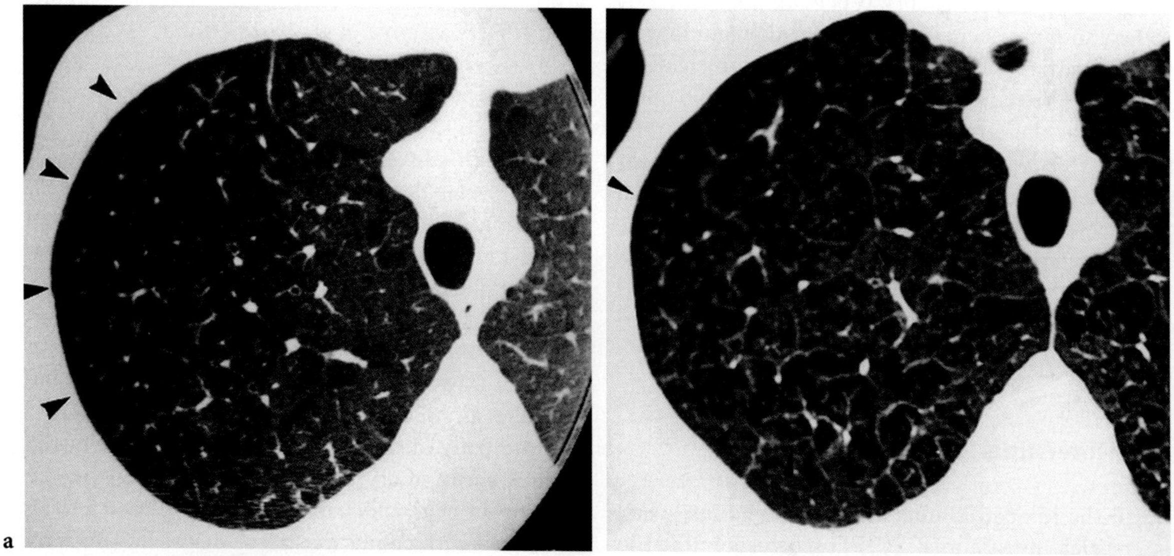

Fig. 4.8a,b. Longitudinal computed tomography (CT) study in a 29-year-old persistent smoker. **a** Initial targeted image of the right lung demonstrates numerous areas of low attenuation in the upper zones (*arrowheads*), suggestive of emphysema. There are a few thickened interlobular septa. **b** Follow-up CT at 6 years demonstrating extensive emphysema (*arrowheads*) and more prominent interlobular septa. Images reproduced with permission of Professor Martine Remy-Jardin and the Radiological Society of North America (REMY-JARDIN et al. 2002)

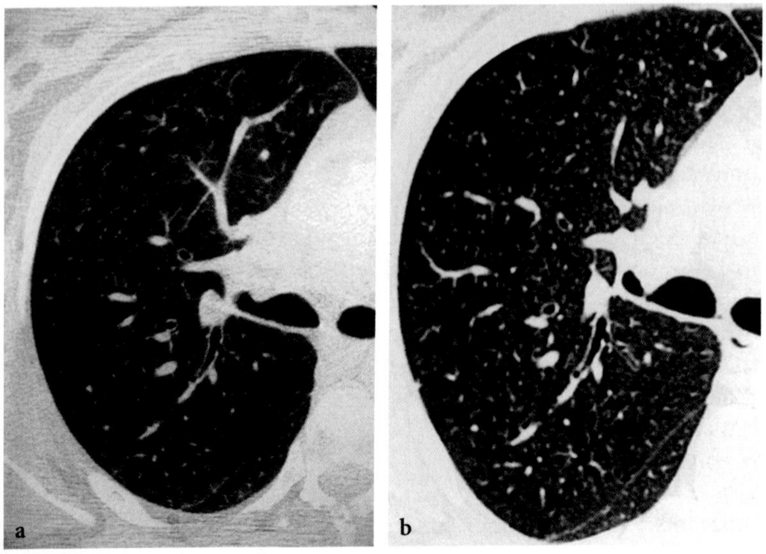

Fig. 4.9a,b. Longitudinal computed tomography (CT) study in a 34-year-old persistent and current smoker. **a** Initial CT study, targeted to right upper zone demonstrates faint parenchymal micronodules. **b** At the 6-year follow-up study, there is replacement of the micronodular pattern by low attenuation lesions of emphysema. Images reproduced with permission of Professor Martine Remy-Jardin and the Radiological Society of North America (Remy-Jardin et al. 2002)

tion, largely because there are variations in the definition of the type and presence of interstitial fibrosis. For example, it is notable that the prevalence of current or ex-smokers in extant series of "idiopathic pulmonary fibrosis" [which admittedly predate the recent re-classification of the idiopathic interstitial pneumonias (Travis et al. 2002)] varies widely from 41% to 83% (Ryu et al. 2001).

By recognising purer histological entities, the recent consensus classification of the idiopathic interstitial pneumonias (Travis et al. 2002) is likely to lead to more accurate data about the aetiology of the interstitial pneumonias, particularly in cigarette smokers. As regards RBILD and DIP, there is no question about the strong aetiological link to cigarette smoke. Thus, whilst both histological patterns appear in the new classification of the idiopathic interstitial pneumonias, the suggestion has been made that the collective term "smoking-related interstitial lung disease" should be used for these entities when there is an appropriate smoking history (Moon et al. 1999).

4.8.1 Usual Interstitial Pneumonia

Of all the idiopathic interstitial pneumonias, usual interstitial pneumonia (UIP) [corresponding to the clinical entity of idiopathic pulmonary fibrosis (IPF)], is the most common (Travis et al. 2002). Review of previous reports indicate the high prevalence smoking in patients with cryptogenic fibrosing alveolitis: 74% of the 220 subjects reported by Turner-Warwick and colleagues were either current or ex-smokers (Turner-Warwick et al. 1980). However, such historical data were undoubtedly confounded by classification issues and would have included some patients with non-specific interstitial pneumonia (NSIP) and DIP. Recently, it has been shown in a multicentre study that more patients with IPF than controls had a smoking history, with a relative risk of 1.6 (Baumgartner et al. 1997). Against this, the most recent published evidence suggests that there may be a potential protective effect of smoking in patients with IPF (Flaherty et al. 2002; King et al. 2001).

4.8.2 Non-Specific Interstitial Pneumonia

Following the description by Katzenstein and Fiorelli in 1994, there has been an increasing interest in and acceptance of NSIP as a recognised histological subtype of the idiopathic interstitial pneumonias (Katzenstein and Fiorelli 1994; Bjoraker et al. 1998; Daniil et al. 1999; Nicholson et al. 2000; Travis et al. 2000). Whilst some cases of the NSIP pattern are truly idiopathic and probably represent the clinical entity of cryptogenic fibrosing alveolitis/IPF (Flaherty et al. 2001), many others are known to be associated with connective tissue disorders (Bouros et al. 2002; Douglas et al. 2001), extrinsic allergic alveolitis or acute lung injury (Katzenstein and Fiorelli 1994). As with UIP, the exact relationship of NSIP with smoking is not entirely clear. However, at a recent workshop, a number of cases of NSIP were examined in which smoking was strongly implicated as an aetiological agent (Professor A.G. Nicholson, personal communication).

4.8.3 Other Idiopathic Interstitial Pneumonias and Diffuse Lung Disorders

There are no reports to date of associations between smoking and the histological entities of organising pneumonia, diffuse alveolar damage or lymphocytic interstitial pneumonia. A minor caveat is the finding of elements of organising pneumonia as a secondary reparative reaction to some other diseases, including LCH. Finally, although the pathophysiological mechanisms are unclear, mention must be made of the putative associations between smoking and cases of intra-alveolar haemorrhage (Donaghy and Rees 1983; Murin et al. 2000) and, more recently (principally in reports from Japan), of the potential link with pulmonary eosinophilia (Nakajima et al. 2000; Shintani et al. 2000; Miki et al. 2002).

4.9 Summary

Interest in the aetiological role of cigarette smoking in diseases other than lung cancer, emphysema and chronic bronchitis has increased recently. LCH, DIP and RBILD are most certainly associated with smoking. For the radiologist, some knowledge of the histopathological features of these disorders is helpful in interpreting thin-section CTs of cigarette smokers. The fine morphological detail seen on thin-section CT provides a unique and non-invasive insight into not only the pathology but also the pathogenesis and natural history of these intriguing disorders.

References

Aberle DR, Hansell DM, Brown K, Tashkin DP (1990) Lymphangiomyomatosis: CT, chest radiographic, and functional correlations. Radiology 176:381-387

Aguayo SM, Kane MA, King TE Jr, Schwarz MI, Grauer L, Miller YE (1989) Increased levels of bombesin-like peptides in the lower respiratory tract of asymptomatic cigarette smokers. J Clin Invest 84:1105-1113

Akira M, Yamamoto S, Hara H, Sakatani M, Ueda E (1997) Serial computed tomographic evaluation in desquamative interstitial pneumonia. Thorax 52:333-337

Amir G, Ron N (1999) Pulmonary pathology in Gaucher's disease. Hum Pathol 30:666-670

Anderson LG, Talal N (1971) The spectrum of benign to malignant lymphoproliferation in Sjogren's syndrome. Clin Exp Immunol 9:199-221

Auerbach O, Stout AP, Hammond EC, Garfinkel L (1963) Smoking habits and age in relation to pulmonary changes. N Engl J Med 269:1045

Austin JHM, Müller NL, Friedman PJ, Hansell DM, Naidich DP, Remy-Jardin M et al (1996) Glossary of terms for computed tomography of the lungs: recommendations of the nomenclature committee of the Fleischner society. Radiology 200:327-331

Bartecchi CE, Mackenzie TD, Schrier RW (1994) The human cost of tobacco use. N Engl J Med 330:907-912

Baumgartner KB, Samet JM, Stidley CA, Colby TV, Waldron JA (1997) Cigarette smoking: a risk factor for idiopathic pulmonary fibrosis. Am J Respir Crit Care Med 155:242-248

Bjoraker JA, Ryu JH, Edwin MK, Myers JL, Tazelaar HD, Schroeder DR et al (1998) Prognostic significance of histopathologic subsets in idiopathic pulmonary fibrosis. Am J Respir Crit Care Med 157:199-203

Bouros D, Wells AU, Nicholson AG, Colby TV, Polychronopoulos V, Pantelidis P et al (2002) Histopathologic subsets of fibrosing alveolitis in patients with systemic sclerosis and their relationship to outcome. Am J Respir Crit Care Med 165:1581-1586

Brauner MW, Grenier P, Mouelhi MM, Mompoint D, Lenoir S (1989) Pulmonary histiocytosis X: evaluation with high-resolution CT. Radiology 172:255-258

Brauner MW, Grenier P, Tijani K, Battesti J-P, Valeyre D (1997) Pulmonary Langerhans cell histiocytosis: evolution of lesions on CT scans. Radiology 204:497-502

Britton J, Bates C, Channer K, Cuthbertson L, Godfrey C, Jarvis M et al (eds) (2000) Tobacco Advisory Group of the Royal College of Physicians. Nicotine addiction in Britain: a report of the tobacco advisory group of the Royal College of Physicians, vol 6. Lavenham, Sudbury, pp 1-189

Burns BF, Colby TV, Dorfman RF (1983) Langerhans' cell granulomatosis (histiocytosis X) associated with malignant lymphomas. Am J Surg Pathol 7:529-533

Burrows B, Fletcher CM, Heard BE, Jones NL, Wootliff JS (1966) The emphysematous and bronchial types of chronic airways obstruction: a clinicopathological study of patients in London and Chicago. Lancet i:830-835

Cardoso WV, Sekhon HS, Hyde DM, Thurlbeck WM (1993) Collagen and elastin in human pulmonary emphysema. Am Rev Respir Dis 147:975-981

Carilli AD, Kotzen LM, Fischer MJ (1973) The chest roentgenogram in smoking females. Am Rev Respir Dis 107:133-136

Carrington CB, Gaensler EA, Coutu RE, Fitzgerald MX, Gupta RG (1978) Natural history and treated course of usual and desquamative interstitial pneumonia. N Engl J Med 298:801-809

Casolaro MA, Bernaudin J-F, Saltini C, Ferrans VJ, Crystal RG (1988) Accumulation of Langerhans' cells on the epithelial surface of the lower respiratory tract in normal subjects in association with cigarette smoking. Am Rev Respir Dis 137:406-411

Colby TV, Carrington CB (1995) Interstitial lung disease. In: Thurlbeck WM, Churg AM (eds) Pathology of the lung. Thieme Medical, New York, pp 589-737

Colby TV, Lombard C (1983) Histiocytosis X in the lung. Hum Pathol 14:847-856

Colby TV, Swensen SJ (1996) Anatomic distribution and histopathologic patterns in diffuse lung disease: correlation with HRCT. J Thorac Imaging 11:1-26

Collins J, Stern EJ (1997) Ground-glass opacity at CT: the ABCs. AJR Am J Roentgenol 169:355-367

Copley SJ, Wells AU, Müller NL, Rubens MB, Cleverley J, Hollings NJ et al The discriminatory value of high resolution CT in obstructive pulmonary disease. Radiology (in press)

Corrin B, Dewar A, Rodriguez-Roisin R, Turner-Warwick M (1985) Fine structural changes in cryptogenic fibrosing alveolitis and asbestosis. J Pathol 147:107-119

Daniil ZD, Gilchrist FC, Nicholson AG, Hansell DM, Harris J, Colby TV et al (1999) A histologic pattern of nonspecific interstitial pneumonia is associated with a better prognosis than usual interstital pneumonia in patients with cryptogenic fibrosing alveolitis. Am J Respir Crit Care Med 160:899-905

Desai SR, Nicholson AG, Stewart S, Twentyman OM, Flower CDR, Hansell DM (1997) Benign pulmonary lymphocytic infiltration and amyloidosis: computed tomographic and pathologic features in three cases. J Thorac Imaging 12:215-220

Dick JA, Morgan WKC, Muir DFC, Reger RB, Sargent N (1992) The significance of irregular opacities on the chest roentgenogram. Chest 102:251-260

Doherty MJ, Pearson MG, O'Grady EA, Pellegrini V, Calverley PMA (1997) Cryptogenic fibrosing alveolitis with preserved lung volumes. Thorax 52:998-1002

Donaghy M, Rees AJ (1983) Cigarette smoking and lung haemorrhage in glomerulonephritis caused by autoantibodies to glomerular basement membrane. Lancet 17:1390-1393

Douglas WW, Tazelaar HD, Hartman TE, Hartman RP, Decker PA, Schroeder DR et al (2001) Polymyositis-dermatomyositis-associated interstitial lung disease. Am J Respir Crit Care Med 164:1182-1185

Etienne B, Bertocchi M, Gamondes J-P, Thévenet F, Boudard C, Wiesendanger T et al (1998) Relapsing pulmonary Lamgerhans cell histiocytosis after lung transplantation. Am J Respir Crit Care Med 157:288-291

Fartoukh M, Humbert M, Capron F, Maître S, Parent F, Le Gall C et al (2000) Severe pulmonary hypertension in histiocytosis X. Am J Respir Crit Care Med 161:216-223

Favara BE, Feller AC (1997) Contemporary classification of histiocytic disorders. Med Pediatr Oncol 29:157-166

Feigen DS, Friedman PJ (1980) Chest radiography in desquamative interstitial pneumonitis: a review of 37 patients. AJR Am J Roentgenol 134:91-99

Fichtenbaum CJ, Kleinman GM, Haddad RG (1990) Eosinophilic granuloma of the lung presenting as a solitary pulmonary nodule. Thorax 45:905-906

Flaherty KR, Travis WD, Colby TV, Toews GB, Kazerooni EA, Gross BH et al (2001) Histopathologic variability in usual and nonspecific interstitial pneumonias. Am J Respir Crit Care Med 164:1722-1727

Flaherty KR, Toews GB, Travis WD, Colby TV, Kazerooni EA, Gross BH et al (2002) Clinical significance of histological classification of idiopathic interstitial pneumonia. Eur Respir J 19:275-283

Foster WL Jr, Pratt PC, Roggli VL, Godwin JD, Halvorsen RA Jr, Putman CE (1986) Centrilobular emphysema: CT-pathologic correlation. Radiology 159:27-32

Fraig M, Shreesha U, Savici D, Katzenstein AL (2002) Respiratory bronchiolitis: a clinicopathologic study in current smokers, ex-smokers, and never-smokers. Am J Surg Pathol 26:647-653

Frasca JM, Auerbach O, Carter HW, Parks VR (1983) Morphologic alterations induced by short-term cigarette smoking. Am J Pathol 111:11-20

Friedman PJ, Liebow AA, Sokoloff J (1981) Eosinophilic granuloma of lung: clinical aspects of primary pulmonary histiocytosis in the adult. Medicine 60:385-396

Fromm GB, Dunn LJ, Harris JO (1980) Desquamative interstitial pneumonitis: characterization of free intraalveolar cells. Chest 77:552-554

Gaensler EA, Goff AM, Prowse CM (1966) Desquamative interstitial pneumonia. N Engl J Med 274:113-128

Gishen P, Saunders AJS, Tobin MJ, Hutchinson DCS (1982) Alpha1-antitrypsin deficiency: the radiological features of pulmonary emphysema in subjects of Pi type Z and Pi type SZ. A survey by the British Thoracic Association. Clin Radiol 33:371-377

Goddard PR, Nicholson EM, Laszlo G, Watt I (1982) Computed tomography in pulmonary emphysema. Clin Radiol 33:379-387

Gückel C, Hansell DM (1998) Imaging the "dirty lung": has high resolution computed tomography cleared the smoke? Clin Radiol 53:717-722

Hamadeh MA, Atkinson J, Smith LJ (1992) Sulfasalazine-induced pulmonary disease. Chest 101:1033-1037

Hansell DM, Moskovic E (1991) High-resolution computed tomography in extrinsic allergic alveolitis. Clin Radiol 43:8-12

Hapke EJ, Seal RME, Thomas GO, Hayes M, Meek JC (1968) Farmer's lung: a clinical, radiographic, functional and serological correlation of acute and chronic stages. Thorax 23:451-468

Hartman TE, Primack SL, Swensen SJ, Hansell DM, McGuinness G, Müller NL (1993) Desquamative interstitial pneumonia: thin-section CT findings in 22 patients. Radiology 187:787-790

Hartman TE, Primack SL, Kang E-Y, Swensen SJ, Hansell DM, McGuinness G et al (1996) Disease progression in usual interstitial pneumonia compared with desquamative interstitial pneumonia: assessment with serial CT. Chest 110:378-382

Hautamaki RD, Kobayashi DK, Senior RM, Shapiro SD (1997) Macrophage elastase is required for cigarette smoke-induced emphysema in mice. Science 277:2002-2004

Hayhurst MD, Flenley DC, McLean A, Wightman AJA, Macnee W, Wright D et al (1984) Diagnosis of pulmonary emphysema by computerized tomography. Lancet 2:320-322

Herbert A, Sterling G, Abraham J, Corrin B (1982) Desquamative interstitial pneumonia in an aluminum welder. Hum Pathol 13:694-699

Heyneman LE, Ward S, Lynch DA, Remy-Jardin M, Johkoh T, Müller NL (1999) Respiratory bronchiolitis, respiratory bronchiolitis-associated interstitial lung disease, and desquamative interstitial pneumonia: different entities or part of the spectrum of the same disease process? AJR Am J Roentgenol 173:1617-1622

Holt RM, Schmidt RA, Godwin JD, Raghu G (1993) High resolution CT in respiratory bronchiolitis-associated interstitial lung disease. J Comput Assist Tomogr 17:46-50

Honda O, Johkoh T, Ichikado K, Tomiyama N, Maeda M, Mihara N et al (1999) Differential diagnosis of lymphocytic interstitial pneumonia and malignant lymphoma on high-resolution CT. AJR Am J Roentgenol 173:71-74

Howarth DM, Gilchrist GS, Mullan BP, Wiseman GA, Edmonson JH, Schomberg PJ (1999) Langerhans cell histiocytosis: diagnosis, natural history, management, and outcome. Cancer 85:2278-2290

Janoff A (1985) Elastases and emphysema: current assessment of the protease-antiprotease hypothesis. Am Rev Respir Dis 132:417-433

Johkoh T, Müller NL, Pickford HA, Hartman TE, Ichikado K, Akira M et al (1999a) Lymphocytic interstitial pneumonia: thin-section CT findings in 22 patients. Radiology 212:567-572

Johkoh T, Müller NL, Cartier Y, Kavanagh PV, Hartman TE, Akira M et al (1999b) Idiopathic interstitial pneumonias: diagnostic accuracy of thin-section CT in 129 patients. Radiology 211:555-560

Johnston IDA, Prescott RJ, Chalmers JC, Rudd RM (1997) British Thoracic Society study of cryptogenic fibrosing alveolitis: current presentation and initial management. Thorax 52:38-44

Kambouchner M, Basset F, Soler P (1996) Tridimensional features of pulmonary Langerhans' cell granulomatosis (PLCG) lesions. Mod Pathol 9:157(A)

Katsura S, Martin CJ (1967) The roentgenologic diagnosis of anatomic emphysema. Am Rev Respir Dis 96:700-706

Katzenstein AA, Fiorelli RF (1994) Non-specific interstitial pneumonia/fibrosis: histologic features and clinical significance. Am J Surg Pathol 18:136-147

Kerley P (1936) Discussion on emphysema. Proc R Soc Med 29:1307-1324

King TE Jr (1993) Respiratory bronchiolitis-associated interstitial lung disease. Clin Chest Med 14:693-698

King TE Jr, Costabel U, Cordier JF, doPico GA, du Bois RM, Lynch D et al (2000) Idiopathic pulmonary fibrosis: diagnosis and treatment. International consensus statement. Am J Respir Crit Care Med 161:646-664

King TE Jr, Schwarz MI, Brown K, Tooze JA, Colby TV, Waldron JA Jr et al (2001) Idiopathic pulmonary fibrosis: relationship between histopathologic features and mortality. Am J Respir Crit Care Med 164:1025-1032

Koss MN, Hochholzer L, Langloss JM, Wehunt WD, Lazarus AA (1986) Lymphoid interstitial pneumonia: clinicopathological and immunopathological findings in 18 cases. Pathology 19:178-185

Lacronique J, Roth C, Battesti J-P, Basset F, Chretien J (1982) Chest radiological features of pulmonary histiocytosis X: a report based on 50 adult cases. Thorax 37:104-109

Lang MR, Fiaux GW, Gillooly M, Stewart JA, Hulmes DJS, Lamb D (1994) Collagen content of alveolar wall tissue in emphysematous and non-emphysematous lungs. Thorax 49:319-326

Laws JW, Heard BE (1962) Emphysema and the chest film: a retrospective radiological and pathological study. Br J Radiol 35:750-761

Lichtenstein L (1953) Histiocytosis X. Integration of eosinophilic granuloma of bone, 'Letterer-Slwe disease' and 'Schuller-Christian disease' as related manifestations of a single nosologic entity. Arch Pathol 56:84-102

Liebow AA, Steer A, Billingsley JG (1965) Desquamative interstitial pneumonia. Am J Med 39:369-404

Marten K, Hansell DM (2005) Imaging of macrophage-related lung diseases. Eur Radiol (Epub ahead of print)

Miki K, Miki M, Okano Y, Nakamura Y, Ogushi F, Ohtsuki Y et al (2002) Cigarette smoke-induced acute eosinophilic pneumonia accompanied with neutrophilia in the blood. Intern Med 41:993-996

Miller GJ, Beadnell HMSG, Ashcroft MT (1968) Diffuse pulmonary fibrosis and blackfat-tobacco smoking in Guyana. Lancet 2:259-260

Mogulkoc N, Veral A, Bishop PW, Bayindir Ü, Pickering CAC, Egan JJ (1999) Pulmonary Langerhans' cell histiocytosis: radiologic resolution following smoking cessation. Chest 115:1452-1455

Moon J, du Bois RM, Colby TV, Hansell DM, Nicholson AG (1999) Clinical significance of respiratory bronchiolitis on open lung biopsy and its relationship to smoking related interstitial lung disease. Thorax 54:1009-1014

Moore ADA, Godwin JD, Müller NL, Naidich DP, Hammar SP, Buschman DL et al (1989) Pulmonary histiocytosis X: comparison of radiographic and CT findings. Radiology 172:249-254

Murin S, Bilello KS, Matthay R (2000) Other smoking-affected pulmonary diseases. Clin Chest Med 21:121-137

Myers JL, Veal CF, Shin MS, Katzenstein AA (1987) Respiratory bronchiolitis causing interstitial lung disease: a clinicopathologic study of six cases. Am Rev Respir Dis 135:880-884

Nakajima M, Manabe T, Sasaki T, Niki Y, Matsushima T (2000) Acute eosinophilic pneumonia caused by cigarette smoking. Intern Med 39:1131-1132

Neumann MP, Frizzera G (1986) The coexistence of Langerhans' cell granulomatosis and malignant lymphoma may take different forms: report of seven cases with a review of the literature. Hum Pathol 17:1060-1065

Nicholson AG, Colby TV, du Bois RM, Hansell DM, Wells AU (2000) The prognostic significance of the histologic pattern of interstitial pneumonia in patients with the clinical entity of cryptogenic fibrosing alveolitis. Am J Respir Crit Care Med 162:2213-2217

Nicklaus TM, Stowell DW, Christiansen WR, Renzetti AD Jr (1966) The accuracy of the roentgenologic diagnosis of chronic pulmonary emphysema. Am Rev Respir Dis 93:889-899

Niewoehner DE, Hoidal JR (1982) Lung fibrosis and emphysema: divergent responses to a common injury? Science 217:359-360

Niewoehner DE, Kleinerman J, Rice DB (1974) Pathological changes in the peripheral airways of young cigarette smokers. N Engl J Med 291:755-758

O'Donnell AE, Tsou E, Awh C, Fallat ME, Patterson K (1987) Endobronchial eosinophilic granuloma: a rare cause of total lung atelectasis. Am Rev Respir Dis 136:1478-1480

Pai U, Tomashefski JF (2002) Occult pulmonary eosinophilic granuloma: an incidental finding in the lungs of cigarette smokers. Am J Clin Pathol 99:335(A)

Park JS, Brown KK, Tuder RM, Hale VA, King TE Jr, Lynch DA (2002) Respiratory bronchiolitis-associated interstitial lung disease: radiologic features with clinical and pathologic correlation. J Comput Assist Tomogr 26:13-20

Patchevsky AS, Israel HL, Hoch WS, Gordon G (1973) Desquamative interstitial pneumonia: relationship to interstitial fibrosis. Thorax 28:680-693

Pomeranz SJ, Proto AV (1986) Histiocytosis X: unusual-confusing features of eosinophilic granuloma. Chest 89:88-92

Rappaport DC, Weisbrod GL, Herman SJ, Chamberlain DW (1989) Pulmonary lymphangioleiomyomatosis: high-resolution CT findings in four cases. AJR 152:961-964

Remy-Jardin M, Remy J, Boulenguez C, Sobaszek A, Edme J-L, Furon D (1993a) Morphologic effects of cigarette smoking on airways and pulmonary parenchyma in healthy adult volunteers: CT evaluation and correlation with pulmonary function tests. Radiology 186:107-115

Remy-Jardin M, Remy J, Gosselin B, Becette V, Edme J-L (1993b) Lung parenchymal changes secondary to cigarette smoking: pathologic-CT correlations. Radiology 186:643-651

Remy-Jardin M, Remy J, Wallaert B, Müller NL (1993c) Subacute and chronic bird breeder hypersensitivity pneumonitis: sequential evaluation with CT and correlation with lung function tests and bronchoalveolar lavage. Radiology 189:111-118

Remy-Jardin M, Edme JL, Boulenguez C, Remy J, Mastora I, Sobaszek A (2002) Longitudinal follow-up study of smoker's lung with thin-section CT in correlation with pulmonary function tests. Radiology 222:261-270

Ryu JH, Colby TV, Hartman TE, Vassallo R (2001) Smoking-related interstitial lung diseases: a concise review. Eur Respir J 17:122-132

Shapiro SD, Goldstein NM, McGarry-Houghton A, Dobayashi DK, Delley D, Belaaouaj A (2003) Neutrophil elastase contributes to cigarette smoke-induced emphysema in mice. Am J Pathol 163:2329-2335

Sherrier RH, Chiles C, Roggli V (1989) Pulmonary lymphangioleiomyomatosis: CT findings. AJR 153:937-940

Shintani H, Fujimura M, Yasui M, Ueda K, Kameda S, Noto M et al (2000) Acute eosinophilic pneumonia caused by cigarette smoking. Intern Med 39:66-68

Silver SF, Müller NL, Miller RR, Lefcoe MS (1989) Hypersensitivity pneumonitis: evaluation with CT. Radiology 173:441-445

Simon G (1964) Radiology and emphysema: Skinner Lecture, 1963. Clin Radiol 15:293-306

Snider GL, Kleinerman J, Thurlbeck WM, Bengali ZH (1985) The definition of emphysema: report of a National Heart, Lung, and Blood Institute, Division of Lung Diseases workshop. Am Rev Respir Dis 132:182-185

Soler P, Bergeron A, Kambouchner M, Groussard O, Brauner M, Grenier P et al (2000) Is high-resolution computed tomography a reliable tool to predict the histopathological activity of pulmonary Langerhans cell histiocytosis. Am J Respir Crit Care Med 162:264-270

Tazi A, Montcelly L, Bergeron A, Valeyre D, Battesti J-P, Hance AJ (1998) Relapsing nodular lesions in the course of adult pulmonary Langerhans cell histiocytosis. Am J Respir Crit Care Med 157:2007-2010

Thurlbeck WM (1995) Chronic airflow obstruction. In: Thurlbeck WM, Churg AM (eds) Pathology of the lung. Thieme Medical, New York, pp 739-825

Thurlbeck WM, Simon G (1978) Radiographic appearance of the chest in emphysema. AJR 130:429-440

Thurlbeck WM, Henderson JA, Fraser RG, Bates DV (1970) Chronic obstructive lung disease: a comparison between clinical, roentgenologic, functional and morphologic criteria in chronic bronchitis, emphysema, asthma and bronchiectasis. Medicine 49:81-145

Tomashefski JF, Khiyami A, Kleinerman J (1991) Neoplasms associated with pulmonary eosinophilic granuloma. Arch Pathol Lab Med 115:499-506

Tonelli M, Stern EJ, Glenny RW (1997) HRCT evident fibrosis in isolated pulmonary emphysema. J Comput Assist Tomogr 21:322-323

Travis WD, Borok Z, Roum JH, Zhang J, Feuerstein I, Ferrans VJ et al (1993) Pulmonary Langerhans cell granulomatosis (histiocytosis X): a clinicopathologic study of 48 cases. Am J Surg Pathol 17:971-986

Travis WD, Matsui K, Moss J, Ferrans VJ (2000) Idiopathic nonspecific interstitial pneumonia: prognostic significance of cellular and fibrosing patterns. Survival comparison with usual interstitial pneumonia and desquamative interstitial pneumonia. Am J Surg Pathol 24:19-33

Travis WD, King TE Jr, the Multidisciplinary Core Panel (2002) American Thoracic Society/European Respiratory Society international multidiscplinary consensus classification of idiopathic interstitial pneumonias. Am J Respir Crit Care Med 165:277-304

Turner-Warwick M, Burrows B, Johnson A (1980) Cryptogenic fibrosing alveolitis: clinical features and their influence on survival. Thorax 35:171-180

Vassallo R, Ryu JH, Colby TV, Hartman T, Limper AH (2000) Pulmonary Langerhans'-cell histiocytosis. N Engl J Med 342:1969-1978

Vassallo R, Ryu JH, Schroeder DR, Decker PA, Limper AH (2002) Clinical outcomes of pulmonary Langerhans'-cell histiocytosis in adults. N Engl J Med 346:484-490

Vassallo R, Jensen EA, Colby TV, Ryu JH, Douglas WW, Hartman TE et al (2003) The overlap between respiratory bronchiolitis and desquamative interstitial pneumonia in pulmonary Langerhans cell histiocytosis: high-resolution CT, histologic, and functional correlations. Chest 124:1199-1205

Vedal S, Welsh EV, Miller RR, Müller NL (1988) Desquamative interstitial pneumonia: computed tomographic findings before and after treatment with corticosteroids. Chest 93:215-217

Von Essen S, West W, Sitorius M, Rennard SI (1990) Complete resolution of roentgenographic changes in a patient with pulmonary histiocytosis X. Chest 98:765-767

Warren CPW (1977) Extrinsic allergic alveolitis: a disease commoner in non-smokers. Thorax 32:567-569

Weiss W (1969) Cigarette smoking and diffuse pulmonary fibrosis. Am Rev Respir Dis 99:67-72

Wells AU, King AD, Rubens MB, Cramer D, du Bois RM, Hansell DM (1997) Lone cryptogenic fibrosing alveolitis: a functional-morphologic correlation based on the extent of disease on thin-section computed tomography. Am J Respir Crit Care Med 155:1367-1375

WHO chronicles (1982) Smoking and health in Asia, vol 36, pp 156-159

Wiggins J, Strickland B, Turner-Warwick M (1990) Combined cryptogenic fibrosing alveolitis and emphysema: the value of high resolution computed tomography in assessment. Respir Med 84:365-369

Youkeles LH, Grizzanti JN, Liao Z, Chang CJ, Rosenstreich DL (1995) Decreased tobacco-glycoprotein-induced lymphocyte proliferation *in vitro* in pulmonary eosinophilic granuloma. Am J Respir Crit Care Med 151:145-150

Yousem SA, Colby TV, Chen YY, Chen WG, Weiss LM (2001) Pulmonary Langerhans' cell histiocytosis: molecular analysis of clonality. Am J Surg Pathol 25:630-636

Yousem SA, Colby TV, Gaensler EA (1989) Respiratory bronchiolitis-associated interstitial lung disease and its relationship to desquamative interstitial pneumonia. Mayo Clin Proc 64:1373-1380

Zeid NA, Muller HK (1995) Tobacco smoke induced lung granulomas and tumors: association with pulmonary Langerhans cells. Pathology 27:247-254

5 Silicosis

Clara Gaik Cheng Ooi and Hiroaki Arakawa

CONTENTS

5.1 Introduction 177
5.2 Pathogenesis 177
5.3 Pathology 178
Classic (Nodular) Silicosis 178
Mixed Dust Fibrosis 178
Silicoproteinosis 178
5.4 Clinical Features 179
5.5 Radiological Evaluation 180
5.5.1 Chest Radiograph 180
5.5.2 Computed Tomography/ Thin-Section Computed Tomography 182
5.5.3 Radiological–Clinical Correlation Using CT Techniques 187
5.6 Complications 188
5.7 Differential Diagnosis 189
5.8 Future Developments 189
References 191

5.1 Introduction

Silicosis is an occupational lung disease caused by inhalation of silica, a ubiquitous mineral found in abundance in the earth's crust, composed of regular molecules of silicon dioxide (SiO_2). Certain occupations predispose the individual to high concentrations of silica, which is fibrogenic to the lungs, resulting in radiographic and pathological abnormalities. Workers engaged in occupations such as tunneling, mining, sandblasting and quarrying are inevitably exposed to the mineral, due to its ubiquity in the earth's crust. Other occupations, such as work with gemstones, including jade polishers (White et al. 1991; Gupta et al. 1991; Ng et al. 1985), foundry and pottery workers (Landrigan et al. 1986; Rees et al. 1992; Epstein et al. 1984) and glass and silica bricks workers (Landrigan et al. 1986), are associated with silica exposure. The diagnosis of silicosis is based on the typical radiographic appearance of diffuse nodules or reticulonodular pattern in the presence of a strong occupational exposure to silica. The International Labour Organization (ILO) 2000 International Classification of Radiographs of the Pneumoconiosis is the most commonly accepted classification of extent of involvement of the pneumoconiosis and one in which the presence or absence of pneumoconiosis is established in workers exposed to mineral dust including silica (Geneva, International Labour Office 2000; Davies 1974). Standard reference radiographs are available from the ILO office with standard nomenclature to describe the changes.

C. G. C. Ooi, MD
Department of Diagnostic Radiology, University of Hong Kong, Queen Mary Hospital, Pokfulam Road, Pokfulam, Hong Kong SAR, China
H. Arakawa, MD
Department of Radiology, Dokkyo University School of Medicine, 880, Mibu, Tochigi, 321-0293 Japan

5.2 Pathogenesis

The role of macrophages in the pathogenesis of silicosis has been extensively studied (Davis and Gemsa 1996; Harmsen et al. 1985; Corry et al. 1984; Lehnert et al. 1986; Graham 1992). Inhaled crystalline silica smaller than 5 μm are deposited in the small airways and alveoli from which they are ingested within 48 h of deposition by alveolar macrophages or tissue macrophages, if they penetrate the interstitium. Free particulate silica that are not ingested by macrophages enter the perivascular lymphatic channels to be translocated to the draining mediastinal lymph nodes as free particles or within macrophages (Davis and Gemsa 1996; Harmsen et al. 1985; Corry et al. 1984; Absher et al. 1992; Lauweryns and Baert 1977). In vivo and in vitro studies have shown that these silica-exposed macrophages release fibroblast growth factors that facilitate the accumulation of fibroblasts and fibroblast products, which induce inflammatory and fibrogenic reaction in the interstitium, alveoli and lymph nodes (Lauweryns and Baert 1977; Brown et al. 1988; Jagirdar et al. 1996; Dubois et al. 1989; Lugano et al. 1984; Hunninghake et al. 1986; Bitterman et al. 1983; Schmidt et al. 1984; Kampschmidt et al. 1986). Other inflammatory cells recruited in the lung in addition to the macrophages include lymphocytes, particularly T-helper cells and neutrophils.

5.3 Pathology

Classic (Nodular) Silicosis

Nodular silicosis is characterized by the presence of small rounded nodules of 3–6 mm in the lung parenchyma (Gibbs and Wagner 1998; Weill et al. 1994).

The nodules of silicosis are well defined and located in the perivascular and peribronchiolar interstitium as well as in the paraseptal and subpleural interstitium (Fig. 5.1) and are preferentially distributed in the upper lobes. The silicotic nodule starts as a central zone of mononuclear cells surrounded by fibroblasts and collagen tissue. With time, the central zone becomes hypocellular, with concentric laminar deposition of reticulin, proteins, phospholipids and collagen in the periphery, giving a whorled appearance (Fig. 5.1). Adjacent vessels and bronchioles may become involved and destroyed by these nodules, with occlusion of their lumen.

Conglomeration of the nodules frequently occurs to form large masses of progressive massive fibrosis (PMF), usually in the upper lobes where nodular profusion is highest. The lower lobes are less frequently involved. PMF lesions sometimes cross the interlobar fissure to form elongated masses from lung apex to the lower lobe. Although conglomeration usually occurs in heavily dust-laden lung with a high profusion of nodules, its development does not always parallel nodular profusion. Cavitation of PMF masses occurs as a result of ischemic necrosis and mycobacterial infection.

Hilar and mediastinal lymph nodes are enlarged and pigmented, with a whorled appearance similar to that found in the silicotic nodule. Calcification is also a frequent finding. Features characterized on imaging, particularly on computed tomography (CT), will reflect these pathological changes in the lungs and lymph nodes.

Mixed Dust Fibrosis

Although the radiographic characteristics of mixed dust fibrosis have not been a subject of interest in recent literature, this entity is frequently described in pathology textbooks and is of some clinical importance within the context of lung damage in silica-exposed workers (Gibbs and Wagner 1998; Weill et al. 1994). Exposure to high content (more than 18% of total dust deposited in lung) of free crystalline silica results in classic silicosis, while mixed dust fibrosis develops in the presence of low silica content (less than 18% of total dust deposited in lung) (Nagelschmidt 1960), particularly with simultaneous inhalation of other minerals such as non-fibrous silicate (mica, kaolin, coal, talc, fuller's earth, etc.). These non-fibrous silicates augment the strong fibrotic effect of crystalline silica (Gibbs and Wagner 1998). Instead of a well-defined, whorled appearance found in the silicotic nodule, the lesions in mixed dust fibrosis are characterized by irregular shaped fibrotic nodules (often called stellate nodules) and a predilection of the fibrotic lesion to extend into the surrounding pulmonary interstitium (Fig. 5.2). The stellate nodules are less fibrotic with less collagen and are more cellular than silicotic nodules. Calcification in the nodule is rarely observed. Depending on the proportion of crystalline silica in the inhaled dust, mixed dust fibrosis and silicotic nodules coexist in the same lung, thus forming a spectrum of pathological findings (Honma et al. 2004). The nodules of mixed dust fibrosis are also located within the center of the secondary pulmonary lobule and in the subpleural and paraseptal interstitium, with upper lobe predominance.

Silicoproteinosis

The principal finding in silicoproteinosis is the presence of surfactant protein filling the alveolar spaces, as is seen in acquired form of alveolar proteinosis (Gibbs and Wagner 1998). Silicotic nodules are sparse and poorly demarcated or absent, probably because of a short period of time after exposure (Hoffman et al. 1973; Roeslin et al. 1980). There is diffuse alveolar wall thickening and fibrosis, as is seen in acquired form of proteinosis (Heppleston and Young 1972).

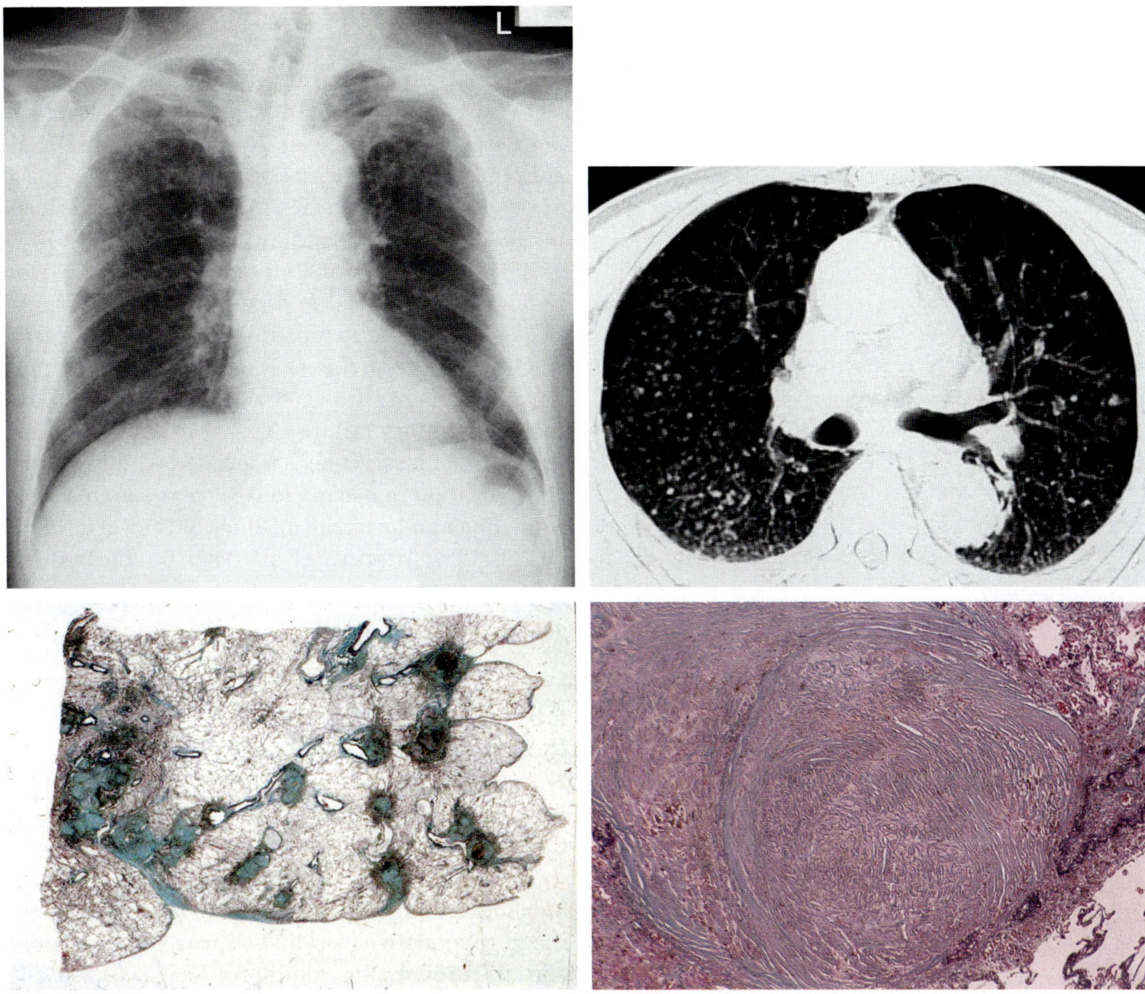

Fig. 5.1a–d. Classic silicosis in 74-year-old retired metal ore miner. **a** Posterior–anterior chest radiograph shows multiple calcified small nodules predominantly in upper lung zones. The size and profusion of the nodules are r/r and 2/2 according to the International Labour Organization classification. **b** Spiral computed tomography image (10-mm thickness) shows multiple small nodules that are most predominant in the posterior half of upper lobes. The nodules are separated with similar distance with each other, which is compatible with the centrilobular localization of silicotic nodules. **c** Photomicrograph of autopsied lung specimen (Elastic–Goldner stain) shows silicotic nodules with or without calcification along the interlobular septa and in the centrilobular areas as well as in the subpleural interstitium. The nodules are separated with equal distance with each other, suggesting a centrilobular localization. **d** Photomicrograph of a silicotic nodule shows a typical whorled appearance

5.4 Clinical Features

Unlike other inhalational occupational lung diseases, lung changes in silicosis can often progress even after the individual is removed from the dusty environment that initiated the fibrogenic lung disease (Nozaki and Sawada 1959; Lee et al. 2001). Whilst most patients are asymptomatic initially, dyspnea on exertion and then at rest is common. A relationship between severity of dyspnea and radiographic abnormalities has been documented (Ooi et al. 2003b; Koskinen 1985). With progressive lung damage, pulmonary hypertension and right heart failure eventually supervenes. Emphysema is common in silicosis and has been attributed as the major cause of cor pulmonale and disability rather than fibrosis by some investigators (Murray et al. 1993). Several studies evaluating airflow obstruction in silica-exposed workers have suggested a relationship between silica dust exposure and reduction in lung function irrespective of radiographic evidence

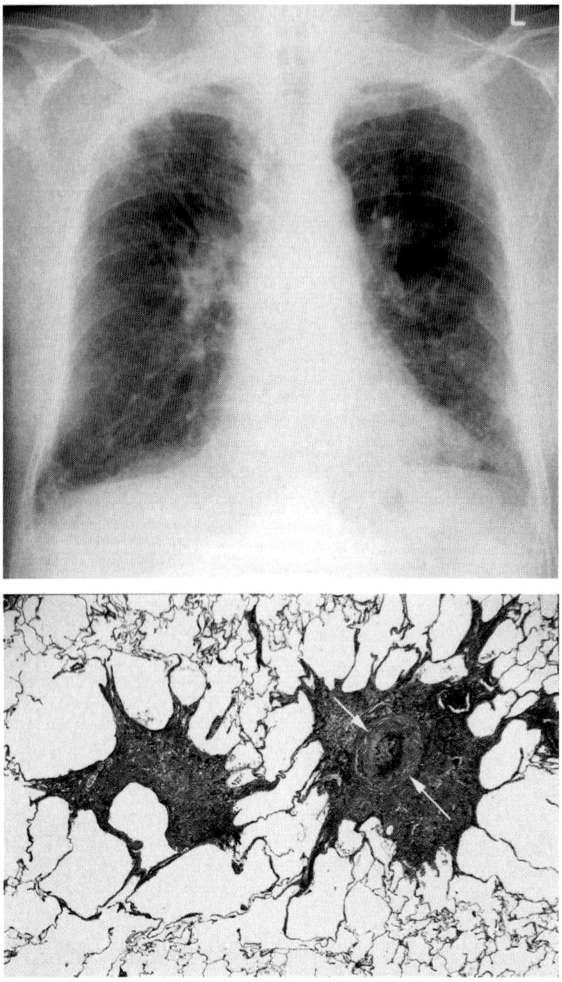

a

b

Fig. 5.2a,b. A 72-year-old retired tunnel worker with silicotic nodules and mixed dust fibrosis. **a** Posterior–anterior chest radiograph shows ill-defined multiple small nodules and reticular opacities in both upper lobes. **b** Photomicrograph obtained at autopsy performed 2 years after chest radiograph shows two pneumoconiotic nodules with stellate appearance. The left nodule shows irregular shape without whorled appearance (*arrows*) typical of silicotic nodule. The right nodule also shows irregular shape but has a central whorled appearance of silicotic nodule. Emphysema is identified around the nodules

of silicosis or fibrosis (Lee et al. 2001; Engholm and von Schamlensee 1982; Johnson et al. 1985; Neukirch et al. 1994).

The three main clinical presentations of silicosis are classic silicosis, accelerated silicosis and silicoproteinosis. Classic silicosis is the most common presentation, in which patients remain asymptomatic until after an interval of 10–20 years of continuous silica exposure, by which time radiographic evidence is present. With accelerated silicosis, the exposure time after which the disease becomes clinically evident is much shorter, ranging from 5 years to 10 years of exposure, and the rate of disease progression noticeably faster. Clinical presentation as early as 1 year after exposure and death within 5 years has been reported (Jiang et al. 2001; Elmes 1994). High concentrations of dust in a relatively confined space are thought to predispose the individual to this form of silicosis (Michel and Morris 1964; Theron et al. 1964). However, for all intents and purposes, the radiographic, clinical and pathological features of this entity are nearly indistinguishable from classic silicosis. Silicoproteinosis is another acute and progressive form of silicosis that often results in death from respiratory failure (Bailey et al. 1974). This variant of silicosis is also associated with high dust concentration in occupations such as sandblasting, tunneling and quartzite milling (Bailey et al. 1974; Oleru 1987; Hughes et al. 1982; Buechner and Ansari 1969).

5.5 Radiological Evaluation

5.5.1 Chest Radiograph

The chest radiograph remains the most convenient imaging modality by which silicosis is diagnosed and its progression monitored (Fig. 5.3). In the ILO classification of radiographs, the radiographic opacities are characterized by their size and shape. Small rounded opacities are described as “p”, “q” or “r”, according to their size (1.5 mm, 1.5–3 mm or 3–10 mm, respectively) (Fig. 5.1, Fig. 5.3, and Fig. 5.4), while irregular opacities of similar size are respectively denoted as “s”, “t” and “u”. Profusion of nodules is a measure of the concentration of small opacities per unit area or zone of lung, determined from comparison of patient’s chest radiograph with standard radiographs provided by the ILO. There are 12 categories of profusion, which represent a continuum of changes ranging from normal to severe profusion (Liddell 1963; Liddell and Lindars 1969). These can be grouped into 4 broad categories, based on the degree obscuration of vascular lung markings by the nodules: category 0 (0/0, 0/0, 0/1), when small opacities are absent or less than category 1; category 1 (1/0, 1/1, 1/2), when small opacities are present in small numbers with normal lung markings (Fig. 5.3); category 2 (2/1, 2/2, 2/3), when numerous small opacities are present and when lung markings are

a
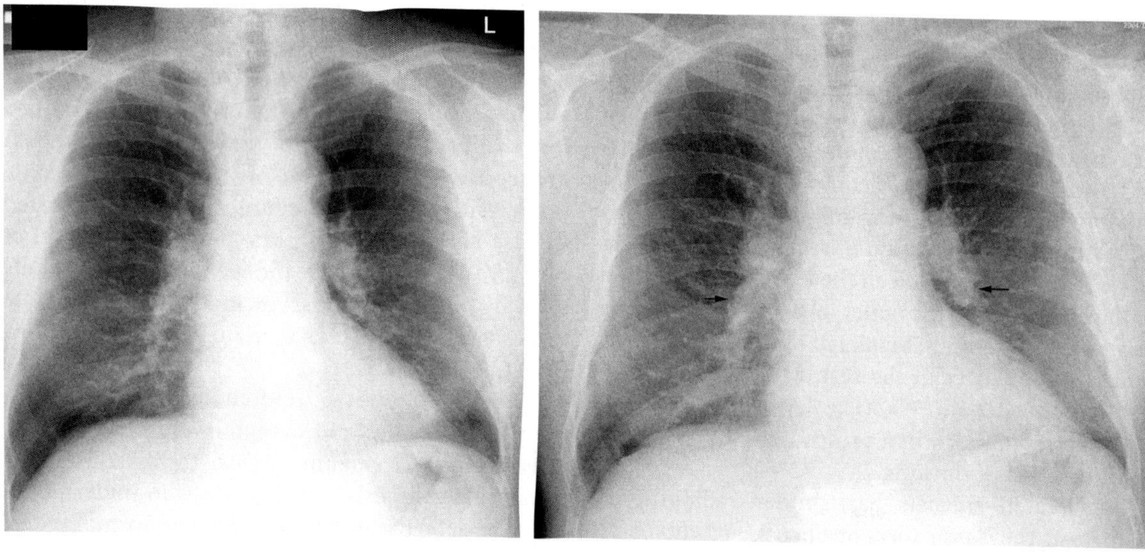
b

Fig. 5.3a,b. A 67-year-old old retired tunnel worker. **a** Posterior–anterior (PA) chest radiograph obtained in 2000 showing small nodules predominantly on the upper lobe. The nodule size and profusion are p/p and 1/1 respectively. **b** PA chest radiograph obtained in 2004 show progression in the profusion of the nodules from 1/1 to 2/2. There is also more prominent egg-shell calcification of enlarged hilar lymph nodes (*arrows*)

partially obscured) (Fig. 5.1, Fig. 5.4) and category 3 (3/2, 3/3, 3/+), when very numerous small opacities totally obscure normal vascular markings (Fig. 5.4). Patients with scores 1/0 or greater are considered to have pneumoconiosis. A separate classification for large opacities (>1 cm in diameter) also exists: *A* denotes one or more opacities greater than 1 cm but each less than 50 mm; *B* indicates one or more opacities greater than A and the combined area is less than the right upper zone and *C* is used when one or more opacities has a combined area greater than the area of the right upper zone.

On the chest radiograph, the nodules in simple silicosis are well defined and small, ranging from 1 mm to 10 mm in diameter. These are present diffusely in the lungs with posterior and upper zone predominance (Bergin et al. 1986). Nodule calcification is present in up to 20% of cases on the chest

a
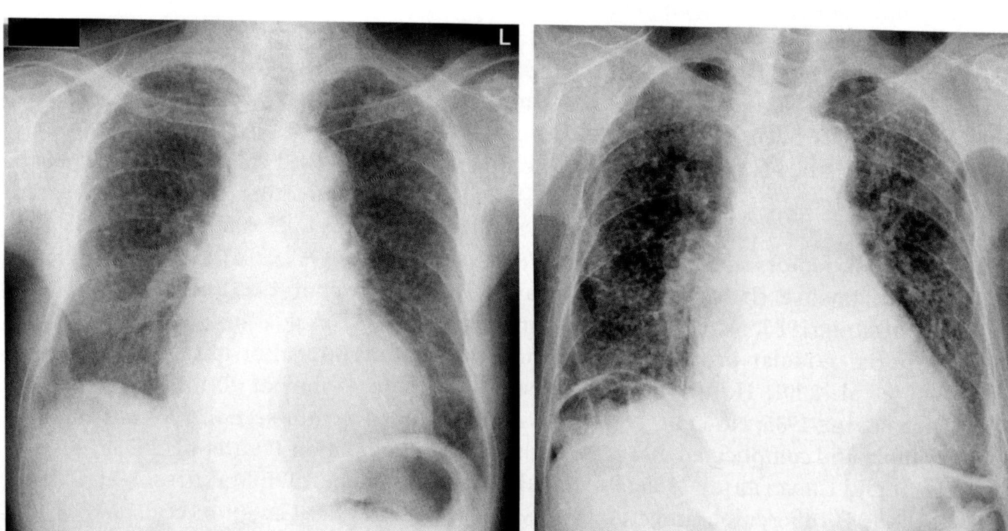
b

Fig. 5.4a,b. Chest radiographs of two retired metal ore miners illustrating different categories of profusion of "r"-size nodules. **a** Posterior–anterior (PA) chest radiograph shows multiple nodules in both lungs. The nodule profusion category is 2/2. **b** PA chest radiograph shows more severe nodular profusion of category 3/3 radiograph, although the incidence is higher with CT. In "complicated silicosis" or PMF, there is conglomeration of nodules to form aggregates greater than 1 cm in diameter (Fig. 5.5). These PMF lesions are usually found in the upper zones with smooth or irregular borders. They commonly start off at the outer two-thirds of the lung, migrating centrifugally with time towards the hilum, resulting in paracicatricial emphysema between the PMF and the pleura, with volume loss in the upper lobes. With increasing severity of PMF and shrinkage of the upper lobes, reduced nodularity in the rest of the lungs will be noted (Gupta et al. 1991) (Fig. 5.5). Unilateral PMF is uncommon and, when present, can be mistaken for carcinoma of the lung.

Accelerated silicosis has similar radiographic features as the classic form of silicosis, except for its earlier onset and rapid rate of progression, which is truncated to a period of between 5 years and 10 years. Silicoproteinosis is a variant characterized by rapid and progressive involvement of the lungs with bilateral air space opacities similar to that found in alveolar proteinosis. The rate of progression ranges from a few months to a couple of years, usually culminating in death in a few years (Buechner and Ansari 1969; Dees et al. 1978).

Lymph node involvement in silicosis reflects the pathogenesis of the disease, and hilar lymphadenopathy on the chest radiograph is therefore common. "Eggshell" calcification of lymph nodes has become synonymous with silicosis, since they were first described over half a century ago and are mainly referable to the hilar lymph nodes (Fig. 5.3), although abdominal lymph nodes have also been described as bearing eggshell calcification (Jacobson et al. 1967; Jacobs et al. 1956; Gross et al. 1980). Its presence in coal and metal miners has been attributed to the concomitant exposure to silica (Jacobson et al. 1967).

Radiographic progression in silicosis is associated with the following risk factors: duration and concentration of silica exposure (Hughes et al. 1982; Saiyed and Chatterjee 1985; Ng et al. 1987; Miller et al. 1998), initial nodular profusion on chest radiograph (Lee et al. 2001; Hughes et al. 1982; Saiyed and Chatterjee 1985; Ng et al. 1987; Miller et al. 1998), simple and complicated disease (Lee et al. 2001; Saiyed and Chatterjee 1985; Ng et al. 1987; Miller et al. 1998), tuberculous infection (Jorgensen 1986), age at initial radiograph (Lee et al. 2001; Hughes et al. 1982), race (Lee et al. 2001; Hughes et al. 1982) and time interval between radiographs (Lee et al. 2001; Hughes et al. 1982). Workers who are exposed to high concentration and longer duration of dust exposure with complicated disease or tuberculous infection and who are younger at initial radiograph, are non-Caucasians and had longer duration between radiographic follow-up are reported to be more likely to have radiographic progression than their counterparts. Complicated disease on initial chest radiograph and interval of radiographic follow were independent determinants of radiographic progression in 37% of 141 granite workers with silicosis exposed to high levels of silica (Lee et al. 2001).

There are, however, limitations associated with the use of the chest radiograph in the assessment of lung changes in pneumoconiosis. This is exemplified by Epler and his colleagues, who undertook a study to determine the prevalence of normal roentgenograms in chronic diffuse infiltrative lung diseases (Epler et al. 1978). Of 458 cases of biopsy-proven chronic interstitial lung disease, 10% had a normal chest radiograph. To further illustrate the point, Kipen et al. evaluated 138 autopsy specimens with histological evidence of parenchymal fibrosis obtained from insulation workers who had died of lung cancer (Kipen et al. 1987): in 25 (18%) cases, there was no radiographic evidence of parenchymal fibrosis. Underestimation of disease, missed diagnosis and greatest inter-observer error are particularly common in subtle disease with lower categories of nodular profusion (Bégin et al. 1991; Rockoff and Schwartz 1988).

5.5.2 Computed Tomography/Thin-Section Computed Tomography

The superiority of CT, and thin-section CT over the chest radiograph in evaluating interstitial and parenchymal lung disease is well established (Epler et al. 1978; Bégin et al. 1991; Hansell and Kerr 1991; Ooi et al. 1997; Muller et al. 1989). Prior to the advent of multi-slice CT, CT evaluation of silicosis was performed using conventional or spiral CT scans comprising contiguous 7-mm or 10-mm section thickness supplemented by thin-section CT scans obtained with 1–2 mm collimation (Ooi et al. 2003b; Bergin et al. 1986; Bégin et al. 1991; Mathieson et al. 1989; Remy-Jardin et al. 1990; Gevenois et al. 1994). These CT techniques allowed clearer depiction of nodules, pleural calcification and conglomeration of nodules than the chest radiograph. Due to superimposition of lesions, 7 mm or 10 mm conventional or spiral CT

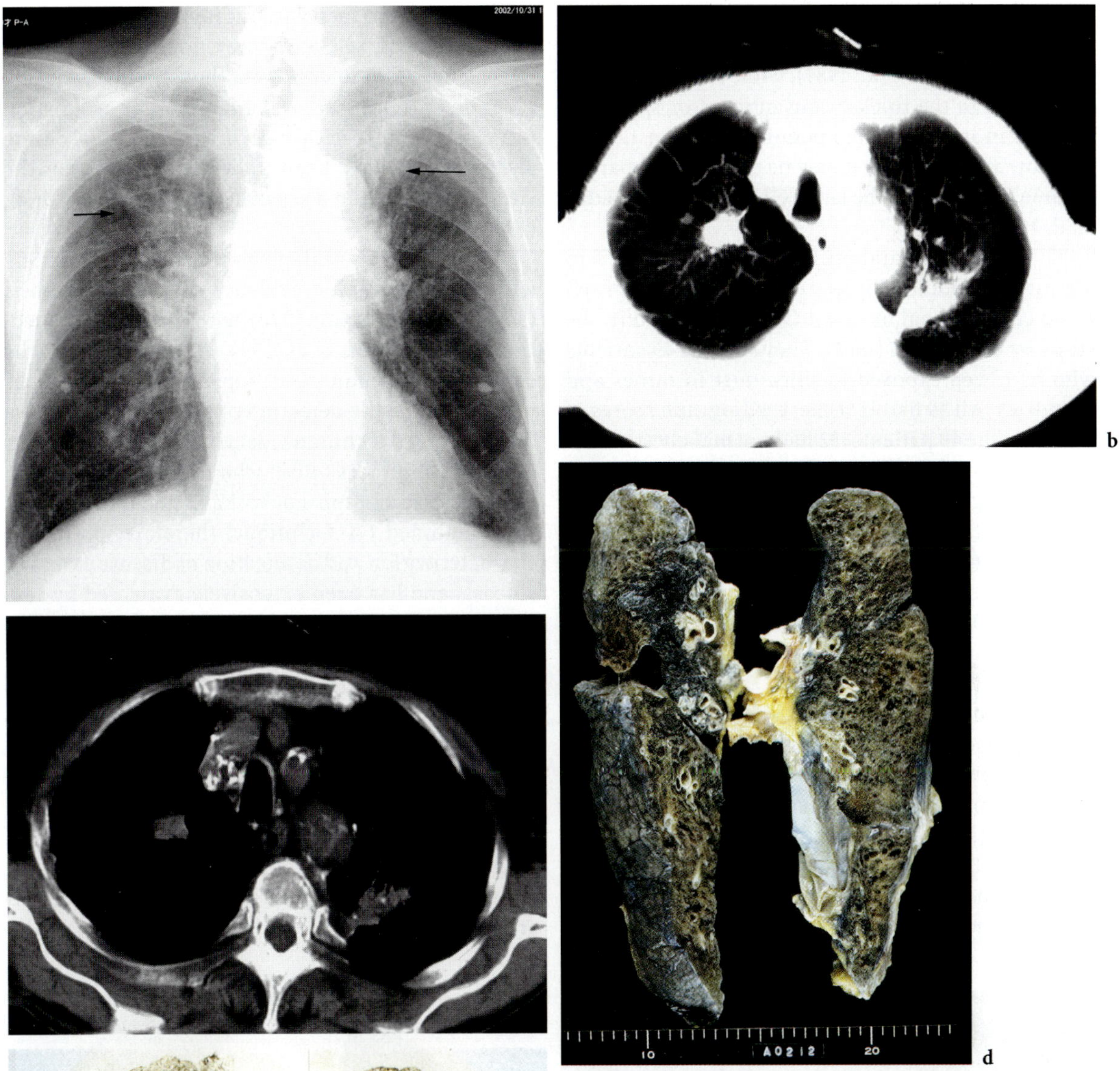

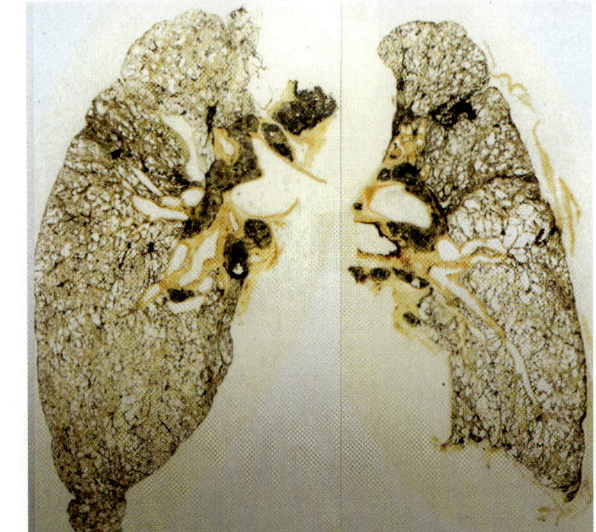

Fig. 5.5a–e. Complicated silicosis in a 79-year-old retired tunnel worker. **a** Posterior–anterior chest radiograph shows bilateral large opacities in the upper lung zones near the pulmonary hila (*arrows*) compatible with the diagnosis of complicated silicosis. Note that there is bilateral hilar lymphadenopathy with reduced background nodulation. **b** Spiral computed tomography image (10-mm thickness) shows bilateral larger nodules with irregular shape, suggesting progressive massive fibrosis (PMF). There are paracicatricial emphysema around the PMF in the right lung. **c** Mediastinal window image shows punctuate calcification in the PMF as well as in the mediastinal lymph nodes. **d** Macroscopic lung image in coronal section reveals black-pigmented PMF in the right upper lung zone adjacent to and contiguous with the right hilar lymphadenopathy. There is moderate centrilobular emphysema but sparse silicotic nodules. **e** Gough–Wentworth whole-lung section clearly demarcates the PMF as well as silicotic nodules with pigmentation. Note that there are advanced emphysematous changes around the PMF in both upper lobes

sections are advocated as the best technique to identify micronodules clustered around vascular structures (Mathieson et al. 1989), while thin-section CT is superior to the thicker conventional or spiral CT sections in imaging small nodules less than 1.5 mm with low attenuation that may be obscured by partial volume averaging in the latter CT techniques (Bégin et al. 1988, 1991).

The superiority and utility of thin-section CT in identifying nodules not seen on the chest radiograph or on conventional or spiral CT is illustrated in the study by Bégin et al. (1991). They studied 49 patients who had been exposed to silica dust in mines and foundries. All 49 had ILO chest radiograph scores of 0 or 1. Of the 49 patients, 32 had normal chest radiographs, 6 were categorized as having indeterminate chest radiographs and 13 had abnormal chest radiographs. Of the 32 patients with normal chest radiographs, 13 (41%) cases were identified using either CT or thin-section CT to have silicosis. In addition, a further 10% of cases were diagnosed to have silicosis only on the thin-section CT scan (Bégin et al. 1991).

Early confluence of nodules and emphysema that are not obvious on the chest radiograph can be demonstrated on conventional or spiral CT and thin-section CT (Ooi et al. 2003b; Bergin et al. 1986; Bégin et al. 1991) (Fig. 5.6). In a study of 76 men with silicosis, Ooi et al. determined that 26 had simple silicosis based on their chest radiographs; the remaining 50 men had radiographic evidence of PMF (Ooi et al. 2003b). Of the 26 men with radiographic evidence of simple silicosis, 10 (38.5%) were found to have early confluence of nodules greater than 1.5 cm, denoting PMF, on CT (Ooi et al. 2003b). A similar proportion (40%) of workers with PMF diagnosed on CT were also noted to have been under-represented on the chest radiograph in a separate study by Bégin et al. (1988).

Gevenois et al. studied the lungs of 40 coal miners without radiographic evidence of pneumoconiosis (ILO profusion score <1/0) with CT and thin-section CT (Gevenois et al. 1994). They noted that the combined technique was superior to either technique alone in the detection of pulmonary nodules. The combined technique identified micronodules in 16 of the 40 miners (40%) who were determined on the chest radiograph not to have pneumoconiosis. The combined CT technique, therefore, optimizes characterization and delineation of disease extent in silicosis and has been extensively evaluated by several workers in the study of pneumoconiosis (Ooi et al. 2003b; Bergin et al. 1986; Bégin et al. 1991; Mathieson et al. 1989; Remy-Jardin et al. 1990; Gevenois et al. 1994). However, with the advent of multi-slice CT, it is now possible to retrospectively reconstruct the acquired data into any slice thickness and algorithm necessary to evaluate the lungs in silicosis (Fig. 5.7).

On CT and thin-section CT, the silicotic nodules are well defined, ranging from 2 mm to 5 mm, and are found predominantly in the centrilobular and

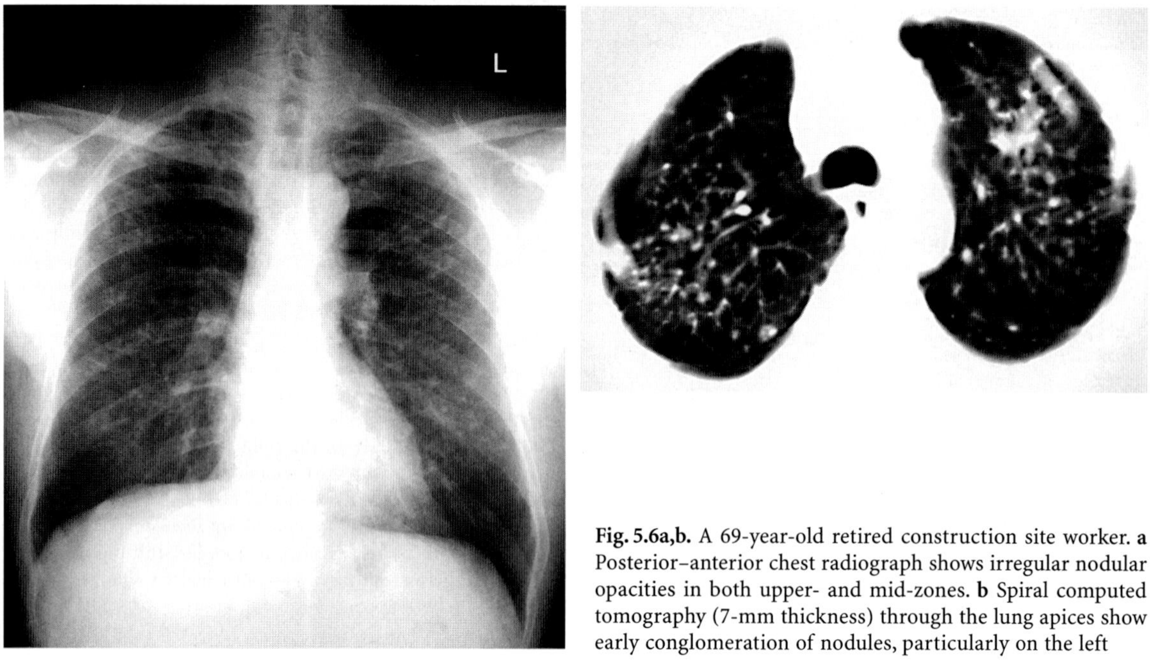

a b

Fig. 5.6a,b. A 69-year-old retired construction site worker. **a** Posterior–anterior chest radiograph shows irregular nodular opacities in both upper- and mid-zones. **b** Spiral computed tomography (7-mm thickness) through the lung apices show early conglomeration of nodules, particularly on the left

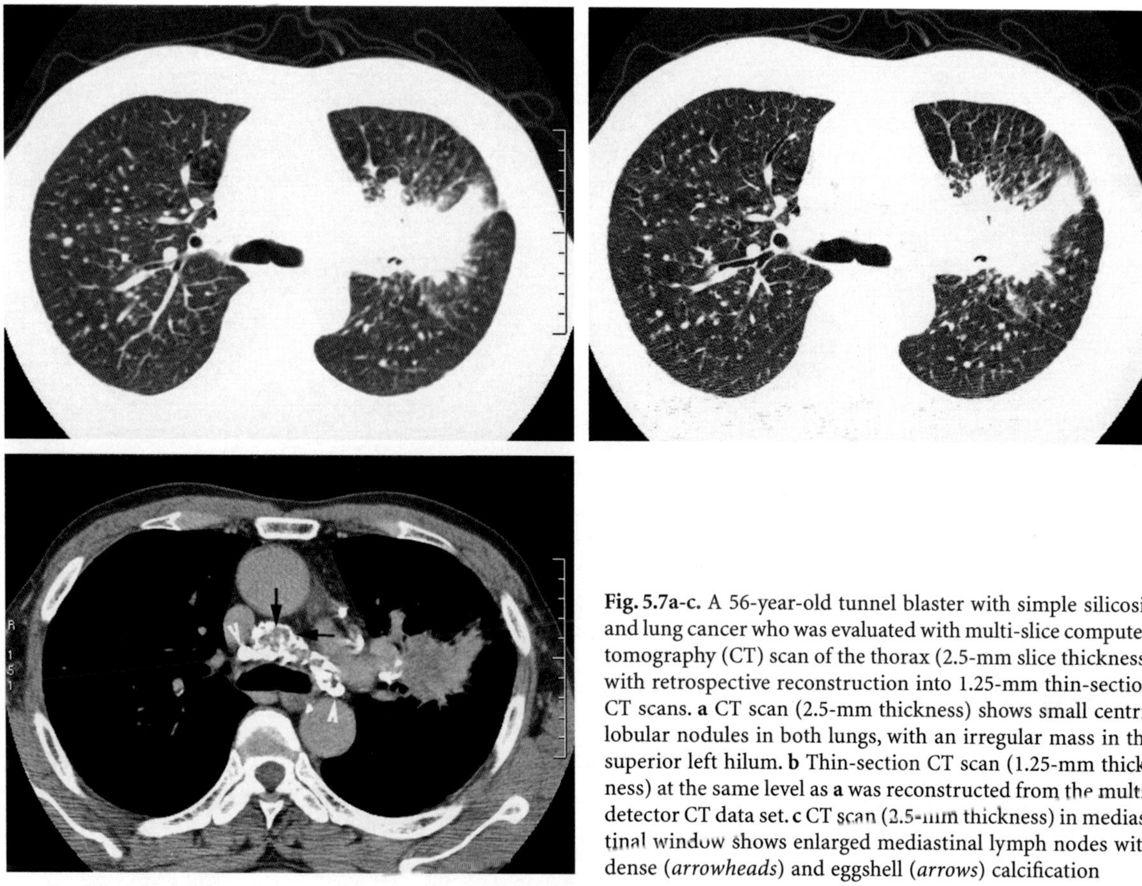

Fig. 5.7a-c. A 56-year-old tunnel blaster with simple silicosis and lung cancer who was evaluated with multi-slice computed tomography (CT) scan of the thorax (2.5-mm slice thickness) with retrospective reconstruction into 1.25-mm thin-section CT scans. **a** CT scan (2.5-mm thickness) shows small centrilobular nodules in both lungs, with an irregular mass in the superior left hilum. **b** Thin-section CT scan (1.25-mm thickness) at the same level as **a** was reconstructed from the multidetector CT data set. **c** CT scan (2.5-mm thickness) in mediastinal window shows enlarged mediastinal lymph nodes with dense (*arrowheads*) and eggshell (*arrows*) calcification

subpleural distribution (Fig. 5.1 and Fig. 5.8). Usually diffuse and bilateral with posterior lung dominance, the nodules in milder cases may be confined to the upper lobes, with sparing of the lower zones. Conglomerate masses or PMF appear as mass-like consolidation, usually with irregular margins and associated with adjacent paracicatricial emphysema and lung parenchymal architectural distortion (Fig. 5.5, Fig. 5.9 and Fig 5.10). The PMF lesions are usually found in the apical and posterior segments of the upper and lower lobes. Cavitation of the PMF lesions occurs as a result of ischemic necrosis or tuberculous infection (Fig. 5.9). Calcification when present may be punctuate, linear or massive (Akira 2002) (Fig. 5.5). Paracicatricial emphysema (Fig. 5.9, Fig. 5.10) has been observed to be more prominent in patients with silicosis compared with coal workers' pneumoconiosis (Remy-Jardin et al. 1990). In their review of thin-section CT scans in 55 patients with type-p pneumoconiosis, Akira et al. found intralobular areas of low attenuation with a central dot, which corresponded to irregular fibrosis around and along the respiratory bronchioles and to focal areas of centrilobular emphysema in two post-mortem specimens (Akira et al. 1989). Nevertheless, there is still debate whether centrilobular emphysema (Fig. 5.10) found in silicosis is due to silica dust per se, exposure to other dust, such as coal and asbestos, or to concomitant smoking (Bégin et al. 1991, 1995; Kinsella et al. 1990). Some studies have reported that emphysema in silicosis occurs independently of smoking (Gevenois et al. 1998; American Thoracic Society Committee of the Scientific Assembly of Environmental and Occupational Health 1997; Hnizdo et al. 1994), while other investigators believe that silicosis per se without PMF does not contribute to emphysema (Bégin et al. 1991, 1995; Akira et al. 1989; Kinsella et al. 1990; Gevenois et al. 1998).

Hilar and mediastinal lymph nodes are generally enlarged and may calcify. Ooi et al. reviewed CT scans of 41 men with silicosis for distribution and pattern of calcification of mediastinal lymph nodes in six lymph node stations (Ooi et al. 2003a). All patients had enlarged lymph nodes in at least two lymph node stations, with calcification found in nearly 50% of lymph node stations. Hyperdense lymph node (Fig. 5.8) was present in one-third of

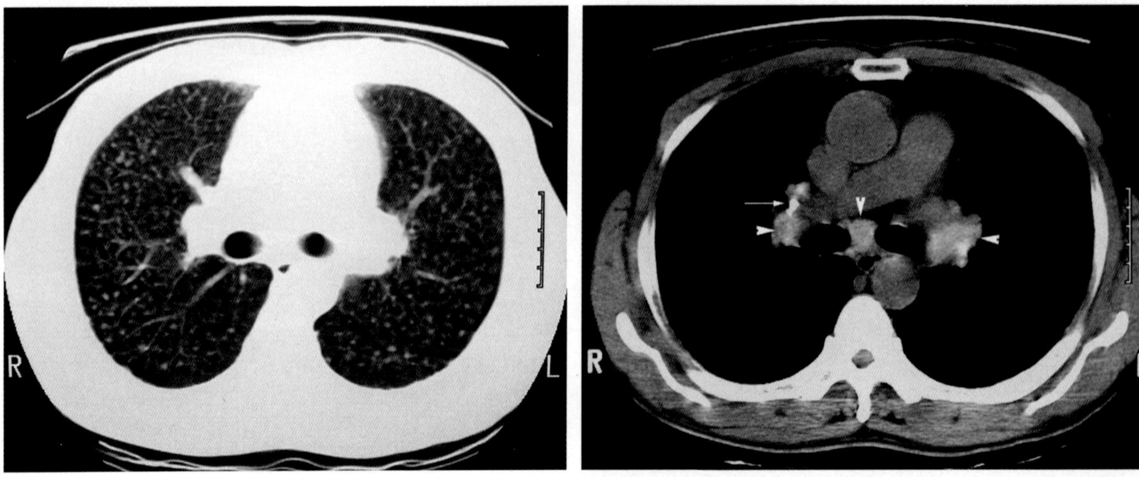

a b

Fig. 5.8a,b. A 78-year-old retired construction site worker. **a** Computed tomography (CT) scan (7-mm thickness) through the upper lobes shows typical silicotic nodules in a centrilobular distribution. **b** CT scan in mediastinal window shows densely calcified (*arrow*) and hyperdense (*arrowheads*) lymph nodes in the mediastinum and hila

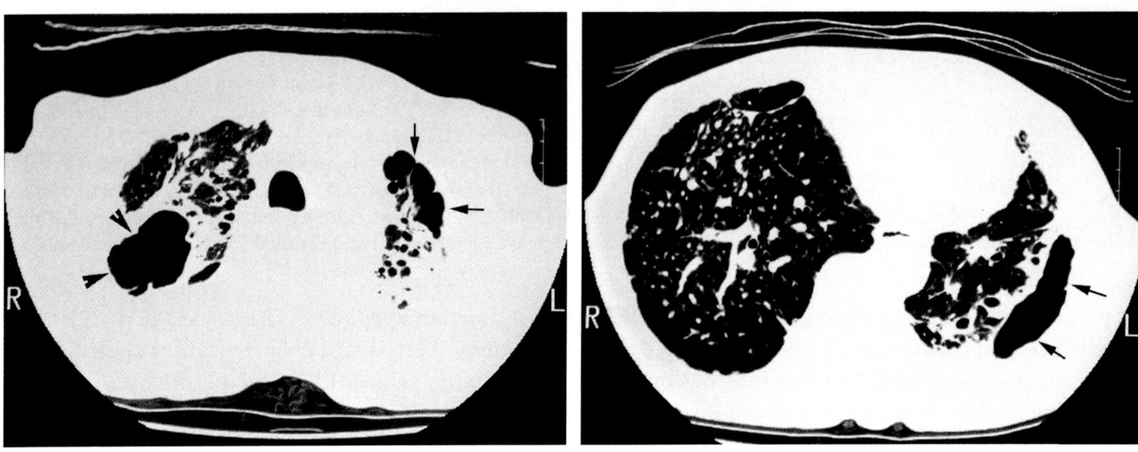

a b

Fig. 5.9a,b. A 74-year-old retired tunnel blaster with progressive massive fibrosis (PMF) complicated by tuberculosis. **a** Thin-section CT scan through the lung apices shows a cavitating PMF lesion (*arrowheads*) in the right upper lobe secondary to *mycobacterium tuberculosis* infection. Note paracicatricial emphysema (*arrows*) surrounding the left PMF lesion and traction bronchiectasis in both lung apices. **b** Thin-section CT scan through the lower lobes shows a loculated pneumothorax (*arrows*) at the lateral aspect of the left lower lobe secondary to ruptured paracicatricial emphysema

lymph node stations, most frequently in the subcarinal region. The predominant type of calcification was the uniformly dense calcified lymph node (53.4%) (Fig. 5.7 and Fig. 5.8) followed by the speckled variety (26.4%). Central, eccentric and eggshell calcification (Fig. 5.7) was rare (4.3, 7.7 and 5.2%, respectively).

Thin-section CT appearances of silicoproteinosis have been described only in occasional case reports (Marchiori et al. 2001). In addition to diffuse ground-glass opacities that typify idiopathic alveolar proteinosis, the presence of centrilobular poorly defined nodules and consolidation in the dorsal portion of lower lobes serve to differentiate silicoproteinosis from the former. Bilateral hilar lymphadenopathy is another discriminating feature found in silicoproteinosis. The pathological basis for the centrilobular nodules and peripheral consolidation has not been disclosed, although ground-glass opacity has been attributed to the accumulation of excess alveolar surfactant protein.

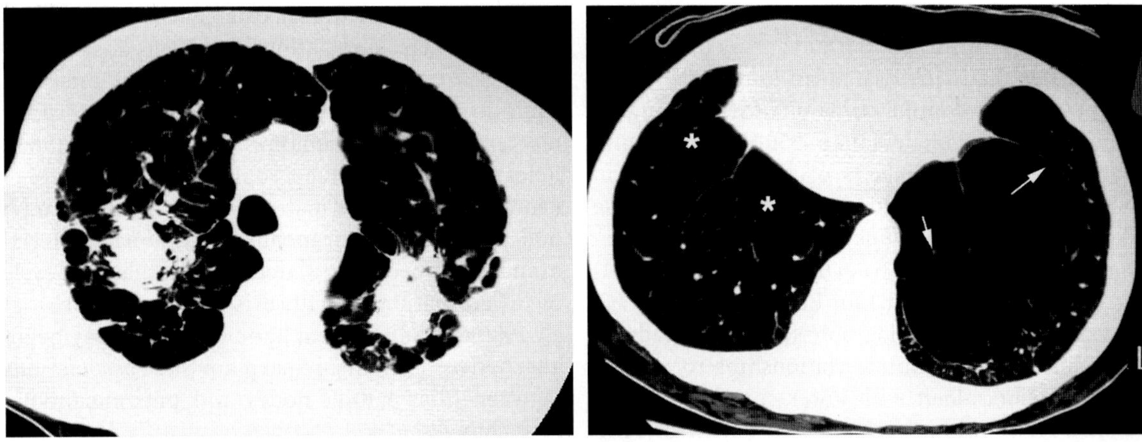

Fig. 5.10a,b. A 68-year-old retired construction site worker. **a** Thin-section CT scan through the upper lobes shows bilateral progressive massive fibrosis (PMF) with surrounding paracicatricial emphysema. **b** Thin-section CT scan through the lower lobes shows confluent centrilobular emphysema (*asterisks*) in the right lower lobes and bullae in the left lower lobe (*arrows*)

5.5.3 Radiological–Clinical Correlation Using CT Techniques

Most studies that have evaluated the utility of CT in silicosis have largely applied the ILO classification, with some modifications, to grade nodular profusion on CT (Bergin et al. 1986; Bégin et al. 1987, 1991, 1995; Kinsella et al. 1990; Ooi et al. 2003a; Talini et al. 1995). Although some previous studies have shown a poor relationship between nodular profusion and lung function (Bergin et al. 1986), other workers have described associations between deteriorating lung function and nodular profusion and coalescence, respectively (Ooi et al. 2003b; Bégin et al. 1988; Kinsella et al. 1990; Gevenois et al. 1998; Talini et al. 1995). Bégin et al. investigated the relationship between lung function, airflow limitation and lung injury assessed on the chest radiograph and CT scans in 94 silica-exposed workers in the foundry and granite industries (Bégin et al. 1988). Workers who had radiographic or CT evidence of coalescence of nodules and conglomerate masses had significant reductions in lung volume, impaired gas exchange and airflow obstruction compared with their counterparts who did not show lung function impairment.

In their study on 17 patients with silicosis and 6 controls, Bergin et al. graded CT scans for nodular profusion and extent of emphysema and measured mean lung attenuation (Bergin et al. 1986). Although there was a significant correlation between ILO radiographic scores of nodular profusion and mean lung attenuation and visual CT scores, there was poor correlation between radiographic and CT scores of nodular profusion and lung function. There was, however, a significant relationship between extent of emphysema graded on CT and indices of airflow obstruction ($r>0.66$, $P<0.001$) and diffusing capacity ($r=0.71$, $P<0.001$).

Emphysema in silicosis can arise from a number of factors, including cigarette smoking, exposure to silica and other dusts such as coal and asbestos and the presence of PMF, as discussed above. To address this issue, Kinsella et al. stratified 30 silica exposed workers into two groups: one group comprised 18 workers who were ex-smokers or current smokers, and the second group consisted of 12 workers who were lifetime non-smokers (Kinsella et al. 1990). Comparison was made between the two groups with respect to extent of emphysema and nodules, respectively, on CT. Extent of emphysema was the strongest independent predictor of lung function impairment, while extent of nodules was a weaker independent predictor of diffusing capacity only. This study also showed that in the absence of PMF, smokers had worse emphysema and lung-function impairment than non-smokers. There was no such difference in the group with PMF. The authors, in agreement with other investigators, concluded that in the absence of PMF, silicosis was not associated with significant emphysema (Bégin et al. 1991, 1995; Akira et al. 1989; Kinsella et al. 1990; Gevenois et al. 1998).

In 2003, Ooi et al. further explored the relationship between nodular profusion, PMF, emphysema and lung function in 76 silica-exposed men (Ooi et al. 2003b). Nodular profusion on CT was evaluated visually and also quantitatively by application of attenuation threshold to isolate areas of attenuation greater than -100 HU. Mean lung density was also obtained and emphysema quantified using an attenuation threshold less than -950 HU. Visual and quantitative CT parameters of nodular profusion and extent of PMF and emphysema showed inverse relationships with lung function indices: the correlation coefficients ranged from 0.47 to 0.63, ($P<0.001$) and 0.41 to 0.61 ($P<0.001$) for FEV_1 and FEV_1/FVC, respectively. Chest radiograph scores for nodular profusion showed similar relationships to indices of obstruction, albeit with lower correlation coefficients. After multiple regression, extent of PMF and emphysema remained significant independent determinants of FEV_1 and FEV_1/FVC, while mean lung attenuation was an independent predictor of lung volume and diffusing capacity. Smoking and duration of silica exposure exerted no independent effects on lung function. Although there were no significant differences with respect to age, duration of silica exposure and cigarette consumption among workers with simple silicosis and PMF, those with PMF had significantly impaired lung function and higher radiological scores compared with their counterparts. Abnormal FEV_1 and FVC (<70% predicted) were also observed in one-third of workers with simple silicosis, consistent with the result of a recent meta-analysis that found an association between silica exposure and airflow obstruction, even in non-smokers (American Thoracic Society Committee of the Scientific Assembly of Environmental and Occupational Health 1997; Hnizdo et al. 1994; Oxman et al. 1993; Becklake et al. 1987).

Ooi et al. also evaluated the relationship between mediastinal lymph node attenuation with severity of nodular profusion and PMF on CT and lung function in 41 men with silica exposure. Increasing lymph node attenuation was directly related to severity of nodular profusion and PMF and inversely related to diffusion coefficient (Ooi et al. 2003a). Men with more severe nodular profusion also had a greater number of calcified lymph node stations, while men with larger numbers of calcified lymph node stations had significantly reduced diffusion coefficients compared with those with fewer calcified lymph node stations. These relationships imply that mediastinal lymph nodes in silicosis increase in attenuation and calcification with severity of lung disease and functional impairment and concur with the findings of Friedetzky et al., who determined that changes in lymph nodes occurred in tandem with lung changes in rats induced with silicosis (Friedetzky et al. 1998). Similar associations between dust-related changes in the hilar lymph nodes and pneumoconiotic lung disease were also found in a postmortem study of 123 coalminers (Seal et al. 1986). Release of dust-laden macrophages from rupture of necrotic collagenous material from affected lymph nodes into adjacent bronchus or pulmonary arterial branch have been postulated to perpetuate the cycle of inflammation and fibrosis in silicosis (Seal et al. 1986). Impaired lymphatic clearance may be an alternative mechanism to explain these associations between hilar lymph nodes and pneumoconiotic lung changes.

5.6 Complications

There are a few diseases that may complicate silicosis; these are primarily Caplan's syndrome, tuberculosis, carcinoma and connective tissue disease. The two most serious complications, lung cancer and tuberculosis, may affect the prognosis and natural history of the underlying disease.

Caplan's syndrome, also known as rheumatoid pneumoconiosis, was initially identified in coal workers' pneumoconiosis but is now known to occur in silicosis as well (Honma and Vallyathan 2002). The incidence of this disease ranges from 0.48% to 0.74% (Honma and Vallyathan 2002). The rheumatoid pneumoconiotic nodules are similar to necrobiotic nodules seen in rheumatoid arthritis and are described as either classic or silicotic type based on their pathological findings (Honma and Vallyathan 2002). The classic type corresponds to the original Caplan's cases, showing large nodules characterized by uniform necrosis and associated with little background pneumoconiotic nodules. The silicotic type consists of multiple smaller nodules, with the necrotic area retaining some characteristics of a silicotic nodule. In both types, a layer of palisaded inflammatory cells surrounds the peripheral zone of the nodules. On the chest radiograph, rheumatoid pneumoconiosis presents with multiple well-defined nodules ranging from 5 mm to 5 cm distributed throughout both lung fields with peripheral predominance (Caplan 1953). Characteristically, these nodules appear suddenly within a few months during the follow-up of those patients. On CT, the rheumatoid pneumoconiotic nodules are well defined and may cavitate and calcify (Arakawa et al. 2003). However, it may be impossible to distinguish silicotic-type nodules of rheumatoid pneumoconiosis from silicotic nodules per se.

It is well established that silicosis predisposes to tuberculous infection, although this predisposition is dependent on the prevalence of tuberculosis in the population from which the workers originate (Becklake 1992). Workers with more severe disease in terms of nodular profusion and PMF are at greatest risk of acquiring tuberculosis, which in turn is associated with an increased likelihood of radiographic progression (Lee et al. 2001). Cavitation of PMF lesions (Fig. 5.9), unusually rapid advancement in nodular profusion or size and presence of tree-in-bud opacities on CT, indicating endobronchial infection, are pointers to the development of silicotuberculosis (Lee and Im 1995; Kuhlman et al. 1994; Solomon 2001). In cases of indolent nodular tuberculosis, it may be impossible to isolate the tubercle bacilli in the sputum, in which case polymerase chain reaction has been advocated as a means of identifying the organism (Cheng et al. 1993).

The association between silicosis and lung cancer is also well documented. Silica has been recognized as a probable human carcinogen [International Agency for Research on Cancer (IARC) type 2A] since 1987 (IARC monographs; 1987). In 1997 (IARC monographs; 1997) the classification of silica was changed from 2A (probable human carcinogen) to type 1 (known human carcinogen). The risk is greatest for workers with established silicosis compared with those with silica exposure, who have a reduced albeit still elevated risk of lung cancer (Chiyotani et al. 1990; Smith et al. 1995; Tsuda et al. 2002).

The strength of the association between silicosis and connective tissue disease varies with the type of connective tissue disorder. The risk of developing systemic sclerosis, particularly in workers with high exposure to silica dust, is well established, although such casual associations between silicosis, rheumatoid arthritis and systemic lupus erythematosis are less widely reported (Rosenman 1999; Sluis-Cremer et al. 1985, 1986; Sanchez-Roman et al. 1993)

5.7 Differential Diagnosis

A similar centrilobular and subpleural distribution of nodules may be noted in sarcoidosis and lymphangitis carcinomatosis, although a careful review of the clinical history may provide useful pointers for and against these other diseases. In addition, on thin-section CT, there are a few distinguishing features, such as beaded septa and fissures and reticular opacities, which are usually not found in silicosis. Clustering of nodules around parahilar regions and bronchi are also more commonly found with sarcoidosis.

5.8 Future Developments

Despite the considerable debate over the role of emphysema, nodule coalescence and PMF in the development of airflow obstruction in silicosis, the ILO classification does not provide classification of emphysema, although it recognizes the presence of bulla, which it denotes as "bu" (Geneva, International Labor Office 2000). There is, however, no system for quantifying bullous change. The chest radiograph is also significantly insensitive in evaluating the extent or severity of emphysema in comparison with CT and thin-section CT, which are techniques that allow quantification of severity and extent of both emphysema and lung nodules. There is also no current consensus on the size of PMF in the pneumoconiosis. Although the ILO radiographic classification recognizes the presence of PMF when a single opacity in the radiograph exceeds 1 cm in diameter (Geneva, International Labor Office 2000; Bégin et al. 1988), the College of American Pathologists defines PMF in coal workers pneumoconiosis as lesions larger than 2 cm (Gamsu 1991; Kleinerman et al. 1979).

There is, therefore, a need for a standardized, reproducible and internationally accepted CT/thin-section CT classification system for the pneumoconiosis in the English language, such as the ILO classification for the chest radiograph. There has been a recent multi-center study involving an international panel of experts who have applied a coding sheet for CT/thin-section CT lung appearances developed by a task group on Diagnostic Radiology in Occupational and Environmental Diseases (Hering 2004; Hering and Kraus 2005). This coding sheet is a descriptive classification of CT and thin-section CT appearances of parenchymal and pleural abnormalities found in occupational and environmentally related diseases. In this system, not only is the presence of each abnormality found in each lung zone and the pleura described, but also, at the same time, the severity and extent of silicotic nodules, PMF, diffuse interstitial fibrosis (i.e., reticular opacities and ground-glass opacity) and emphysema are quantified based on the reference images. The establishment of a reproducible CT/thin-section CT classification system would, therefore, standardize the reporting and documentation of abnormalities found in the CT/thin-section CT evaluation of pneumoconiosis.

Other imaging techniques that are currently available to evaluate the chest include magnetic resonance imaging (MRI) and positron emission tomography (PET), although the utility of both techniques has not been substantially evaluated or validated in silicosis. Matsumoto et al. evaluated MR appearances in 17 patients with 34 PMF lesions, 11 of whom had silicotuberculosis (Matsumoto et al. 1998b). They classified signal intensity pattern on T1- and T2-weighted images (WI) and the pattern of contrast enhancement. The most common signal change of PMF lesions was isointensity (70%) on T1-WI and hypointensity (68%) on T2-WI relative to skeletal muscle. In 41% of lesions, focal hyperintense areas were noted within the PMF lesions, which corresponded to low density areas on CT, suggestive of necrosis. Rim enhancement was present in a little over half (53%) of all cases. Diffuse enhancement was noted in only 2 of 34 PMF lesions; the remaining lesions did not enhance reflecting the hypovascular nature of the hyaline collagenous tissue without formation of new capillaries or cellular reaction that comprise PMF lesions in silicosis (Spencer 1985). The authors hypothesized that the rim enhancement described above was due to collapsed alveoli caused by emphysema (Matsumoto et al. 1998b). The same authors also described MRI features of lung cancer occurring in a patient with PMF (Matsumoto et al. 1998a) as a high-signal intensity area separate from the fibrotic mass, which appeared as a low-signal intensity area, on both T1- and T2-weighted images. MRI, particularly with gadolinium enhancement, may therefore be potentially useful in differentiating lung cancer from the fibrous tissue in the PMF lesions. Other uses of MRI may lie in imaging complications of silicosis that involve the central vessels, such as pulmonary artery stenosis, with MR angiography being a less invasive modality than conventional angiography (Mahnaken et al. 2001).

The utility of PET-CT in silicosis has not been thoroughly investigated, but increased uptake has been described in both PMF lesions and also in enlarged mediastinal and hilar lymph nodes in silicosis (O'Connell and Kennedy 2004) (Fig. 5.11). Whether this will present problems when there is a concomitant lung cancer arising in a silicosis patient, particularly one complicated by PMF, remains unclear, although Bandoh et al. have described the utility of PET in identifying malignancy in the set-

a

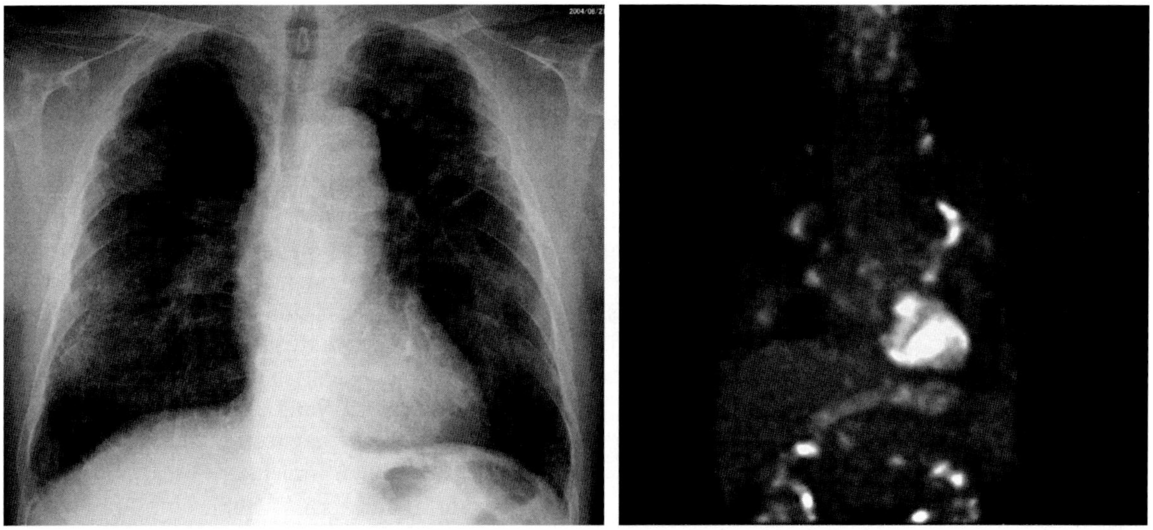

b

Fig. 5.11a,b. A 71-year-old retired metal ore miner. **a** Chest radiograph shows multiple conglomerated masses in both upper and lower lobes with diffuse pleural thickening adjacent to the masses bilaterally. Silicotic nodules are also present especially around the masses. **b** F-18 Fluorodeoxyglucose (FDG) positron emission tomography image with maximum intensity projection shows increased uptake of FDG in the progressive massive fibrosis lesions. The high uptake in the upper lobe lesions is indistinguishable from that of pulmonary neoplasm. The uptake in the lower lobe lesions is less prominent. Weak uptake is also identified in bilateral hilar lymph nodes and left supraclavicular node ting of pneumoconiosis (Bandoh et al. 2003). A new PET tracer, a fluorinated analog of proline amino acid, cis-4-[(18)F]fluoro-L-proline (FP), was tested for potential use in PET for detection and evaluation of pulmonary response to respirable crystalline silica in experimental rabbits (Wallace et al. 2003). The results were promising, with increased uptake noted in the lungs of silicotic animals compared with controls. This suggests that FP PET imaging may have the potential sensitivity to detect active fibrosis in silicosis and other lung diseases.

References

Absher MP, Hemenway DR, Leslie KO et al (1992) Intrathoracic distribution and transport of aerosolized silica in the rat. Exp Lung Res 18:743-757

Akira M (2002) High resolution CT in the evaluation of occupational and environmental disease. Radiol Clin North Am 40:43-59

Akira M, Higashihara T, Yokoyama K et al (1989) Radiographic type p pneumoconiosis: high-resolution CT. Radiology 171:117-123

American Thoracic Society Committee of the Scientific Assembly of Environmental and Occupational Health (1997) Adverse effects of crystalline silica exposure. Am J Respir Crit Care Med 155:761-765

Arakawa H, Honma K, Shida H et al (2003) Computed tomography findings of Caplan syndrome. J Comput Assist Tomogr 27:758-760

Bailey WC, Brown M, Buechner HA et al (1974) Silico-mycobacterial disease in sandblasters. Am Rev Respir Dis 110:115-125

Bandoh S, Fujita J, Yamamoto Y et al (2003) A case of lung cancer associated with pneumoconiosis diagnosed by fluorine-18 fluorodeoxyglucose positron emission tomography. Ann Nucl Med 17:597-600

Becklake MR (1992) The mineral dust diseases. Tuber Lung Dis 73:13-20

Becklake MR, Irwig L, Kielkowski D et al (1987) The predictors of emphysema in South African gold miners. Am Rev Respir Dis 135:1234-1241

Bégin R, Bergeron D, Samson L et al (1987) CT assessment of silicosis in exposed workers. Am J Roentgenol 148:509-514

Bégin R, Ostiguy G, Cantin A et al (1988) Lung function in silica-exposed workers. A relationship to disease severity assessed by CT scan. Chest 94:539-545

Bégin R, Ostiguy G, Fillion R et al (1991) Computed tomography in the early detection of silicosis. Am Rev Respir Dis 44:697-705

Bégin R, Filion R, Ostiguy G (1995) Emphysema in silica- and asbestos-exposed workers seeking compensation. A CT scan study. Chest 108:647-655

Bergin CJ, Müller NL, Vedal S et al (1986) CT in silicosis: correlation with plain films and pulmonary function tests. Am J Roentgenol 146:477-483

Bitterman PB, Rennard SI, Adelberg S et al (1983) Role of fibronectin as a growth factor for fibroblasts. J Cell Biol 97:1925-1932

Brown GP, Monicj M, Hunninghake GW (1988) Fibroblast proliferation induced by silica-exposed human alveolar macrophages. Am Rev Respir Dis 138:85-89

Buechner HA, Ansari A (1969) Acute silico-proteinosis. A new pathologic variant of acute silicosis in sandblasters, characterized by histologic features resembling alveolar proteinosis. Dis Chest 55:274-278

Caplan A (1953) Certain unusual radiological appearances in the chest of coal-miners suffering from rheumatoid arthritis. Thorax 8:29-37

Cheng SJ, MA Y, Pan YX (1993) A study on the diagnosis of pulmonary tuberculosis and silicotuberculosis by PCR. Zhonghua Jie He He Hu Xi Za Zhi 16:221-224

Chiyotani K, Saito K, Okubo T et al (1990) Lung cancer risk among pneumoconiosis patients in Japan, with special reference to silicotics. IARC Sci Publ 97:95-104

Corry D, Kulkarni P, Lipscomb MF (1984) The migration of bronchoalveolar macrophages into hilar lymph nodes. Am J Pathol 115:321-328

Davies D (1974) Disability and coal workers pneumoconiosis. BMJ 2:652

Davis GS, Gemsa D (1996) Immunopathogenesis of silicosis. In: Immunopathology of lung disease. Edited by Kradin RL and Robinson BWS. Butterworth-Heinemann, Oxford, pp 445-467

Dees PM, Suratt P, Winn W (1978) The radiographic finding in acute silicosis. Radiology 126:359

Dubois CM, Bissonnette E, Rola-Pleszczynski M (1989) Asbestos fibers and silica particles stimulate rat alveolar macrophages to release tumour necrosis factor. Autoregulatory role of leukotriene B4. Am Rev Respir Dis 139:1257-1264

Elmes PC (1994) Inorganic dusts. In: Raffle PAB, Adams PH Baxter PJ, Lee WR (eds) Hunter's diseases of occupations, 8th edn. Arnold, London

Engholm G, von Schamlensee G (1982) Bronchitis and exposure to manmade mineral fibers in nonsmoking construction workers. Eur J Respir Dis [Suppl] 118:73-88

Epler GR, McCloud TC, Gaensler EA et al (1978) Normal chest roentgenogtrams in chronic diffuse infiltrative lung disease. N Engl J Med 298:943-939

Epstein DM, Miller WO, Bresnitz EA et al (1984) Application of ILO classification to a population without industrial exposure: findings to be differentiated from pneumoconiosis. AJR 142:53-58

Friedetzky A, Garn H, Kirchner A et al (1998) Histopathological changes in enlarged thoracic lymph nodes during the development of silicosis in rats. Immunobiology 199:119-132

Gamsu G (1991) Computed Tomography and High Resolution Computed Tomography of Pneumoconioses. Journal of Occupational Medicine 33:794-796

Geneva, International Labor Office (2000) International Labor Office Guidelines for the use of ILO International Classification of Radiographs of Pneumoconiosis. Occupational safety and health series no 22

Gevenois PA, Pichot E, Dargent F et al (1994) Low grade coal worker's pneumoconiosis. Comparison of CT and chest radiography. Acta Radiol 35:351-356

Gevenois PA, Sergent G, de Maertelaer V et al (1998) Micronodules and emphysema in coal mine dust or silica exposure: relation with lung function. Eur Respir J 12:1020-1024

Gibbs AR, Wagner JC (1998) Disease due to Silica. In: Churg A,

Green FHY, (eds) Pathology of occupational lung disease, 2nd edn. Williams and Wilkins, Baltimore, pp 209-234

Graham WH (1992) Silicosis. Clin Chest Med 13:253-267

Gross BH, Schneider HJ, Protos AV (1980) Eggshell calcification of lymph nodes: an update. Am J Roentgenol 135:1265-1268

Gupta BN, Rastogi SK, Husain T et al (1991) A study of respiratory morbidity and pulmonary function among solderers in the electronics industry. Am Ind Hyg Assoc J 52:45-51

Hansell DM, Kerr IH (1991) The role of high resolution computed tomography in the diagnosis of interstitial lung disease. Thorax 46:77-84

Harmsen AG, Muggenburg BA, Snipes MB et al (1985) The role of macrophages in particle translocation from lungs to lymph nodes. Science 230:1277-1280

Heppleston AG, Young AE (1972) Alveolar lipo-proteinosis: an ultrastructural comparison of the experimental and human forms. J Pathol 107:107-117

Hering KG (2004) Standardized CT/HRCT-classification of the German Federal Republic for work and environmental related thoracic diseases. Radiologe 44:500-511

Hering KG, Kraus T (2005) Coding CT-Classification in Occupational and environmental respiratory diseases. In Kusaka Y, Hering KG, Parker JE (eds) International classification of HRCT for occupational and environmental respiratory diseases. Springer, Berlin Heidelberg New York

Hnizdo E, Sluis-Cremer GK, Baskind E et al (1994) Emphysema and airway obstruction in non-smoking South African gold miners with long exposure to silica dust. Occup Environ Med 51:557-563

Hoffmann EO, Lamberty J, Pizzolato P et al (1973) The ultrastructure of acute silicosis. Arch Pathol 96:104-107

Honma K, Vallyathan V (2002) Rheumatoid pneumoconiosis: a comparative study of autopsy cases between Japan and North America. Ann Occup Hyg 46S:265-267

Honma K, Abraham JL, Chiyotani K et al (2004) Proposed criteria for mixed-dust pneumoconiosis: definition, descriptions, and guidelines for pathologic diagnosis and clinical correlation. Hum Pathol 35:1515-1523

Hughes JM, Jones RN, Gilson JC et al (1982) Determinants of progression in sandblasters' silicosis. Ann Occup Hyg 26:701-712

Hunninghake GW, Hemken C, Brady M et al (1986) Immune interferon is a growth factor for human lung fibroblasts. Am Rev Respir Dis 134:1025-1028

IARC Monographs on the evaluation of the carcinogenic risks of chemicals to humans, silica and some silicates (1987) Volume 42, IARC, Lyon, France

IARC Monographs on the evaluation of carcinogenic risks to humans (1997) Volume 68, IARC, Lyon, France

Jacobs LG, Gerstl B, Hollander AG et al (1956) Intraabdominal egg-shell calcification due to silicosis. Radiology 67:527-530

Jacobson G, Felson B, Pendergrass EP et al (1967) Egg shell calcification in coal and metal workers. Semin Roentgenol 2:276-281

Jagirdar J, Bégin R, Dufresne A et al (1996) Transforming growth factor-b in silicosis. Am J Respir Crit Care Med 154:1076-1081

Jiang CQ, Xiao LW, Lam TH et al (2001) Accelerated silicosis in workers exposed to agate dust in Guangzhou, China. Am J Ind Med 40:87-91

Johnson A, Moira CY, Maclean L et al (1985) Respiratory abnormalities among workers in an iron and steel foundry. Br J Ind Med 42:94-100

Jorgensen HS (1986) Silicosis in the iron-ore mine in Kiruna, Sweden, and the future need for silicosis control. Arch Occup Environ Health 58:251-257

Kampschimdt RF, Worthingrton ML, Mesecher MI (1986) Release of interleukin-1 (IL-1) and IL-1-like factors from rabbit macrophages with silics. J Leukoc Biol 39:123-132

Kinsella M, Müller N, Vedal S et al (1990) Emphysema in silicosis. A comparison of smokers with nonsmokers using pulmonary function testing and computed tomography. Am Rev Respir Dis 141:1497-1500

Kipen HM, Lilis R, Suzuki Y et al (1987) Pulmonary fibrosis in asbestos insulation workers with lung cancer. A radiological and histopathological evaluation. Br J Ind Med 44:96-100

Kleinerman J, Green F, Harley RA et al (1979) Pathology standards for coal worker's pneumoconiosis. Arch Pathol Lab Med 103:375-432

Koskinen H (1985) Symptoms and clinical findings in patients with silicosis. Scand J Environ Health 11:101-106

Kuhlman JE, Deutsch JH, Fishman EK, Siegelman SS (1990) CT features of thoracic mycobacterial disease. Radiographics. 10:413-431

Landrigan PJ, Cherniack MG, Lewis FA et al (1986) Silicosis in a grey iron foundry. The persistence of an ancient disease. Scand J Work Environ Health 12:32-39

Lauweryns JM, Baert JH (1977) Alveolar clearance and the role of pulmonary lymphatics. Am Rev Respir Dis 115:625-683

Lee HS, Poon WH, Ng TP (2001) Radiological progression and its predictive risk factors in silicosis. Occup Environ Med 58:467-471

Lee KS, Im JG (1995) CT in adults with tuberculosis of the chest. Characteristic findings and role in management. Am J Roentgenol 164:1361-1367

Lehnert BE, Valdez YE, Stewart CC (1986) Translocation of particles to the tracheobronchial lymph nodes after lung deposition: kinetics and particle-cell relationships. Exp Lung Res 10:245-266

Liddell FDK (1963) An experiment in film reading. Br J Ind Med 20:300

Liddell FDK, Lindars DC (1969) An elaboration of the ILO classification of simple pneumoconiosis. Br J Ind Med 26:89

Lugano EM, Dauber JH, Elias JA et al (1984) The regulation of lung fibroblast proliferation by alveolar macrophages in experimental silicosis. Am Rev Respir Dis 129:767-771

Mahnaken AH, Breuer C, Haage P (2001) Silicosis-induced pulmonary artery stenosis: demonstration by MR angiography and perfusion MRI. Br J Radiol 74:859-861

Marchiori E, Ferreira A, Muller NL (2001) Silicoproteinosis: high-resolution CT and histologic findings. J Thorac Imaging 16:127-129

Mathieson JR, Mayo JR, Staples CA et al (1989) Chronic diffuse infiltrative lung disease: comparison of diagnostic accuracy of CT and chest radiography. Radiology 171:111-116

Matsumoto S, Miyake H, Oga M et al (1998a) Diagnosis of lung cancer in a patient with pneumoconiosis and progressive massive fibrosis using MRI. Eur Radiol 8:615-617

Matsumoto S, Mori H, Miyake H et al (1998b) MRI signal characteristics of progressive massive fibrosis in silicosis. Clin Radiol 53:510-514

Michel RD, Morris JF (1964) Acute Silicosis. Arch Intern Med 113:850-855

Miller BG, Hagen S, Love RG et al (1998) Risks of silicosis in coal workers exposed to unusual concentrations or respirable quartz. Occup Environ Med 55:52-58

Muller NL, Mawson JB, Mathieson JR et al (1989) Sarcoidosis: correlation of extent of disease at CT with clinical, functional, and radiographic findings. Radiology 171:613-618

Murray J, Reid G, Kielkowski D et al (1993) Cor pulmonale and silicosis: a necropsy based case control study. Br J Ind Med 50:544-548

Nagelschmidt G (1960) The relation between lung dust and lung pathology in pneumoconiosis. Br J Ind Med 17:247-259

Neukirch F, Cooreman J, Korobaeff M et al (1994) Silica exposure and chronic airflow limitation in pottery workers. Arc Environ Health 49:459-464

Ng TP, Allan WG, Tsin TW et al (1985) Silicosis in jade workers. Br J Ind Med 42:761-764

Ng TP, Chan Sl, Lam KP (1987) Radiographic progression and lung function in silicosis: a ten year follow up study. BMJ 295:164-168

Nozaki S, Sawada Y (1959) Progress of simple pulmonary silicosis in retired miners. Jpn J Clin Tuberc 18:154

O'Connell M, Kennedy M (2004) Progressive massive fibrosis secondary to pulmonary silicosis appearance on F-18 fluorodeoxyglucose PET/CT. Clin Nucl Med 29:754-755

Oleru UG (1987) Respiratory and nonrespiratory morbidity in a titanium oxide paint factory in Nigeria. Am J Ind Med 12:173-180

Ooi GC, Ngan H, Peh WC et al (1997) Systemic lupus erythematosus patients with respiratory symptoms: the value of HRCT. Clin Radiol 52:775-781

Ooi CG, Khong PL, Cheng RS et al (2003a) The relationship between mediastinal lymph node attenuation with parenchymal lung parameters in silicosis. Int J Tuberc Lung Dis 7:1199-1206

Ooi GC, Tsang KWT, Cheung TF et al (2003b) Qualitative and quantitative CT evaluation in 76 men with silicosis: a clinical radiological correlative study. Radiology 228:816-825

Oxman AD, Muir DCF, Shannon HS et al (1993) Occupational dust exposure and chronic obstructive pulmonary disease. Am Rev Respir Dis 148:38-48

Rees D, Cronje R, du Toit RS (1992) Dust exposure and pneumoconiosis in a South African pottery. 1. Study objectives and dust exposure. Br J Ind Med 49:459-464

Remy-Jardin M, Degreef JM, Beuscart R et al (1990) Coal worker's pneumoconiosis: CT assessment in exposed workers and correlation with radiographic findings. Radiology 177:363-371

Rockoff SD, Schwartz A (1988) Roentgenographic underestimation of early asbestosis by International Labor Organization classification. Chest 93:108-109

Roeslin N, Lassabe-Roth C, Morand G et al (1980) La siilicoproteinose aique. Arch Mal Prof 41:15-18

Rosenmen KD, Moore-Fuller M, Reilly MJ (1999) Connective tissue disease and silicosis. Am J Ind Med 35:375-381

Saiyed HN, Chatterjee BB (1985) Rapid progression of silicosis in slate pencil workers. II. A follow up study. Am J Ind Med 8:135-142

Sanchez-Roman J, Wichmann I, Salaberri J et al (1993) Multiple clinical and biological autoimmune manifestations in 50 workers after occupational exposure to silica. Ann Rheum Dis 52:534-538

Schmidt JA, Oliver CN, Lepe-Zuniga JL et al (1984) Silica-stimulated monocytes release fibroblast proliferation factors identical to interleukin 1. A potential role for interleukin 1 in the pathogenesis of silicosis. J Clin Invest 73:1462-1472

Seal RME, Cockcroft A, Kung I et al (1986) Central lymph node changes and progressive massive fibrosis in coalworkers. Thorax 41:531-537

Sluis-Cremer GK, Hessel PA, Nizdo EH et al (1985) Silica, silicosis, and progressive systemic sclerosis. Br J Ind Med 42:838-843

Sluis-Cremer GK, Hessel PA, Hnizdo E et al (1986) Relationship between silicosis and rheumatoid arthritis. Thorax 41:596-601

Smith AH, Lopipero PA, Barroga VR (1995) Meta-analysis of studies of lung cancer among silicotics. Epidemiology 6:617-624

Solomon A (2001) Silicosis and tuberculosis, part 2. A radiographic presentation of nodular tuberculosis and silicosis. Int J Occup Environ Health 7:54-57

Spencer H (1985) Pathology of the lung: the Pneumoconiosis and other occupational lung diseases. Pergamon, Oxford

Talini D, Paggiaro PL, Falaschi F et al (1995) Chest radiography and high resolution computed tomography in the evaluation of workers exposed to silica dust: relation with functional findings. Occup Environ Med 52:262-267

Theron CP, Walters LG, Webster I (1964) The international classification of radiographs of the pneumoconiosis: Based on the findings in 100 decreased white South African gold miners: an evaluation. Med Proc (Johannesburg) 10:352

Tsuda T, Mino Y, Babazono A et al (2002) A case-control study of lung cancer in relation to silica exposure and silicosis in a rural area in Japan. Ann Epidemiol 12:285-287

Wallace WE, Gupta NC, Hubbs AF (2003) Cis-4-[F-18] fluoro-L-proline PET imaging of pulmonary fibrosis in a rabbit model. J Nucl Med 44:43-44

Weill H, Jones RN, Parkes WR (1994) Silicosis and related diseases. In: Parkes WR (ed) Occupational lung disorders, 3rd edn. Butterworth-Heinemann, Oxford, pp 285-339

White NW, Chetty R, Bateman ED (1991) Silicosis among gemstone workers in South Africa: tiger's-eye pneumoconiosis. Am J Ind Med 19:205-213

6 Coal Worker's Pneumoconiosis

Johny A. Verschakelen and Pierre Alain Gevenois

CONTENTS

6.1 Introduction 195
6.2 Radiographic Features of CWP 196
6.2.1 Pulmonary Small Opacities 196
6.2.2 Pulmonary Massive Fibrosis 196
6.3 CT in the Diagnosis of CWP 198
6.4 CT Features of CWP 200
6.4.1 Pulmonary Nodular Opacities 200
6.4.2 Subpleural Micronodules 201
6.4.3 Progressive Massive Fibrosis 201
6.4.4 Hilar and Mediastinal Lymph Nodes 203
6.5 Relationship Between Imaging and Lung Function 203
6.6 Associated Disorders 204
6.6.1 Pulmonary Emphysema 204
6.6.2 Caplan's Syndrome 204
References 204

6.1 Introduction

Pneumoconiosis is the term applied to interstitial lung disease resulting from chronic exposure to airborne mineral dust, its inhalation and deposition and the tissue reaction of the host to its presence. Pneumoconiosis due to coal dust – and coal mine dust – is known as "coal worker's pneumoconiosis" (CWP). Nevertheless, the inhalation and retention in the lung of dust composed predominantly of carbon – often termed "anthracosis" – is seen in many individuals, particularly those who smoke or live in a city or industrial environment. Microscopically, this material is recognized as dense black particles, mostly 1–2 µm in size, within macrophages adjacent to terminal or proximal respiratory bronchioles and in the pleura (Fraser et al. 1999). In the lung, this deposit of anthracotic pigment unassociated with fibrosis is termed "coal macule". This anthrocotic material is also commonly present in bronchopulmonary, hilar and mediastinal lymph nodes, to which it characteristically imparts a distinct blackness on gross examination. In these lesions, associated fibrosis or emphysema is invariably minimal or absent, except when associated with cigarette smoking, and it is generally believed that the presence of such particles is of no pathological or functional significance. Although the coal macule is characteristic of CWP, identical lesions can be found in individuals from other environments, and the simple presence of a macule does not constitute definite evidence of occupational dust exposure.

Environmental anthracosis is caused by the inhalation of small amount of dust. Inhalation of large amounts of carbonaceous material, however, can be associated with significant pulmonary disease. The pathological appearances and behaviour of this pneumoconiosis are similar whether it is the result of exposure to coal or other carbonaceous material (Parkes 1994). This disease is, thus, not limited to coal miners, but as the most important occupation in terms of the number of individuals affected is coal mining, the resulting disease has been called "coal workers' pneumoconiosis". Workers involved in production of graphite, carbon black and carbon electrodes are affected less often.

In coal mining, the nature of coal and its potential to cause pneumoconiosis vary widely from mine to mine and from coal field to coal field (Brichet et al. 2002). The carbon content has an influence on the risk of CWP: the higher the content, the greater the risk (Seaton et al. 1995). Silica contamination increases the pneumoconiosis risk meaningfully. It is generally accepted that the higher the content of free silica in the inhaled particles, the higher the likelihood of pneumoconiosis and the more accelerated its course. Overall, carbon content and the degree of silica contamination are probably the principal factors that account for

J. A. Verschakelen, MD, PhD
Department of Radiology, K. U. Leuven, Herestraat 49, 3000 Leuven, Belgium
P. A. Gevenois, MD, PhD
Clinic of Chest Imaging, Department of Radiology, Hôpital Erasme, Université Libre de Bruxelles, Route de Lennik 808, 1070 Brussels, Belgium

observed variability in risk between one coal mine and another (Brichet et al. 2002). Local geographic variation consequently exerts considerable influence, and the risk of pneumoconiosis is particularly increased when coal seems are thin and separated by silica-containing rock. Pneumoconiosis in coal miners may, thus, represent a mixed picture of CWP and silicosis.

CWP can be divided into a simple form with multiple small rounded pulmonary nodules and a complicated form with large masses, also called progressive massive fibrosis (PMF). The complication occurs in about 30% of patients who have diffuse bilateral small opacities and may develop after exposure to coal dust has ceased and may progress in the absence of further exposure (Morgan 1984).

6.2 Radiographic Features of CWP

CWP is generally first recognized from the plain chest radiograph, which is critical also in evaluation disease progression and compensation. Since the 1990s, computed tomography (CT) has played a major complementary role for the diagnosis and the compensation of CWP, including its complications.

6.2.1 Pulmonary Small Opacities

On chest radiograph, the characteristic lesions of CWP are pulmonary small rounded opacities that predominate in the upper part of the lungs (Fig. 6.1). In a minority of cases, they are confined to the lower lung fields. By reference to the ILO International Classification of Radiographs of Pneumoconioses (International Labour Office 2002), small opacities are smaller than 1 cm in diameter. Calcification of pulmonary nodules is identified radiologically in 10–20% of older coal miners (Fig. 6.2) (Fraser et al. 1999).

There are moderate to good correlations between the radiographic profusion of small opacities and the pathology grade of pneumoconiosis, but the sensitivity of radiography to detect mild to moderate grades of CWP is low (Vallyathan et al. 1996).

6.2.2 Pulmonary Massive Fibrosis

On chest radiograph, PMF appears as large opacities, arbitrarily larger than 1 cm in diameter. The threshold of 1 cm refers to the ILO Classification that defines large opacities but not PMF. However, histopathological classification considers that a lesion larger than 2 cm in diameter corresponds to a PMF (Kleinerman et al. 1979). The appearance of large opacities indicates the development of complicated pneumoconiosis. PMF opacities vary greatly in shape as well in size. They typically start near the periphery of the lung and are manifested as a mass. They can be ill or well defined. These lesions range from 1 cm in diameter to the volume of a whole lobe in aggregate.

PMF opacities are more commonly seen in the upper than in the lower halves of the lung fields. They may be unilateral or bilateral and, if the latter,

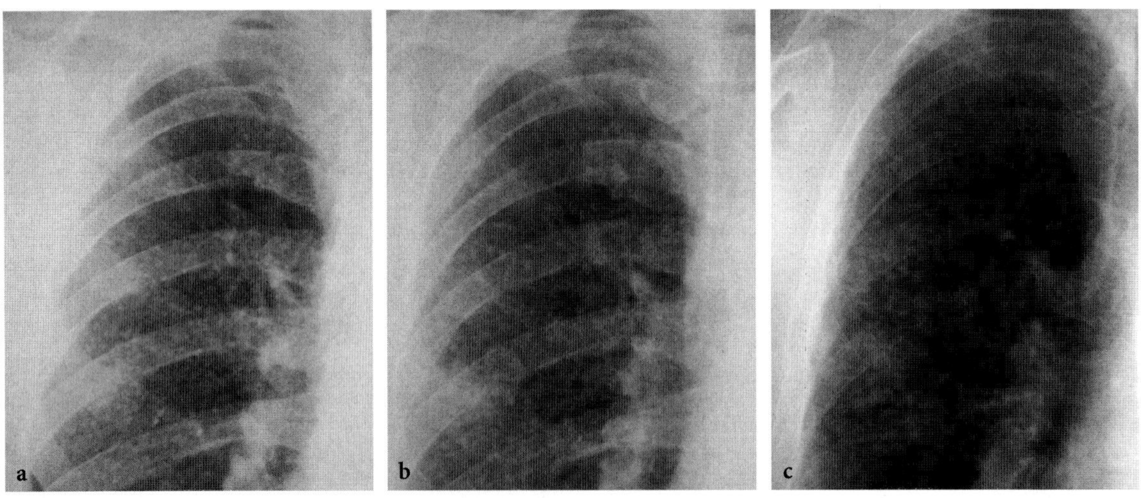

Fig. 6.1a–c. Coal worker's pneumoconiosis: three postero-anterior chest radiographs obtained at 7-year intervals in a coal miner showing increasing profusion of small round opacities

may be distributed roughly symmetrically or asymmetrically (Fig. 6.3). In a minority of cases, they are confined to the lower lung fields. Normally there is a background of small opacities with PMF, but in a minority of cases this is absent (PARKES 1994), at least on chest radiographs. Particularly when unilateral, a large mass may closely simulate pulmonary carcinoma. PMF can produce shrinkage of adjacent lung with hyperexpansion of the lower lobes (Fig. 6.4), signs of bullous emphysema, distortion of the lung and shift of the trachea and mediastinum to the affected side caused by fibrotic scarring (Fig. 6.5).

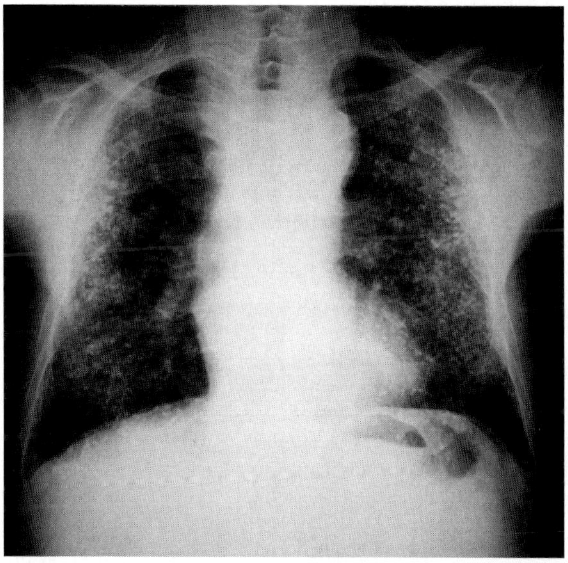

Fig. 6.2. Coal worker's pneumoconiosis: postero-anterior chest radiograph showing calcified small round opacities in a coal miner

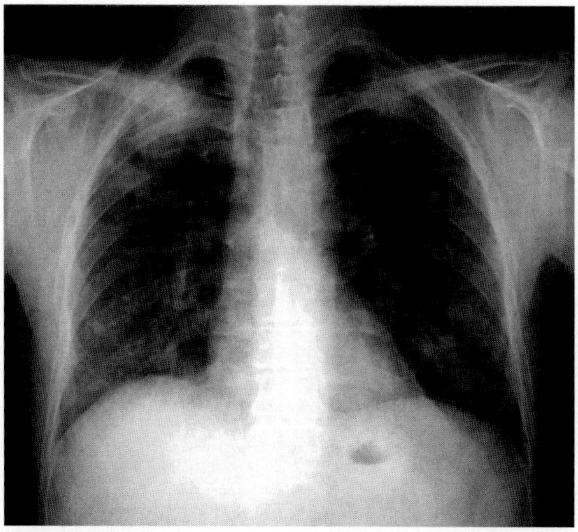

Fig. 6.3. Coal worker's pneumoconiosis: postero-anterior chest radiograph showing progressive massive fibrosis as a large opacity, approximately 6 cm in diameter, in the right upper lung field. Confluence is also visible on the left upper lung field

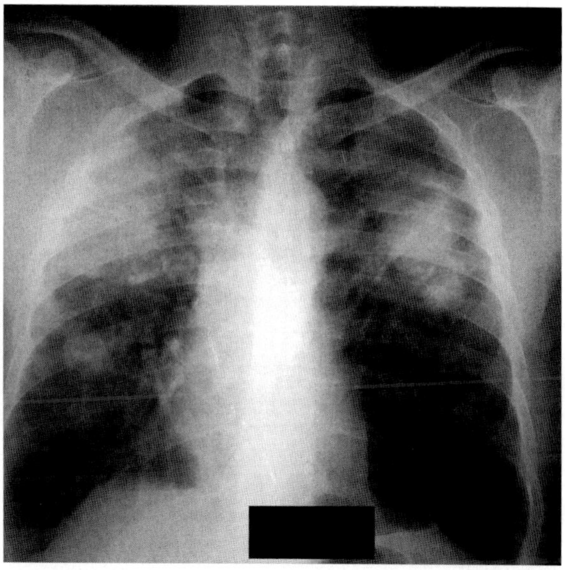

Fig. 6.4. Coal worker's pneumoconiosis: postero-anterior chest radiograph showing progressive massive fibrosis that produces shrinkage of adjacent lung with hyperexpansion of the lower lobes

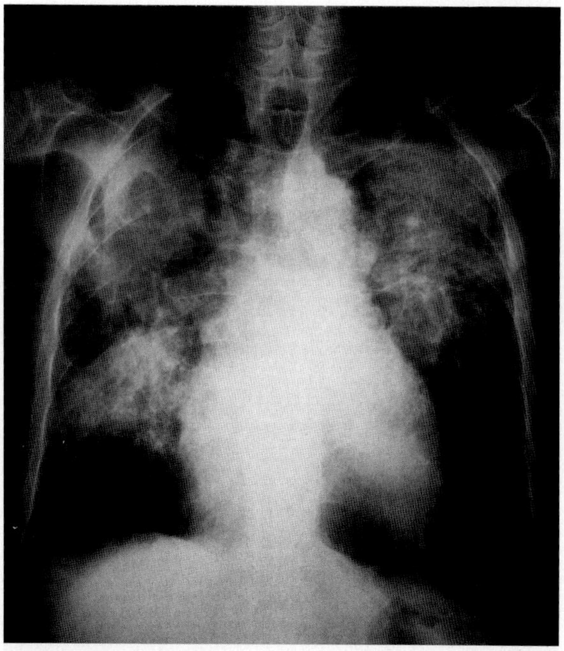

Fig. 6.5. Coal worker's pneumoconiosis: postero-anterior chest radiograph showing progressive massive fibrosis that produces shift of the trachea to the right side caused by fibrotic scarring

PMF opacities can cavitate. The development of a cavity within a PMF lesion is indicated by a well-defined, circumscribed translucency (Fig. 6.6) in which there may be a fluid level (Fig. 6.7) (PARKES 1994). In most cases, the cavity vanishes, and appearances return wholly or partly to normal.

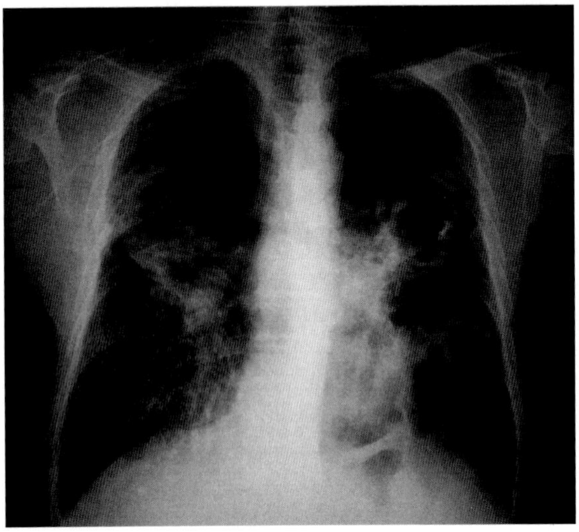

Fig. 6.6. Coal worker's pneumoconiosis: postero-anterior chest radiograph showing cavities within progressive massive fibrosis lesions indicated by a well-defined and circumscribed translucencies

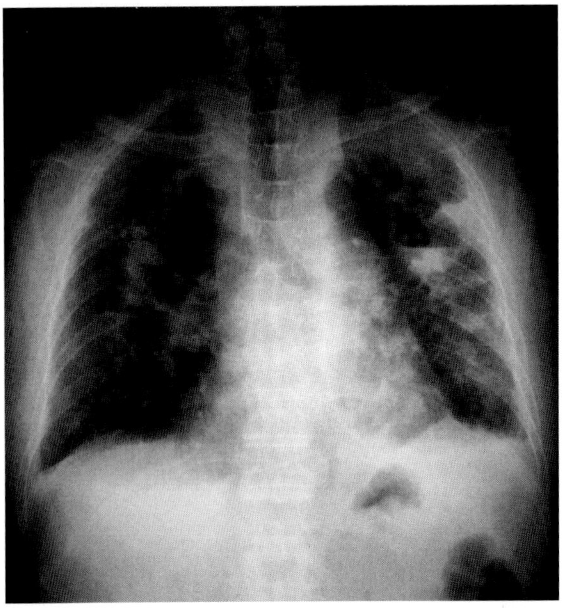

Fig. 6.7. Coal worker's pneumoconiosis: postero-anterior chest radiograph showing cavities within progressive massive fibrosis lesions with fluid levels

6.3 CT in the Diagnosis of CWP

Although many of the disorders in patients with silicosis and CWP can be detected on a chest radiograph, CT and thin-section CT have shown to be superior to chest radiography in depicting lung parenchymal, airway and pleural abnormalities (REMY-JARDIN et al. 1990b; VALLYATHAN et al. 1996). It has been documented that CT is useful to rule out CWP in patients with opacities on chest radiograph consistent with the diagnosis of CWP (GEVENOIS et al. 1994). In addition, CT also shows better the mediastinal changes and can be very helpful to depict complications. The cross-sectional format of CT allows a better recognition of the axial distribution of the disease, while coronal reformations generated from spiral CT can more accurately show the craniocaudal distribution (Fig. 6.8). In addition,

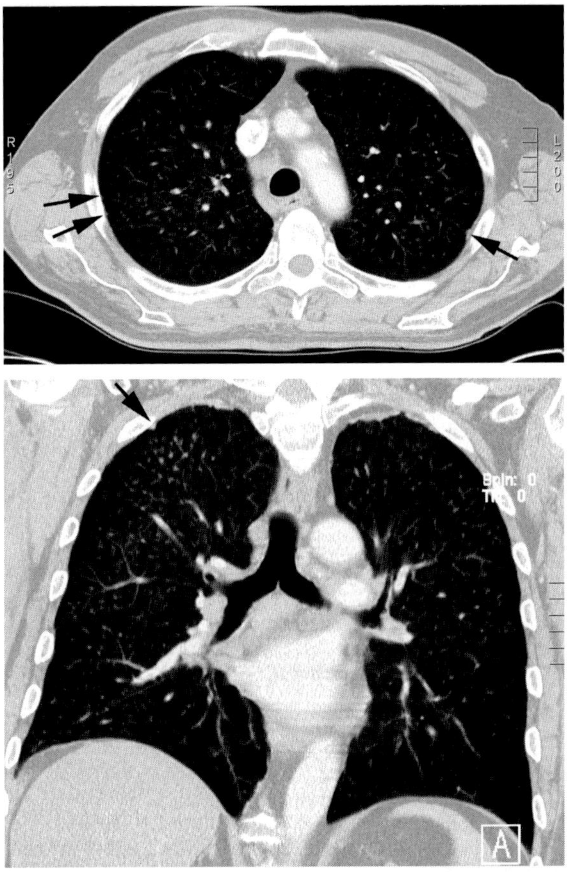

a

b

Fig. 6.8a,b. Coal worker's pneumoconiosis: computed tomography scan showing mild micronodular lung and subpleural involvement. **a** Axial view with slice thickness of 1 mm. **b** Coronal reconstruction with slice thickness of 3 mm. Micronodules are seen in the upper part of the right lung. Notice also the presence of a few subpleural micronodules (*arrows*) because of their higher density resolution, CT scans may detect parenchymal changes that are below the resolution of conventional chest radiographs. Moreover, with CT and especially with thin-section CT, a detailed analysis of the lung parenchymal changes becomes possible, and thin-section CT can often depict whether a disease has a predominant vascular, airway or lymphatic distribution or whether the disease is predominantly located in the interstitial tissue. This is particularly helpful in the diagnosis of CWP. Indeed, after inhalation, the predominant deposition of dust particles is in and around the respiratory bronchioles, which have an intralobular location. Many of the inhaled particles are cleared by the macrophages in the airway walls or evacuated by the mucociliary transport mechanism (International Commission on Radiological Protection Task Group on Lung Dynamics 1966), but a variable fraction penetrates the respiratory epithelium and moves through the lung, where it is destined for slow removal via the lymphatic system or for long-term retention (Gurney and Schroeder 1988). Thus, further distribution of the lesions largely depends on the lymphatic clearance of the lung, and the lung zones with poorest lymph flow are most severely affected (Dock 1946; Goodwin and Desprez 1983; Gurney 1991; Gurney and Schroeder 1988; Remy-Jardin et al. 1992). The main driving force for lymph flow is the pulmonary artery pressure. Since there is a vertical, gravity-dependent difference in pulmonary artery pressure, lymphatic flow is more pronounced in the bottom of the lung than in the top. In addition, because the main pulmonary artery is inclined to the left, higher blood flow and lymphatic flow occur in the left upper lobe than in the right (Dollery et al. 1961). It is also believed that respiratory excursion increases lymphatic flow because the chest wall motion "milks" the lymphatic vessels passively (Valberg et al. 1985). However, this is not a uniform process, since the posterior chest wall shows a lesser outward excursion than the lateral and in particular the anterior chest wall (Gurney 1991). The result of these regional differences in lymphatic flow is that there is a predilection for dust retention in the upper and posterior part of the lungs, especially on the right side (Green 1988). The removal of the dust particles by the lymphatics occurs via two intercommunicating networks of lymph flow. One part is removed centripetally along the bronchovascular bundles toward the hilum, while another part is first removed centrifugally in the pleural network before reaching the hilar lymph nodes. This probably explains why dust retention changes are often seen in the subpleural areas and in the peripheral interlobular septa in addition to peribronchovascular locations (Gurney 1991; Gurney and Schroeder 1988) (Fig. 6.9).

Although silicosis and CWP are two distinct diseases, with differing histological features resulting from the inhalation of different inorganic dusts, the CT appearances of both entities are quite similar, so that the two disease entities cannot be easily or reliably distinguished in individual cases (Webb et al. 2001). In addition, both pneumoconioses can be observed among miners, although silicosis is seen in a wide range of other trades, such as stone cutting, quarrying, tunnelling, ceramics and a variety of other small industries employing forms of silica.

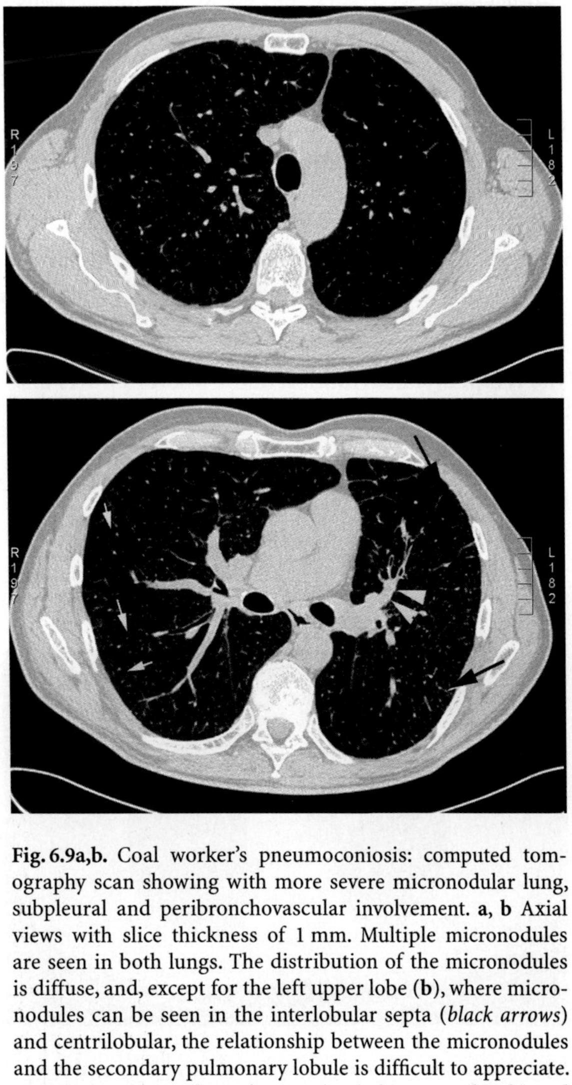

a

b

Fig. 6.9a,b. Coal worker's pneumoconiosis: computed tomography scan showing with more severe micronodular lung, subpleural and peribronchovascular involvement. **a, b** Axial views with slice thickness of 1 mm. Multiple micronodules are seen in both lungs. The distribution of the micronodules is diffuse, and, except for the left upper lobe (**b**), where micronodules can be seen in the interlobular septa (*black arrows*) and centrilobular, the relationship between the micronodules and the secondary pulmonary lobule is difficult to appreciate. Notice also the peribronchovascular (*white arrowheads*) and the subpleural micronodules, as well as focal emphysema surrounding some of the micronodules (*white arrows*)

6.4 CT Features of CWP

6.4.1 Pulmonary Nodular Opacities

The characteristic lesions of CWP are pulmonary nodular opacities. By extension of histopathological criteria, these opacities are usually called micronodules when smaller than 7 mm in diameter and nodules when between 7 mm and 20 mm. Lesions larger than 20 mm are not considered as nodules anymore but as a sign of PMF (Kleinerman et al. 1979; Roggli and Shelbourne 1987). When lung involvement is mild, usually only a few micronodules are seen. At this stage, these micronodules are almost exclusively distributed in the upper zones of the lung and show a posterior and right-sided predominance (Fig. 6.8). The relationship between these nodules and the secondary pulmonary lobule is not always easy to determine, but sometimes CT may show their predominant intralobular and, to a lesser degree, septal distribution. When involvement is more severe, the number and size of these micronodules increase, and the distribution becomes more diffuse over the lung, although the typical predominance in the upper zones of the lung as well as the right-sided predominance remains. In many cases, the lymphatic distribution of the micronodules also becomes more evident with nodular opacities in the interlobular septa in the subpleural areas and around the bronchovascular bundles (Fig. 6.9). In a next step, these micronodules may grow and merge, and nodules will develop (Fig. 6.10).

It has been suggested that thick slices (5–10 mm) should be used to depict these micronodules because these slices take advantage of the superposition of lesions (Leung et al. 1991; Remy-Jardin et al. 1991) and allow a better distinction between micronodules and tubular vessels. Thin slices (1 mm) can, however, depict smaller micronodules that are obscured at thick-slice studies because of partial volume averaging and can also show other early changes that are attributed to CWP. Indeed, sometimes thin-section CT is able to demonstrate intralobular ill-defined punctuate opacities that correspond to early irregular fibrosis around the respiratory bronchioles (Akira et al. 1989) and to dilated respiratory bronchioles and focal collections of coal-dust-laden macrophages within the wall of these respiratory bronchioles and adjacent alveoli (Remy-Jardin et al. 1992) (Fig. 6.11). The earlier described micronodules and nodules consist of dust-laden macrophages that are surrounded by a fibrotic stroma composed of collagen and reticulin. These fibrotic stroma, containing collagen and reticulin zones, usually have enlarged airspaces at their periphery that are responsible for the usually irregular borders of these nodules seen at both CT and thin-section CT.

In coal miners whose lung residue contains 18% or more of quartz, the pathological lesions are those of silicosis (Morgan 1984), i.e. nodules consisting of a fibrous laminar core with variable calcification and hyalinization and a dust laden cellular peripheral zone of variable width (Kleinerman et al. 1979; Morgan 1984). Although these nodules are usually more sharply defined and arise more frequently in the region of the respiratory bronchioli, CT is not

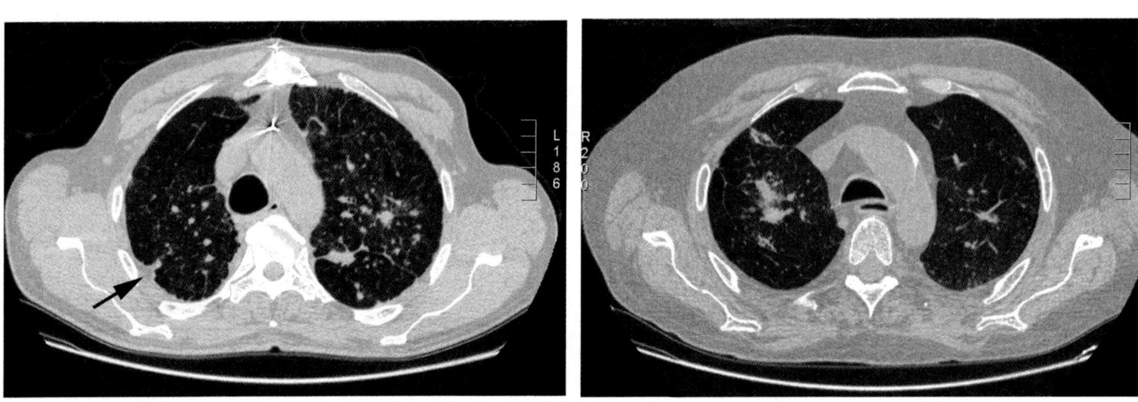

a b

Fig. 6.10a,b. Coal worker's pneumoconiosis: computed tomography scan showing micronodular and nodular lung and subpleural involvement. **a,b** Axial views with slice thickness of 5 mm. Micronodules grow and merge, and nodules develop (*arrows*). Notice also the subpleural focal area of increased opacity (**a**) "pseudo plaque", which should be differentiated from real pleural plaques related to asbestos exposure (*arrow*)

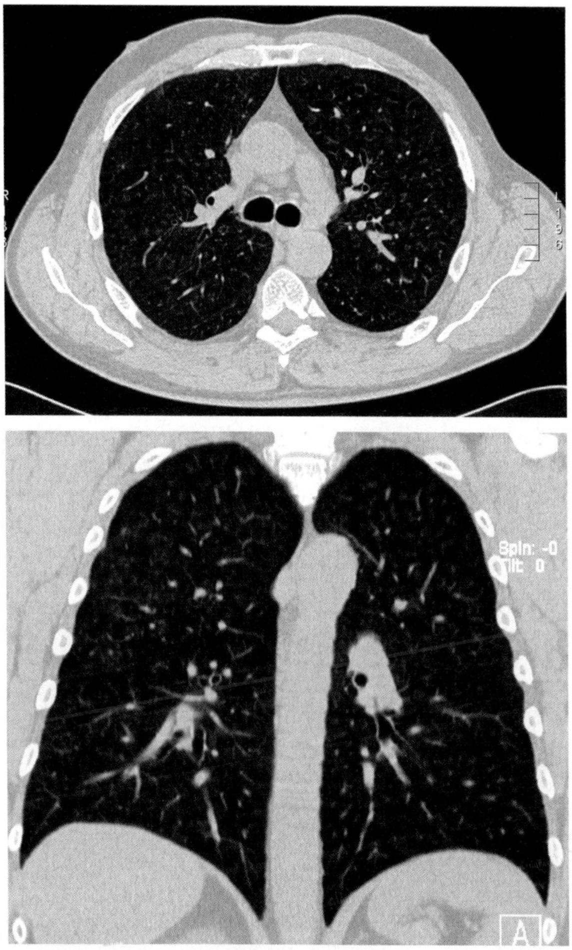

a b

Fig. 6.11a,b. Coal worker's pneumoconiosis: computed tomography scan showing early changes (axial view with slice thickness of 1 mm: coronal reconstruction with slice thickness of 3 mm). Intralobular ill-defined punctuate opacities are seen

able to distinguish these from the nodules seen after inhalation of coal-mine dust containing no or little free silica.

6.4.2 Subpleural Micronodules

Subpleural micronodules are closely related to the subpleural lymphatic system and present on CT as rounded, hemispheric or triangular opacities with a diameter less than 7 mm (Remy-Jardin et al. 1992) in the peripheral and fissural subpleural areas (Fig. 6.8, Fig 6.9). These micronodules are seen in the majority of coal miners with radiographic evidence of CWP, although with thin-section CT, they are often depicted in miners without radiographic changes. Pathologically, they correspond to focal areas of coal-dust-laden macrophages surrounded by a fibrotic stroma composed of collagen and reticulin. Often, there is also localized visceral pleural thickening (Remy-Jardin et al. 1990a), while calcifications are seen in 36% of patients (Remy-Jardin et al. 1990b). The distribution of these subpleural micronodules is similar to the distribution of the intrapulmonary nodules and is also a reflection of the phenomenon that the lung zones that have the poorest lymph flow are most severely affected (Dock 1946; Goodwin and Desprez 1983; Gurney 1991; Gurney and Schroeder 1988). In patients with mild parenchymal involvement, subpleural micronodules are predominantly seen in the upper zones of the lung, often only in the posterior areas and are unilateral and right sided (Remy-Jardin et al. 1992). In patients with more severe disease, they are more numerous and occur both in upper and lower lung zones, and, although they are seen bilaterally, there is often a posterior and right-sided predominance (Remy-Jardin et al. 1992) (Fig. 6.10). It should be emphasized, however, that isolated subpleural micronodules cannot be considered as an early sign of CWP, because they are also observed in healthy urban living adults, especially in smokers and ex-smokers (Remy-Jardin et al. 1993; Roggli and Shelbourne 1987).

The subpleural micronodules can merge, and subpleural focal linear areas of increased opacity develop (Fig. 6.10). These "pseudo plaques" have a diameter of less than 7 mm and should be differentiated from real "plaques", which are focal areas of fibrous thickening on the parietal pleura and occur in response to asbestos exposure. The differential diagnosis is based on the distribution of these pleural abnormalities: asbestos exposure-related plaques are usually located in the dorsal and posterior part of the chest when involvement is mild and extend towards the anterior chest wall when diseases become more pronounced. Sometimes the "pseudo plaque" is separated from the chest wall by small emphysematous areas and then presents as a tubular opacity parallel to the chest wall (Remy-Jardin et al. 1992).

6.4.3 Progressive Massive Fibrosis

PMF presents as large oval or rounded masses with a diameter of at least 2 cm (Fig. 6.12). It is seen in some miners but does not develop in every coal miner exposed to respirable dust. It is formed either by the aggregation and fusion of groups of smaller fibrotic nodules or by the enlargement of single nodules in the lung. When formed by the aggregation and fusion of smaller nodules, PMF has irregular borders (Fig. 6.12) and is associated with disruption of the surrounding lung parenchyma, leading to the typical scar emphysema (Fig. 6.13). Enlargement of single nodules is a less frequently observed cause of PMF and can be recognized on CT by the fact that the nodular opacities have regular borders and lack surrounding scar emphysema (Remy-Jardin et al. 1992). When the lesions develop centrally, they tend to contract towards the hilum; whereas, peripheral lesions are often seen with a thickening of the overlying extrapleural fat. The lesions of PMF have a typical predilection for the upper and posterior portions of the lung (Lyons and Campbell 1981) but

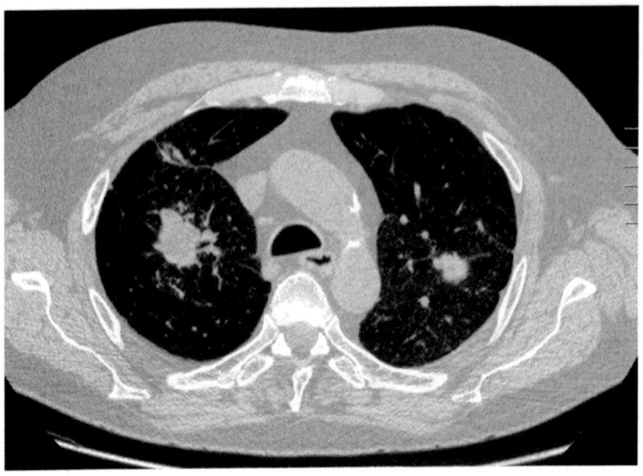

Fig. 6.12. Coal worker's pneumoconiosis: computed tomography scan showing early stage progressive massive fibrosis (axial view with slice thickness of 5 mm). Lung opacities larger than 20 mm are considered as a sign of progressive massive fibrosis. Notice the irregular borders

a b c d

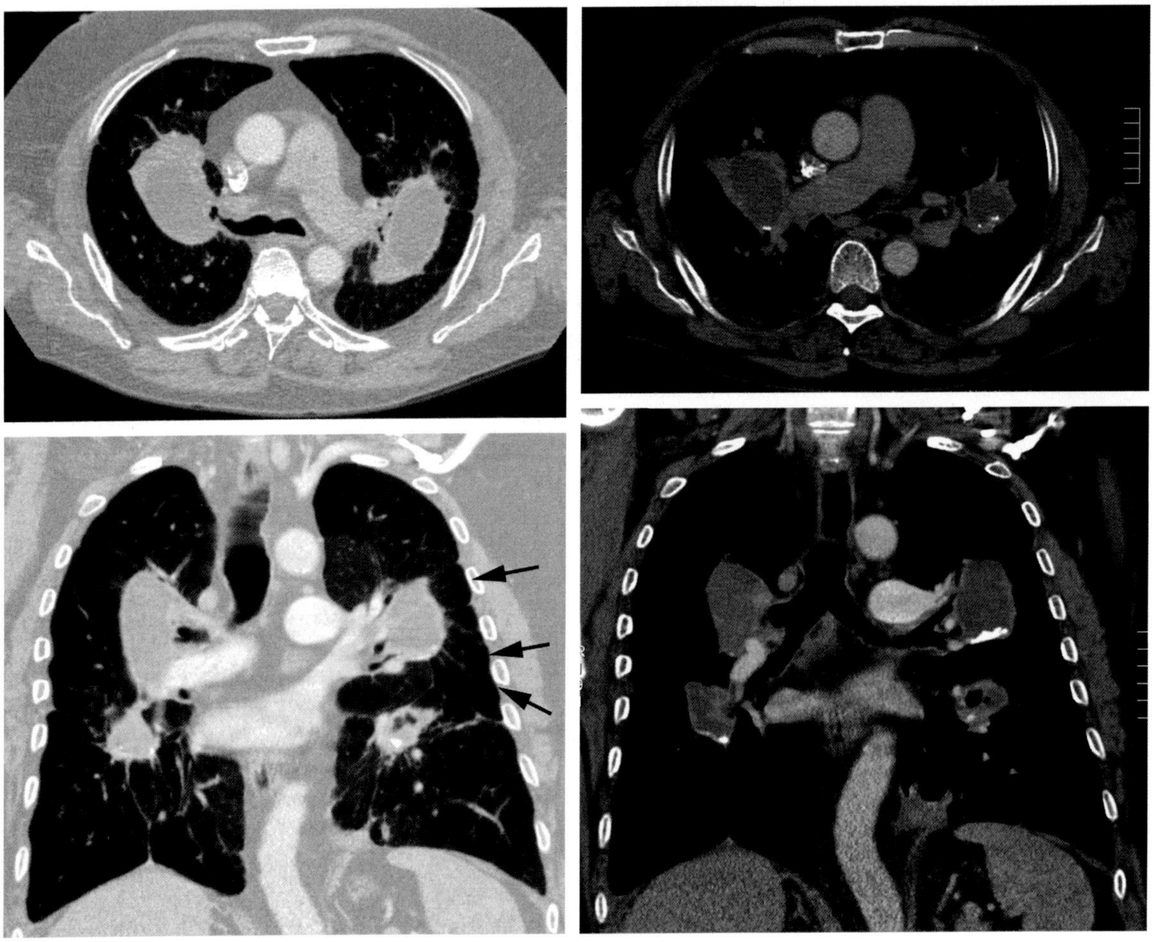

Fig. 6.13a–d. Coal worker's pneumoconiosis: computed tomography scan showing advanced progressive massive fibrosis (PMF). **a, b** Axial views with slice thickness of 5 mm. **c, d** Coronal reconstructions with slice thickness of 3 mm. Large lesions of PMF that are typically located in the upper and posterior portions of the lung. There is disruption of the surrounding lung parenchyma with scar emphysema (**c**, *arrows*). Notice the calcifications and hypodense areas within the fibrotic masses

can be observed in the posterior part of the lower zones of the lung as well (Fig. 6.13). Various types of calcifications can occur, but they are mostly punctuated rather than linear or massive (Fig. 6.13).

When these lesions of PMF become larger, irregular areas of aseptic necrosis can occur. These areas present as hypodense areas within the mass (Fig. 6.13) and can cavitate, producing excavated masses, sometimes with air-fluid levels. These excavated masses may be complicated by infections such as tuberculosis or intracavitary aspergilloma. These infections can, in turn, induce severe bronchial hypervascularization with risk of bronchial bleeding. CT is indicated when haemoptysis occurs in coal workers, because it can detect this complication. However, in the case of massive haemoptysis, a bronchial arteriography and embolization may be necessary.

6.4.4 Hilar and Mediastinal Lymph Nodes

Enlarged mediastinal and hilar lymph nodes are often seen in coal miners, especially when large areas of PMF are also present (Seal et al. 1986) (Fig. 6.14). Enlarged lymph nodes can be found in all mediastinal sites, but the internal mammary and superior diaphragmatic nodes are less frequently involved. Necrosis can occur, but a typical feature of these lymph nodes is eggshell calcification, although punctuate or massive calcification may also occur (Remy-Jardin et al. 1992; Webb et al. 2001) (Fig. 6.14).

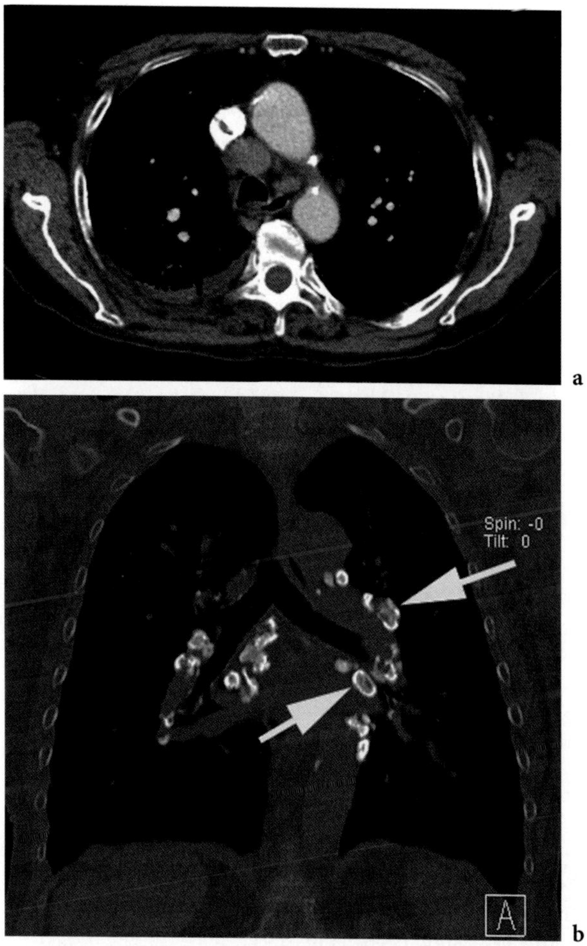

Fig. 6.14a,b. Coal worker's pneumoconiosis: computed tomography scan showing enlarged mediastinal and hilar lymph nodes. **a** Axial view with slice thickness of 5 mm. **b** Coronal reconstruction with slice thickness of 3 mm. A typical feature of the enlarged lymph nodes is eggshell calcification (*arrows*)

6.5 Relationship Between Imaging and Lung Function

There are clear and consistent relationships between dust exposure and ventilatory function in smoking and non-smoking coal miners, but dust effect on ventilatory function is independent of the presence or absence of radiological CWP (Coggon and Taylor 1998; Oxman et al. 1993). Particularly, micronodules detected by CT scanning do not, by themselves, have an influence on the pulmonary function, but associated chronic obstructive pulmonary disease, whatever its cause, is the major determinant of the impaired lung function (Collins et al. 1993; Gevenois et al. 1998).

Pneumoconiotic micronodules detected using CT correspond to dust deposits with more or less fibrotic reaction at the level of respiratory bronchioles, where particle deposition is maximal (Parkes 1994). This kind of small airways lesion can exist without airflow limitation detected by classical manoeuvres (FEV_1 and FEV_1/VC), which are more likely to reflect preacinar airway alterations. Morphological changes at the level of respiratory bronchioles can, however, be associated with abnormalities of other indices, such as inert gas washout tests when the FEV_1/VC ratio is within normal range (Churg et al. 1985; Van Muylem et al. 1992).

Occupational exposure to coal-mine dust has an adverse effect on pulmonary function tests, independently of the presence of CT evidence of pneumoconiosis (Nemery et al. 1987; Parkes 1994). Medico-legal experts and compensation boards or organizations should be aware that a decision to compensate lung function abnormalities only on the basis of the presence of micronodules on CT scans has no scientific basis. In other words, since the function impairment does not depend on the micronodules detected by CT scans, the search for their presence in workers with a normal chest radiograph or low radiological grades according to the ILO Classification seems to have little relevance for a decision on compensation. In this context, micronodules detected by CT should only be considered as a marker of exposure.

6.6 Associated Disorders

6.6.1 Pulmonary Emphysema

Focal emphysema is the form most commonly associated with coal mining, which constitutes a 1–2 mm zone of tissue destruction around the coal-dust macula. Focal emphysema differs from centrilobular emphysema only through its association with the macula and in its often limited extent (Attfield and Wagner 1996) (Fig. 6.9).

Two major forms of pulmonary emphysema can be detected using CT in patients with CWP: bullous changes around PMF, considered as paracicatricial emphysema (Fig. 6.6), and irregular emphysematous lesions characterized by areas of low attenuation without definable walls that, when nodular opacities are present, are considered to be features of CWP (Remy-Jardin et al. 1992).

6.6.2 Caplan's Syndrome

The syndrome, as first described by Caplan, is defined as multiple, large (0.5–5 cm diameter), round, radiographic opacities frequently associated with evidence of cavity formation or calcification, usually unaccompanied by the small opacities of simple pneumoconiosis, in coal miners with rheumatoid arthritis (Caplan 1959). This concept has been broadened to the occurrence of radiographic opacities in the absence of rheumatoid arthritis but associated with circulating rheumatoid factor (Caplan et al. 1962). Rheumatoid arthritis may precede or succeed the appearance of lung lesions by a number of years and, in some cases, never develops (Parkes 1994). The appearances of simple CWP or PMF may have been present for years when additional changes develop in relation to the development of rheumatoid arthritis, but there is no evident relationship between the severity of the rheumatoid disease when present and the extent of Caplan's syndrome (Brichet et al. 2002).

Radiographically, it may be difficult to differentiate Caplan's nodules, PMF, tuberculosis and other infective granulomatous disorders (Remy-Jardin et al. 1992). Typical Caplan nodules are discrete, up to 3 cm in diameter, although they may be larger, and they are sometimes formed into composite groups. They are distributed at random in the lungs, and cavitary necrosis is fairly common in one or more lesions. However, PMF are also discrete, but they are smaller than Caplan nodules, they predominate in the upper lung field and central necrosis is rare (Parkes 1994).

References

Akira M, Higashihara T, Yokoyama K, Yamamoto S, Kita N, Morimoto S, Ikezoe J, Kozuka T (1989) Radiographic type p pneumoconiosis: high resolution CT. Radiology 171:117–123

Attfield M, Wagner GR (1996) Coal. In: Harber H, Schenker MB, Balmes JR (eds) Occupational and environmental respiratory disease. Mosby, St. Louis, pp 362–372

Brichet A, Desurmont S, Wallaert B (2002) Coal worker's pneumoconiosis. In: Hendrick DJ, Burge PS, Beckett WS, Churg A (eds) Occupational disorders of the lung. WB Saunders, London, pp 129–141

Caplan A (1959) Certain unusual radiological appearances in the chest of coal miners suffering rheumatoid arthritis. Thorax 8:29–37

Caplan A, Payne RB, Withey JL (1962) A broader concept of Caplan's syndrome related to rheumatoid factors. Thorax 17:205–212

Churg A, Wright JL, Wiggs B, Pare PD, Lazar N (1985) Small airways disease and mineral dust exposure: prevalence, structure, and function. Am Rev Respir Dis 131:139–143

Coggon D, Taylor AN (1998) Coal mining and chronic obstructive pulmonary disease: a review of the evidence. Thorax 53:398–407

Collins L, Willing S, Bretz R, Harty M, Lane E, Anderson WH (1993) High-resolution CT in simple coal worker's pneumoconiosis. Chest 104:1156–1162

Dock W (1946) Apical localization of phtysis. Am Rev Tuberc 53:297–305

Dollery CT, West JB, Wilcken DEL, Hugh-Jones P (1961) A comparison of the pulmonary blood flow between the left and right lungs in normal subjects and patients with congenital heart disease. Circulation 24:617–625

Fraser RS, Müller NL, Colman N, Paré PD (1999) Diagnosis of diseases of the chest, 4nd edn. Saunders, Philadelphia

Gevenois PA, Pichot E, Dargent F, Dedeire S, Vande Weyer R, De Vuyst P (1994) Low grade coal worker's pneumoconiosis: comparison of CT and chest radiography. Acta Radiol 35:351–356

Gevenois PA, Sergent G, De Maertelaer V, Gouat F, Yernault JC, De Vuyst P (1998) Micronodules and emphysema in coal mine dust or silica exposure: relation with lung function. Eur Respir J 12:1020–1024

Goodwin RA, Desprez RM (1983) Apical localization of pulmonary tuberculosis, chronic pulmonary histoplasmosis and progressive massive fibrosis of the lung. Chest 83:801–805

Green FHY (1988) Coal workers' pneumoconiosis and pneumoconiosis due to other carbonaceous dusts. In: Churg A, Green FHY (eds) Pathology of occupational lung disease. Igaku-Shoin, New York, pp 89–154

Gurney JW (1991) Cross-sectional physiology of the lung. Radiology 178:1–10

Gurney JW, Schroeder BA (1988) Upper lobe lung disease: physiologic correlates. Radiology 167:359–366

International commission on radiological protection task group on lung dynamics: deposition and retention models for internal dosimetry of the human respiratory tract (1966) Health Phys 12:173–207

International Labour Office (ILO) (2002) Guidelines for the use of the ILO International Classification of Radiographs of Pneumoconioses, revised edition 2000. Occupational Safety and Health Series, No. 22 (Rev.) International Labour Office, Geneva

Kleinerman J, Green F, Harley RA, Lapp L, Laqueur W, Naeye RL, Pratt P, Taylor G, Wiot J, Wyatt J (1979) Pathology standards for coal worker's pneumoconiosis. Report of the Pneumoconiosis Committee of the College of American Pathologists to the National Institute for Occupational Safety and Health. Arch Pathol Lab Med 103:375–432

Leung AN, Staples CA, Muller NL (1991) Chronic diffuse infiltrative lung disease: comparison of diagnostic accuracy of high-resolution CT and conventional CT. AJR Am J Roentgenol 157:693–696

Lyons JP, Campbell H (1981) Relation between progressive massive fibrosis, emphysema and pulmonary dysfunction in coal worker's pneumoconiosis. Br J Ind Med 38:125–129

Morgan WKC (1984) Coal workers' pneumoconiosis. In: Morgan WKC, Seaton A (eds) Occupational lung diseases. WB Saunders, Philadelphia, pp 377–448

Nemery B, Brasseur L, Veriter C, Frans A (1987) Impairment of ventilatory function and pulmonary gas exchange in non-smoking coal miners. Lancet 2:1427–1430

Oxman AD, Muir DCF, Shannon HS, Stock SR, Hnizdo A, Lange HJ (1993) Occupational dust exposure and chronic obstructive pulmonary disease – a systematic overview of the evidence. Am Rev Respir Dis 148:38–48

Parkes WR (1994) Pneumoconiosis associated with coal and other carbonaceous materials. In: Parkes WR (ed) Occupational lung disorders, 3rd edn. Butterworth-Heinemann, Oxford, pp 340–410

Remy-Jardin M, Beuscart R, Sault MC, Marquette CH, Remy J (1990a) Subpleural micronodules in diffuse infiltrative lung diseases: evaluation with thin section CT scans. Radiology 177:133–139

Remy-Jardin M, Degreef J-M, Beuscart R, Voisin C, Remy J (1990b) Coal worker's pneumoconiosis: CT assessment in exposed workers and correlation with radiographic findings. Radiology 177:363–371

Remy-Jardin M, Remy J, Deffontaines C, Duhamel A (1991) Assessment of diffuse infiltrative lung disease: comparison of conventional CT and high resolution CT. Radiology 181:157–162

Remy-Jardin M, Remy J, Farre I, Marquette CH (1992) Computed tomographic evaluation of silicosis and coal worker's pneumoconiosis. Radiol Clin North Am 30:1155–1176

Remy-Jardin M, Remy J, Boulenguez C, Sobaszek A, Edme JL, Furon D (1993) Morphologic effects of cigarette smoking on airways and pulmonary parenchyma in healthy adult volunteers: CT evaluation and correlation with pulmonary function tests. Radiology 186:107–115

Roggli VL, Shelbourne JD (1987) Mineral pneumoconiosis. In: Dail DH, Hammar SP (eds) Pulmonary pathology, 2nd edn, Springer, Berlin Heidelberg New York, pp 867–900

Seal RME, Cockcroft A, Kung I, Wagner JC (1986) Central lymph node changes and progressive massive fibrosis in coal workers. Thorax 41:531–537

Seaton A (1995) Coal workers' pneumoconiosis. In: Morgan WKC, Seaton A (eds) Occupational lung diseases. WB Saunders, Philadelphia, pp 374–406

Valberg PA, Wolff RK, Mauderly JL (1985) Redistribution of retained particles: effect of hyperpnea. Am Rev Respir Dis 131:273–280

Vallyathan V, Brower PS, Green FHY, Attfield MD (1996) Radiographic and pathologic correlation of coal workers' pneumoconiosis. Am J Respir Crit Care Med 154:741–748

Van Muylem A, De Vuyst P, Yernault JC, Paiva M (1992) Inert gas single-breath washout and structural alteration of respiratory bronchioles. Am Rev Respir Dis 146:1167–1172

Webb WR, Muller NL, Naidich DP (2001) High-resolution CT of the lung, 3rd edn. Lippincott-Raven, Philadelphia, pp 259–353

7 Asbestosis

Susan J. Copley

CONTENTS

7.1 Introduction 207
7.2 Clinical Features 207
7.3 Chest Radiography 208
7.4 Computed Tomography 210
7.4.1 Background 210
7.4.2 Technique 210
7.4.3 CT findings 210
7.4.4 CT–Histopathological Correlation 213
7.4.5 Sensitivity and Specificity of CT 213
7.4.6 Distinction Between Pleural and Parenchymal Disease 216
7.4.7 CT as a Screening Tool 216
7.5 Radiological–Functional Correlation 217
7.6 Summary 218
References 219

7.1 Introduction

Asbestosis is defined as diffuse interstitial pulmonary fibrosis due to the inhalation of asbestos fibers (American Thoracic Society 1986). The process requires the inhalation of considerable numbers of asbestos fibers, usually occurring after prolonged exposure (Anonymous 1997; Rosenberg 1997). The diagnosis of asbestosis is important as the individual may be eligible for compensation. As there is no accepted treatment for the condition, the diagnosis is often made by referring to clinical criteria, without resorting to open lung biopsy (Weill 1987). Imaging findings are therefore pivotal to the diagnosis of asbestosis.

Initially, the American Thoracic Society (ATS) guidelines published in 1986 advocated caution in making the diagnosis of asbestosis if radiographic changes were not present (American Thoracic Society 1986). However, the most recent (2004) ATS guidelines recognise the increased sensitivity of computed tomography (CT) as a marker of structural pulmonary change (American Thoracic Society 2004). The recent guidelines also require evidence of causation as demonstrated by one or more of the following: occupational and environmental exposure (with plausible latency), markers of exposure (e.g. pleural plaques) and recovery of asbestos fibers (includes sampling with bronchoalveolar lavage) (American Thoracic Society 2004). Evidence of functional impairment is now not required for diagnosis of asbestosis by the ATS, but functional data are considered important as part of a complete evaluation. Evidence of functional impairment includes one or more of the following: symptoms and signs (including crackles), change in ventilatory function (restrictive pattern), impaired gas exchange, detection of inflammation (e.g. by bronchoalveolar lavage) and data from exercise testing.

7.2 Clinical Features

Individuals with asbestosis initially present with shortness of breath on exertion, which becomes progressively more severe and eventually present at rest when the disease is advanced. Dyspnoea is commonly the most disabling symptom, although a dry cough is also a feature of more advanced disease and may become more distressing than breathlessness (Parkes 1994). Dyspnoeic individuals may also experience thoracic pain due to respiratory muscle fatigue.

Typically, clinical examination reveals late inspiratory crepitations which may be pan-inspiratory in advanced disease (Parkes 1994). Crepitations occur bilaterally at the lung bases and may precede symptoms and radiographic abnormalities. Digital clubbing is less common than in idiopathic pulmo-

S. J. Copley, MB.BS, MD, MRCP, FRCR
Consultant Radiologist and Honorary Clinical Lecturer, Radiology Department, Hammersmith Hospital, Du Cane Road, London, W12 0HS, UK

nary fibrosis (IPF) and tends to be present only in advanced cases. The clinical features of clubbing and haemoptysis also raise the possibility of a coexisting lung cancer.

These clinical features are not specific for asbestosis and are similar to symptoms and signs of other fibrotic lung diseases such as IPF, although progression tends to be slower and more insidious in asbestosis. The difficulty in distinguishing these features from other fibrotic lung diseases makes an accurate exposure history vital.

7.3 Chest Radiography

Traditionally, chest radiographic features of diffuse interstitial fibrosis have been regarded as crucial for the diagnosis of asbestosis (American Thoracic Society 1986; Weill 1987). Characteristically, a bilateral basal reticulonodular pattern is seen (Parkes 1994). Small irregular opacities, which may differ in size, are seen in early disease and are denoted by the symbols *s*, *t* and *u* of the International Labour Office (ILO) classification (International Labour Office 2002) (Fig. 7.1a,b), although mixed irregular and rounded opacities are sometimes present (American Thoracic Society 2004). As the disease progresses, the fine reticular pattern may become coarser and result in honeycombing, and the distribution may extend to the middle and upper zones (Fig. 7.2) (American Thoracic Society 2004). Thickening of interlobular septa may occur giving rise to Kerley B lines (Selikoff 1978), although, as with other causes of pulmonary fibrosis, these are not a consistent feature. The cardiac outline often becomes irregular, and basal volume loss is seen as depression of the horizontal fissure. The rare finding of predominantly upper lobe pleuroparenchymal fibrosis in a small minority of individuals exposed to asbestos has been described in the absence of mycobacterium tuberculosis infection or lung cancer (Hillerdal 1990). However, conventionally, if the fibrosis is upper or mid zone in distribution, asbestosis is less likely than other causes (Parkes 1994).

The previously described characteristic radiographic features may be increasingly uncommon in the developed world as advanced radiographic asbestosis becomes a rarity. A recent study by OHAR et al. observed that, in a large number of cases (over 3,000) of asbestosis, the majority had normal or 'low' (i.e. <1/1) ILO profusion scores, with extensive fibrosis being rare. The authors also found that a normal or even obstructive defect was commoner

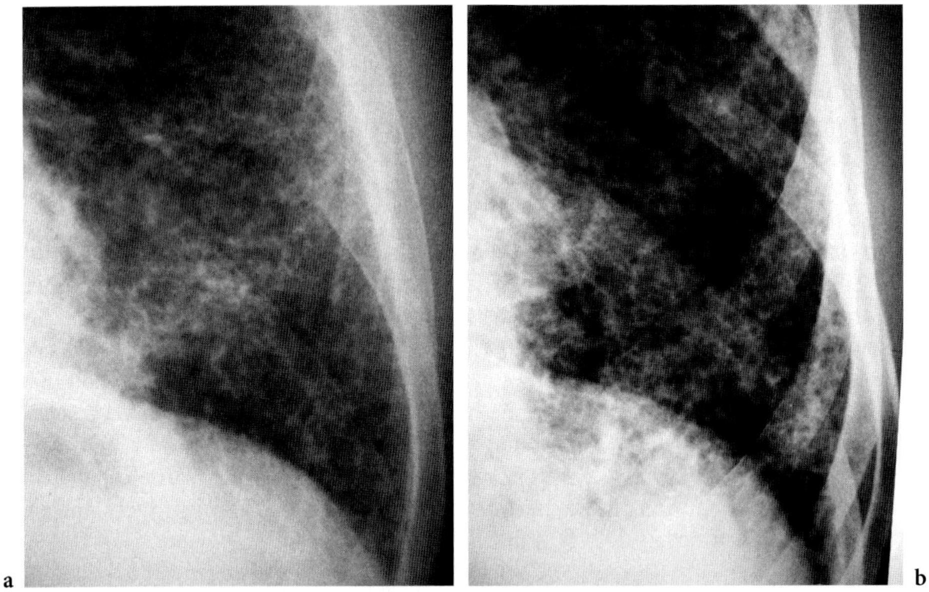

Fig. 7.1a,b. Coned views of sample radiographs showing examples of the International Labour Office (ILO) classification irregular opacities 's' (**a**) and 't' (**b**) commonly seen in asbestosis. Reproduced with permission from ILO International Classification of Radiographs of Pneumoconioses (revised 1980), Set of Standard Films (profusion score 3/3, s/s and profusion score 3/3, t/t). Copyright (c) 2000 International Labour Organization. The ILO shall accept no responsibility for any inaccuracy, errors or omissions or for the consequences arising from the use of the Radiographs

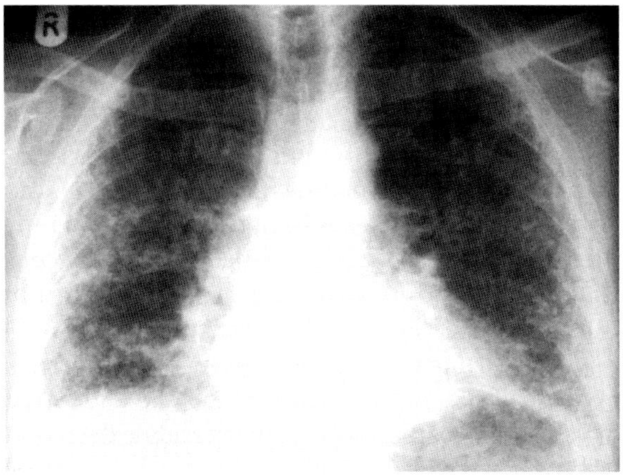

Fig. 7.2. A radiograph showing advanced asbestosis with a bilateral basal coarse reticulonodular pattern extending to the mid zones, reduction in lung volumes and irregular cardiac and diaphragmatic outlines. The patient was a 73-year old who had worked as a ship fitter for 30 years cutting asbestos sheets (courtesy of Dr. Robin Rudd, London)

than a restrictive defect on lung function testing (Ohar et al. 2004). However, the study was hampered by a lack of thin-section CT data given that, in a population with a significant smoking history, early emphysema may not have been radiographically apparent (De Vuyst et al. 2004).

A disadvantage of the chest radiograph, as with other causes of diffuse interstitial lung disease, is that the radiograph may be normal in individuals with asbestosis (Epler et al. 1978; Kipen et al. 1987). In a radiographic study of 138 cases of asbestosis with histopathological correlation, Kipen et al. found that 18% of cases had no radiographic features of parenchymal fibrosis despite histopathological fibrosis, and in 7% both pleural and parenchymal disease was undetectable on chest radiography (Kipen et al. 1987). Furthermore, Rockoff and Schwartz evaluated the ILO classification (1980) for the detection of early asbestosis and found that there was a 10–20% probability of a normal radiographic interpretation despite significant histopathological asbestosis (Rockoff and Schwartz 1988). The authors concluded that, in individuals exposed to asbestos, the ILO classification of 'normal' should not be misconstrued as the absence of parenchymal disease.

The most recent ATS guidelines (2004) recognise the distinction between radiographs "that are suggestive but not presumptively diagnostic (0/1) and those that are presumptively diagnostic but not unequivocal (1/0)" (American Thoracic Society 2004). Given that opacity profusion is part of a continuous spectrum, an arbitrary dividing point may be taken to separate radiographs that are 'positive' for asbestosis from those that are negative (American Thoracic Society 2004; International Labour Office 2002). However, in extensive disease, a radiograph showing characteristic signs of asbestosis in the presence of an appropriate history of exposure is considered to be sufficient for the diagnosis without further imaging techniques such as CT (American Thoracic Society 2004).

As well as problems with sensitivity, chest radiography is also limited by the fact that the radiographic features are not specific for asbestosis and are similar to IPF and other interstitial lung diseases. The presence of pleural plaques are obvious pointers to the diagnosis. However, pleural disease is not always present or detectable using radiography (Gamsu et al. 1995; Staples et al. 1989). Furthermore, small irregular opacities are not specific for asbestosis, or even fibrosis, as they may be related to age and cigarette smoking (Barnhart et al. 1990; Dick et al. 1992; Hnizdo and Sluis-Cremer 1988) and have also been described in a variety of other surprisingly diverse processes including bronchiectasis and emphysema (Friedman et al. 1988). Additionally, workers may have occupational exposures to a combination of dusts (e.g. silica and asbestos) (American Thoracic Society 2004). Thin-section CT may be useful to more accurately identify coexisting pneumoconiosis in the same individual, for example, upper lobe rounded opacities characteristic of silicosis and lower lobe honeycombing indicating asbestosis.

Other disadvantages of the chest radiograph (including the ILO system) are significant inter- and intraobserver variability for both pleural and parenchymal disease (Amandus et al. 1974; Bourbeau and Ernst 1988; Reger and Morgan 1970). Technical factors such as exposure may also affect ILO interpretation: if a radiograph is overexposed, small discrete opacities tend to be classified in a lower category, whereas with underexposed films the reverse is true (Reger et al. 1972; Wise and Oldham 1963). Additionally, individuals with asbestosis may have extensive coexisting pleural disease, which obscures the lung parenchyma, further decreasing radiographic sensitivity.

However, despite these disadvantages, the chest radiograph remains an important epidemiological tool and is central to the diagnosis of asbestosis in many countries where access to CT is limited. Moreover, chest radiography is relatively specific in the context of a combination of pleural plaques and advanced parenchymal disease in an individual with an appropriate history of asbestos exposure. However, in early asbestosis and with extensive coexisting pleural disease which obscures the lung parenchyma, chest radiography is clearly insensitive, hence the increasing interest in techniques such as thin-section CT.

7.4 Computed Tomography

7.4.1 Background

The technique of thin-section (or high-resolution) CT has revolutionised the approach to all interstitial lung diseases, including asbestosis. Several studies have shown that by comparison with chest radiography, thin-section CT is more sensitive, has greater observer agreement and is more accurate in the diagnosis of infiltrative lung diseases (Grenier et al. 1991; Mathieson et al. 1989; Padley et al. 1991). Despite traditional reliance on chest radiography, it is unsurprising that thin-section CT, therefore, has an increasingly central role in the diagnosis and medicolegal assessment of asbestosis in many countries.

The particular relevance of transaxial imaging for evaluating the lung parenchyma in patients with a combination of asbestosis and pleural disease was first recognised by Kreel in the mid 1970s (Kreel 1976). Due to the lack of superimposed structures, CT provided information about the lung parenchyma that would have been radiographically cryptic. In another early study by Katz and Kreel (1979), it was found that even conventional CT (contiguous thick 10-mm sections) was more sensitive for both diffuse pleural thickening and early asbestosis than chest radiography.

7.4.2 Technique

Despite the early studies using conventional CT, the use of thin (1–3 mm thickness) interspaced sections has been advocated to maximise sensitivity, particularly in subjects with early disease (Gevenois et al. 1994). However, small pleural plaques may be missed with thin interspaced sections, with some authors suggesting the use of additional contiguous sections for the detection of plaques when the lung parenchyma is normal in asbestos-exposed subjects (Gevenois et al. 1994). The ATS guidelines (2004) state that CT sections should be obtained with at least 2-cm intervals to allow a more accurate assessment of pleural abnormalities (American Thoracic Society 2004). There has been recent interest in the use of low dose multidetector helical CT with contiguous 5-mm reconstructions as opposed to thin interspaced sections for the detection of asbestos-related pleuroparenchymal disease, with no apparent loss of diagnostic accuracy and the additional advantage of increased pulmonary nodule detection (Remy-Jardin et al. 2004).

The use of additional prone sections may be helpful to distinguish the normal dependent increase in attenuation from early infiltrative lung disease (Lynch 1995; Webb et al. 1993), and the ATS (2004) criteria state prone views should be obtained in all cases (American Thoracic Society 2004). For purposes of compensation, some experts prefer images on both lung and soft tissue windows for assessment of the pleura; however, in practice, pleural disease is usually apparent on the lung windows alone (Copley et al. 2001).

7.4.3 CT findings

In early disease, subpleural branching nodular X and Y structures are seen (Fig. 7.3) and, as the disease

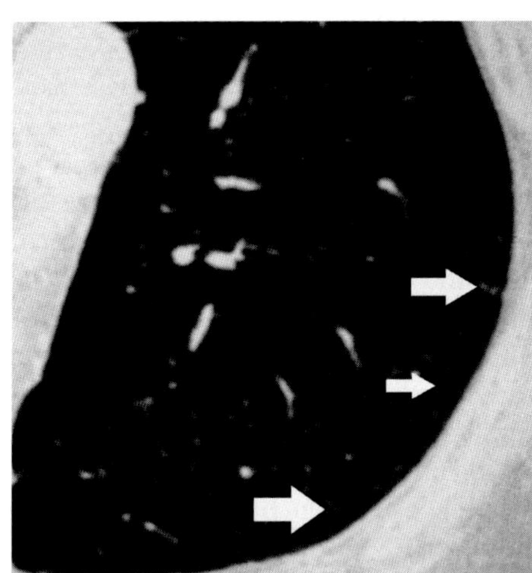

Fig. 7.3. Prone thin-section computed tomography in an individual with early asbestosis showing small subpleural dots (*arrows*) which correlate histopathologically with areas of peribronchiolar fibrosis

becomes more advanced, these become more confluent to produce pleural-based nodular irregularities (Fig. 7.4) (AKIRA et al. 1991). On subsequent serial CT examinations, ground glass opacity (Fig. 7.5), subpleural curvilinear areas (Fig. 7.6) and honeycombing (Fig. 7.7) become apparent (AKIRA et al. 1991). Ground glass opacity is defined as increased attenuation of the lung without obscuration of the underlying bronchovascular margins (AUSTIN et al. 1996). Subpleural curvilinear lines are linear densities usually within 1 cm of the pleura and parallel to the chest wall (YOSHIMURA et al. 1986). Honeycombing is defined as cystic air spaces, usually 0.3–1.0 cm in diameter, with well-defined walls (AUSTIN et al. 1996). The other thin-section CT findings that have been described in asbestosis include: intralobular lines (Fig. 7.8), thickened interlobular septal lines (Fig. 7.9), parenchymal bands of fibrosis (Fig. 7.10) and architectural distortion (ABERLE et al. 1988a; AKIRA et al. 1991; GAMSU et al. 1995). Intralobular or core lines occur when the interlobular interstitium is thickened and appear as fine branching structures arising about 1 cm from the pleural surface but often not in contact with the pleura (ABERLE

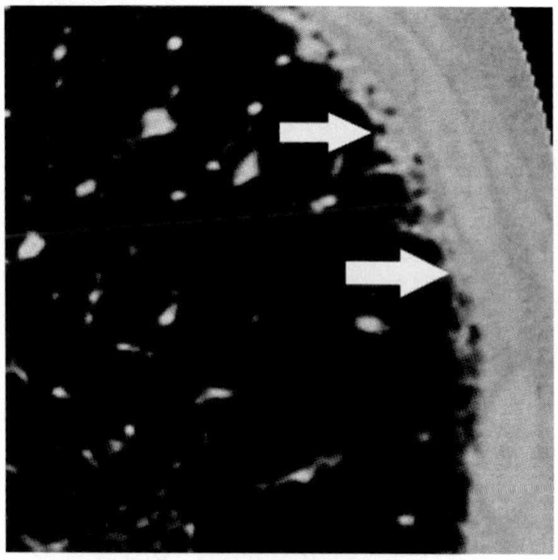

Fig. 7.4. Coned thin-section computed tomography in a different individual showing more extensive disease where there are more confluent pleurally based nodules (*arrows*)

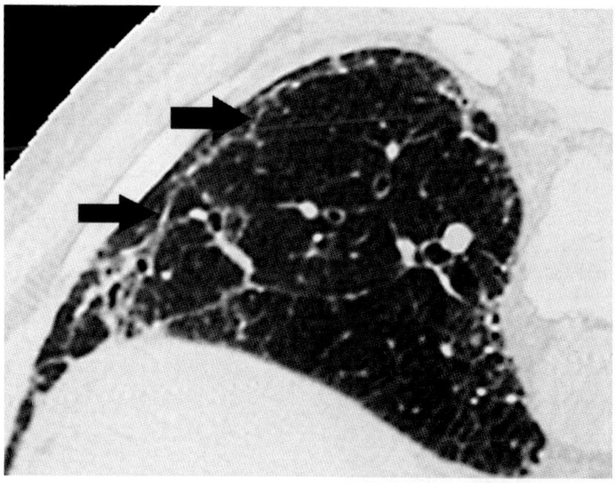

Fig. 7.6. Prone thin-section computed tomography of an individual with early asbestosis showing a subpleural curvilinear line (*arrows*)

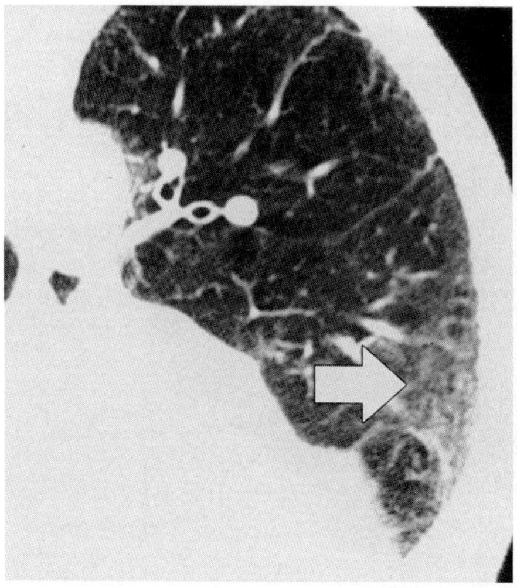

Fig. 7.5. Supine thin-section computed tomography of an asbestos miner showing an area of ground glass opacity (*arrow*) defined as increased attenuation of the lung parenchyma without obscuration of underlying bronchovascular structures

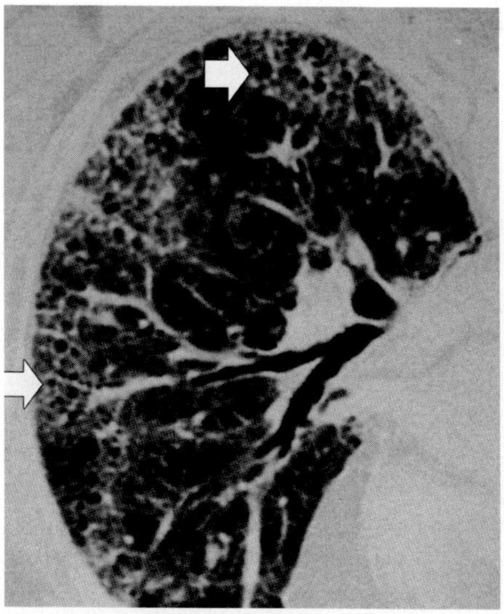

Fig. 7.7. Prone thin-section computed tomography of an asbestos miner showing areas of subpleural peripheral honeycombing (small cystic spaces a few millimetres in diameter) (*arrows*)

et al. 1988b). When numerous they appear as a fine reticular pattern. Septal lines correspond with thickening of the interlobular septa which contain venules and lymphatics and often contact the pleural surface (Austin et al. 1996). Parenchymal bands are defined as linear nontapering densities 2–5 cm in length, extending through the lung to contact the pleural surface, often with distortion of the lung parenchyma and terminate at sites where the pleura is thickened (Aberle et al. 1988b). Although parenchymal bands have been described in asbestosis, they are usually associated with pleural thickening and most authorities now believe them to be a parenchymal manifestation of pleural thickening (Section 7.4.6). These abnormalities commonly have a peripheral and basal distribution. Areas of decreased attenuation, so called 'mosaic attenuation', reflecting small airways disease, have also been described on thin-section CT in individuals with asbestosis (Fig. 7.11) (Akira et al. 1991, 2003).

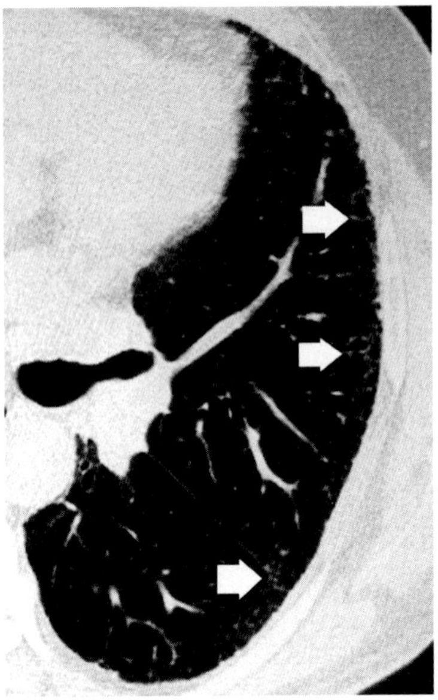

Fig. 7.8. Supine thin-section computed tomography of an individual with asbestosis showing a subpleural reticular pattern due to thickened intralobular structures (*arrows*)

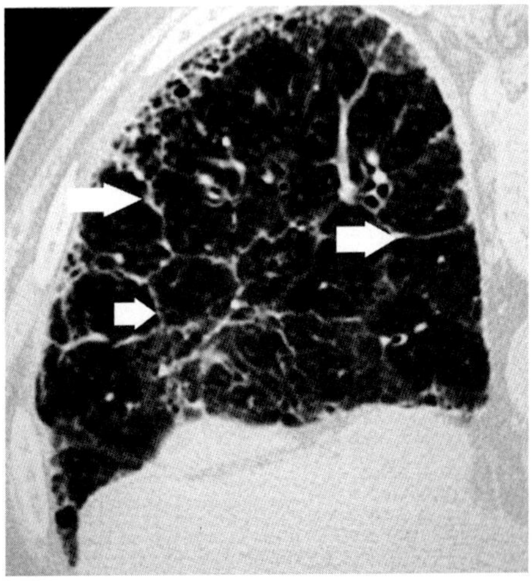

Fig. 7.9. Prone thin-section computed tomography of an asbestos miner with subpleural honeycombing and thickened interlobular septal lines (*arrows*)

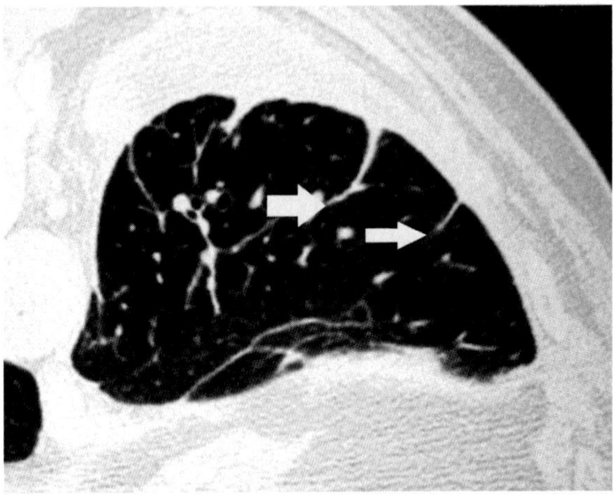

Fig. 7.10. Prone thin-section computed tomography of an asbestos-exposed individual showing multiple parenchymal bands (*arrows*) arising from an area of pleural thickening

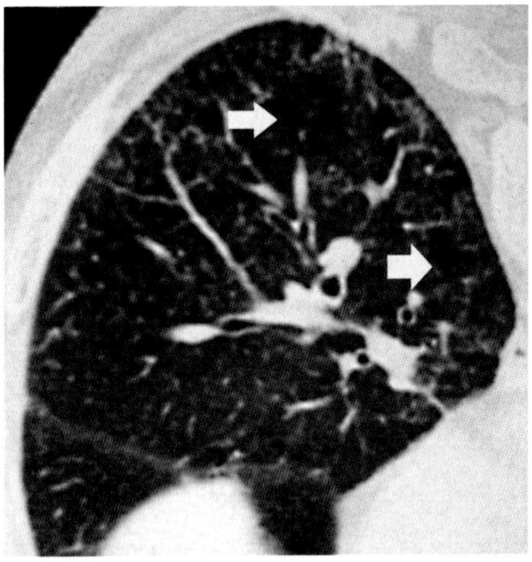

Fig. 7.11. Prone inspiratory thin-section computed tomography of an asbestos miner showing areas of differing attenuation with regions of pulmonary parenchyma which appear blacker than adjacent areas (*arrows*), an indirect sign of small airways disease. The difference may be accentuated on end-expiratory sections (not shown)

Pleural thickening and plaques are almost invariably demonstrated in asbestosis with CT (ABERLE et al. 1988a; GAMSU et al. 1995), but conversely the presence of isolated pleural plaques on CT do not predict asbestosis (REN et al. 1991). Ancillary findings of enlarged reactive mediastinal lymph nodes are often seen in asbestos-related pleuroparenchymal disease (SAMPSON and HANSELL 1992).

The issue of whether asbestos causes emphysema (areas of parenchymal destruction and distortion on CT) is controversial. BEGIN et al. studied individuals exposed to asbestos and silicosis with ILO category 0 or 1 chest radiographs, and found the prevalence of emphysema on thin-section CT was increased in individuals with both conditions, even in lifetime non-smokers (BEGIN et al. 1995). The lifetime non-smokers had more paracicatricial emphysema than smokers or ex-smokers, but all types–including centrilobular, paraseptal and panacinar–were seen. Whilst these findings support the theory that emphysema is associated with asbestosis in the absence of cigarette smoking, this and more recent studies are not conclusive and more confirmatory studies are required (CHURG 1998; HUUSKONEN et al. 2004).

7.4.4 CT–Histopathological Correlation

In an exquisitely detailed study of serial CT scans of asbestos-exposed individuals with histopathological correlation, AKIRA et al. (1991) found that the earliest thin-section CT features of asbestosis were lower zones subpleural centrilobular 'dots' or branching structures often connected with the most peripheral branch of the pulmonary artery (Fig. 7.3), which correlated histopathologically with peribronchiolar fibrosis (Fig. 7.12a, b). These subpleural isolated dots became more confluent on sequential examinations to produce pleurally based nodules (Fig. 7.4) correlating histopathologically with subpleural fibrosis (Fig. 7.13) (AKIRA et al. 1991).

In another meticulous study of more extensive asbestosis, AKIRA et al. correlated inflated postmortem lung specimens with in vitro CT (AKIRA et al. 1990). The observed CT findings of thickened interlobular and intralobular lines, pleural-based opacities, parenchymal bands, subpleural curvilinear shadows, ground glass attenuation, traction bronchiectasis and honeycombing correlated well with histopathological fibrosis (AKIRA et al. 1990). In particular, intralobular lines corresponded with peribronchiolar fibrosis, which was more severe in the subpleural regions. However, interlobular lines and ground glass attenuation were not specific for fibrosis as these findings also represented areas of oedema histopathologically (AKIRA et al. 1990). In a larger study with CT–histopathological correlation, GAMSU et al. described interstitial lines, parenchymal bands and architectural distortion of secondary pulmonary lobules as the commonest CT abnormalities in cases of histopathologically confirmed asbestosis (GAMSU et al. 1995).

7.4.5 Sensitivity and Specificity of CT

Several studies have shown that by comparison with chest radiography, thin-section CT is more sensitive

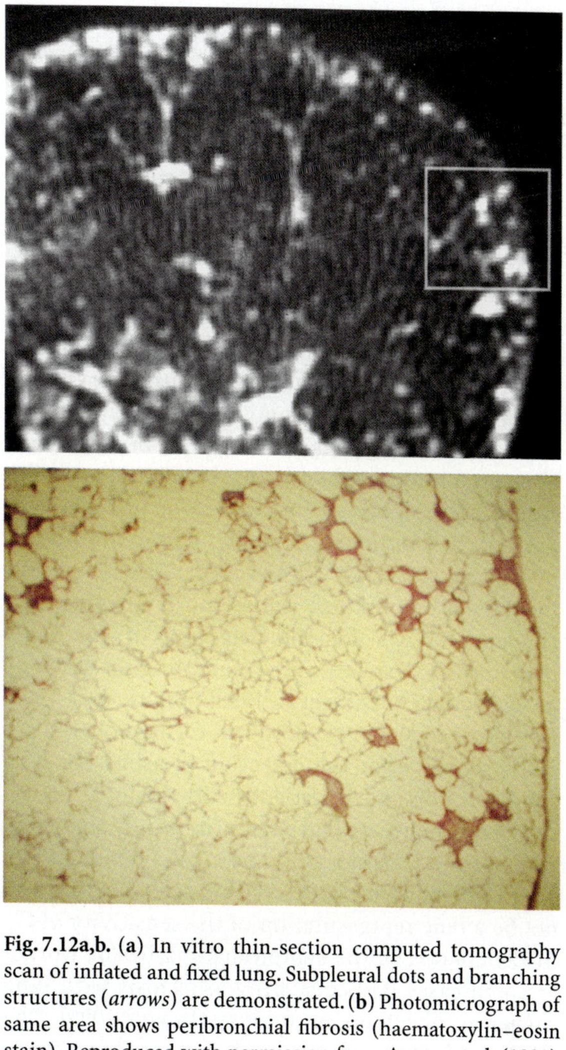

a

b

Fig. 7.12a,b. (**a**) In vitro thin-section computed tomography scan of inflated and fixed lung. Subpleural dots and branching structures (*arrows*) are demonstrated. (**b**) Photomicrograph of same area shows peribronchial fibrosis (haematoxylin–eosin stain). Reproduced with permission from AKIRA et al. (1991)

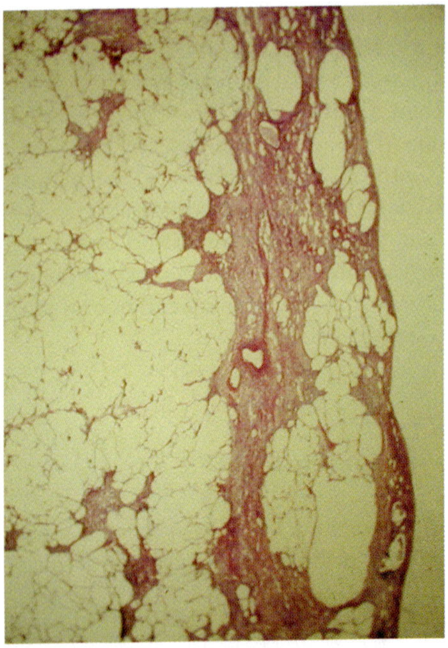

Fig. 7.13. Photomicrograph shows subpleural fibrosis which corresponds with pleurally based nodularity on thin-section computed tomography (e.g. Fig. 7.4). Reproduced with permission from AKIRA et al. (1991)

for the detection of parenchymal fibrosis in asbestos-exposed subjects (ABERLE et al. 1988a; GAMSU et al. 1989, 1995; OKSA et al. 1994; STAPLES et al. 1989). AKIRA et al. found parenchymal abnormalities consisting of thickened interlobular and intralobular lines, pleural-based nodules, subpleural curvilinear lines, ground glass attenuation and honeycombing in a group of patients with normal or minimally abnormal radiographs (AKIRA et al. 1991). Similar results were obtained in a group of patients with normal chest radiographs and lung function studied by NERI et al. (1994). Thin-section CT, with supplementary prone images, is also more sensitive than conventional CT for the detection of parenchymal fibrosis despite limited 'sampling' of the lung parenchyma (ABERLE et al. 1988b; BEGIN et al. 1993; GEVENOIS et al. 1994). However, CT is probably not 100% sensitive for the detection of asbestosis as a small proportion of patients with histopathologically proven disease had normal or mildly abnormal thin-section CTs in a study by GAMSU et al. (1995). The study may have suffered from selection bias and not be a true representation of the sensitivity of CT in the context of the symptomatic asbestos worker as some cases had coexisting asbestosis with lung cancer at lobectomy or autopsy (LYNCH 1995). The clinical relevance of such mild and possibly asymptomatic disease is unknown. Another drawback of the study was that the thin-section CT features were recorded by consensus of two radiologists, whereas the histopathological grading was performed by a single histopathologist, despite known problems with interobserver agreement for semiquantitative histopathological grading in other infiltrative lung diseases such as IPF (ASHCROFT et al. 1988; CHERNIACK et al. 1991). However, all the cases with a 'normal' or mildly abnormal thin-section CT were graded as having histopathologically mild or moderate fibrosis, and some of the near-normal thin-section CTs had limited individual thin-section CT features of asbestosis such as interstitial lines and architectural distortion. In an invited commentary, Lynch concluded that, despite pressures on the radiologist to state definitively whether or not an individual has asbestosis, there will inevitably be cases with very early histopathological disease (which may not be functionally significant) where the CT findings are equivocal (LYNCH 1995).

The specificity of individual CT features for asbestosis is more controversial, as many studies are limited by lack of histopathological proof of the diagnosis (ABERLE and BALMES 1991). Initially YOSHIMURA et al. proposed that the subpleural curvilinear line, representing 'fibrosing bronchioloalveolitis', was characteristic of asbestosis (Fig. 7.6) (YOSHIMURA et al. 1986). However, this feature was later described in a variety of patients without asbestos exposure and, although commonly seen is asbestosis, is no longer considered pathognomonic (ABERLE et al. 1988b; ARAI et al. 1990; BERGIN et al. 1994; PILATE et al. 1987). Furthermore, in a study evaluating the thin-section CT scans of non-asbestos exposed patients investigated for a variety of indications such as recurrent malignancy and infection, a significant proportion had individual features described in asbestosis such as parenchymal bands, subpleural increased density, thickened interlobular septal lines and honeycomb lung (BERGIN et al. 1994). GAMSU et al. showed that a cumulative score taking into account the number of individual features of asbestosis increased specificity for the diagnosis of asbestosis and discarded subpleural increased density as a useful sign in asbestosis because of the lack of specificity (GAMSU et al. 1995). The cumulative score and a subjective grading of the profusion and severity of abnormalities were similar for suggesting the presence of disease, and the authors concluded that a combination of the various types of abnormalities and the severity should be taken into account when suggesting the diagnosis of asbestosis on CT (GAMSU et al. 1995).

Of all the infiltrative lung diseases, the parenchymal features of asbestosis are most similar to IPF. The histopathological features are also similar, and asbestosis most closely resembles the histopathological subtype of usual interstitial pneumonia (UIP) apart from the presence of ferruginous or asbestos bodies in asbestosis (Churg 1998). The thin-section CT features of a subpleural basal honeycomb pattern are common to both (Al-Jarad et al. 1992) and often the presence or absence of pleural plaques or diffuse pleural thickening is relied on to discriminate between the two conditions. However, pleural plaques and thickening are not always ubiquitous in asbestosis and sometimes an individual with IPF may have had a limited exposure to asbestos in the past, resulting in coexisting plaques (Gaensler et al. 1991). Important differences such as the differences in prognosis and eligibility for compensation highlight the need for accurate differentiation, wherever possible. Al-Jarad et al. found that ground glass opacities were commoner in IPF and rare in asbestosis, whereas the converse was true for thick band-like opacities (Al-Jarad et al. 1992). Akira et al. found that subpleural dot-like or branching opacities, subpleural curvilinear lines, mosaic perfusion and parenchymal bands were commoner in asbestosis, whereas visible intralobular bronchioles, bronchiolectasis within fibrotic consolidation and honeycombing were commoner in IPF (Akira et al. 2003). In contrast to the Al-Jarad study, ground glass opacification and thickened interlobular septa occurred with equal frequency, which may have been due to inclusion of a different spectrum of histopathological subtypes of IPF. The authors concluded that, in early disease, it may be possible to discern the effects of fibrosis on the subpleural secondary pulmonary lobule, with asbestosis having initially centrilobular densities due to deposition of fibers via airways, whereas immunologically mediated IPF is more widespread resulting in traction effects on the bronchioles (Akira et al. 2003). In these studies, the frequency of individual thin-section CT features were assessed and no attempt was made to differentiate between the histopathological subgroups of IPF. A subsequent study examined differences in the 'quality' of fibrosis rather than individual CT features and included biopsy-proven cases of UIP and non-specific pneumonitis (NSIP) (Copley et al. 2003). The authors found that the thin-section CT pattern of asbestosis closely resembled that of UIP but differed markedly from NSIP, after controlling for disease extent (Fig. 7.14a, b and c) (Copley et al. 2003).

Certainly no individual CT feature can be regarded as specific for asbestosis, but a constellation of features which are bilateral and multifocal with a coexisting appropriate occupational history is often diagnostic (Gamsu et al. 1995). The lack of

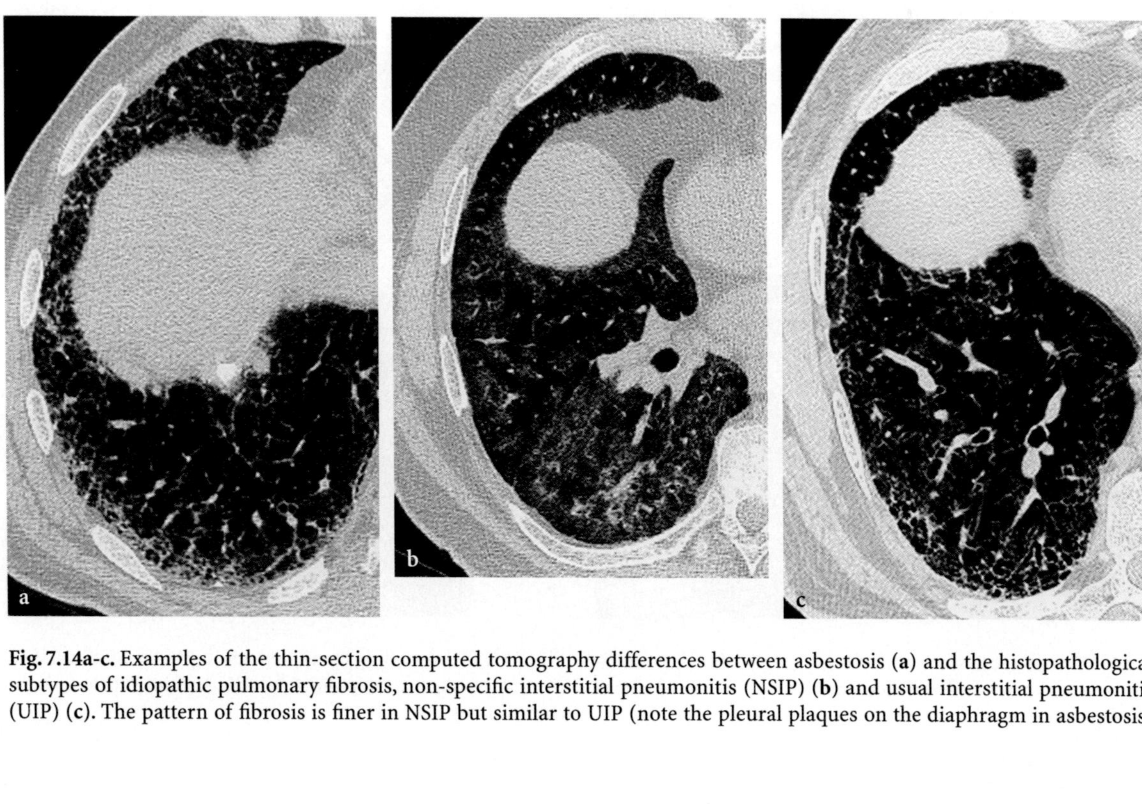

Fig. 7.14a-c. Examples of the thin-section computed tomography differences between asbestosis (**a**) and the histopathological subtypes of idiopathic pulmonary fibrosis, non-specific interstitial pneumonitis (NSIP) (**b**) and usual interstitial pneumonitis (UIP) (**c**). The pattern of fibrosis is finer in NSIP but similar to UIP (note the pleural plaques on the diaphragm in asbestosis)

standardised interpretation of CT compared with the chest radiograph is a potential problem. Despite this, studies of interobserver agreement have shown good agreement for CT by comparison with chest radiography (Begin et al. 1993; Huuskonen et al. 2001). It has been suggested that a CT classification system analogous to the ILO system for radiographs would be a useful addition, but, as yet, none has been universally adopted (American Thoracic Society 2004; Kraus et al. 1997).

7.4.6 Distinction Between Pleural and Parenchymal Disease

The distinction between asbestos-related parenchymal and pleural disease is important as the magnitude of compensation may be much greater with asbestos-induced interstitial fibrosis. The pleural features of asbestos exposure are covered in detail in Chap. 5, but there are several parenchymal features that are a feature of adjacent pleural disease and should not be confused with widespread interstitial fibrosis (Peacock et al. 2000). Parenchymal bands are defined as linear opacities, several millimetres wide and up to 5 cm long which extend to the pleura (often the pleura is thickened at the site of contact; Fig. 7.10) (Austin et al. 1996). When multiple and radiating from a single point on the pleura, the term 'crow's feet' is sometimes used (Fig. 7.15) (Solomon 1991). The features are due to adjacent visceral pleural thickening and are not regarded as a defining feature of asbestosis (Gevenois et al. 1998). Moreover, parenchymal bands are non-specific for asbestos exposure and seen in a variety of conditions with a pleural reaction such as infection or trauma (Gevenois et al. 1998; Solomon 1991). Rounded atelectasis or folded lung is again a parenchymal feature of adjacent pleural thickening (Chap. 2.5). Thin-section CT of pleural plaques may show adjacent short interstitial lines within the lung parenchyma (Fig. 7.16). The significance of these lines is unknown due to a lack of CT–histopathological correlation, but appearances are similar to mechanical effects on the lung parenchyma due to adjacent osteophyte formation (Otake et al. 2002). Therefore, because pleural disease (plaques and thickening) can cause distortion of immediately adjacent lung, the parenchymal features of asbestosis are more convincing in areas unrelated to pleural disease.

7.4.7 CT as a Screening Tool

The advent of helical or spiral CT has led to further reductions in scan time so the entire thorax can be imaged in a single breath hold. The technique has evolved due to advances in slip ring technology enabling continuous rotation of the X-ray beam and detectors around the patient who is positioned on a table that moves perpendicularly to the gantry (Naidich et al. 1999). Furthermore, the combina-

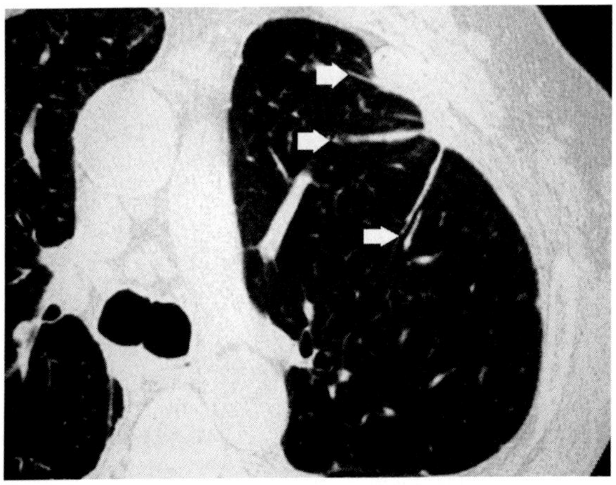

Fig. 7.15. Thin-section computed tomography showing multiple parenchymal bands arising from a single point of thickened pleura likened to 'crow's feet' (*arrows*)

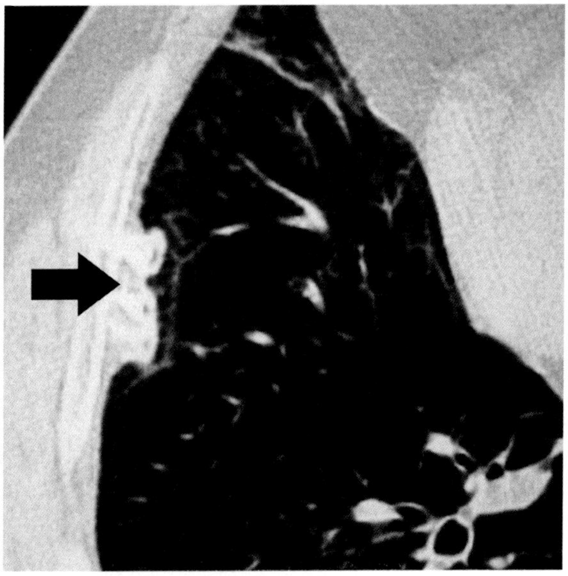

Fig. 7.16. Thin-section computed tomography of a calcified pleural plaque (*arrow*) showing adjacent interstitial parenchymal lines

tion of low-dose CT techniques and single breath-hold scanning capabilities has led to relatively recent interest in the use of CT as a mass screening method for patients with a high risk of developing lung cancer (Diederich and Wormanns 2004; Itoh et al. 1998; Kaneko et al. 1996). The effective dose for this technique is approximately ten times that of a chest radiograph for an entire thorax (Kaneko et al. 1996). The technique may ultimately prove to be of relevance to asbestos-exposed populations, given the increased risk of malignancy. The use of limited thin-section CT for large-scale screening in the asbestos-exposed workforce to detect asbestosis is more controversial because of the additional cost and radiation burden (Aberle 1991; Lozewicz et al. 1989). Although variations occur between centres, the cost for a thin-section CT examination is comparable to a four-view series of chest radiographs (Gamsu 1989). It may also be possible to substantially lower the radiation dose by reducing the mAs without loss of image quality and diagnostic accuracy (Majurin et al. 1994). With greater understanding of the specificity of thin-section CT and widespread standardisation of technique and image interpretation, the additional information given may outweigh the cost and potential increased radiation dose (Aberle 1991).

7.5 Radiological–Functional Correlation

'Uncomplicated' asbestosis results in a restrictive pattern of lung function abnormality which is discussed in Chap. 3.3. The vital capacity and total lung capacity are reduced, whereas the residual volume is normal resulting in an increased residual volume/total lung capacity ratio; the diffusing capacity (DLco) is also usually reduced (Williams and Hugh-Jones 1960).

Traditionally, chest radiography is the mainstay of radiological evaluation in asbestos-exposed individuals and has historically provided some valuable pathophysiological insights in conditions such as pulmonary oedema (Pistolesi et al. 1985). Studies of asbestos-exposed individuals have correlated radiographic features with physiological indices including exercise data with varying success (Becklake et al. 1970; Lee et al. 2003; Miller et al. 1992). However, the chest radiograph is a relatively insensitive means of correlating morphology with function in the pneumoconioses and in other causes of diffuse interstitial lung disease (Carrington 1976; Gaensler et al. 1972; Turner-Warwick et al. 1980). Furthermore, CT scoring systems are more sensitive and specific with better intra- and inter-observer agreement than radiographic systems based on the ILO classification system (Huuskonen et al. 2001).

Individuals with asbestosis may have other coexisting histopathological processes also contributing to a functional deficit, such as emphysema (many workers are also cigarette smokers), small airways disease and diffuse pleural thickening, in addition to the defining presence of interstitial fibrosis (Gibson 1996; Kilburn and Warshaw 1990). Concurrent emphysema in interstitial lung disease may be impossible to detect radiographically but has a major confounding effect on pulmonary function indices, with a paradoxical preservation of lung volumes and disproportionate reduction in DLco (Wells et al. 1997). The difficulties in separating out the different functional components are well recognised (Gibson 1996). These additional conditions may have a separate and patchy distribution to the predominantly lower zone interstitial fibrosis (for example, upper zone centrilobular emphysema) or may not be sampled by lung biopsy (for example, diffuse pleural thickening). Therefore, CT has the potential to give a more universal assessment of the relative proportions of fibrosis, emphysema, small airways disease and diffuse pleural thickening than histopathological examination of a lung biopsy specimen. The relevance of morphological–functional correlations in an asbestos-exposed population largely relates to medicolegal implications: it is important to establish what degree of disability is a result of 'compensatable' interstitial fibrosis (asbestosis) or diffuse pleural thickening and how much is ascribable to currently non-compensatable emphysema.

A variety of studies have shown that thin-section CT is more sensitive than chest radiography at detecting emphysema (Kuwano et al. 1990; Staples et al. 1989), interstitial fibrosis (Lozewicz et al. 1989; Staples et al. 1989) and pleural disease (Aberle et al. 1988b; Friedman et al. 1988). Several studies have correlated physiological indices with CT morphology in asbestos-exposed individuals (Aberle et al. 1988a; Dujic et al. 1992; Jarad et al. 1992; Neri et al. 1996; Schwartz et al. 1994; Sette et al. 2004; Staples et al. 1989). Aberle et al. were the first to correlate thin-section CT appearances with lung function in asbestos-exposed individuals and found significant inverse correlations between 'probability scores' for asbestosis and percentage predicted forced vital capacity (FVC) and single-breath diffusing capacity (Aberle et al. 1988a). Probability scores were derived from a combination of thin-section CT features including honeycombing. Furthermore, although pleural disease was assessed, this was not correlated with pulmonary function and no attempt was made to identify coexisting emphysema, a limitation common to other studies (Dujic et al. 1992; Neri et al. 1996). A longitudinal study by Schwartz et al. in 117 subjects exposed to asbestos showed that TLC was negatively independently related to diffuse pleural thickening and that DLco was also negatively independently related to honeycombing on thin-section CT (Schwartz et al. 1994).

Jarad et al. performed multivariate analyses in their study of asbestos workers and found strong independent relationships between functional indices and the thin-section CT extent of fibrosis, emphysema and diffuse pleural thickening (Jarad et al. 1992). The thin-section CT scoring system used by Jarad et al. was based on the ILO (1980) classification system for pneumoconioses (International Labour Office 1980). More recently, Sette et al. used a scoring system based on that used by Gamsu et al. (1995) for the extent of disease in asbestos workers (Sette et al. 2004). The scoring system was based on a combination of a semi-quantitative and severity score and a qualitative score based on individual CT features described in asbestos (Gamsu et al. 1995). Using this system, CT was found to be useful in assessing the likelihood of gas exchange impairment at rest and during exercise (Sette et al. 2004); however, the effects of coexisting diffuse pleural thickening and emphysema were not evaluated.

Another approach for the CT quantification of the extent of parenchymal disease in the pneumoconioses is the objective measurement of lung density using computer-assisted methods (Eterovic et al. 1993; Hartley et al. 1994; Wollmer et al. 1987). Despite the drawback of a small study group, Eterovic et al. found that in 22 patients with early or advanced asbestosis, the CT density score correlated well with indices of pulmonary function (Eterovic et al. 1993). In a larger study including individuals with IPF and asbestosis, Hartley et al. found that measures of grey scale density of the lung parenchyma were most strongly correlated with TLC, DLco and FVC (Hartley et al. 1994). The limitations of the study by Hartley et al. were that emphysema and pleural disease were not quantified. There are established computer-assisted methods for the quantification of emphysema (Bankier et al. 1999; Park et al. 1999; Remy-Jardin et al. 1996) and pleural disease (Copley et al. 2001); so, theoretically, a study examining the relationships of objective measures of CT extent of the different processes would be possible in the future. However, the main advantage of a subjective scoring system over objective methods, is speed and ease of application (Gurney et al. 1992).

A recent study has been undertaken to identify independent relationships between individual pulmonary function indices and thin-section CT variables with prospective testing of the relationships in a separate group with asbestosis (Copley 2000). The study showed that, despite the variable combination of pathological processes in patients with asbestosis, strong correlations were seen between the extent of individual CT features and the degree of functional impairment. The strongest relationships were observed between the extent of fibrosis and TLC and DLco; the circumference of diffuse pleural thickening and FVC and TLC and the extent of emphysema and Kco. The functional indices that correlated best with the extent of the combined pathological processes on multivariate analysis were TLC and DLco. The derived multivariate equations were validated definitively by their strikingly accurate prediction of pulmonary function indices in a prospective study group. In asbestos-exposed individuals, the definition of the functional consequences of asbestos, as opposed to smoking, is a significant medicolegal problem, because emphysema is not generally compensatable. Until now, no robust method has been developed for this purpose, and the degree of physiological impairment attributed to asbestos exposure in smokers is often estimated arbitrarily or based on the intensity and number of years of asbestos exposure (Guidotti 2002). Using multivariate techniques, the combination of CT features most closely linked to individual pulmonary function indices has been identified and tested in a separate group. Thus, for a given reduction in TLC or DLco, the proportion of the deficit ascribable to fibrosis, pleural thickening and emphysema can be preliminarily quantified (Copley 2000).

7.6 Summary

Despite the advantages of chest radiography in terms of cost and availability, CT is increasingly useful in the context of investigation of an asbestos-exposed individual. The limitations of chest radiography to diagnose asbestosis are now well recognised by most authorities (American Thoracic Society 2004; Ross 2003) and nowadays thin-section CT plays an increasingly central role in the clinical and medicolegal assessment of individuals with suspected asbestos-induced parenchymal lung disease (Kim and Lynch 2002). Thin-section CT is most useful in the context of a normal or equivocal chest radiograph, where there is unexplained functional deficit or when there is extensive pleural disease which obscures the lung parenchyma (Aberle 1991). Further advantages are the potential to demonstrate asbestos-related malignancies or non-asbestos-induced lung disease, such as emphysema due to cigarette smoking.

References

Aberle DR (1991) High-resolution computed tomography of asbestos-related diseases. Semin Roentgenol 26:118-131

Aberle DR, Balmes JR (1991) Computed tomography of asbestos-related pulmonary parenchymal and pleural diseases. Clin Chest Med 12:115-131

Aberle DR, Gamsu G, Ray CS (1988a) High-resolution CT of benign asbestos-related diseases: clinical and radiographic correlation. AJR Am J Roentgenol 151:883-891

Aberle DR, Gamsu G, Ray CS et al (1988b) Asbestos-related pleural and parenchymal fibrosis: detection with high-resolution CT. Radiology 166:729-734

Akira M, Yamamoto S, Yokoyama K et al (1990) Asbestosis: high-resolution CT-pathologic correlation. Radiology 176:389-394

Akira M, Yokoyama K, Yamamoto S et al (1991) Early asbestosis: evaluation with high-resolution CT. Radiology 178:409-416

Akira M, Yamamoto S, Inoue Y et al (2003) High-resolution CT of asbestosis and idiopathic pulmonary fibrosis. AJR Am J Roentgenol 181:163-169

Al-Jarad N, Strickland B, Pearson MC et al (1992) High resolution computed tomographic assessment of asbestosis and cryptogenic fibrosing alveolitis: a comparative study. Thorax 47:645-650

Amandus HE, Pendergrass EP, Dennis JM et al (1974) Pneumoconiosis: inter-reader variability in the classification of the type of small opacities in the chest roetgenogram. AJR Am J Roentgenol 122:740-743

American Thoracic Society (1986) Medical section of the American Lung Association: the diagnosis of nonmalignant diseases related to asbestos. Am Rev Respir Dis 134:363-368

American Thoracic Society (2004) Diagnosis and initial management of nonmalignant diseases related to asbestos. Am J Respir Crit Care Med 170:691-715

Anonymous (1997) Asbestos, asbestosis, and cancer: the Helsinki criteria for diagnosis and attribution. Scand J Work Environ Health 23:311-316

Arai K, Takashima T, Matsui O et al (1990) Transient subpleural curvilinear shadow caused by pulmonary congestion. J Comput Assist Tomogr 14:87-88

Ashcroft T, Simpson JM, Timbrell V (1988) Simple method of estimating severity of pulmonary fibrosis on a numerical scale. J Clin Pathol 41:467-470

Austin JH, Müller NL, Friedman PJ et al (1996) Glossary of terms for CT of the lungs: recommendations of the Nomenclature Committee of the Fleischner Society. Radiology 200:327-331

Bankier AA, de Maertelaer V, Keyzer C et al (1999) Pulmonary emphysema: subjective visual grading versus objective quantification with macroscopic morphometry and thin-section CT densitometry. Radiology 211:851-858

Barnhart S, Thornquist M, Omenn GS et al (1990) The degree of roentgenographic parenchymal opacities attributable to smoking among asbestos-exposed subjects. Am Rev Respir Dis 141:1102-1106

Becklake MR, Fournier-Massey G, McDonald JC et al (1970) Lung function in relation to chest radiographic changes in Quebec asbestos workers. I. Methods, results and conclusions. Bull Physiopathol Resp (Nancy) 6:637-659

Begin R, Ostiguy G, Filion R et al (1993) Computed tomography in the early detection of asbestosis. Br J Ind Med 50:689-698

Begin R, Filion R, Ostiguy G (1995) Emphysema in silica- and asbestos-exposed workers seeking compensation. A CT scan study. Chest 108:647-655

Bergin C, Castellino RA, Blank N et al (1994) Specificity of high-resolution CT findings in pulmonary asbestosis: do patients scanned for other indications have similar findings? AJR Am J Roentgenol 163:551-555

Bourbeau J, Ernst P (1988) Between and within-reader variability in the assessment of pleural abnormality using the ILO 1980 international classification of pneumoconioses. Am J Ind Med 14:537-543

Carrington CB (1976) Structure and function in sarcoidosis. Ann NY Acad Sci 278:265-283

Cherniack RM, Colby TV, Flint A et al (1991) Quantitative assessment of lung pathology in idiopathic pulmonary fibrosis. The BAL Cooperative Group Steering Committee. Am Rev Respir Dis 144:892-900

Churg A (1998) Non-neoplastic disease caused by asbestos. In: Churg A, Green FHY (eds) Pathology of occupational lung disease. Williams and Wilkins, Baltimore, pp 277-338

Copley SJ (2000) Computed tomographic-functional relationships in asbestos-induced pleural and parenchymal disease. MD Thesis, University of London, UK

Copley SJ, Wells AU, Rubens MB et al (2001) Functional consequences of pleural disease evaluated with chest radiography and CT. Radiology 220:237-243

Copley SJ, Wells AU, Sivakumaran P et al (2003) Asbestosis and idiopathic pulmonary fibrosis: a comparison of the thin-section CT features. Radiology 229:731-736

De Vuyst P, Gevenois PA, van Muylem A et al (2004) Changing patterns in asbestos-induced lung disease. Chest 126:999

Dick JA, Morgan WK, Muir DF et al (1992) The significance of irregular opacities on the chest roentgenogram. Chest 102:251-260

Diederich S, Wormanns D (2004) Impact of low-dose CT on lung cancer screening. Lung Cancer 45:S13-S19

Dujic Z, Tocilj J, Boschi S et al (1992) Biphasic lung diffusing capacity: detection of early asbestos induced changes in lung function. Br J Ind Med 49:260-267

Epler GR, McLoud TC, Gaensler EA et al (1978) Normal chest roentgenograms in chronic diffuse infiltrative lung disease. N Engl J Med 298:934-939

Eterovic D, Dujic Z, Tocilj J et al (1993) High resolution pulmonary computed tomography scans quantified by analysis of density distribution: application to asbestosis. Br J Ind Med 50:514-519

Friedman AC, Fiel SB, Fisher MS et al (1988) Asbestos-related pleural disease and asbestosis: a comparison of CT and chest radiography. AJR Am J Roentgenol 150:269-275

Gaensler EA, Carrington CB, Coutu RE et al (1972) Pathological, physiological, and radiological correlations in the pneumoconioses. Ann NY Acad Sci 200:574-607

Gaensler EA, Jederlinic PJ, Churg A (1991) Idiopathic pulmonary fibrosis in asbestos-exposed workers. Am Rev Respir Dis 144:689-696

Gamsu G (1989) High-resolution CT in the diagnosis of asbestos-related pleuroparenchymal disease. Am J Ind Med 16:115-117

Gamsu G, Aberle DR, Lynch D (1989) Computed tomography in the diagnosis of asbestos-related thoracic disease. J Thorac Imaging 4:61-67

Gamsu G, Salmon CJ, Warnock ML et al (1995) CT quantification of interstitial fibrosis in patients with asbestosis: a comparison of two methods. AJR Am J Roentgenol 164:63-68

Gevenois PA, De Vuyst P, Dedeire S et al (1994) Conventional and high-resolution CT in asymptomatic asbestos-exposed workers. Acta Radiol 35:226-229

Gevenois PA, de Maertelaer V, Madani A et al (1998) Asbestosis, pleural plaques and diffuse pleural thickening: three distinct benign responses to asbestos exposure. Eur Respir J 11:1021-1027

Gibson GJ (1996) Alveolar diseases. In: Clinical tests of respiratory function, 2nd edn. Chapman and Hall Medical, London, pp 223-247

Grenier P, Valeyre D, Cluzel P et al (1991) Chronic diffuse interstitial lung disease: diagnostic value of chest radiography and high-resolution CT. Radiology 179:123-132

Guidotti TL (2002) Apportionment in asbestos-related disease for purposes of compensation. Ind Health 40:295-311

Gurney JW, Jones KK, Robbins RA et al (1992) Regional distribution of emphysema: correlation of high-resolution CT with pulmonary function tests in unselected smokers. Radiology 183:457-463

Hartley PG, Galvin JR, Hunninghake GW et al (1994) High-resolution CT- derived measures of lung density are valid indexes of interstitial lung disease. J Appl Physiol 76:271-277

Hillerdal G (1990) Pleural and parenchymal fibrosis mainly affecting the upper lobes in persons exposed to asbestos. Respir Med 84:129-134

Hnizdo E, Sluis-Cremer GK (1988) Effect of tobacco smoking on the presence of asbestosis at postmortem and on the reading of irregular opacities on roentgenograms in asbestos-exposed workers. Am Rev Respir Dis 138:1207-1212

Huuskonen O, Kivisaari L, Zitting A et al (2001) High-resolution computed tomography classification of lung fibrosis for patients with asbestos-related disease. Scan J Work Environ Health 27:106-112

Huuskonen O, Kivisaari L, Zitting A et al (2004) Emphysema findings associated with heavy asbestos-exposure in high resolution computed tomography of Finnish construction workers. J Occup Health 46:266-271

International Labour Office (1980) International Labour Office guidelines for the use of the ILO international classification of the radiographs of pneumoconioses, revised edition 1980. International Labour Office Occupational Health and Safety Series, no 22 (rev 80), Geneva

International Labour Office (2002) International Classification of Radiographs of Pneumoconioses. Revised edition 2000. International Labour Office Occupational Health and Safety Series, no 22, Geneva

Itoh S, Ikeda M, Isomura T et al (1998) Screening helical CT for mass screening of lung cancer: application of low-dose and single-breath-hold scanning. Radiat Med 16:75-83

Jarad NA, Wilkinson P, Pearson MC et al (1992) A new high resolution computed tomography scoring system for pulmonary fibrosis, pleural disease, and emphysema in patients with asbestos related disease. Br J Ind Med 49:73-84

Kaneko M, Eguchi K, Ohmatsu H et al (1996) Peripheral lung cancer: screening and detection with low-dose spiral CT versus radiography. Radiology 201:798-802

Katz D, Kreel L (1979) Computed tomography in pulmonary asbestosis. Clin Radiol 30:207-213

Kilburn KH, Warshaw R (1990) Pulmonary functional impairment associated with pleural asbestos disease. Circumscribed and diffuse thickening. Chest 98:965-972

Kim JS, Lynch DA (2002) Imaging of nonmalignant occupational lung disease. J Thorac Imaging 17:238-260

Kipen HM, Lilis R, Suzuki Y et al (1987) Pulmonary fibrosis in asbestos insulation workers with lung cancer: a radiological and histopathological evaluation. Br J Ind Med 44:96-100

Kraus T, Raithel HJ, Lehnert G (1997) Computer-assisted classification system for chest X-ray and computed tomography findings in occupational lung disease. Int Arch Occup Environ Health 69:482-486

Kreel L (1976) Computer tomography in the evaluation of pulmonary asbestosis. Preliminary experiences with the EMI general purpose scanner. Acta Radiol 17:405-412

Kuwano K, Matsuba K, Ikeda T et al (1990) The diagnosis of mild emphysema. Correlation of computed tomography and pathology scores. Am Rev Respir Dis 141:169-178

Lee YC, Singh B, Pang SC et al (2003) Radiographic (ILO) readings predict arterial oxygen desaturation during exercise in subjects with asbestosis. Occup Environ Med 60:201-206

Lozewicz S, Reznek RH, Herdman M et al (1989) Role of computed tomography in evaluating asbestos related lung disease. Br J Ind Med 46:777-781

Lynch DA (1995) CT for asbestosis: value and limitations. AJR Am J Roentgenol 164:69-71

Majurin ML, Varpula M, Kurki T et al (1994) High-resolution CT of the lung in asbestos-exposed subjects. Comparison of low-dose and high-dose HRCT. Acta Radiol 35:473-477

Mathieson J, Mayo JR, Staples CA et al (1989) Chronic diffuse infiltrative lung disease: comparison of diagnostic accuracy of CT and chest radiography. Radiology 171:111-116

Miller A, Lilis R, Godbold J et al (1992) Relationship of pulmonary function to radiographic interstitial fibrosis in 2,611 long-term asbestos insulators. An assessment of the International Labour Office profusion score. Am Rev Respir Dis 145:263-270

Naidich DP, Webb WR, Müller NL et al (1999) Principles and techniques of thoracic computed tomography and magnetic resonance. In: Naidich DP, Zerhouni EA, Siegelman SS (eds) Computed tomography and magnetic resonance of the thorax. Lippincott-Raven, Philadelphia, pp 1-37

Neri S, Antonelli A, Falaschi F et al (1994) Findings from high resolution computed tomography of the lung and pleura of symptom free workers exposed to amosite who had normal chest radiographs and pulmonary function tests. Occup Environ Med 51:239-243

Neri S, Boraschi P, Antonelli A et al (1996) Pulmonary function, smoking habits, and high resolution computed tomography (HRCT) early abnormalities of lung and pleural fibrosis in shipyard workers exposed to asbestos. Am J Ind Med 30:588-595

Ohar J, Sterling DA, Bleeker E et al (2004) Changing patterns in asbestos-induced lung disease. Chest 125:744-753

Oksa P, Suoranta H, Koskinen H et al (1994) High-resolution computed tomography in the early detection of asbestosis. Int Arch Occup Environ Health 65:299-304

Otake S, Takahashi M, Ishigake T (2002) Focal pulmonary interstitial opacities adjacent to thoracic spine osteophytes. AJR Am J Roentgenol 179:893-896

Padley SP, Hansell DM, Flower CD et al (1991) Comparative accuracy of high resolution computed tomography and chest radiography in the diagnosis of chronic diffuse infiltrative lung disease. Clin Radiol 44:222-226

Park KJ, Bergin CJ, Clausen JL (1999) Quantitation of emphysema with three-dimensional CT densitometry: comparison with two-dimensional analysis, visual emphysema scores, and pulmonary function test results. Radiology 211:541-547

Parkes WR (1994) An approach to the differential diagnosis of asbestosis and nonoccupational diffuse interstitial pulmonary fibrosis. In: Parkes WR (ed) Occupational lung disorders. Butterworths, London, pp 505-535

Peacock C, Copley SJ, Hansell DM (2000) Asbestos-related benign pleural disease. Clin Radiol 55:422-432

Pilate I, Marcelis S, Timmerman H et al (1987) Pulmonary asbestosis: CT study of subpleural curvilinear shadow. Radiology 164:584

Pistolesi M, Miniati M, Milne ENC et al (1985) The chest roentgenogram in pulmonary edema. Clin Chest Med 6:315-344

Reger RB, Morgan WK (1970) On the factors influencing the consistency in the radiologic diagnosis of pneumoconiosis. Am Rev Respir Dis 102:905-915

Reger RB, Smith CA, Kibelstis JA, Morgan WK (1972) The effect of film quality and other factors on the roentgenographic categorization of coal worker's pneumoconiosis. Am J Roentgenol Radium Nucl Med 115:462-472

Remy-Jardin M, Remy J, Gosselin B et al (1996) Sliding thin slab, minimum intensity projection technique in the diagnosis of emphysema: histopathologic-CT correlation. Radiology 200:665-671

Remy-Jardin M, Sobaszek A, Duhamel A et al (2004) Asbestos-related pleuroparenchymal disease: evaluation with low-dose four-detector row spiral CT. Radiology 233:182-190

Ren H, Lee DR, Hruban RH et al (1991) Pleural plaques do not predict asbestosis: high-resolution computed tomography and pathology study. Mod Pathol 4:201-209

Rockoff SD, Schwartz A (1988) Roentgenographic underestimation of early asbestosis by International Labor Organization classification. Analysis of data and probabilities. Chest 93:1088-1091

Rosenberg DM (1997) Asbestos-related disorders. A realistic perspective. Chest 111:1424-1426

Ross RM (2003) The clinical diagnosis of asbestosis in this century requires more than a chest radiograph. Chest 124:1120-1128

Sampson C, Hansell DM (1992) The prevalence of enlarged lymph nodes in asbestos-exposed individuals: a CT study. Clin Radiol 45:340-342

Schwartz DA, Davis CS, Merchant JA et al (1994) Longitudinal changes in lung function among asbestos-exposed workers. Am J Respir Crit Care Med 150:1243-1249

Selikoff IJ (1978) Prevalence, diagnosis and course of the asbestoses. In: Selikoff IJ (ed) Asbestosis and disease. Academic Press, New York, pp 207-237

Sette A, Neder JA, Nery LE et al (2004) Thin-section CT abnormalities and pulmonary gas exchange impairment in workers exposed to asbestos. Radiology 232:66-74

Solomon A (1991) Radiological features of asbestos-related visceral pleural changes. Am J Ind Med 19:339-355

Staples CA, Gamsu G, Ray CS et al (1989) High resolution computed tomography and lung function in asbestos-exposed workers with normal chest radiographs. Am Rev Respir Dis 139:1502-1508

Turner-Warwick M, Burrows B, Johnson A (1980) Cryptogenic fibrosing alveolitis: clinical features and their influence on survival. Thorax 35:171-180

Webb WR, Stern EJ, Kanth N et al (1993) Dynamic pulmonary CT: findings in healthy adult men. Radiology 186:117-124

Weill H (1987) Diagnosis of asbestos-related disease. Chest 91:802-803

Wells AU, King AD, Rubens MB et al (1997) Lone cryptogenic fibrosing alveolitis: a functional-morphologic correlation based on extent of disease on thin-section computed tomography. Am J Respir Crit Care Med 155:1367-1375

Williams R, Hugh-Jones P (1960) The significance of lung function changes in asbestosis. Thorax 15:109-119

Wise ME, Oldham PD (1963) Effect of radiographic technique on readings of categories of simple pneumoconiosis. Br J Ind Med 20:145-153

Wollmer P, Jakobsson K, Albin M et al (1987) Measurement of lung density by X-ray computed tomography. Relation to lung mechanics in workers exposed to asbestos cement. Chest 91:865-869

Yoshimura H, Hatakeyama M, Otsuji H et al (1986) Pulmonary asbestosis: CT study of subpleural curvilinear shadow. Work in progress. Radiology 158:653-658

8 Non-Malignant Asbestos-Related Pleural Disorders

Pierre Alain Gevenois and Paul De Vuyst

CONTENTS

8.1 Pleural Plaques 223
8.1.1 Histopathology 224
8.1.2 Physiopathology 224
8.1.3 Significance 225
8.1.4 Imaging 225
8.1.4.1 Radiography 225
8.1.4.2 Computed Tomography 228
8.2 Benign Asbestos Pleural Effusion 228
8.2.1 Imaging 230
8.3 Diffuse Pleural Thickening 230
8.3.1 Physiopathology 231
8.3.2 Significance 232
8.3.3 Imaging 232
8.3.3.1 Radiography 232
8.3.3.2 Computed Tomography 232
8.4 Pericarditis 233
8.5 CT Protocols for Imaging of Non-Malignant Asbestos-Related Pleural Disorders 233
References 235

The word asbestos is a collective term that refers to a family of fibrous hydrous silicate minerals, including a serpentine (chrysotile) and amphiboles (crocidolite, amosite, tremolite). Because of its heat resistance and insulating properties, asbestos has been extensively used in most industrialized countries. The health effects of asbestos were described early in the 20th century, but it was only in the last few decades of this century that an intense medical and political debate was started, resulting in the ban of the use of these minerals in many countries and increasing restrictions in others. Even if the use of asbestos has dramatically decreased, leading to a virtual disappearance of severe cases of asbestosis (lung fibrosis), pleural manifestations are and will still frequently be diagnosed in the next decades. This is due to the very long latency between asbestos exposure and its manifestations and to the extensive use of thin-section computed tomography (CT) in the surveillance of exposed workers. In addition, malignant and non-malignant pleural diseases can be induced with low cumulative exposures, and many workers are still exposed to asbestos materials remaining in buildings.

The pleura, principally the parietal pleura, is a main target for asbestos fibers and is involved far more often than the lung parenchyma, despite the fact that the lung is the first organ reached by inhaled fibers. The precise mechanisms of translocation of fibers toward the pleura and the physiopathology of pleural fiber-induced diseases are still not well understood.

The non-malignant forms of asbestos-related pleural disorders include pleural plaques, benign pleural effusion, and diffuse pleural thickening. Although circumscribed pleural plaques and diffuse pleural thickening are considered under this broad category of asbestos-related pleural fibrosis, these processes are distinct entities that are likely to involve different pathogenic mechanisms and have different clinical consequences (Schwartz 1991).

8.1 Pleural Plaques

Pleural plaques are the most common thoracic lesions found in persons exposed to asbestos (Hillerdal and Lindgren 1980). These lesions predominantly involve the parietal pleura and are not associated with adhesions between the visceral and parietal pleural layers, unless there has been a complicating pleurisy or a surgical exploration (Schwartz 1991). Pleural plaques are most commonly found on the posterior wall of the lower half of the pleural spaces, laterally on the costal pleura, over the vertebrae, on the mediastinum, on the central part of the diaphragm,

P.A. Gevenois, MD, PhD
Clinic of Chest Imaging, Department of Radiology, Hôpital Erasme, Université Libre de Bruxelles, Brussels, Belgium
P. De Vuyst, MD, PhD
Department of Respiratory Medicine, Hôpital Erasme, Université Libre de Bruxelles, Brussels, Belgium

and, more rarely, close to the costochondral junctions on the anterior wall (Roberts 1971). They are almost never located at the apices of the pleural cavities or in the costophrenic angles. Plaques also can be found on the pericardium. Pleural plaques are most often multiple and bilateral but unilateral asbestos-related plaques have been reported in up to 25–35% of asbestos-exposed patients with plaques (Fisher 1985; Gevenois et al. 1998; Neri et al. 1994). They have also been described to occur on the visceral pleura, within the interlobar fissures (Rockoff 1987; Sargent et al. 1981; Solomon et al. 1979), and exceptional cases of calcification within the fissures have been reported (Sargent et al. 1981; Rockoff 1987; Remy-Jardin et al. 2004).

8.1.1 Histopathology

Macroscopically, pleural plaques are discrete, raised, and irregularly shaped areas (Roberts 1971). They vary in size from a few millimeters to 10 cm. The thinner plaques are only slightly raised above the pleural surface, while the thicker plaques are either smooth or show a fine or coarse nodularity. Most of the plaques have a leathery consistency, but as pleural plaques tend to calcify with time, more heavily calcified plaques are brittle and can be fractured (Roberts 1971).

Microscopically, the pleural plaques consist of undulating dense fibrous bands of avascular collagen, lying parallel to the surface (Roberts 1971). They are relatively acellular with only occasional spindle-shaped fibroblasts, do not contain histologically visible asbestos bodies (Meurman 1968; Roberts 1971), and are covered with a normal mesothelium (Gefter and Conant 1988).

8.1.2 Physiopathology

The mechanism of the induction of pleural plaques is unknown, but they are so frequent that they probably represent the "normal" tissular reaction to the abnormal presence of fibers in the lung or in the pleura. Indeed, in animal studies, the development of plaques requires a normal immune response, whereas less well-organized pleural reactions occur when the immunity is modified by cytotoxic agents (Sahn and Antony 1984).

In contrast with the fact that pleural plaques are specifically associated with asbestos exposure, mineralogical studies have rarely detected such fibers in the parietal pleura. Boutin et al. (1996) hypothesized that the distribution of asbestos fibers in the pleura is heterogeneous and that these are concentrated in certain areas, probably derived from Wang's pores and/or milky spots present at the surface of the parietal pleura. These structures are connected with the subpleural lymphatic network and are involved in the physiological clearance mechanisms of the pleural space (Kanazawa et al. 1979). In humans, milky spots are almost invisible on healthy pleura. However, direct examination of the pleura using thoracoscopy or autopsy frequently visualizes foci of anthracosis near lymphatic vessels of the parietal pleura (Boutin et al. 1991). They are found in more than 90% of urban dwellers at autopsy (Mitchev et al. 2002). They contain macrophages and lymphocytes. The pigmentation of these "black spots" is due to accumulation of inhaled exogenous dusts (coal, soot), and they are mainly located in the posterior and lower part of the costovertebral gutter and on the diaphragm (Mitchev et al. 2002). Most importantly, it has been shown that asbestos fibers, including long carcinogenic amphibole fibers, are heterogeneously distributed in the parietal pleural and that they concentrate in these black spots, whereas few or no fibers are detected in macroscopically normal pleural areas. The accumulation of fibers in these black spots make them possible starting points for asbestos-induced lesions of the parietal pleura (Fig. 8.1). The correspondence between the number, type, and dimensions of fibers in black spots and in the respective lungs is consistent with a mechanism of direct migration of fibers from the alveoli into the pleural cavity through the

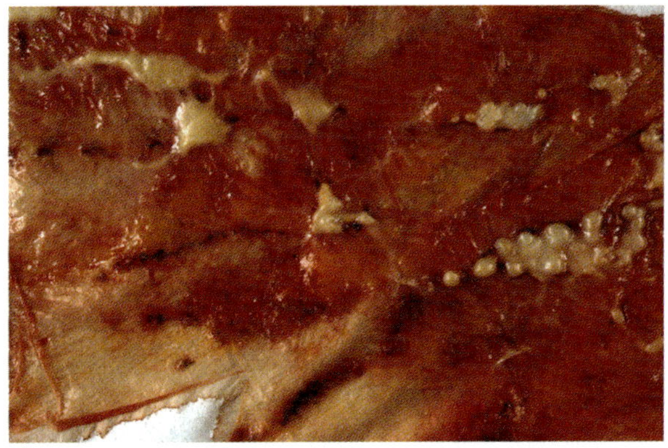

Fig. 8.1. Macroscopic aspect of the parietal pleura of a past heating worker exposed to asbestos, coal, and soot dusts (autopsy specimen). Pleural plaques are visible in close contact with foci of anthracosis ("black spots")

visceral pleural and absorption by the parietal pleura through Wang stoma and/or milky spots (Boutin et al. 1991). In rats, Rey et al. observed that after intratracheal instillation, crocidolite and chrysotile fibers pass into the pleural space (Rey et al. 1993). Another possible pathway for rapid dissemination of short fibers is the bloodstream (Monchaux et al. 1982), as the glomerular vascular structure of milky spots may facilitate the uptake of circulating fibers. Kanazawa et al. demonstrated that asbestos fibers concentrated only in milky spots (Kanazawa et al. 1979) after subcutaneous or intravenous injection in mice. Finally, fibers could also migrate via the lymphatic system pathway (Taskinen et al. 1973; Hillerdal 1980). This pathway is responsible for translocation of inhaled particles such as silica or coal into lymphoid tissue, particularly in regional lymph nodes (Dodson et al.1990; Roggli and Benning 1990). Further, whatever the pathway(s), once fibers have reached the parietal pleura, they could initiate a prolonged process of fibroblast stimulation and collagen formation (Hillerdal 1980; Rey et al. 1993; Boutin et al. 1996). Another hypothesis involves the possible role of pro-inflammatory cytokines, which are produced in the lung exposed to asbestos and could reach the pleura. This could lead to inflammatory and fibrotic reactions of the pleura, without a direct contact between the fibers and the target organ (Adamson et al. 1994).

8.1.3 Significance

The clinical significance of pleural plaques is their importance as a marker of asbestos exposure in individuals or populations. Asbestos exposure is indeed the far most important if not the sole cause of typical plaques. Their presence indicates a potential risk of developing a more severe asbestos-related disease but otherwise has no clinical impact, except the psychological consequences of fearing such diseases (Hillerdal 1987; Sison et al. 1989). However, a pleural plaque is not a "premalignant" lesion and does not evolve in mesothelioma.

The possible increased risk for bronchogenic carcinoma in patients with pleural plaques is still a matter of debate (Smith 1984). Epidemiological studies are difficult to conduct, as they should adequately control for asbestos fiber type, duration and intensity of asbestos exposure, as well as cigarette smoking habits, race, gender, and exposure to other potential carcinogens (Smith 1984). Nevertheless, it seems that there is no difference in the incidence of lung cancer between individuals with pleural plaques and controls matched for exposure but without pleural plaques. It should be reminded that pleural plaques are not pulmonary lesions and that the parietal pleura is anatomically very far from the bronchi, where asbestos-related cancers may develop (Wain et al. 1984).

As a summary, the presence or absence of plaques does not appear to modify the risk for mesothelioma or lung cancer among individuals who have the same level and type of exposure.

Plaques may occur after low cumulative or short exposures, but in occupationally exposed groups, the prevalence of plaques increases with increasing dose as asbestos inhaled. While the overall incidence of pleural plaques increases with dose, there is not a linear correlation between plaque extent and total dust exposure. The prevalence continues to increase more than 40 years after first exposure to asbestos and is not affected by smoking (Harries et al. 1972; Lilis et al. 1991). The progression of plaques is most directly related to the length of time from initial exposure rather than the dose of ongoing exposure (Gefter and Conant 1988). The latency period between exposure to asbestos and development of pleural plaques, as detected by chest radiography, varies greatly, with a mean of approximately 33 years, and it is very infrequent to observe pleural plaques after less than 10 years of latency (Hillerdal 1978).

Pleural plaques are generally asymptomatic, but thoracic pain has been reported in cases with extensive plaques. Several studies based on chest radiographs have reported mild impairment of pulmonary restriction in subjects with pleural plaques, but pieces of evidence suggest that concomitant parenchyma fibrosis is the principle determinant of restrictive lung function seen in persons with asbestos-related pleural plaques. Recently, using CT to quantify the surface area of pleural plaques, Van Cleemput et al. clearly demonstrated that neither their presence nor their extent is correlated with lung function parameters (Van Cleemput et al. 2001).

8.1.4 Imaging

8.1.4.1 Radiography

On chest radiographs, the earliest radiographic change suggesting a pleural plaque is a thin line of soft tissue density adjacent to the seventh or eighth ribs, which often may be mistaken as a companion shadow (Fletcher and Edge 1970). At a more advanced stage, pleural plaques appear as bilateral uneven opacities, situated mainly in the flanks – between the fifth and the tenth ribs – and/or the middle portions of the diaphragm, from few millimeters to approximately 1-cm thick, which may contain calcifications with clear costophrenic angles (Hillerdal and Lindgren 1980; Rosenstock and Hudson 1986). The radiographic appearance of plaques varies, depending on their orientation to the X-ray beam; when seen in profile (parallel to the beam), they are denser with more distinct borders than when seen *en face* (at right angles to the beam) (Rosenstock and Hudson 1986). On chest radiograph, the pleural plaque is identified as a localized area of increased density along the peripheral chest wall, intervening between the lung air lucency and the chest wall. They range from several millimeters to many centimeters in length but rarely extend more than four interspaces in length. Pleural plaques may also be seen *en face*. In this instance, they often appear to be a nodule with irregular margins. These radiographic findings are illustrated in Figures 8.2–8.4.

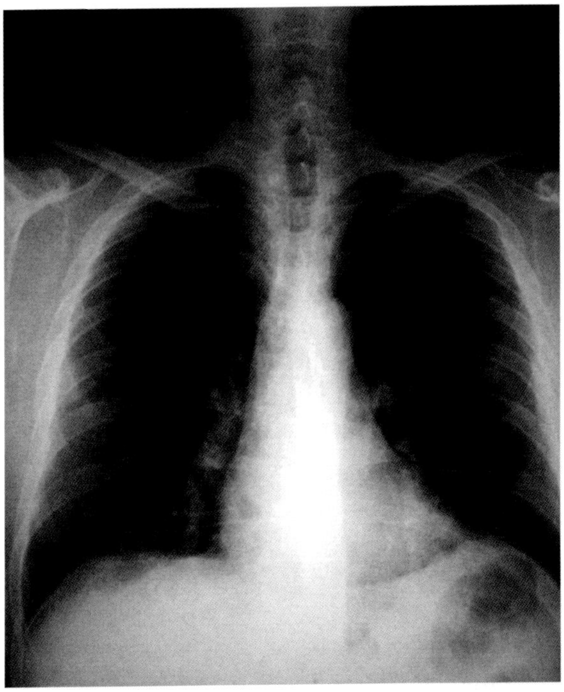

Fig. 8.2. Postero-anterior chest radiograph shows non-calcified pleural plaques appearing as bilateral uneven opacities with clear costophrenic angles

The diagnostic performance of radiography for the detection of pleural plaques must be examined relative to the gold standard of plaque detection – autopsy (Gefter and Conant 1988). Depending on the diagnostic criteria used, 15–50% of plaques found at visual inspection of the pleural cavity at autopsy or at surgical operation can be diagnosed from chest radiograph. Radiographic detection of pleural plaques is greatly influenced by their calcium content, and detection of non-calcified plaques depends on their thickness, as plaques less than 3-mm thick at autopsy are not detectable radiographically (Svenes et al. 1986).

Plaques must be differentiated from normal anatomic structures, such as costal slips of the origins

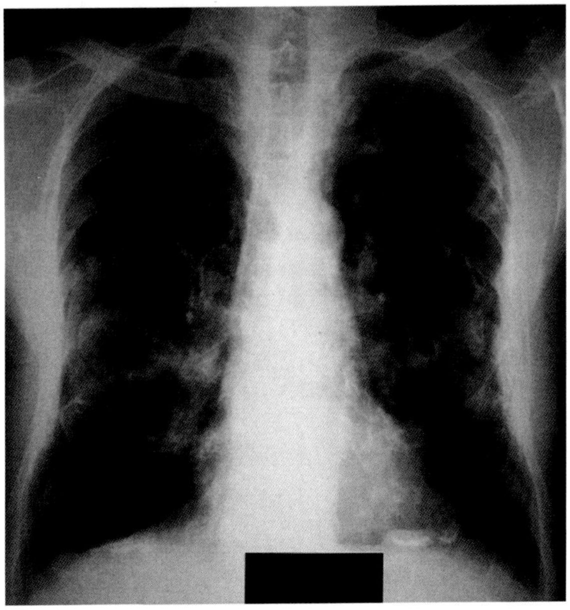

Fig. 8.3. Postero-anterior chest radiograph shows calcified pleural plaques appearing as bilateral dense opacities

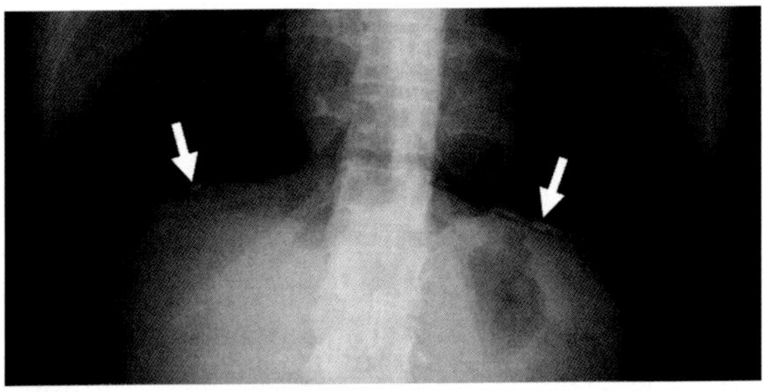

Fig. 8.4. Postero-anterior chest radiograph shows diaphragmatic calcified pleural plaques seen in profile (*arrows*), parallel to the X-ray beam

of the anterior serratus and external oblique muscles that may cause a prominent rhythmic sequence of shadows between successive intercostal spaces (Sargent et al. 1977). Another normal shadow that should not be confused with pleural plaques is the so-called companion shadow, which parallels the medial surface of the first three or four ribs and is most prominent along the second rib (Fig. 8.5) (Gefter and Conant 1988). This shadow characteristically tapers as it projects inferiorly, usually becoming imperceptible below the level of the fourth intercostal interspace (Sargent et al. 1977). This opacity is thought to represent a combination of intercostal muscles and fatty tissue. Rib fracture callus and early pleural metastatic disease may also mimic pleural plaques (Fig. 8.6) (Gefter and Conant 1988).

In addition, extrapleural fat pads may mimic pleural thickening. Generally, they increase in size and extent in obese patients and also vary with nutritional status; however, they can be quite extensive, even in patients without excess body fat (Sargent et al. 1984). They are often accompanied by prominent pericardial fat pads and the mediastinal widening of lipomatosis. Extrapleural fat usually accumulates in a posterior distribution, often with symmetric and smooth, wavy contours. It is generally not focal but diffuse, extending from the apices to the base, parallels the chest wall, and is often of greatest thickness over the lung apices, an unusual distribution for asbestos-related pleural disorder (Fig. 8.7) (Sargent et al. 1984). Calcification is helpful if present to distinguish plaques from extrapleural fat pads, but calcification occurs in only 15% of pleural plaques on plain films (Sargent et al. 1984). In some cases, pleural plaques may occur in areas of extrapleural fat deposition, which can be extremely confusing on the plain film (Gefter and Conant 1988).

Radiography, thus, has some limitations. A first limitation is that thin pleural plaques may be overlooked, especially if non-calcified and if viewed *en face*. Autopsy studies have shown that the plain radiograph demonstrates only a small percentage of pleural plaques detected by autopsy (Hourihane et al. 1966; Svenes et al. 1986). Oblique films, which bring off-midline, *en face* plaques into profile, have been suggested to increase the detection of plaques on radiographs. However, the routine use of oblique views has certain limitations. Normal peripheral densities, such as companion shadows and slips of the internal intercostal muscles, become more apparent and erroneously may be identified as pleural plaques (McLoud et al. 1985). Oblique films are,

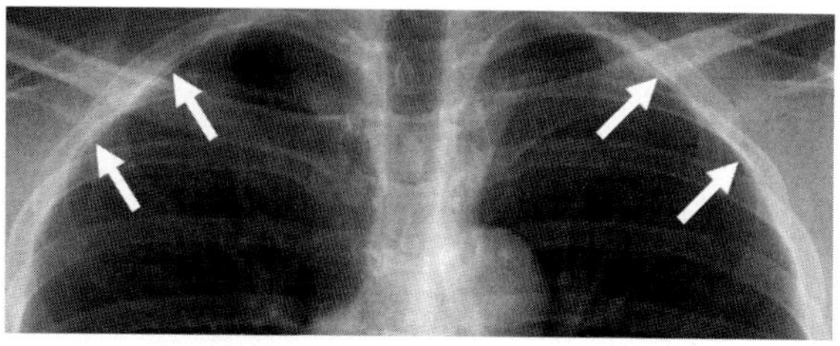

Fig. 8.5. Postero-anterior chest radiograph shows the so-called companion shadow (*arrows*), which parallels the medial surface of the first three or four ribs and is most prominent along the second rib

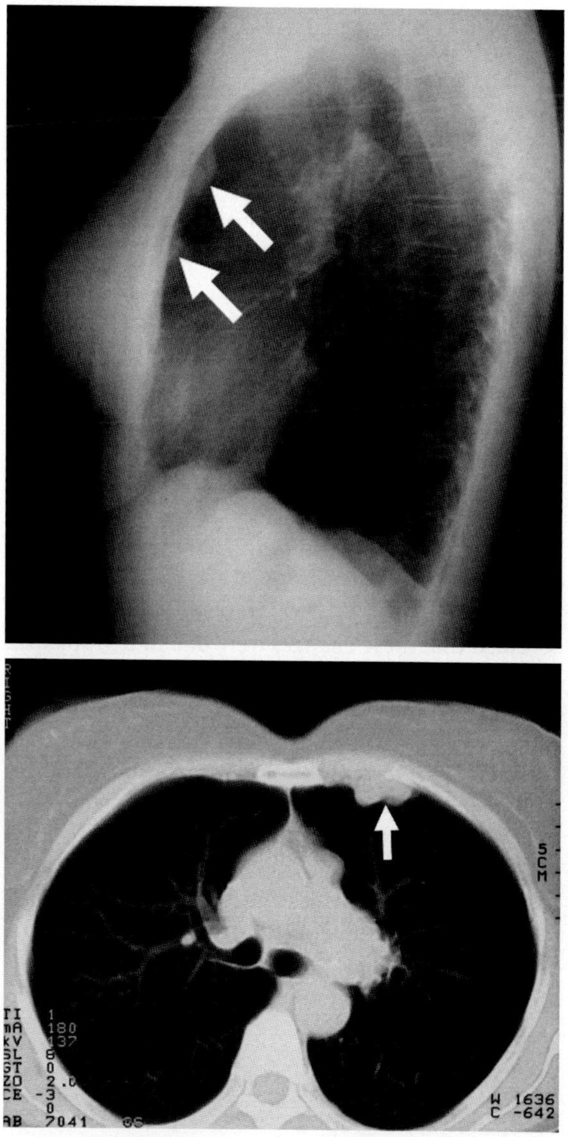

Fig. 8.6a,b. Lateral chest radiograph (**a**) and computed tomography scan of the chest (**b**) show smooth pleural thickening (*arrows*) in a patient with left renal carcinoma and homolateral pleural metastasis

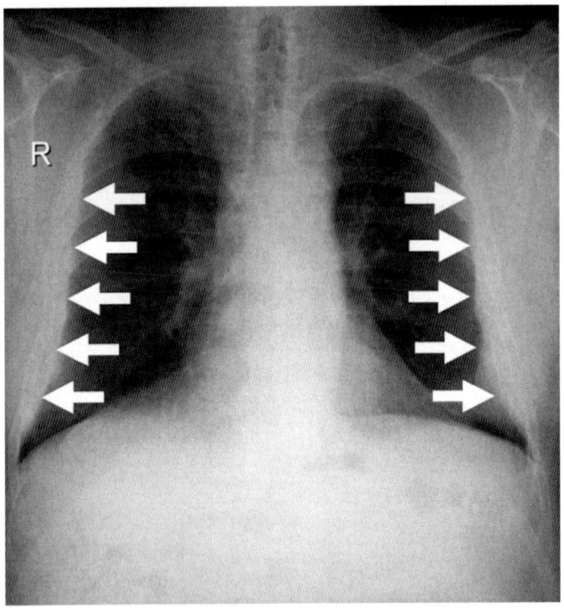

Fig. 8.7. Postero-anterior chest radiograph shows extrapleural symmetric and smooth fat pads, with wavy contours, mimicking pleural thickening (*arrows*)

thus, no longer recommended. A second limitation is that normal thoracic structures, such as muscles or fat pads, may be confused with pleural plaques. Sargent et al. reported that, in a study group of 31 patients with known asbestos exposure who were studied by CT because of uncertainty as to whether the pleural changes observed on the radiographs were due to plaques or extrapleural fat pads, CT revealed that these changes were due to extrapleural fat in 48% of them (Sargent et al. 1984). This study clearly illustrates the insufficient specificity of chest radiography. A third limitation of radiography is a considerable interreader variability, the proportion of agreement between two *B* readers ranging from 68% to 93% when pleural plaques are searched on frontal views (Frumkin et al. 1990). Interestingly, the interreader variability increases with the use of oblique views. All these limitations largely explain that the major role currently played by CT is the assessment of asbestos-related pleural abnormalities.

8.1.4.2 Computed Tomography

On CT, pleural plaques are visible as single or multiple discrete irregular or smooth lines or as small masses of various thickness and length, which may contain calcifications, and are often separated by a thin fat layer from underlying rib or muscle (Figs. 8.8–8.13).

No study has investigated the diagnostic performance of CT in detecting pleural plaques by comparison with autopsy as the method of reference, but more plaques are detected using CT than radiography and, except for obviously calcified plaques, CT eliminates false-positive diagnoses of asbestos-related pleural disease caused by extrapleural fat (Friedman et al. 1988). CT is, thus, now widely recommended to detect pleural plaques in asbestos-exposed workers and plays an important role in medico-legal and compensation issues.

To detect pleural plaques with the highest possible sensitivity, CT should consist of contiguous sections without any gap, which can be easily achieved with multidetector CT (MDCT) scanners, the entire thorax being scanned during one breath hold at full inspiration. Sequential modes of scanning with gaps between two successive images acquisition, as has been recommended to investigate the lung parenchyma using thin-section CT obtained with 1- to 3-cm intervals, are insufficient for excluding the presence of plaques (Gevenois et al. 1994; Remy-Jardin et al. 2004).

8.2 Benign Asbestos Pleural Effusion

Among asbestos-related pleural disorders, benign effusion is the most recent to come to our atten-

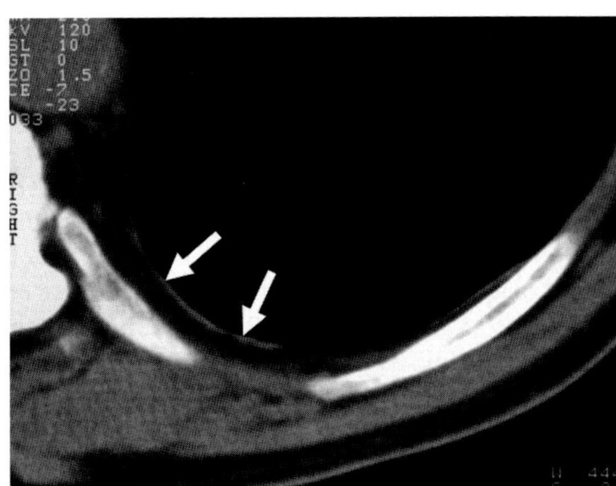

Fig. 8.8. Computed tomography scan of the chest shows posterior pleural plaque appearing as a discrete smooth line of soft tissue attenuation (*arrows*)

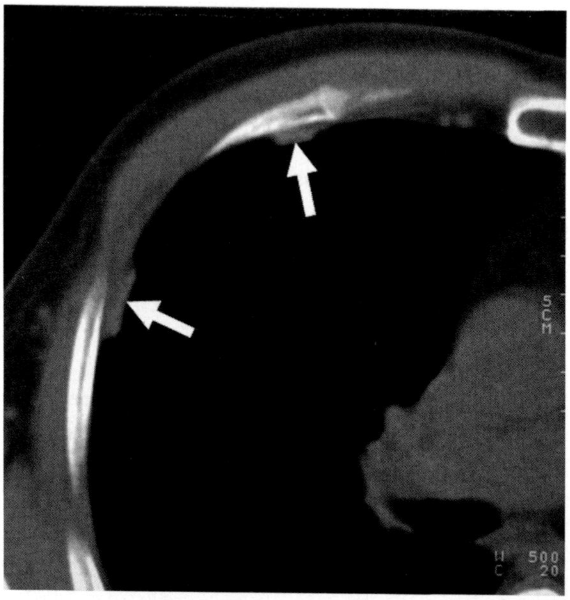

Fig. 8.9. Computed tomography scan of the chest shows anterior and lateral pleural plaques appearing as a discrete smooth line of soft tissue attenuation (*arrows*)

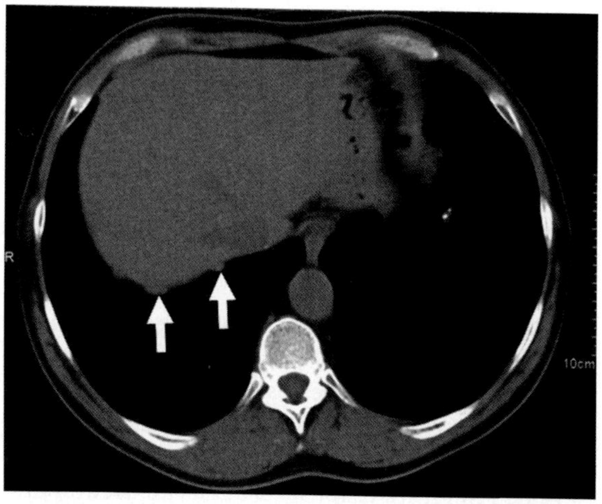

Fig. 8.10. Computed tomography scan of the chest shows diaphragmatic pleural plaque appearing as small masses of soft tissue attenuation (*arrows*)

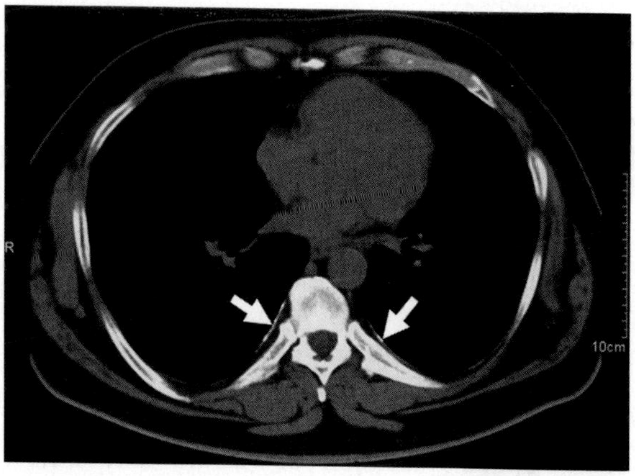

Fig. 8.12. Computed tomography scan of the chest shows posterior calcified pleural plaque appearing as a discrete smooth line of calcium attenuation (*arrows*)

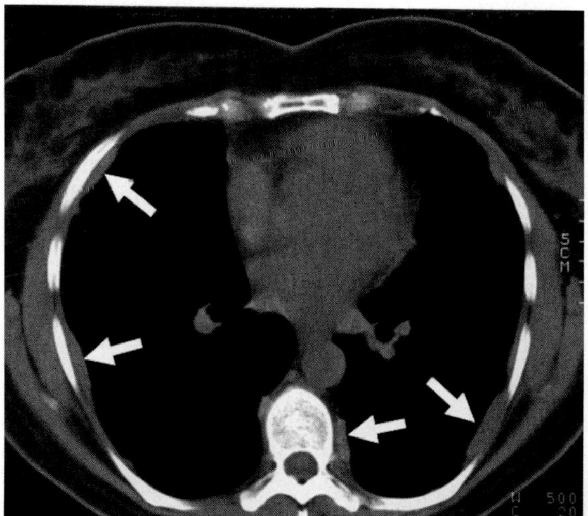

Fig. 8.11. Computed tomography scan of the chest shows extensive anterior-lateral and postero-lateral pleural plaques appearing as smooth lines of soft tissue attenuation (*arrows*)

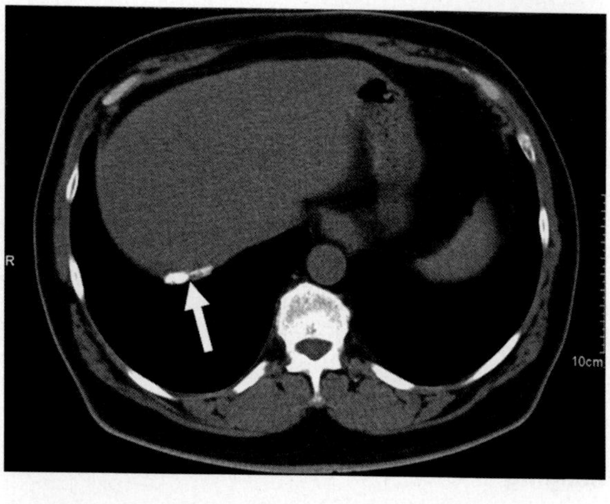

Fig. 8.13. Computed tomography scan of the chest shows calcified diaphragmatic pleural plaque appearing as a discrete line of calcium attenuation (*arrow*)

tion (Gaensler and Kaplan 1971). Benign asbestos effusion is defined by four criteria: direct or indirect exposure to asbestos, an effusion confirmed by a transient pleural change in serial films or by thoracocentesis, lack of evidence of any other cause of pleural effusion, and no malignant tumor detected within 3 years after the effusion (Epler et al. 1982). In asbestos-exposed individuals, thoracoscopy and PET scan are now frequently performed to discriminate benign pleural effusion from mesothelioma.

There is an obvious and positive relationship between exposure to asbestos and prevalence of effusions (Epler et al. 1982). Benign asbestos effusion is virtually the only manifestation seen within the first 10 years after initial exposure, but it can occur many years after exposure to asbestos (Hillerdal and Ozesmi 1987). This contrasts with pleural plaques that are almost absent during the first 10 years after initial exposure.

Benign asbestos pleural effusion may resolve spontaneously, recur on the same side or occur later on the other side. Two-thirds of patients are asymptomatic, and, in those who present symptoms, pleuritic pain is the most frequent (Epler et al. 1982; Hillerdal and Ozesmi 1987), which can be relieved by anti-inflammatory analgesics. Benign asbestos effusion can be associated with cough and/or dyspnea (Epler et al. 1982; Hillerdal and Ozesmi 1987). The acute form may be associated with fever, leukocytosis, high sedimentation rate, and general systemic symptoms (Eisenstadt 1974). Spontaneous resolution of each episode within 1–10 months is usual (Hillerdal and Ozesmi 1987), but the condition may be recurrent, with increasing diffuse pleural thickening after each episode (Gaensler and Kaplan 1971).

Pleural fluid is an exudate, which may contain lymphocytes and mesothelial cells but is more classically associated with eosinophils, up to 50% of total number of nucleated cells (Hillerdal and Ozesmi 1987; Sahn and Heffner 2003). Macroscopically, it appears hemorrhagic in approximately 50% of patients (Hillerdal and Ozesmi 1987), and it is, thus, very important to emphasize that a blood-stained effusion in an asbestos worker does not necessarily imply mesothelioma (Rudd 1996).

8.2.1 Imaging

Benign asbestos pleural effusion may be the sole manifestation of asbestos disease, so that neither plain films nor CT depict specific findings of pleural plaques or asbestosis. Because of very large differences in latency times, coexistent pleural plaques are relatively rare, since they are only present in approximately one-fifth of patients (Epler et al. 1982). As benign asbestos effusion is frequently asymptomatic and can be recurrent, sequelae of a previous unknown episode, such as rounded atelectasis and parenchymal bands, reflecting the visceral pleural fibrosis, can coexist with current pleural effusion (Martensson et al. 1987).

Follow-up radiographs showed blunted costophrenic angles in virtually all cases, and residual diffuse pleural thickening in one-half (Epler et al. 1982) of cases. Follow-up CT scans can disclose diffuse pleural thickening as well, with a possible small amount of remnant fluid within the pleural cavity (Figs. 8.14 and 8.15).

8.3 Diffuse Pleural Thickening

Diffuse pleural thickening involves the visceral pleura or both the visceral and parietal pleura and the subpleural peripheral lung tissue. The word "diffuse" refers to its extent by opposition to circumscribed pleural plaques, but the definitions are numerous. On plain films, McLoud et al. have defined diffuse

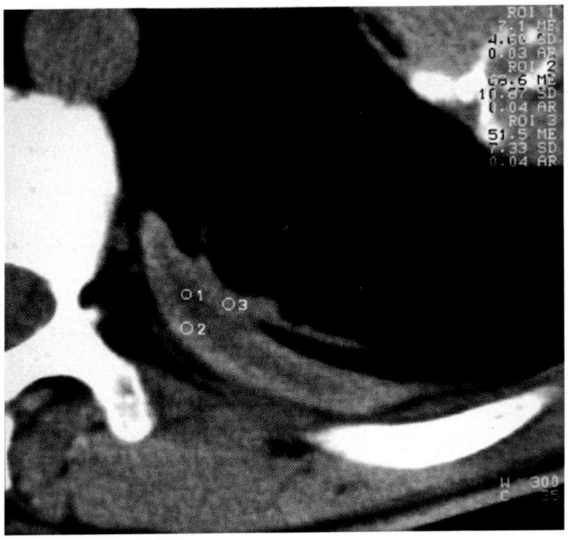

Fig. 8.14. Computed tomography scan of the chest photographed in mediastinal window settings shows a small amount of remnant fluid within the left pleural cavity in a patient who had a benign asbestos pleurisy

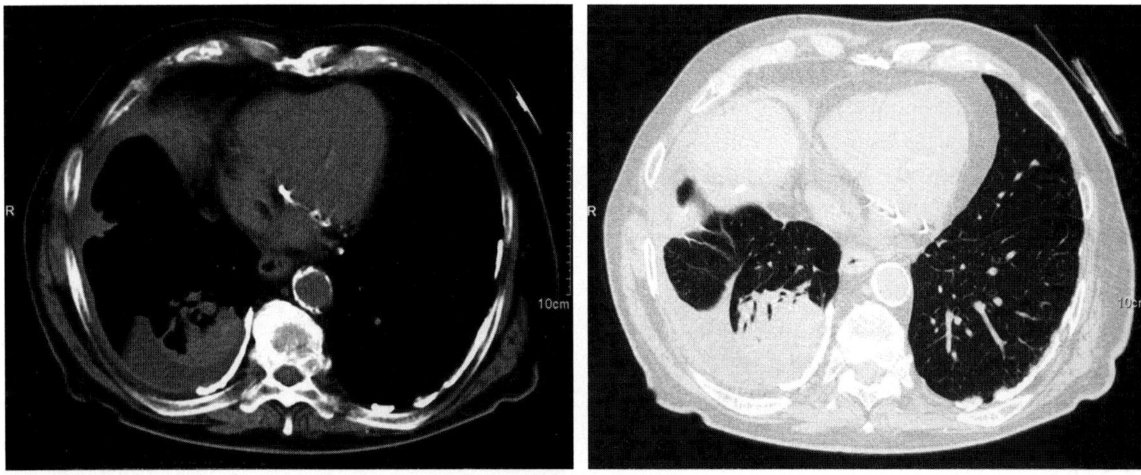

a b

Fig. 8.15a,b. Computed tomography scan of the chest photographed in mediastinal (**a**) and pulmonary (**b**) window settings shows a small amount of remnant fluid within the right pleural cavity in a patient who had a benign asbestos pleurisy. Note the presence of bilateral calcified pleural plaques, and parenchymal bands and rounded atelectasis in the right lower lobe

pleural thickening on its craniocaudal extent as a smooth, non-interrupted pleural density extending over at least one-fourth of the chest wall, with or without costophrenic-angle obliteration (McLoud et al. 1985), while Lynch et al. have defined a pleural thickening as diffuse when it extends craniocaudally more than 8 cm or obliterates the costophrenic angle (Lynch et al. 1988). However, Hillerdal has defined diffuse pleural thickening, independently of its extent, as a thickening that involves the costophrenic angle and the mid- and apical pleural space (Hillerdal 1987). On CT, Lynch et al. have defined diffuse pleural thickening as a continuous sheet of pleural thickening more than 5-cm wide, more than 8 cm in craniocaudal extent, and more than 3-mm thick (Lynch 1989).

With the recent extensive use of CT in asbestos-exposed workers, attention has been paid to lung involvement associated with pleural thickening in the form of parenchymal bands and rounded atelectasis that reflect the fibrosis of the visceral pleura (Solomon 1989; Cohen et al. 1993; Gevenois et al. 1998). These associated findings help us to distinguish visceral pleural fibrosis from parietal pleural plaques and have revealed that visceral pleural fibrosis can be focal.

8.3.1 Physiopathology

Previously, diffuse pleural thickening was usually thought to be secondary to the extension of pulmonary fibrosis (asbestosis) to both the visceral and parietal pleura. With the definition reported above, McLoud et al. have shown that the most common cause of such diffuse pleural thickening was prior benign pleural effusion related to asbestos exposure, accounting for approximately one-third of cases (McLoud et al. 1985). Diffuse pleural thickening is now thought to be the result, in descending order of frequency (Gefter and Conant 1988), of benign asbestos-related effusion, confluent plaques, or extension of parenchymal fibrosis. Pleural thickening often begins on one side, with effusion followed by pleural thickening, to be followed months or years later by a similar episode on the other side (Rudd 1996). Benign asbestos pleural effusion is probably the major, if not the only cause of this particular asbestos-related pleural disorder, characterized by fibrosis of the visceral pleura, often associated with pleural adhesions, and that, radiographically, appears as diffuse pleural thickening. Diffuse pleural thickening tends to progress gradually, mainly during the first 15 years after its onset (de Klerk et al. 1989).

A wide range of fiber counts is observed in association with this condition (Roggli et al. 1986), but the levels in cases with diffuse pleural fibrosis are of similar order of magnitude to those in cases of mild to moderate asbestosis (Rudd 1996, Stephens et al. 1987). Independently of the burden of inhaled fibers, their type plays an important role – diffuse pleural thickening being much more frequent than plaques in crocidolite workers, supporting the role of amphibole fibers in its causation (de Klerk et al. 1989).

8.3.2 Significance

Diffuse pleural thickening is not a specific asbestos-related disorder and, as such, is not a reliable marker of exposure. Moreover, patients who have been exposed to asbestos may have coincidental pleural thickening due to trauma, infection, inflammation, recurrent pneumothorax or drug intake (Herbert 1986; Mossman and Gee 1989). Asbestos-exposed workers can, of course, develop pleural diseases of other origins and could even be at higher risk for developing pleural disease due to ergot drugs (De Vuyst et al. 1997).

The characteristic features of diffuse pleural thickening on lung function testing are a restrictive ventilatory defect, decreased compliance, a reduction in total lung capacity, and impairment of gas transfer characterized by a low carbon monoxide transfer factor with a normal or increased carbon monoxide transfer coefficient (Schwartz et al. 1990). The degree of impairment of lung function correlates with the extent of pleural disease assessed using CT (Al Jarad et al. 1991; Al Jarad N et al. 1992; Schwartz et al. 1993) and is independent of coexisting pleural plaques, parenchymal fibrosis, or rounded atelectasis (Kee et al. 1996); however the two latter lesions may, of course, contribute to loss of lung volume. Unilateral disease may cause disability, although it is less severe than that associated with bilateral disease (Rudd 1996). Interestingly, longitudinal lung function studies showed that initial decrement in lung function is followed by comparatively little change over time, even if diffuse pleural thickening increases radiographically with time (Yates et al. 1996).

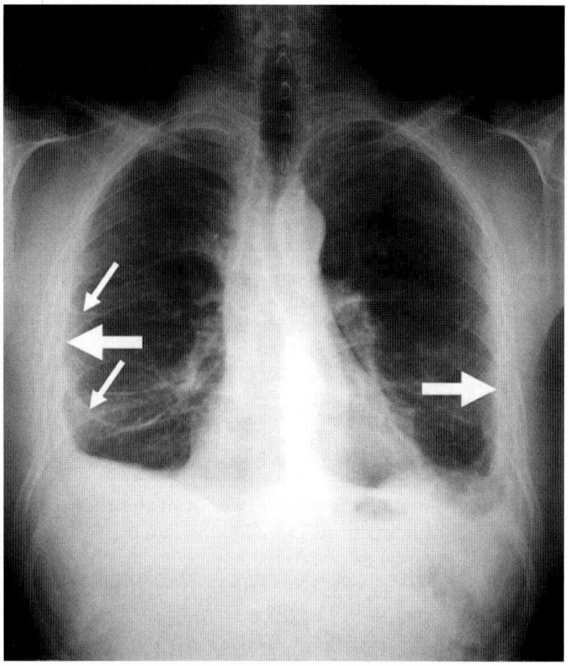

Fig. 8.16. Postero-anterior chest radiograph shows bilateral diffuse pleural thickening with non-interrupted pleural density extending over at least one-fourth of the chest wall (*large arrows*), with parenchymal bands, particularly well visible on the right side (*thin arrows*), and bilateral costophrenic-angle obliteration

8.3.3 Imaging

8.3.3.1 Radiography

The chest radiograph shows pleural thickening along the chest walls. The costophrenic angles are often obliterated and, when the condition is extensive, the diaphragmatic and cardiac contours may be obscured. Fibrous strands extending from thickened pleura may have a "crow's feet" appearance, and rounded atelectasis may be seen (Fig. 8.16). The pleural thickening occasionally involves only or mainly the upper lobes, with a radiological appearance difficult to distinguish from that of past tuberculosis (Olivier and Neville 1988; Hillerdal 1990).

Rounded atelectasis presents as a rounded, sharply marginated, pleural-based mass with a comet tail extension (Mintzer and Cugell 1982) (Figs. 8.17 and 8.18). The mass has an intrapulmonary location, as manifested by an acute angle seen between it and the pleura. Pleural thickening, widest near the mass, is present, and frequently there is thickening of the ipsilateral intralobar fissure (Mintzer et al. 1981; Mintzer and Cugell 1982). When previous chest films are available for comparison, the appearance of the process is frequently static (Mintzer and Cugell 1982).

8.3.3.2 Computed Tomography

CT demonstrates the extent of the pleural thickening more clearly than the plain chest radiograph, particularly in the region of paravertebral gutter, which is very frequently involved and difficult to assess

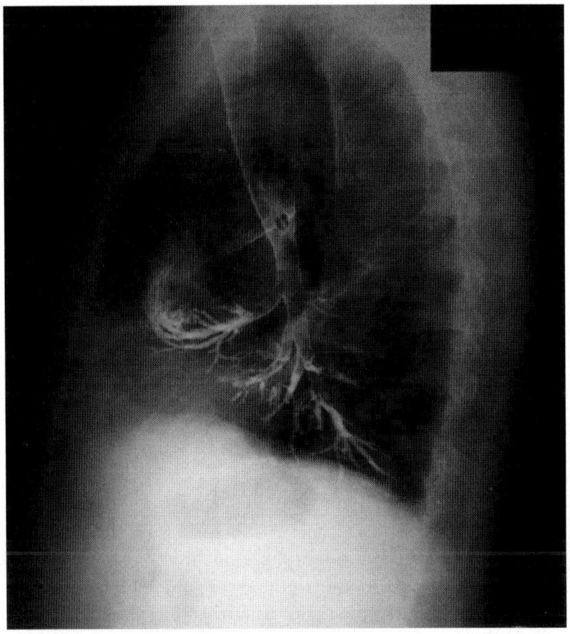

Fig. 8.17. Lateral view of a bronchography shows a rounded atelectasis in the right middle lobe, with the comet tail of bronchi sweeping into the posterior and inferior aspect of the atelectasis

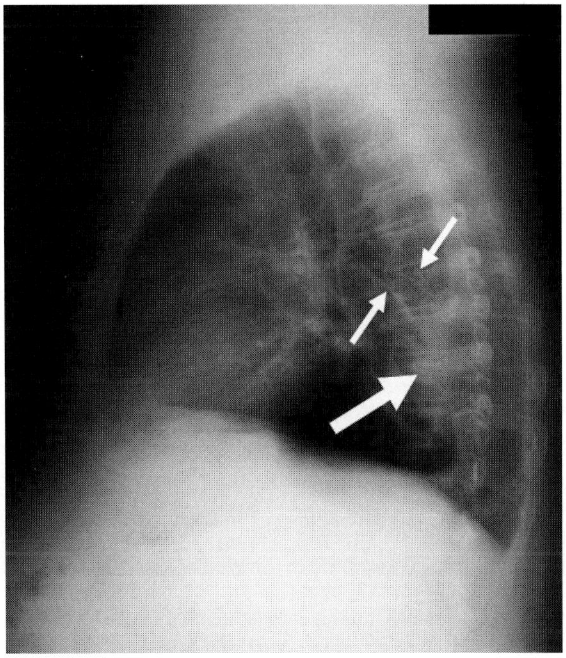

Fig. 8.18. Lateral radiograph shows a posterior rounded atelectasis (*large arrow*) associated with parenchymal bands (*thin arrows*)

on the plain radiograph (Rudd 1996). CT aids differentiation between multiple discrete plaques and diffuse pleural thickening (Al Jarad et al. 1991), and CT is helpful in identifying what may appear to be a mass lesion on the plain radiograph as a parenchymal band or rounded atelectasis (Lynch et al. 1988). More importantly, by detecting rounded atelectasis and parenchymal bands more accurately than the plain chest radiograph, CT will help us in differentiating visceral pleural fibrosis from parietal pleural fibrosis (Lynch et al. 1988; Gevenois et al. 1998).

The signs at CT typical of rounded atelectasis are a mass related to a pleural abnormality, evidence of lung volume loss in the surrounding lung, partial interposition of lung between pleura and mass, and visible comet tail of vessels and bronchi sweeping into the lateral, or medial and lateral, aspect of the mass (Lynch et al. 1988) (Figs. 8.19 and 8.20). When these criteria are fulfilled, no further examination is needed to exclude malignancy (Hillerdal 1989).

Parenchymal bands consist of linear densities 2–5 cm in length, usually contacting the pleural surface and distinguishable from pulmonary blood vessels in that they are thicker, do not taper peripherally, and are often oriented in a direction incompatible with normal vessels (Fig. 8.21) (Aberle et al. 1988).

8.4 Pericarditis

Exposure to asbestos occasionally causes benign pericardial effusion, thickening, and calcification (Figs. 8.22 and 8.23) (Davies et al. 1991). These manifestations are analogous to the effects of asbestos on the pleura, and pericardial disease is usually associated with pleural disease. The pericardial thickening may result in constrictive pericarditis with functional cardiac consequences. Both anatomical and functional aspects of pericardial constriction may be demonstrated by magnetic resonance imaging (Al Jarad et al. 1993).

8.5 CT Protocols for Imaging of Non-Malignant Asbestos-Related Pleural Disorders

Both the expense and the time required to perform CT of the entire thorax have made this examination impractical for examining large asbestos-exposed populations (McLoud 1988). In addition, chest CT protocols have been associated with relatively high radiation doses to patients, which have raised

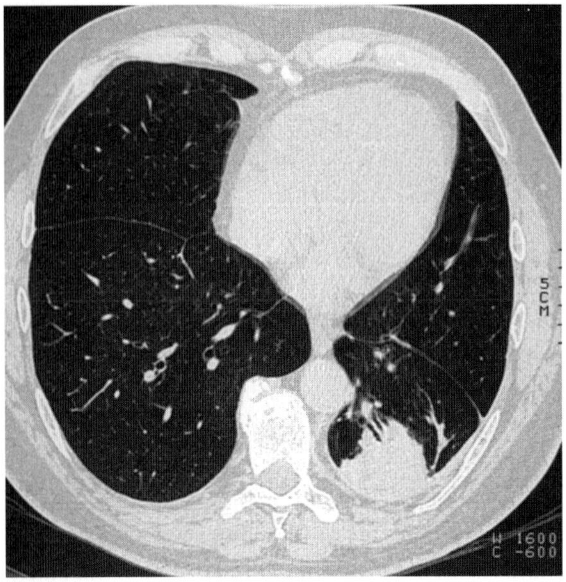

Fig. 8.19. Computed tomography scan of the chest shows a rounded atelectasis in the left lower lobe associated with a left diffuse pleural thickening. Note the backward displacement of the left fissure compared with the right major fissure, as the evidence of lung volume loss in the surrounding lung. Other findings are the partial interposition of lung between the pleura and the mass and the visible comet tail of vessels and bronchi sweeping into the medial and lateral aspect of the mass

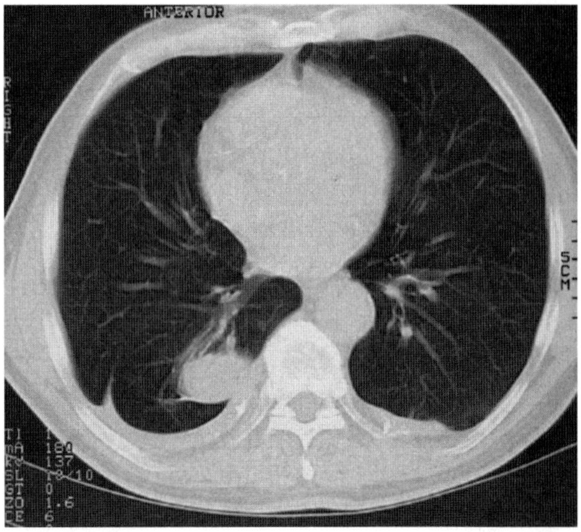

Fig. 8.20. Computed tomography scan of the chest shows a rounded atelectasis in the right lower lobe. Note the backward displacement of the major fissure as the evidence of lung volume loss in the surrounding lung. Other findings are the right calcified diffuse pleural thickening and the left calcified pleural plaque

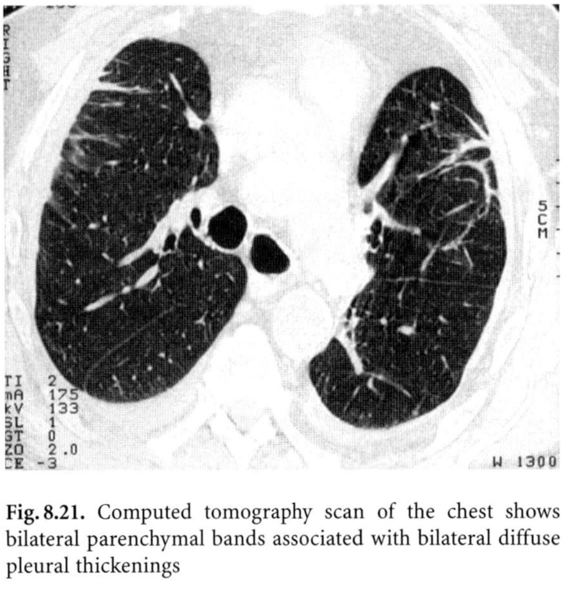

Fig. 8.21. Computed tomography scan of the chest shows bilateral parenchymal bands associated with bilateral diffuse pleural thickenings

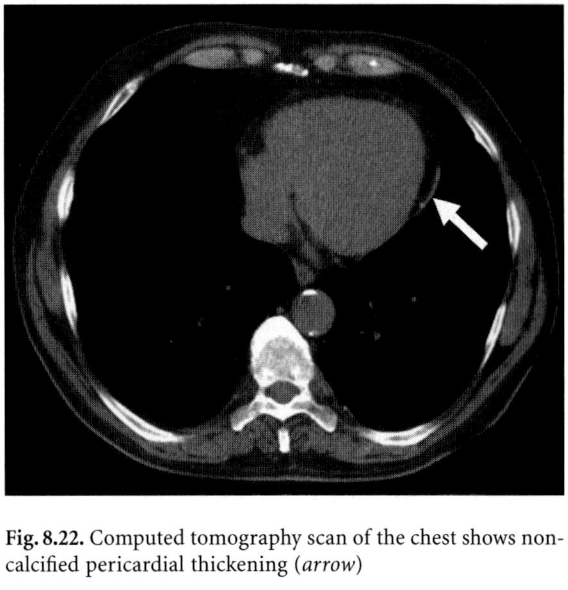

Fig. 8.22. Computed tomography scan of the chest shows non-calcified pericardial thickening (*arrow*)

concern about the potential for induced malignant disease, particularly in screening settings (Remy-Jardin 2004). The introduction of low-dose helical scanning techniques has facilitated renewed interest in the potential usefulness of CT as a first-line imaging technique. Adjustments to scanning parameters at the console, as well as automatic dose modulation systems, are used so that the radiation dose is as low as possible yet sufficient to yield the required image quality (Tack et al. 2003). With use

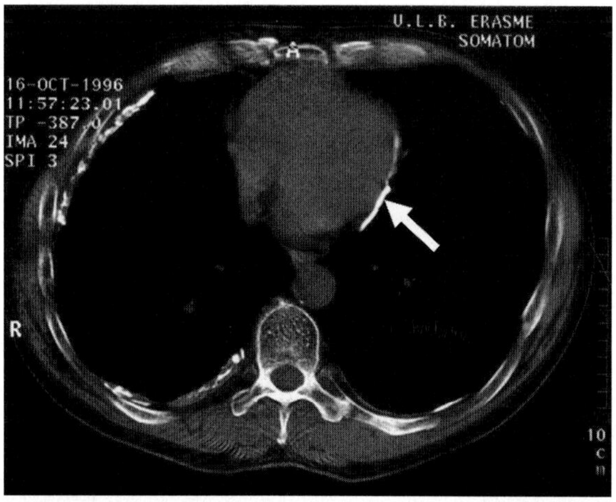

Fig. 8.23. Computed tomography scan of the chest shows calcified pericardial thickening (*arrow*)

of such approaches, M. Remy-Jardin et al. have shown that contiguous 5-mm-thick scans obtained at low-dose MDCT depicts asbestos-related disease as accurately as thin-section CT obtained 30 mm apart, with the great advantage to provide images without any gap between them, a necessary condition for excluding the presence of pleural plaques (Gevenois et al. 1994; Remy-Jardin et al. 2004). The results reported by M. Remy-Jardin et al. suggest, thus, that low-dose helical MDCT should be used for scanning asymptomatic subjects, particularly in screening programs and for medico-legal issues, CT techniques delivering a higher radiation dose, such as thin sections, being only performed in selected subjects who have lung abnormalities that are insufficiently characterized on low-dose images (Remy-Jardin et al. 2004).

References

Aberle DR, Gamsu G, Ray CS (1988) High-resolution CT of benign asbestos-related diseases: clinical and radiographic correlation. AJR Am J Roentgenol 151:883–891

Adamson IY, Bakowska J, Bowden DH (1994) Mesothelial cell proliferation: a non-specific response to lung injury associated with fibrosis. Am J Respir Cell Mol Biol 10:253–258

Al Jarad N, Poulakis N, Pearson MC, Rubens MB, Rudd RM (1991) Assessment of asbestos-induced pleural disease by computed tomography – correlation with chest radiograph and lung function. Respir Med 85:203–208

Al Jarad N, Wilkinson P, Pearson MC, Rudd RM (1992) A new high resolution computed tomography scoring system for pulmonary fibrosis, pleural disease, and emphysema in patients with asbestos related disease. Br J Ind Med 49:73–84

Al Jarad N, Underwood SR, Rudd RM (1993) Asbestos-related pericardial thickening detected by magnetic resonance imaging. Respir Med 87:309–312

Boutin C, Vialat JR, Aelony Y (1991) Practical thoracoscopie. Springer Berlin Heidelberg New York

Boutin C, Dumortier P, Rey F, Viallat JR, De Vuyst P (1996) Black spots concentrate oncogenic asbestos fibers in the parietal pleura. Am J Respir Crit Care Med 153:444–449

Cohen AM, Crass JR, Chung-Park M, Tomashefsky JF Jr (1993) Rounded atelectasis and fibrotic pleural disease: the pathologic continuum. J Thorac Imag 8:309–312

Davies D, Andrews MIJ, Jones JSP (1991) Asbestos induced pericardial effusion and constrictive pericarditis. Thorax 46:429–432

De Klerk NH, Cookson WOC, Musk AW, Armstrong BK, Glancy JJ (1989) Natural history of pleural thickening after exposure to crocidolite. Br J Ind Med 46:461–467

De Vuyst P, Pfitzenmeyer P, Camus P (1997) Asbestos, ergot drugs and the pleura. Eur Respir J 10:2695–2698

Dodson RF, Williams MG, Corn CJ, Brollo A, Bianchi C (1990) Asbestos content of lung tissue, lymph nodes, and pleural plaques from former shipyard workers. Am Rev Respir Dis 142:843–847

Eisenstadt HB (1974) Pleural effusion in asbestosis [letter]. N Engl J Med 290:1025

Epler GR, McLoud TC, Gaensler EA (1982) Prevalence and incidence of benign asbestos pleural effusion in a working population. JAMA 247:617–622

Fisher MS (1985) Asymmetric changes in asbestos-related disease. J Can Assoc Radiol 36:110–112

Fletcher DE, Edge JR (1970) The early radiographic changes in pulmonary and pleural asbestosis. Clin Radiol 21:355–365

Friedman AC, Fiel SB, Fisher MS, Radecki PD, Lev-Toaff AS, Caroline DF (1988) Asbestos-related pleural disease and asbestosis: a comparison of CT and chest radiography. AJR Am J Roentgenol 150:269–275

Frumkin H, Pransky G, Cosmatos I (1990) Radiologic detection of pleural thickening. Am Rev Respir Dis 142:1325–1330

Gaensler EA, Kaplan AI (1971) Asbestos pleural effusion. Ann Intern Med 74:178–191

Gefter WB, Conant EF (1988) Issues and controversies in the plain-film diagnosis of asbestos-related disorders in the chest. J Thorac Imag 3:11–28

Gevenois PA, De Vuyst P, Dedeire S, Cosaert J, Van De Weyer R, Struyven J (1994) Conventional and high-resolution CT in asymptomatic asbestos-exposed workers. Acta Radiol 35:226–229

Gevenois PA, De Maertelaer V, Madani A, Winant C, Sergent G, De Vuyst P (1998) Asbestosis, pleural plaques and diffuse pleural thickening: three distinct benign responses to asbestos exposure. Eur Respir J 11:1021–1027

Harries PG, Mackenzie FA, Sheers G, Kemp JH, Oliver TP, Wright DS (1972) Radiological survey of men exposed to asbestos in naval dockyards. Br J Ind Med 29:274–279

Herbert A (1986) Pathogenesis of pleurisy, pleural fibrosis, and mesothelial proliferation. Thorax 41:176–189

Hillerdal G (1978) Pleural plaques in a health survey material. Frequency, development and exposure to asbestos. Scand J Respir Dis 59:257–263

Hillerdal G (1980) The pathogenesis of pleural plaques and pulmonary asbestosis: possibilities and impossibilities. Eur J Respir Dis 61:129–138

Hillerdal G (1987) Asbestos-related pleural disease. Sem Respir Med 9:65–74

Hillerdal G, Ozesmi M (1987) Benign asbestos pleural effusion: 73 exudates in 60 patients. Eur J Respir Dis 71:113–121

Hillerdal G (1989) Rounded atelectasis: clinical experience with 74 patients. Chest 95:836–841

Hillerdal G (1990) Pleural and parenchymal fibrosis mainly affecting the upper lung lobes in persons exposed to asbestos. Respir Med 84:129–134

Hillerdal G, Lindgren A (1980) Pleural plaques: correlation of autopsy findings to radiographic findings and occupational history. Eur J Respir Dis 61:315–319

Hourihane DO, Lessof L, Richardson PC (1966) Hyaline and calcified pleural plaques as an index of exposure to asbestos: a study of radiological and pathological features of 100 cases with epidemiology. Br Med J 1:1069–1074

Kanazawa K, Roe FJC, Yamamoto T (1979) Milky spots (taches laiteuses) as structures which trap asbestos in mesothelial layers and their significance in the pathogenesis of mesothelial neoplasia. Int J Cancer 23:858–865

Kee ST, Gamsu G, Blanc P (1996) Causes of pulmonary impairment in asbestos-exposed individuals with diffuse pleural thickening. Am J Respir Crit Care Med 154:789–793

Lilis R, Miller A, Godbold J, Chan E, Selikoff IJ (1991) Radiographic abnormalities in asbestos insulators: effects of duration from onset of exposure and smoking. Relationships of dyspnea with parenchymal and pleural fibrosis. Am J Ind Med 20:1–15

Lynch DA, Gamsu G, Ray CS, Aberle DR (1988) Asbestos-related focal lung masses: manifestations on conventional and high-resolution CT scans. Radiology 169:603–607

Lynch DA, Gamsu G, Aberle DR (1989) Conventional and high resolution computed tomography in the diagnosis of asbestos-related diseases. Radiographics 9:523–551

Martensson G, Hagberg S, Pettersson K, Thiringer G (1987) Asbestos pleural effusion: a clinical entity. Thorax 42:646–651

McLoud TC (1988) The use of CT in the examination of asbestos-exposed persons. Radiology 169:862–863

McLoud TC, Woods BO, Carrington CB, Epler GR, Gaensler EA (1985) Diffuse pleural thickening in asbestos-exposed population: prevalence and causes. Am J Roentgenol 144:9–18

Meurman LO (1968) Pleural fibrocalcific plaques and asbestos exposure. Environ Res 2:30–46

Miller WT, Gefter WB, Miller WT Sr (1992) Asbestos-related chest diseases: plain radiographic findings. Semin Roentgenol 27:102–120

Mintzer RA, Cugell DW (1982) The association of asbestos-induced pleural disease and rounded atelectasis. Chest 81:457–460

Mintzer RA, Gore RM, Vogelzang RL, Holz S (1981) Rounded atelectasis and its association with asbestos-induced pleural disease. Radiology 139:567–570

Mitchev K, Dumortier P, De Vuyst P (2002) « Black spots » and hyaline pleural plaques on the parietal pleura of 150 urban necropsy cases. Am J Surg Pathol 26:1198–1206

Monchaux G, Bignon J, Hirsch A, Sebastien P (1982) Translocation of mineral fibers through the respiratory system after injection into the pleural cavity of rats. Ann Occup Hyg 26:309–318

Mossman BT, Gee JBL (1989) Asbestos-related diseases. N Engl J Med 26:1721–1730

Neri S, Antonelli A, Falaschi F, Boraschi P, Baschieri L (1994) Findings from high resolution computed tomography of the lung and pleura of symptom free workers exposed to amosite who had normal chest radiographs and pulmonary function tests. Occup Environ Med 51:239–243

Olivier RM, Neville E (1988) Progressive apical pleural fibrosis: a "constrictive" defect. Br J Dis Chest 82:439–443

Remy-Jardin M, Sobaszek A, Duhamel A, Mastora I, Zanetti C, Remy J (2004) Asbestos-related pleuropulmonary diseases: evaluation with low-dose four-detector row spiral CT. Radiology 233:182–190

Rey F, Viallat JR, Farisse P, Boutin C (1993) Pleural migration of asbestos fibers after intratracheal injection in rats. Eur Respir J 3:145–147

Roberts GH (1971) The pathology of parietal pleural plaques. J Clin Pathol 24:348–353

Rockoff SD (1987) CT demonstration of interlobar fissure calcification due to asbestos exposure. J Comput Assist Tomogr 11:1066–1068

Rockoff SD, Kagan E, Schwartz A, Kriebel D, Hix W, Rohatgi P (1987) Visceral pleural thickening in asbestos exposure. The occurrence and implications of thickened interlobular fissures. J Thorac Imaging 2:58–66

Roggli VL, Benning TL (1990) Asbestos bodies in pulmonary hilar lymph nodes. Mod Pathol 3:513–517

Roggli VL, Pratt PC, Brody AR (1986) Asbestos content of lung tissue in asbestos associated diseases: a study of 110 cases. Br J Ind Med 43:18–28

Rosenstock L, Hudson LD (1986) Nonmalignant asbestos-induced pleural disease. Semin Respir Med 7:197–202

Rudd RM (1996) New developments in asbestos-related pleural disease. Thorax 51:210–216

Sahn SA, Antony VB (1984) Pathogenesis of pleural plaques. Relationship of early cellular response and pathology. Am Rev Respir Dis 130:884–887

Sahn SA, Heffner JE (2003) Pleural fluid analysis. In: Light RW, Lee YCG (eds) Textbook of pleural diseases. Arnold Publisher, London, pp 191–209

Sargent EN, Jacobson G, Gordonson JS (1977) Pleural plaques: a signpost of asbestos dust inhalation. Semin Roentgenol 12:287–297

Sargent EN, Felton JS, Barnes LT (1981) Calcified interlobar pleural plaques: visceral involvement due to asbestos. Radiology 140:634

Sargent EN, Boswell WD, Ralls PW, Markovitz A (1984) Subpleural fat pads in patients exposed to asbestos: distinction from non-calcified pleural plaques. Radiology 152:273–277

Schwartz DA (1991) New developments in asbestos-induced pleural disease. Chest 99:191–198

Schwartz DA, Galvin JR, Dayton CS, Standford W, Merchant JA, Hunninghake GW (1990) Determinants of restrictive lung in asbestos-induced pleural fibrosis. J Appl Physiol 68:1932–1937

Schwartz DA, Galvin JR, Yagla SJ, Speakman SB, Merchant JA, Hunninghake GW (1993) Restrictive lung function and asbestos-induced pleural fibrosis; a quantitative approach. J Clin Invest 91:2685–2692

Sison RF, Hruban RH, Moore GW, Kuhlman JE, Wheeler PS, Hutchins GM (1989) Pulmonary disease associated with pleural "asbestos" plaques. Chest 95:831–835

Smith DD (1984) Plaques, cancer, and confusion. Chest 105:8–9

Solomon A (1989) Computerized tomographic identification of visceral pleural changes other than in interlobar lung fissures. Am J Ind Med 15:557–563

Solomon A, Sluis-Cremer GK, Goldstein B (1979) Visceral pleural plaque formation in asbestosis. Environ Res 19:258

Stephens M, Gibbs AR, Pooley FD, Wagner JC (1987) Asbestos induced diffuse pleural fibrosis: pathology and mineralogy. Thorax 42:583–588

Svenes KB, Borgersen A, Haaversen O, Holten K (1986) Parietal pleural plaques: a comparison between autopsy and x-ray findings. Eur J Respir Dis 69:10–15

Tack D, De Maertelaer V, Gevenois PA (2003) Dose reduction in multidetector CT using attenuation-based online tube current modulation. AJR Am J Roentgenol 181:331–334

Taskinen E, Ahlman K, Wiikeri M (1973) A current hypothesis of the lymphatic transport of inspired dust to the parietal pleura. Chest 64:193–196

Van Cleemput J, De Raeve H, Verschakelen JA, Rombouts J, Lacquet LM, Nemery B (2001) Surface of localized pleural plaques quantitated by computed tomography scanning. Am J Respir Crit Care Med 163:705–710

Wain SL, Roggli VL, Foster WL (1984) Parietal pleural plaques, asbestos bodies, and neoplasia: a clinical, pathologic, and roentgenographic correlation of 25 consecutive cases. Chest 86:707–713

Yates DH, Browne K, Stidolph PN, Nevill E (1996) Asbestos-related bilateral diffuse pleural thickening: natural history of radiographic and lung function abnormalities. Am J Respir Crit Care Med 153:301–306

9 Mesothelioma

Alexander Bankier and Tomas Franquet

CONTENTS

9.1 Epidemiology 239
9.2 Incidence and Frequency 240
9.3 Clinical Symptoms 240
9.4 Chest Radiographic Signs 240
9.5 Computed Tomography 241
9.6 Magnetic Resonance Imaging 245
9.7 Pathology 246
9.8 Diagnosis 247
References 247

The inhalation and deposition of asbestos in the respiratory tract can lead to the following conditions:

1. Asbestos-induced pleural effusion, which may result in pleural thickening
2. Circumscribed pleural thickening, or pleural plaques, which may proceed to pleural calcification
3. Asbestosis, i.e., asbestos-induced lung fibrosis
4. Lung carcinoma
5. Malignant mesothelioma of the pleura and the peritoneum

In general, the term mesothelioma is used to designate both a benign pedunculated pleural tumor associated with hypertrophic osteoarthropathy and a diffuse malignant tumor of the pleura, the peritoneum, the pericardium, or rarely, the tunica vaginalis. Only diffuse malignant mesothelioma is related to asbestos exposure. In this chapter, only diffuse malignant mesothelioma of the pleura will be discussed, and the term "mesothelioma" will be employed as a synonym of diffuse malignant mesothelioma of the pleura.

A. Bankier, MD
Professor, Department of Radiology, Medical University of Vienna, Waehringer Guertel 18–20, 1090 Vienna, Austria
T. Franquet, MD
Professor, Department of Radiology, Section of Thoracic Imaging, Hospital de Sant Pau, Universidad Autonoma de Barcelona, San Antonio M. Claret 167, 08025 Barcelona, Spain

9.1 Epidemiology

Epidemiological studies suggest that over 80% of mesotheliomas are associated with a prior exposure to asbestos (Greenberg and Davies 1974; Milne 1976). Although the close relationship between exposure to asbestos and mesothelioma is now strongly established (Wagner et al. 1960), the tumor has also been associated with other fibrous material, such as erionite and zeolite (Milne 1976). Although some imply that the relationship between the exposure to asbestos and the occurrence of mesothelioma was already known in the 1940s and 1950s, it must be underlined that, at that time, many pathologists denied the existence of mesothelioma and maintained the opinion that mesothelioma was, in fact, a secondary deposit from a primary adenocarcinoma elsewhere in the body (Browne 1983a,b).

The incubation period of mesotheliomas varies between 15 years and 40 years, and most mesotheliomas develop 25–40 years after the first episode of exposure to asbestos (Browne 1983a,b). Once the lungs of the susceptible individual have been primed with a sufficient dose of asbestos, the development of mesothelioma becomes inevitable. Thus, individuals in whom mesotheliomas develop late in their lives might not have been exposed to asbestos for 20–35 years (Greenberg and Davies 1974). Contrary to previous opinions, it has become evident that mesotheliomas do not result from short-lived exposures but that they require average exposures to asbestos ranging from 6 months to 3 years (Milne 1976).

There now is little doubt that mesotheliomas have increased in frequency with the widespread use of asbestos. In 1951, Hochberg noted that, in a series of more than 60,000 autopsies performed in various European and American cities between 1919 and 1949, malignant pleural tumors were found in 0.07% of subjects (Hochberg 1951). Probably, some of these tumors were secondary deposits of primary tumors elsewhere in the body. From 1950 to 1970, malignant pleural tumors were found in 0.24% of 70,000 autopsies performed in similar cities (McDonald and McDonald 1977). Although this increase, per se, is substantial, the overall incidence of mesothelioma remains low.

9.2 Incidence and Frequency

The overall incidence of mesothelioma is indeed low, which is particularly true for the general population. Recent American data indicate that the incidence of mesothelioma is 14–15 individuals per million population for men (Connelly et al. 1987). This amounts to approximately 1750 male individuals per year in the United States. In women, the risk is approximately 2 subjects per million population and year, which amounts to 250 individuals per year. The incidence of mesothelioma shows a birth cohort effect, i.e., the incidence of mesothelioma increases with age but diminishes by 70 years of age. In the period between 1960 to 1983, Canada witnessed an increase in mesotheliomas from 0.5 per million to 2 per million in men (Connelly et al. 1987). No increase in female cases of mesothelioma was observed in the same period. A similar pattern of the development of the incidence of mesothelioma has occurred in Great Britain (Jones et al. 1985). The fact that the incidence in male individuals has been increasing in the United States, Canada, and Great Britain, while that for female individuals has substantially remained the same, confirms that occupational exposure is the primary cause of the observed increase in the incidence of mesotheliomas (Connelly et al. 1987).

9.3 Clinical Symptoms

The first presentation of mesothelioma usually is that of unilateral chest pain. This chest pain often has a pleuritic component. Initially, the pain is transient, but in the further course of disease it may become persistent, tends to migrate centrally, and is no longer worsened by deep breathing or coughing. The patient starts to lose weight and becomes increasingly dyspneic (Elmes and Simpson 1976). Dyspnea is directly related to the size of the tumor and the resulting compression and collapse of the lung. At this stage of disease, the typical radiographic sign of the disease is that of pleural effusion. As the mesothelioma grows, the diseased hemithorax flattens and displays radiographic signs of a fibrothorax. Concomitantly, the mediastinum shifts toward the diseased side. Occasionally, after the pleural effusion has been drained or the patient has undergone open pleural biopsy, seeding of the tract or the scar with tumor cells may occur (Miller et al. 1996). As the tumor further grows, it may compress and invade the great vessels of the thorax and the pericardium. Cardiac arrhythmias are a relatively common finding and tend to persist in the late stages of the disease, when pericardial invasion is far advanced. The heart may also be compressed by varying amounts of pericardial effusion. Death usually occurs within 18–24 months after diagnosis, as a consequence of terminal pneumonia and the involvement of mediastinal and/or hilar vessels. A minority of patients, averaging up to 15%, may show survival times as long as 3–4 years. Although, in its typical form, mesothelioma affects a hemithorax unilaterally, bilateral mesotheliomas have been sporadically reported.

9.4 Chest Radiographic Signs

The classical initial radiographic presentation of mesothelioma is that of a large unilateral pleural effusion (Wang et al. 2004). In a minority of patients, multiple pleura-based lesions might also be visible (Figs. 9.1 and 9.2). Furthermore, some patients display pleural

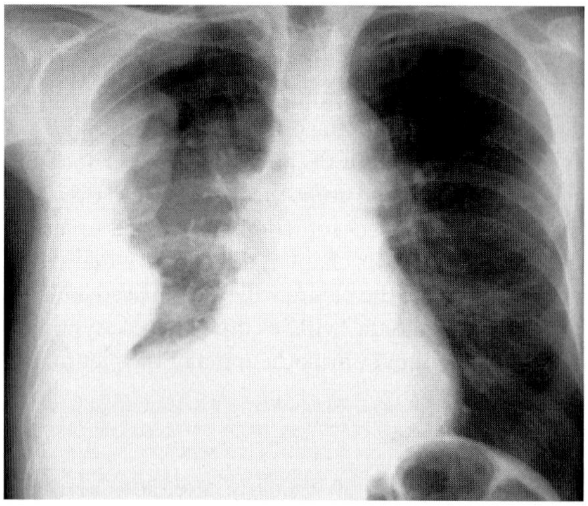

Fig. 9.1. Diffuse nodular pleural thickening in a 63-year-old man with malignant pleural mesothelioma. Frontal chest radiograph shows lobulated smooth thickening along the right lateral chest wall

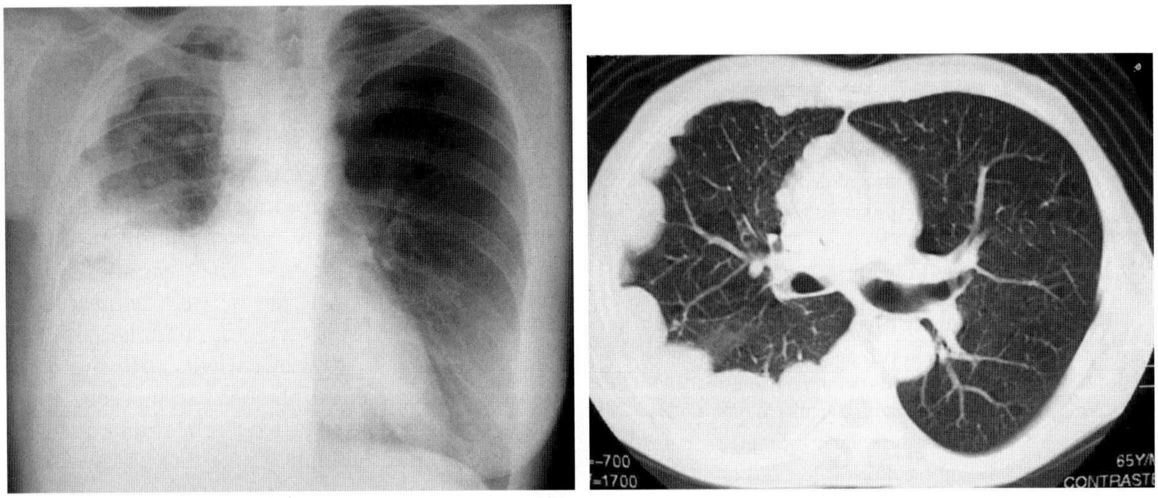

a b

Fig. 9.2a,b. Nodular pleural involvement in a 65-year-old man with malignant pleural mesothelioma. **a** Chest radiograph shows lobulated smooth thickening along the right lateral chest wall. **b** Axial non-enhanced computed tomography scan (lung window) confirms the presence of multiple pleural nodules

plaques, asbestosis, and other potential signs of previous asbestos exposure (Leung et al. 1990). Serial radiographs will invariably show a slow extension of the tumor, sometimes with partial disappearance of pleural fluid, but with signs of destructive growth, such as rib destruction. As the tumor progresses, the remaining pleural fluid may become loculated. In most patients with peritoneal mesothelioma, pulmonary sequels of asbestos exposure can be seen on the chest radiograph but without displaying the typical radiological signs of pleural mesothelioma.

9.5 Computed Tomography

Computed tomography (CT) certainly is the key imaging modality used for the evaluation of mesothelioma. This applies to both the clinical assessment of mesothelioma and the staging of mesothelioma for therapeutic or epidemiological purposes. The morphological descriptors and criteria for the tumor node metastasis staging of mesothelioma are summarized in Tables 9.1–9.3.

Table 9.1. Tumor descriptors for mesothelioma as related to the tumor node metastasis stages (from Rusch et al. 1998 and Rusch 1995)

Descriptor	Region involved	Characteristics
T1a	Limited to the ipsilateral parietal pleura, including the mediastinal and diaphragmatic pleura	No involvement of the visceral pleura
T1b	Ipsilateral parietal pleura, including the mediastinal and diaphragmatic pleura	Scattered tumor foci that also involve the visceral pleura
T2	Each ipsilateral pleural surface	At least one of the following: (a) involvement of the diaphragmatic muscle or (b) a confluent visceral pleural tumor (including fissures) or tumor extension from the visceral pleura into the underlying pulmonary parenchyma
T3	Locally advanced but potentially resectable tumor (each ipsilateral pleural surface)	At least one of the following: (a) involvement of the endothoracic fascia, (b) extension into mediastinal fat, (c) a solitary, completely resectable focus of tumor that extends into the soft tissues of the chest wall, or (d) non-transmural involvement of the pericardium
T4	Locally advanced, technically unresectable tumor (each ipsilateral pleural surface)	At least one of the following: (a) diffuse tumor extension or multiple tumor foci in the chest wall with or without associated rib destruction, (b) direct transdiaphragmatic extension to the peritoneum, (c) direct extension to the mediastinal organs, (e) direct extension to the spine, or (f) extension to the internal surface of the pericardium with or without pericardial effusion or involvement of the myocardium

Table 9.2. Node and metastasis descriptors for mesothelioma as related to the tumor node metastasis classification (from Rusch et al. 1998 and Rusch 1995)

Descriptor	Characteristics
NX	Regional lymph nodes not assessable
N0	No regional lymph node metastases
N1	Metastases in ipsilateral bronchopulmonary or hilar lymph nodes
N2	Metastases in subcarinal or ipsilateral mediastinal lymph nodes, including ipsilateral internal mammary lymph nodes
N3	Metastastes in contralateral mediastinal, contralateral internal mammary, and ipsilateral or contralateral supraclavicular lymph nodes
MX	Distant metastases not assessable
M0	No distant metastases
M1	Distant metastases

Table 9.3. Staging and tumor node metastasis (TNM) classification of mesothelioma (from Rusch et al. 1998 and Rusch 1995)

TNM Classification			
Stage	Tumor	Node	Metastasis
Ia	T1a	N0	M0
Ib	T1b	N0	M0
II	T2	N0	M0
III	Any T3	Any N1 or N2	M0
IV	Any T4	Any N3	Any M1

Major CT findings that suggest the presence of mesothelioma include unilateral pleural effusion, nodular thickening of the pleura, and interlobar pleural thickening (Wang et al. 2004) (Figs. 9.3 and 9.4). Growth of mesothelioma typically leads to progressive tumoral encasement of the lung that may finally result in circumferential pleural thickening and consequently give a rind-like appearance to the pleura (Fig. 9.5). The circumferentially thickened pleura can either be well delineated or, more frequently, display irregular nodular contours (Fig. 9.5). In up to 20% of patients with mesothelioma, calcified pleural plaques can be seen. These plaques can become engulfed by the tumor and may then mimic mesothelioma (Leung et al. 1990). Notably, in advanced disease, the affected hemithorax can be contracted (Fig. 9.6). This contraction eventually results in a mediastinal shift to the diseased side, a narrowing of the intercostal spaces, and an elevation of the ipsilateral diaphragm (Wang et al. 2004).

Given that mesothelioma is a locally aggressive tumor, invasion of the chest wall, the mediastinum, and the diaphragm are frequent. Chest wall invasion may manifest as an obliteration of the extrapleural fat planes, as invasion of intercostal muscles, as displacement of ribs, or as destruction of bones (Fig. 9.7). Despite the high frequency of these latter findings, irregularities of the interface between the chest wall and the tumor are not reliable in predicting chest wall invasion (Patz et al. 1992). Mesothelioma has also been reported to be able to extend into the chest wall via the tracks of biopsy needles, via

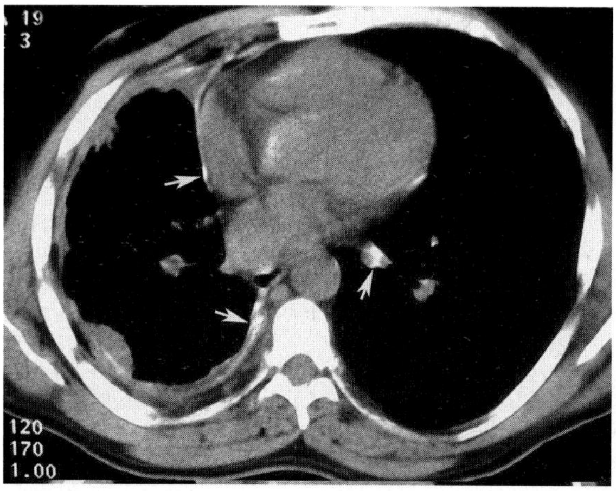

a

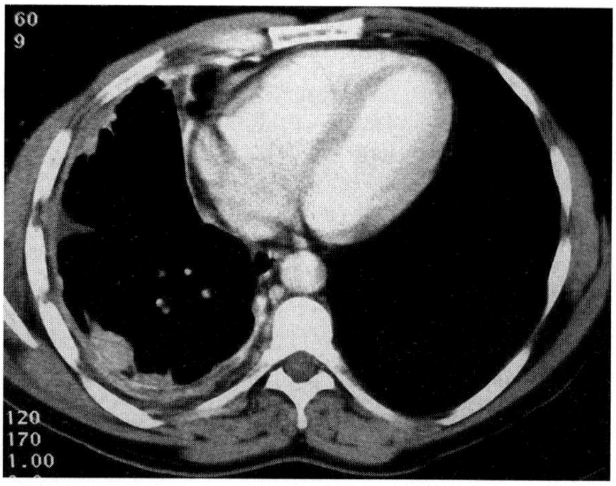

b

Fig. 9.3a,b. Asbestos exposure in a 56-year-old man with malignant pleural mesothelioma. **a** Axial non-enhanced computed tomography scan shows concentric nodular pleural thickening. Bilateral calcified pleural plaques are seen (*arrows*). Note reduction in volume of the affected hemithorax. **b** Axial enhanced computed tomography scan demonstrates that pleural nodules enhance following contrast administration

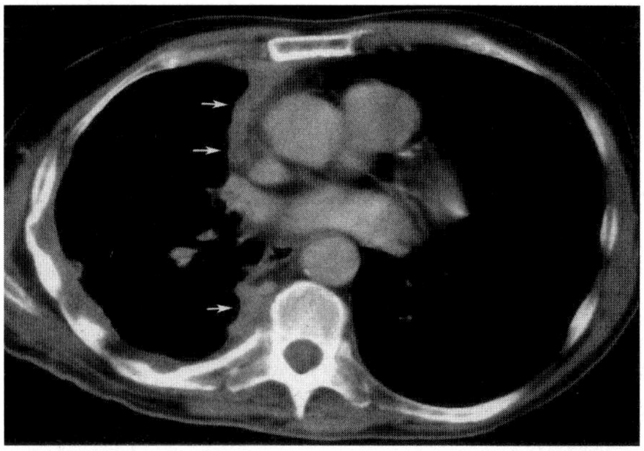

Fig. 9.4. Malignant pleural mesothelioma in a 57-year-old man. Axial contrast-enhanced computed tomography scan shows circumferential extension of the disease along the mediastinal pleura (*arrows*)

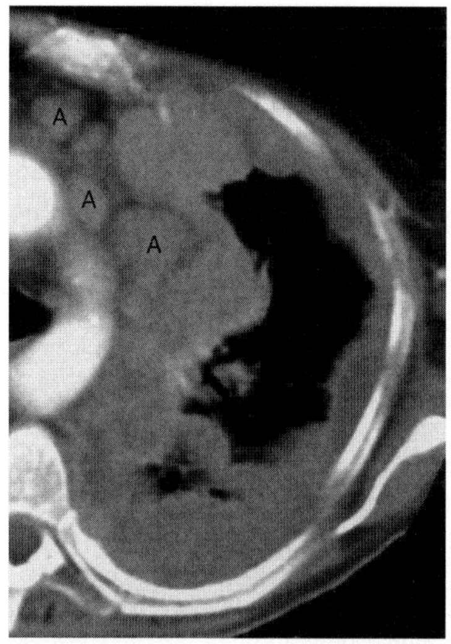

Fig. 9.5. Mediastinal lymphadenopathy in a 49-year-old man with malignant pleural mesothelioma. Localized view of an axial computed tomography scan at the level of the aortic arch shows multiple adenopathies (*A*) and circumferential nodular pleural thickening

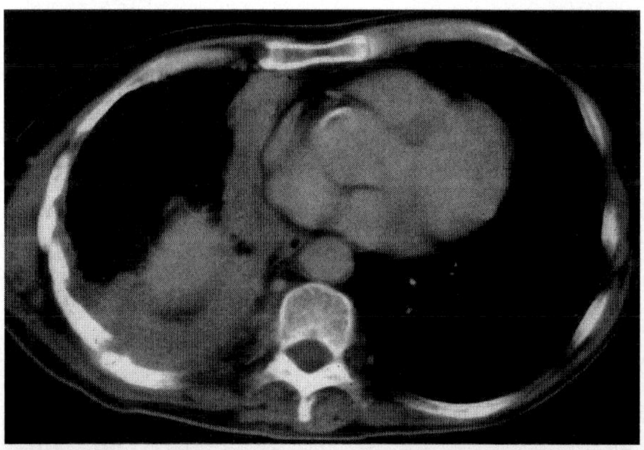

a

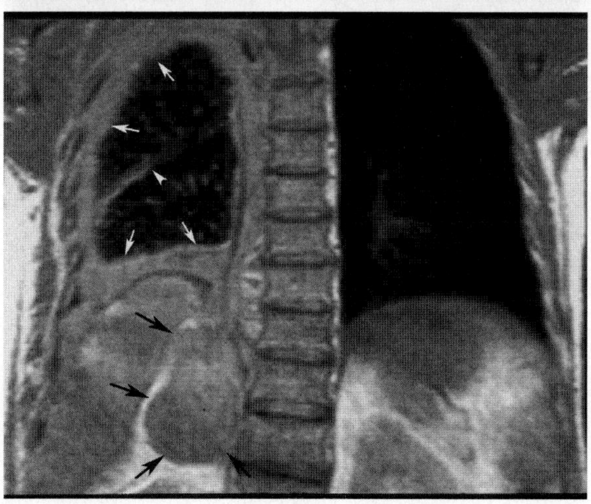

b

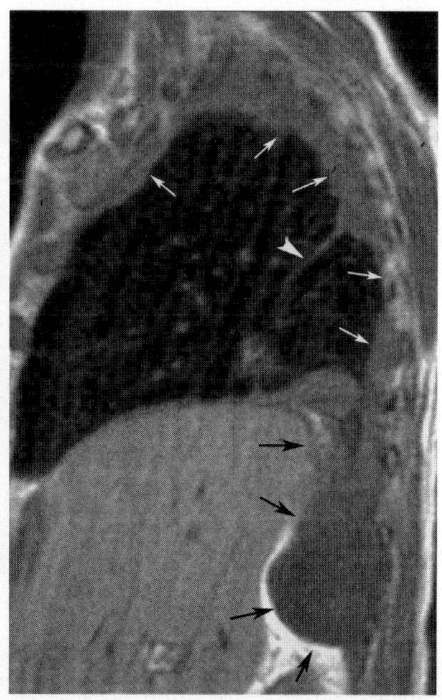

c

Fig. 9.6a–c. Malignant pleural mesothelioma in a 60-year-old man. **a** Axial non-enhanced computed tomography scan at the lung bases shows extension of the disease along the mediastinal pleura. Coronal (**b**) and sagittal (**c**) proton density magnetic resonance images show circumferential pleural thickening (*white arrows*) extending into the right costophrenic sulcus (*black arrows*). The tumor encases the contracted left hemithorax having a rindlike appearance. Note that some of them extend within the major fissure (*arrowheads*)

surgical scars, and via chest tube tracts (Miller et al. 1996). Direct extension of the tumor into vascular and/or mediastinal structures such as the aorta, the superior vena cava, the heart, the esophagus, and the trachea may also occur. Direct tumor extension is frequently accompanied by the obliteration of surrounding fat planes. The presence of a soft-tissue mass that surrounds more than 50% of the circumference of a vascular or other mediastinal structure must be interpreted as being a strong evidence

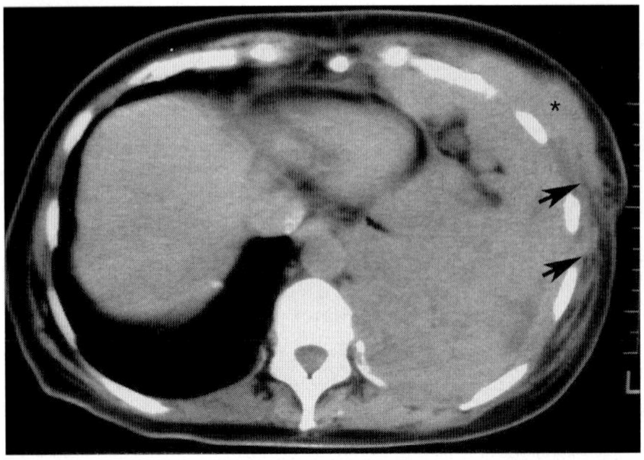

Fig. 9.7. Chest wall invasion in a 59-year-old man with a left-sided malignant pleural mesothelioma. Axial non-enhanced computed tomography scan shows diffuse anterior chest wall involvement by the tumor. Obliteration of extrapleural fat planes (*arrows*) and invasion of the chest wall musculature (*asterisk*) is clearly seen

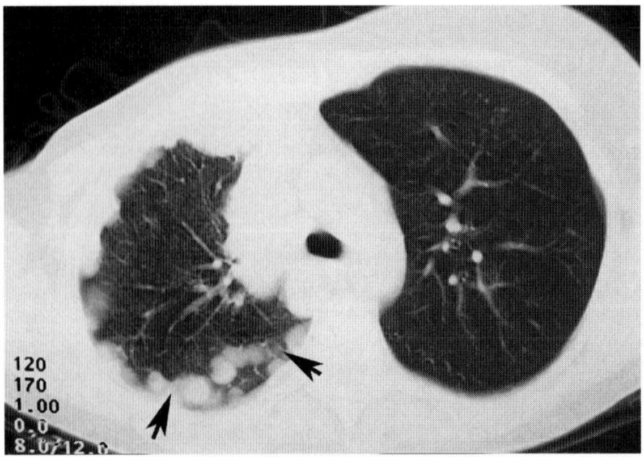

Fig. 9.8. Diffuse nodular pleural thickening in a 58-year-old woman with breast carcinoma. Axial non-enhanced computed tomography scan (lung window) shows multiple pleural nodules. Some of them extend within the major fissure (*arrows*)

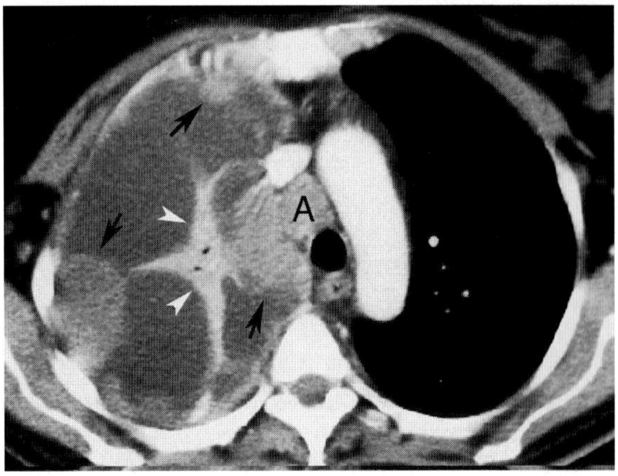

Fig. 9.9. Loculated pleural fluid collections in a 66-year-old man with right-sided malignant pleural mesothelioma. Axial enhanced computed tomography scan shows multiple lenticular fluid collections indicating the presence of loculation. The collapsed right upper lobe (*arrowheads*) enhances following contrast administration. Nodular pleural thickening (*arrows*) and mediastinal adenopathy (*A*) are clearly seen

for invasion and, hence, a strong evidence of high tumor aggressivity (Patz et al. 1992). Mesothelioma may invade the pericardium and can be seen on CT as nodular pericardial thickening or as pericardial effusion (Patz et al. 1992). Transdiaphragmatic extension of mesothelioma is suggested on CT by a soft-tissue mass that encases the hemidiaphragm (Patz et al. 1992). This finding can be particularly well appreciated on coronal reconstructions. However, a clear fat plane between the diaphragm and adjacent abdominal organs and a smooth diaphragmatic contour indicate that the tumor is limited to the thorax (Patz et al. 1992).

Pulmonary metastases from mesothelioma can either manifest as nodules or masses. Less commonly, miliary nodules can be seen on CT. The most important differential diagnosis of such lesions is pleural metastases from other origins (Fig. 9.8). Rarely, CT may also show extrathoracic spread of mesothelioma, for example, direct invasion of the liver or extension to the retroperitoneum and the retrocrural spaces (Kawashima and Libshitz 1990). At autopsy, metastasis to the mediastinal and hilar lymph nodes is present in 40–45% of patients with mesothelioma (Huncharek and Smith 1988) (Fig. 9.9).

Despite the fact that CT is the most commonly used imaging modality for evaluating potential adenopathy, its diagnostic accuracy remains suboptimal, because lymph-node enlargement alone does not prove nodal involvement (Boiselle et al. 1998). In early stages of chest wall involvement and of peritoneal studding, CT may also underestimate the extent of disease (Patz et al. 1996, Rusch et al. 1988). Despite these limitations, CT remains the imaging modality of choice for the initial evaluation of patients with suspected mesothelioma. The introduction of multi-detector-row CT units with multiplanar reformatting capabilities may potentially improve the diagnostic accuracy of tumor detection (Wang et al. 2004). Three-dimensional reconstructions have indeed been shown to improve the staging of neck and lung cancer (Padhani et al. 1995; Franca et al. 2000). Although the staging of mesothelioma using multiplanar reformatting has not been studied in detail, it is conceivable that volumetric CT techniques will further improve the visualization of tumor extent, notably in regions such as the diaphragm, which remains difficult to assess on axial CT sections (WANG et al. 2004).

9.6 Magnetic Resonance Imaging

Based on the use of different pulse sequences and on gadolinium-based contrast enhancement, magnetic resonance (MR) imaging contributed to a improved differentiation between tumor and normal tissue. Therefore, MR imaging can provide valuable staging information, notably in patients with potentially resectable disease. Relative to adjacent chest wall muscle, mesothelioma is typically isointense or slightly hyperintense on T1-weighted images and moderately hyperintense on T2-weighted images. Mesothelioma increases in signal after the intravenous administration of contrast material. The excellent contrast resolution of MR imaging can allow for improved detection of tumor extension, especially to the chest wall and diaphragm, and better prediction of overall tumor resectability (WANG et al. 2004). The anatomical and morphological MR features used to confirm or to exclude local tumor invasion are similar to those used for CT. Tumor extension into the mediastinal fat, the loss of normal fat planes, and tumoral encasement of more than 50% of the circumference of a mediastinal structure are the most important MR findings suggestive of tumor invasion (WANG et al. 2004) (Figs. 9.10 and 9.11).

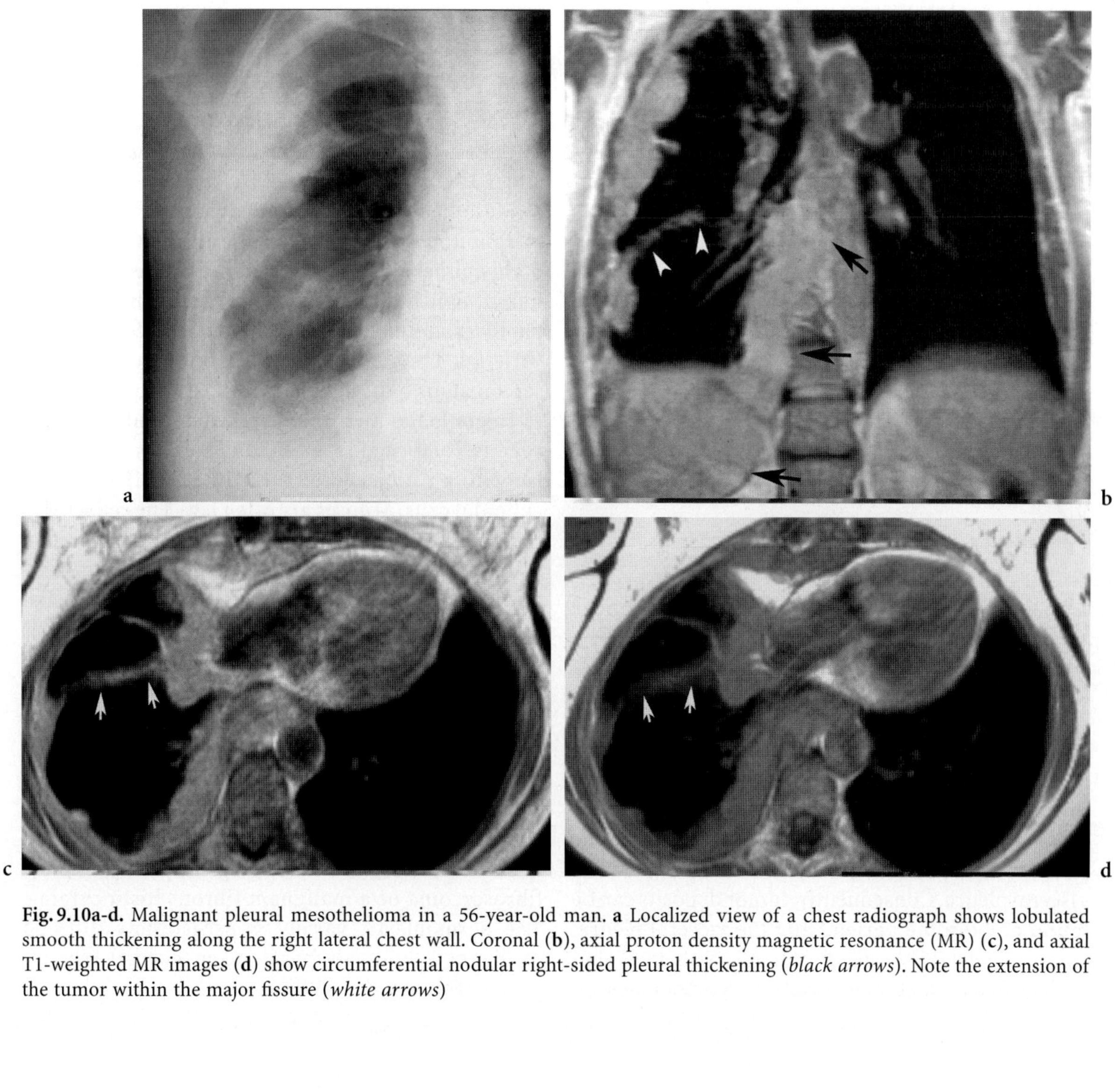

Fig. 9.10a-d. Malignant pleural mesothelioma in a 56-year-old man. **a** Localized view of a chest radiograph shows lobulated smooth thickening along the right lateral chest wall. Coronal (**b**), axial proton density magnetic resonance (MR) (**c**), and axial T1-weighted MR images (**d**) show circumferential nodular right-sided pleural thickening (*black arrows*). Note the extension of the tumor within the major fissure (*white arrows*)

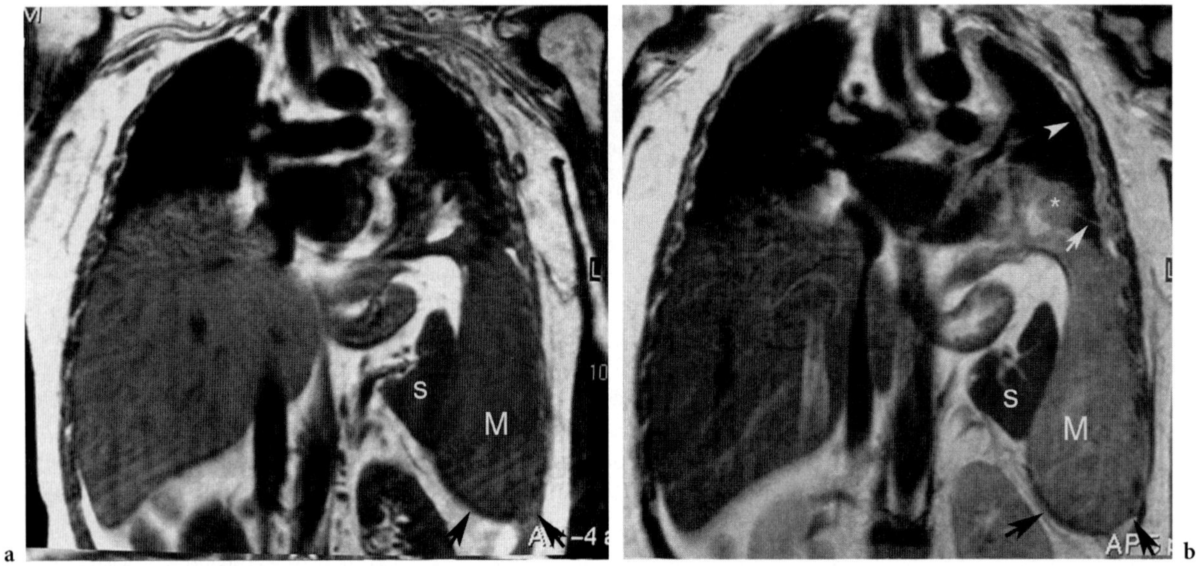

Fig. 9.11a,b. Magnetic resonance (MR) imaging evaluation of malignant pleural mesothelioma. **a** Coronal T1-weighted and **b** coronal T2-weighted MR images show circumferential pleural thickening (*white arrows* in **b**) extending into the left costophrenic sulcus (*black arrows* in **a,b**). *S* spleen, *M* mesothelioma

As shown by a recent study, MR imaging is superior to CT in the detection of two types of invasive growth of mesothelioma: (1) invasion of the diaphragm, and (2) invasion of the endothoracic fascia (Heelan et al. 1999). Another potential application of MR imaging is the evaluation of patients with questionable areas of local tumor extension on CT or in whom intravenous administration of iodinated contrast material is contraindicated (Wang et al. 2004) (Figs. 9.10 and 9.11).

9.7 Pathology

The typical mesothelioma found at autopsy is a firm and hard mass of whitish or grayish tissue that envelops adjacent anatomical structures, including the lung and the mediastinal and hilar vessels. In most cases, the pleural space is obliterated. Gelatinous material is often present in small cysts that are located inside the tumor. Most tumors will spread diffusely, but in some cases they might include areas that are well circumscribed. The tumor starts on the parietal surface of the pleura but soon reaches the visceral pleura. Consequently, tumor deposits can be found on both the parietal and the visceral pleura. Approximately 50% of all patients with mesothelioma will have distant metastases. Lymph nodes are the most common site of metastatic spread, followed by the heart, bones, liver, and adrenal glands (Elmes and Simpson 1976).

Mesotheliomas are separated into epithelial sarcomatous and mixed types. In one-third of all tumors, both epithelial and sarcomatous elements can be found. Epithelial tumors are separated into tubulopapillary, epithelioid, adenomatoid, and desmoplastic varieties. The sarcomatous variants are either fibrosarcomatous or desmoplatic (Miller et al. 1996).

In epithelial mesotheliomas, the tubulupapillary type is composed of branching tubules and papillae with a fibrous core that is lined by flattened or cuboidal cells. Mitoses are often few. The cells lining the papillae can be columnar rather than cuboidal. A minority of epithelial mesotheliomas are composed of cells similar to the reactive mesothelial cells seen in pleural fluids. In this case, a diagnosis of a small primary carcinoma elsewhere in the body must be excluded. Some epithelial mesotheliomas have smaller cells and are difficult to distinguish from carcinomas. Few have a strong dense collagenous stroma with only scattered tumor cells. This is the desmoplastic variant, which is also seen in sarcomatous mesotheliomas. The sarcomatous variant is often cellular and morphologically identical to a fibrosarcoma or a malignant fibrous histiocytoma. The desmoplastic variety is exceedingly difficult to diagnose and to separate from normal reactive pleura (Miller et al. 1996).

9.8 Diagnosis

The diagnostic suspicion of mesothelioma requires a suitable history of exposure to asbestos and a suitable latency period. Because the chest radiograph may appear normal in early stages of the disease, CT should be performed early in the course of the disease to confirm the presence of a pleural pathology and to guide biopsy. Blind needle biopsy of the pleura commonly provides negative results and is seldom helpful. Video-assisted thoracoscopy is another diagnostic option, because it allows both direct visualization of the tumor and sufficient sampling of tissue for the definite diagnosis. In cases where video-assisted thoracoscopy cannot be performed, open lung biopsy remains the ultimate option to establish the diagnosis. A definitive histological proof of mesothelioma is of crucial importance for both patients and their relatives, given that the diagnosis might prompt the claim for compensation.

References

Boiselle PM, Patz EF Jr, Vining DJ, Weissleder R, Shepard JA, McLoud TC (1998) Imaging of mediastinal lymph nodes: CT, MR, and FDG PET. Radiographics 18:1061–1069

Browne K (1983a) Asbestos-related mesothelioma: epidemiological evidence for asbestos as a promoter. Arch Environ Health 38:261–266

Browne K (1983b) The epidemiology of mesothelioma. J Soc Occup Med 33:190–194

Connelly RR, Spirtas R, Myers MH, Percy CL, Fraumeni JF Jr (1987) Demographic patterns for mesothelioma in the United States. J Natl Cancer Inst 78:1053–1060

Elmes PC, Simpson JC (1976) The clinical aspects of mesothelioma. Q J Med 45:427–449

Franca C, Levin-Plotnik D, Sehgal V, Chen GT, Ramsey RG (2000) Use of three-dimensional spiral computed tomography imaging for staging and surgical planning of head and neck cancer. J Digit Imaging 13:24–32

Greenberg M, Davies TA (1974) Mesothelioma register 1967-68. Br J Ind Med 31:91–104

Heelan RT, Rusch VW, Begg CB, Panicek DM, Caravelli JF, Eisen C (1999) Staging of malignant pleural mesothelioma: comparison of CT and MR imaging. AJR Am J Roentgenol 172:1039–1047

Hochberg LA (1951) Endothelioma (mesothelioma) of the pleura; a review with a report of seven cases, four of which were extirpated surgically. Am Rev Tuberc 63:150–175

Huncharek M, Smith K (1988) Extrathoracic lymph node metastases in malignant pleural mesothelioma. Chest 93:443–444

Jones RD, Smith DM, Thomas PG (1985) Mesothelioma in Great Britain in 1968–1983. Br J Cancer 51:47–63

Kawashima A, Libshitz HI (1990) Malignant pleural mesothelioma: CT manifestations in 50 cases. AJR Am J Roentgenol 155:965–969

Leung AN, Muller NL, Miller RR (1990) CT in differential diagnosis of diffuse pleural disease. AJR Am J Roentgenol 154:487–492

McDonald JC, McDonald AD (1977) Epidemiology of mesothelioma from estimated incidence. Prev Med 6:426–442

Miller BH, Rosado-de-Christenson ML, Mason AC, Fleming MV, White CC, Krasna MJ (1996) From the archives of the AFIP. Malignant pleural mesothelioma: radiologic-pathologic correlation. Radiographics 16:613–644

Milne JE (1976) Thirty-two cases of mesothelioma in Victoria, Australia: a retrospective survey related to occupational asbestos exposure. Br J Ind Med 33:115–122

Padhani AR, Fishman EK, Heitmiller RF, Wang KP, Wheeler JH, Kuhlman JE (1995) Multiplanar display of spiral CT data of the pulmonary hila in patients with lung cancer. Preliminary observations. Clin Imaging 19:252–257

Patz EF Jr, Shaffer K, Piwnica-Worms DR, Jochelson M, Sarin M, Sugarbaker DJ Pugatch RD (1992) Malignant pleural mesothelioma: value of CT and MR imaging in predicting resectability. AJR Am J Roentgenol 159:961–966

Patz EF Jr, Rusch VW, Heelan R (1996) The proposed new international TNM staging system for malignant pleural mesothelioma: application to imaging. AJR Am J Roentgenol 166:323–327

Rusch VW, Godwin JD, Shuman WP (1988) The role of computed tomography scanning in the initial assessment and the follow-up of malignant pleural mesothelioma. J Thorac Cardiovasc Surg 96:171–177

Rusch VW (1995) A proposed new international TNM staging system for malignant pleural mesothelioma. From the International Mesothelioma Interest Group. Chest 108:1122–1128

Wagner JC, Sleggs CA, Marchand P (1960) Diffuse pleural mesothelioma and asbestos exposure in the North Western Cape Province. Br J Ind Med 17:260–271

Wang ZJ, Reddy GP, Gotway MB, Higgins CB, Jablons DM, Ramaswamy M, Hawkins RA, Webb WR (2004) Malignant pleural mesothelioma: evaluation with CT, MR imaging, and PET. Radiographics 24:105–119

10 Beryllium-Related Diseases

David A. Lynch

CONTENTS

10.1 Health Effects of Beryllium Disease 249
10.2 Clinical Presentation/Pathology 250
10.3 Imaging Appearances 250
10.4 Comparison of Chronic Beryllium Disease and Sarcoidosis 254
10.5 Beryllium and Lung Cancer 254
10.6 Summary 256
References 256

10.1 Health Effects of Beryllium Disease

There are two distinct types of lung injury related to beryllium exposure: an acute chemical pneumonitis (acute berylliosis) and a chronic granulomatous disease similar to sarcoidosis [chronic beryllium disease (CBD)]. With modern manufacturing safeguards, acute berylliosis has become rare, but chronic beryllium disease remains an important cause of disability in exposed workers. CBD is commonly classified as a pneumoconiosis, because it represents a reaction of the lungs to inhalation of an inorganic dust particle. However, it differs from the classic pneumoconioses in the following ways: (1) it represents a granulomatous hypersensitivity response to inhaled beryllium, and (2) its incidence and severity is not always related to the intensity and duration of exposure; in fact, it may occur with relatively trivial exposure.

Table 10.1. Health effects of beryllium exposure

Condition	Imaging manifestations
Acute berylliosis	Chemical pneumonitis
Beryllium sensitization	None
Chronic beryllium disease	Adenopathy, nodules, ground glass abnormality
Lung cancer	Lung nodules or masses

Inhalation of beryllium in the form of dust, fumes, or vapors can lead to a beryllium-mediated T-cell immune response in exposed workers (Maier 2002a). Such sensitization is detected by abnormal lymphocyte proliferation in response to beryllium. The beryllium lymphocyte proliferation test may be performed on lymphocytes obtained from peripheral blood or from broncho-alveolar lavage fluid, with the latter being more sensitive. Sensitization is found in between 2% and 19% of exposed workers. Up to 30% of sensitized workers progress to biopsy-proven chronic beryllium disease (Newman et al. 2005). Beryllium sensitization may occur after as little as 9 weeks of exposure, while CBD may develop after only 3 months (Newman et al. 2001). However, because the latency may be as long as 40 years, past employment history must be rigorously evaluated in individuals presenting with findings suggestive of this condition. Although the exposure response relationship for beryllium sensitization and CBD is nonlinear, higher exposures may be associated with higher rates of sensitization and CBD (Maier 2002b).

Beryllium sensitization is usually detected during workplace screenings or medical surveillance programs. A diagnosis of beryllium sensitivity requires two abnormal beryllium lymphocyte proliferation test results. If sensitization is detected, a thorough clinical, physiological and radiological evaluation is required, and transbronchial lung biopsy is usually performed. If granulomatous inflammation is found on biopsy, the worker receives the diagnosis of CBD. Beryllium sensitization is diagnosed if the patient has no symptoms or radiological, physiological, or pathological abnormalities attributable to CBD (Maier 2002a). Once sensitization is diagnosed, serial follow-up is usually performed to watch for the development of CBD (Newman, Mroz et al. 2005).

D.A. Lynch, MD
Professor of Radiology and Medicine, Department of Radiology, Box A030, University of Colorado Health Sciences Center, 4200 East Ninth Avenue, Denver, CO 80262, USA

Exposure to beryllium occurs in a variety of high-technology industries (including aerospace, ceramics, dentistry and dental supplies, nuclear weapons and reactors, recycling, telecommunications, and several others) where workers may be at risk for disease from either direct or indirect exposure to the metal. Beryllium machinists may be at highest risk for sensitization and CBD (Newman, Mroz et al. 2005). However, CBD has also been found in communities surrounding beryllium-manufacturing facilities and in office workers with relatively trivial exposure in these plants (Maier 2002a).

10.2 Clinical Presentation/Pathology

Acute berylliosis (Hooper 1981), which usually results from a single intense exposure, is now rare with appropriate workplace protection. It manifests as an acute tracheobronchitis and pulmonary edema.

Before the advent of widespread workplace screening using the beryllium lymphocyte proliferation test results, individuals with CBD presented with chronic respiratory symptoms of cough and progressive shortness of breath, often associated with systemic symptoms of fatigue, night sweats, arthralgias, myalgias, and weight loss (Maier 2002a). These cases were often quite advanced, with crackles on lung examination, clubbing, cyanosis, and evidence of pulmonary hypertension and cor pulmonale. Although some patients still present with more advanced disease, workplace screening with the lymphocyte proliferation test has allowed earlier detection of CBD, often before the onset of symptoms. The clinical significance of CBD diagnosed in this way remains unclear, as it is unclear how many patients with biopsy-proven CBD progress to clinically significant disease (Cullen 2005).

Physiological evaluations of individuals with CBD detected using workplace screening reveals a variety of physiological patterns, including normal, obstructive, restrictive, or mixed spirometric patterns. Diffusion capacity for carbon monoxide may be normal or reduced (Maier 2002a). An important clinical difference between CBD and sarcoidosis is that extrathoracic involvement is rare in CBD.

The histological appearance of chronic beryllium disease is indistinguishable from that of sarcoidosis, with non-caseating granulomas accompanied by mononuclear cell infiltrates and variable interstitial fibrosis (Maier 2002a).The granulomas are primarily found along the bronchovascular bundle, in the bronchial submucosa, in the pulmonary interstitium, and occasionally in regional lymph nodes. However, absence of granulomas on transbronchial or thoracoscopic lung biopsy does not exclude a diagnosis of CBD (Maier 2002a). Diagnostic criteria for chronic beryllium disease include: (1) a history of beryllium exposure; (2) demonstration of a beryllium-specific cell-mediated immune response; and (3) granulomas and/or mononuclear cell infiltrates on biopsy in the absence of infection.

With early diagnosis, no treatment may be needed. With symptomatic, progressive, or impairing chronic beryllium disease, oral corticosteroids are used. Other immunosuppressive agents and lung transplantation should be considered if there is no response to corticosteroids. Removal of sensitized individuals and those with CBD from further beryllium exposure is generally recommended, but it is unclear whether this influences the clinical course of the disease.

10.3 Imaging Appearances

The radiographic and computed tomography (CT) appearances of chronic beryllium disease are similar to those of sarcoidosis, though mediastinal and hilar lymphadenopathy is less common. In a study of 28 patients with CBD, only 15 (54%) had abnormal chest radiographs (Newman et al. 1994). Most of these patients had diffuse symmetric parenchymal abnormality, with relatively mild profusion [Category 1 according to the International Labour Organization (ILO) classification system]. Of these patients, 11 had predominantly round nodules (p, q, or r according to the ILO classification system), while the remaining 4 had small irregular opacities. Typically, the abnormalities predominate in the upper lobes (Fig. 10.1). Hilar or mediastinal adenopathy was seen in 6 cases (21%), always in the presence of parenchymal opacities (Newman, Buschman et al. 1994). Adenopathy without parenchymal abnormality appears to be rare. In advanced disease, there is progressive volume loss and hilar distortion. Conglomerate masses were seen on chest radiographs in 2 (7%) of the 28 cases in the series described above, while 3 (11%) had enlargement of central pulmonary arteries suggesting pulmonary hypertension. Because patients with beryllium exposure may also have had exposure to asbestos, changes of asbestos-related pleural disease or even asbestosis may be found.

On thin-section CT, enlarged lymph nodes are detected in the pulmonary hila in 32% of patients with CBD and in the mediastinum in 25% (Fig. 10.2) (NEWMAN, BUSCHMAN et al. 1994). As with the chest radiograph, adenopathy was found on CT only in the presence of parenchymal abnormalities. The adenopathy may show an amorphous or eggshell pattern of calcification similar to that seen in sarcoidosis and distinct from the more punctuate dense calcification seen in patients with previous tuberculosis or histoplasmosis (Fig. 10.3). Even if not overtly calcified, the nodes may be slightly hyperdense (Fig. 10.4).

Nodules are seen in about 60% of cases, often clustered together around the bronchi, interlobular septa, or in the subpleural region (Fig. 10.5) (NEWMAN, BUSCHMAN et al. 1994). Subpleural clusters of nodules may form pseudo-plaques, and pleural irregularity is found in about 25%. As in sarcoidosis, even small subpleural nodules may be readily visible along the major fissures (Fig. 10.5). Although the nodules are usually well defined and 2–5 mm in size, fine micronodules, quite similar to those found in hypersensitivity pneumonitis, may also be seen (Fig. 10.6).

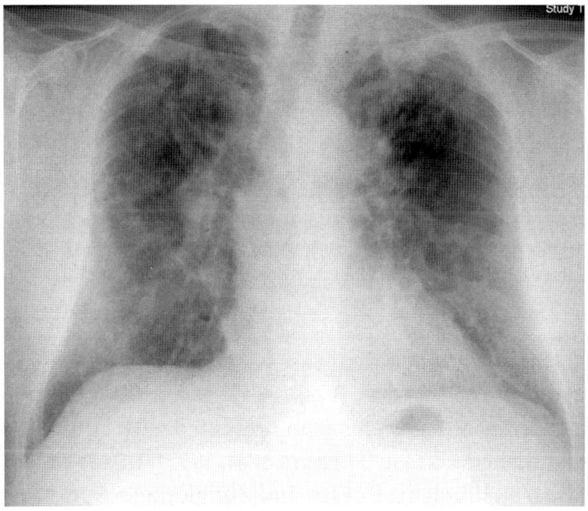

Fig. 10.1. Chest radiograph in a patient with advanced chronic beryllium disease shows abnormality predominating in the upper lobes, consisting of coarse well-defined nodules, which appear to coalesce in areas. Some of the nodules appear calcified. There is moderate upper lobe volume loss with superior hilar retraction and some anatomic distortion. Hilar enlargement is likely due to a combination of adenopathy and pulmonary arterial enlargement due to pulmonary hypertension

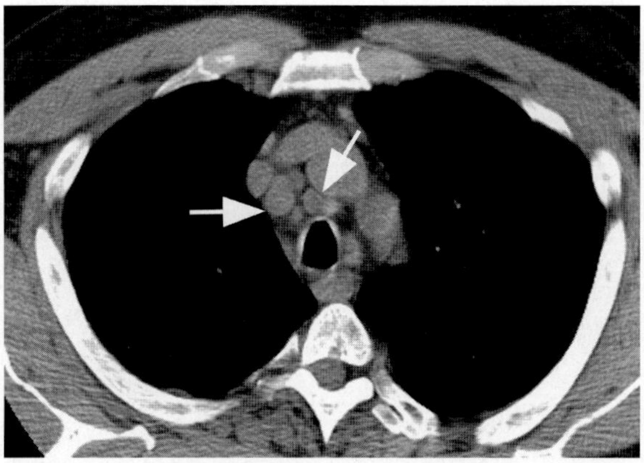

Fig. 10.2. Computed tomography image obtained just above the aortic arch in a patient with chronic beryllium disease shows multiple moderately enlarged pretracheal and paratracheal nodes (*arrows*)

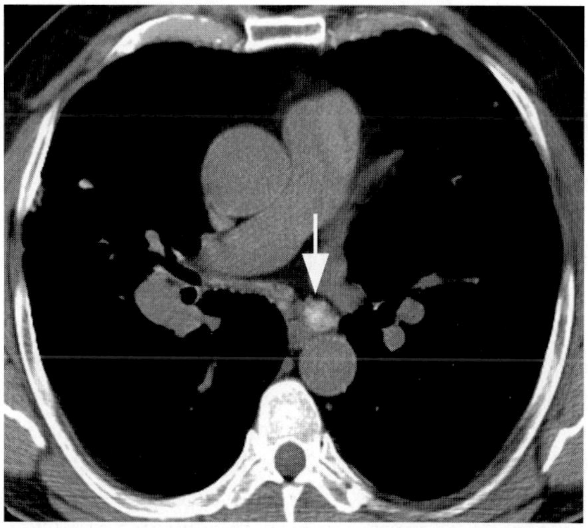

Fig. 10.3. Computed tomography through the subcarinal region in a patient with chronic beryllium disease shows right hilar enlargement due to adenopathy. A mildly enlarged left subcarinal node (*arrow*) shows an amorphous pattern of calcification

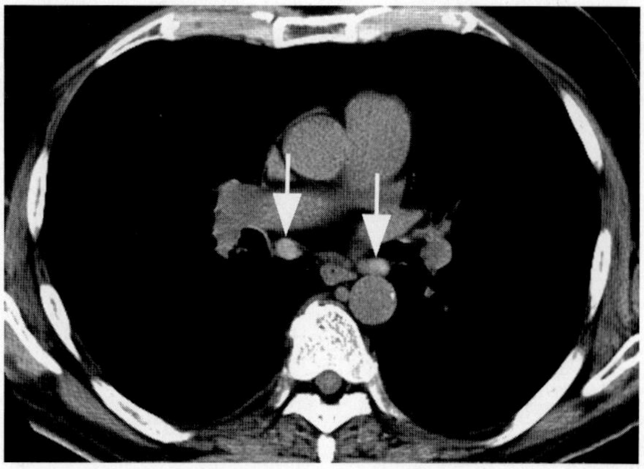

Fig. 10.4. Computed tomography through the subcarinal region in a patient with chronic beryllium disease shows slightly hyperdense, mildly enlarged mediastinal nodes (*arrows*)

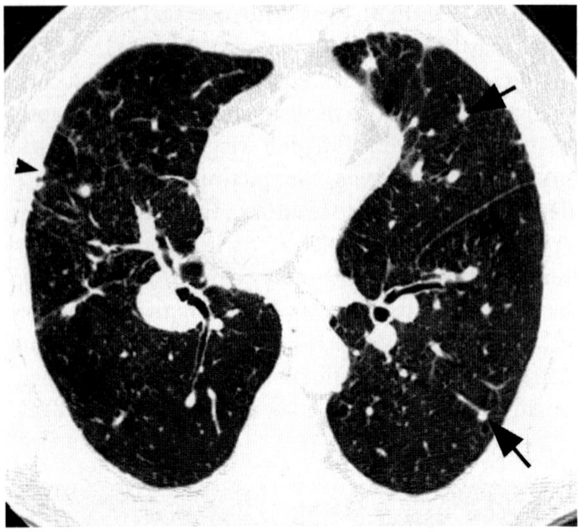

Fig. 10.5. Thin-section computed tomography through the lower lobes shows nodules less than 5 mm in diameter, some of which are peribronchovascular (*arrows*), but most of which are subpleural (*arrowheads*)

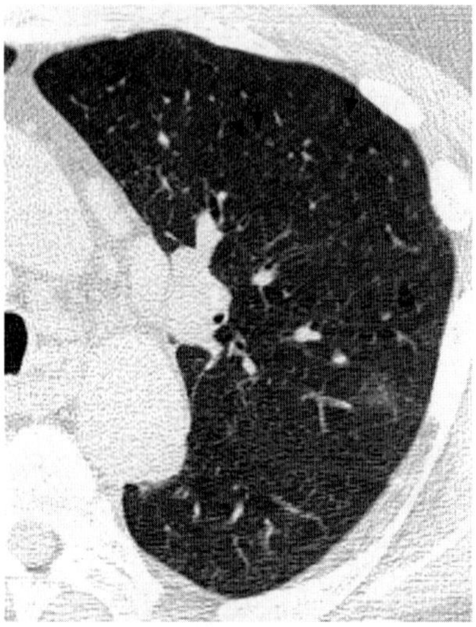

Fig. 10.6. Thin-section CT through the left upper lobe in a patient with chronic beryllium disease shows quite widespread, subtle, fine micronodules (*arrows*). There is a peribronchovascular patch of ground glass abnormality more posteriorly

Ground glass opacity (Fig. 10.7), bronchial wall thickening (Fig. 10.8), and thickening of interlobular septa (Fig. 10.9) are common CT features, found in 32%, 46%, and 50% of cases, respectively (Newman, Buschman et al. 1994). The ground glass abnormality is commonly predominantly peribronchovascular (Fig. 10.6, Fig. 10.8). Bronchial wall thickening, although commonly related to cigarette smoking, appears to be more common in subjects with CBD than in control subjects. Reticular opacity (Fig. 10.10) and architectural distortion (Fig. 10.11) may occur. The prevalence of honeycombing has ranged from 7% in a series including cases detected using medical screening (Newman, Buschman et al. 1994) to 38% in a series of 8 patients who presented with clinically established disease (Harris et al. 1993). In advanced disease, subpleural cysts and conglomerate masses (Fig. 10.11) may be found. Bronchial stenoses may rarely occur (Iles 1981). As with sarcoidosis, the nodules, masses, and adenopathy may show large areas of increased lung attenuation, presumed to represent calcification (Gevenois et al. 1994).

On follow-up evaluation of subjects with CBD, the CT findings of nodules, ground glass abnormal-

a 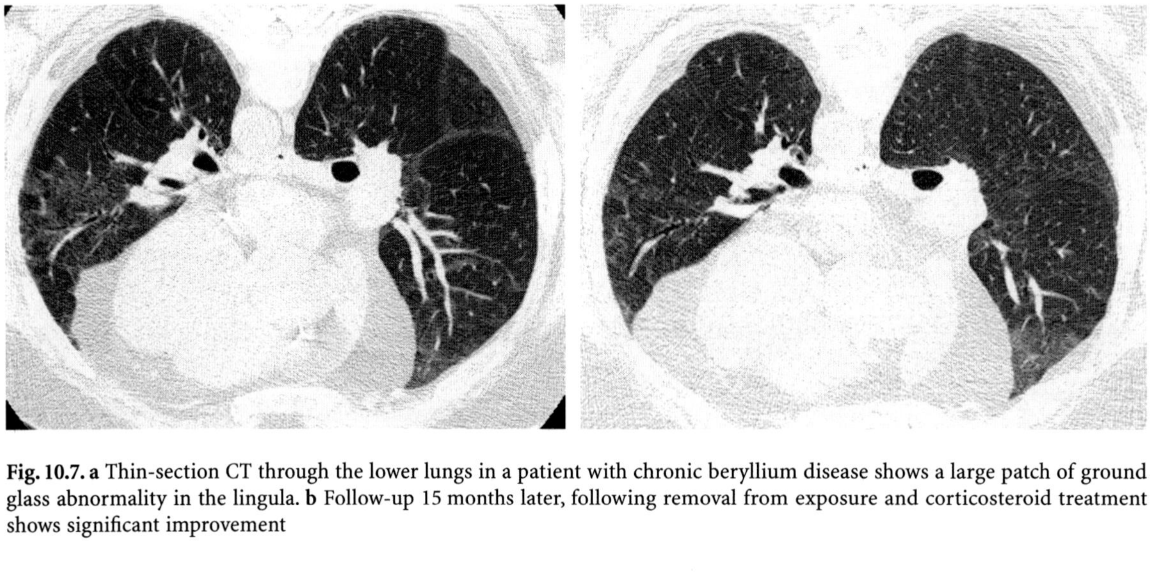 b

Fig. 10.7. a Thin-section CT through the lower lungs in a patient with chronic beryllium disease shows a large patch of ground glass abnormality in the lingula. **b** Follow-up 15 months later, following removal from exposure and corticosteroid treatment shows significant improvement

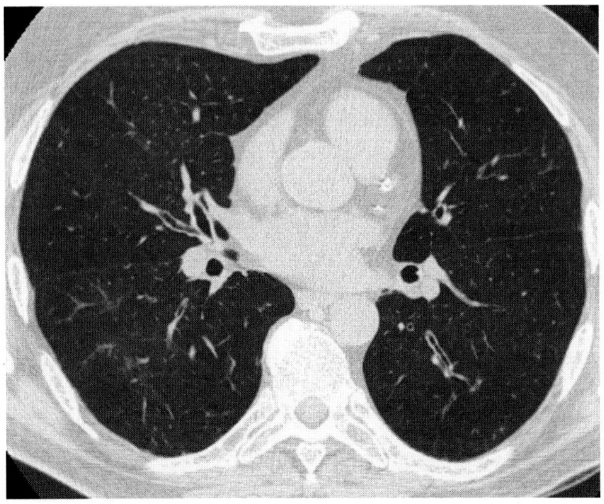

Fig. 10.8. Thin-section computed tomography through the mid-lungs in a patient with chronic beryllium disease shows marked airway wall thickening and mild, predominantly peribronchovascular, ground glass abnormality

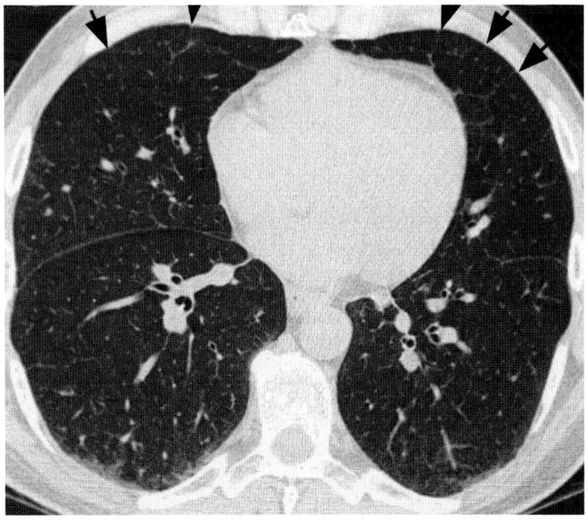

Fig. 10.9. Thin-section computed tomography through the lower lungs in a patient with chronic beryllium disease shows fine anterior septal thickening (*arrows, arrowheads*)

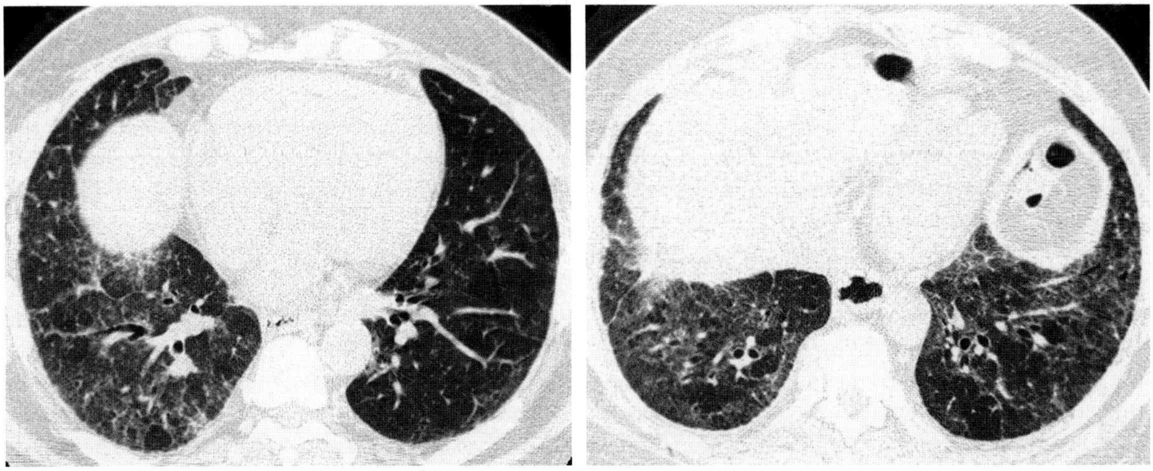

Fig. 10.10. a Thin-section computed tomography through the lung bases in a patient with chronic beryllium disease shows asymmetric reticular and ground glass abnormality. **b** Thin-section computed tomography at a slightly lower level 13 months later shows progression of reticular abnormality, particularly on the left

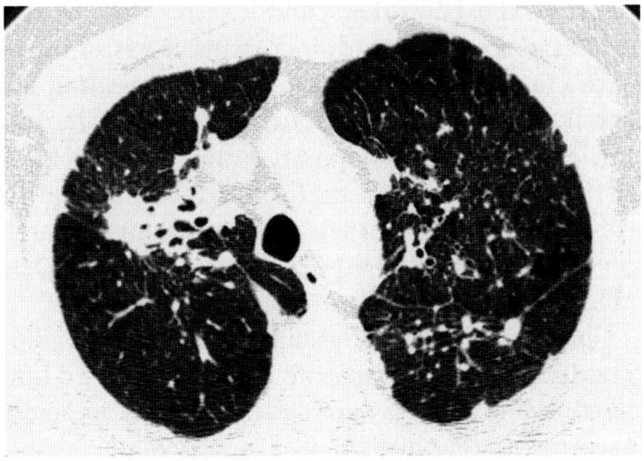

Fig. 10.11. Thin-section computed tomography through the upper lungs in a patient with advanced chronic beryllium disease shows multiple predominantly subpleural nodules, with a conglomerate mass on the right, associated with marked distortion and dilation of segmental bronchi. Anterior displacement of the right major fissure indicates significant upper lobe volume loss. An azygos lobe is present

ity, and septal thickening are commonly reversible (Fig. 10.12). As in sarcoidosis (BRAUNER et al. 1992; MURDOCH and MULLER 1992), architectural distortion, cysts, and honeycombing are usually irreversible.

In the study by Newman et al. cited above, the sensitivity of the chest radiograph for biopsy-proven chronic beryllium disease was approximately 45%, compared with approximately 89% for thin-section CT (NEWMAN, BUSCHMAN et al. 1994). However, 4 study patients who were cigarette smokers had bronchial wall thickening as the sole abnormality on thin-section CT. If this non-specific abnormality was excluded, the sensitivity of thin-section CT for detection of beryllium disease was 75%. In reviewing the 13 patients in this series who presented through medical screening and had normal chest radiographs, CT showed at least one abnormality in 10 (77%) and was entirely normal in the remaining 3. Findings detectable on CT but not on chest radiograph in these cases included ground glass abnormality, septal thickening, and nodules. The prognostic significance of normal or abnormal CT in screen-detected patients with CBD has not been evaluated.

A study by DANILOFF et al. evaluated the interobserver variation of assessment of thin-section CT findings and the relationship between these findings and physiological impairment (DANILOFF et al. 1997). Moderate intra-observer and inter-observer agreement was found for assessment of extent of ground glass abnormality, septal thickening, nodules, and percentage of abnormal lung. Interobserver variation was higher for bronchial wall thickening. All of the thin-section CT measures showed significant inverse correlations with the percent predicted forced expiratory volume in 1 s (FEV_1), while the percentage of abnormal lung correlated inversely with percent predicted values of forced vital capacity and total lung capacity. All measures of CT abnormality correlated significantly with indices of impaired gas exchange on exercise. However, the strength of the correlations was not strong (Spearman rho values between 0.3 and 0.7). These findings are consistent with previous studies evaluating the correlation between CT findings of sarcoidosis and physiological impairment (BRAUNER et al. 1989; MULLER et al. 1989; REMY-JARDIN et al. 1994).

10.4 Comparison of Chronic Beryllium Disease and Sarcoidosis

Although the clinical, histological, and imaging manifestations of chronic beryllium disease are indistinguishable from those of sarcoidosis, it should be noted that extrathoracic manifestations are very uncommon in berylliosis. Also, hilar and mediastinal adenopathy without parenchymal radiographic abnormality is a common radiographic presentation of sarcoidosis but has not been described in berylliosis. Despite these differences, the most important message for the radiologist is that berylliosis must always be considered in the differential diagnosis of sarcoidosis. Listing berylliosis as part of the differential diagnosis of sarcoidosis may lead the clinician to obtain a more detailed occupational history.

10.5 Beryllium and Lung Cancer

Animal studies have demonstrated that beryllium can induce cancer in a number of species (FINCH et al. 1996, NEWMAN 1994). On histological evaluation, these animal tumors were mainly adenocarcinomas or bronchioloalveolar carcinoma (FINCH, HOOVER et al. 1996) (GOTTSCHALL 2002). Several large epidemiological studies have reported an increased risk for lung cancer in beryllium-exposed workers, with increased standardized mortality ratios (SMR) of 1.37 to 1.97 in beryllium production workers and as high as 3.14 for individuals who have had acute beryllium disease (INFANTE et al. 1980; WAGONER et al. 1980) (MANCUSO and EL-ATTAR 1969; MANCUSO 1970; MANCUSO 1980). A study of cases from the US Beryllium Case Registry supported an increased risk for lung cancer in those with chronic beryllium disease (SMR: 1.57) and those with acute beryllium disease (SMR: 2.32) (STEENLAND and WARD 1991). In workers at beryllium-processing plants, the SMR for lung cancer was increased at 1.26, even after allowing for the effects of smoking (WARD et al. 1992). Most, if not all, of these studies dealt with heavily exposed workers, and it seems that the risk of cancer increases with increasing levels of exposure (SANDERSON et al. 2001). Data regarding the carcinogenic risks of lighter exposure levels remain unclear. However, the quality of the evidence from the animal and human studies cited above was sufficient to allow the International Agency for Research on Cancer (IARC) to list beryllium as a known carcinogen in humans (GOTTSCHALL 2002).

Lung cancer should be suspected on chest radiographs or CT of patients with CBD if there is a dominant nodule or mass and if adenopathy is markedly asymmetric (Fig. 10.13).

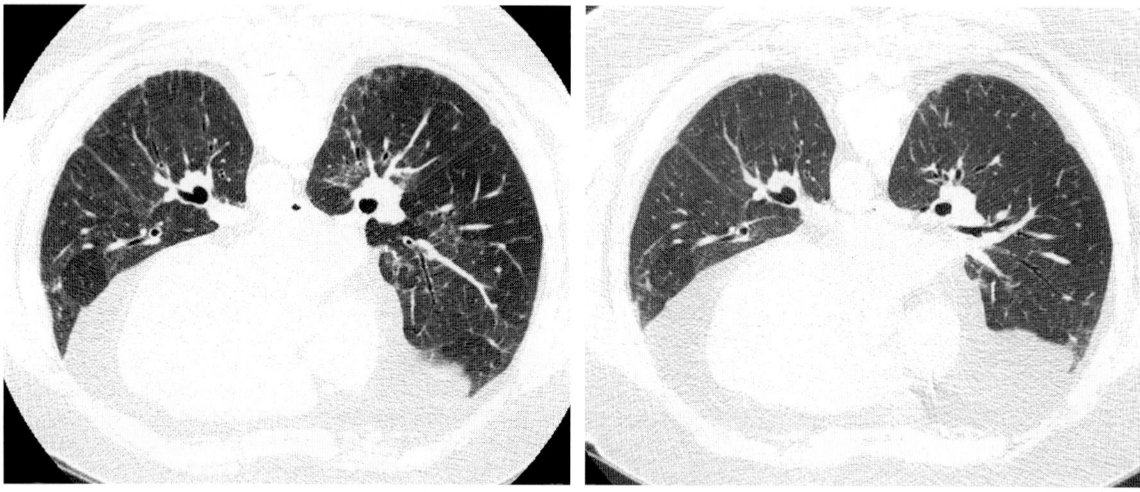

Fig. 10.12. **a** Prone high resolution computed tomography (CT) through the lower lungs in a patient with chronic beryllium disease shows moderate interlobular septal thickening and ground glass abnormality. **b** Follow-up CT 15 months later shows decrease in ground glass abnormality and septal thickening

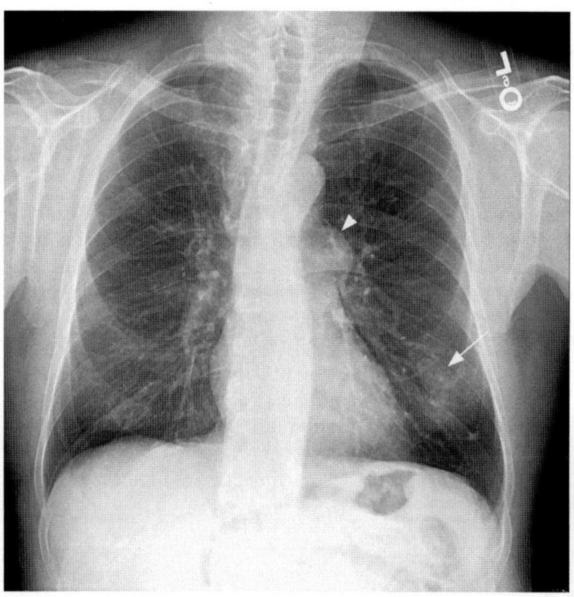

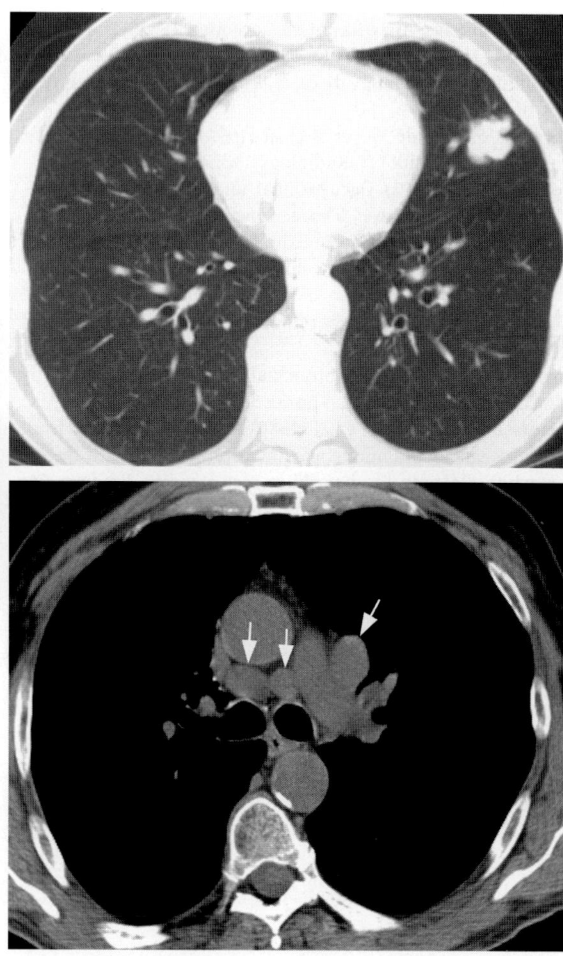

Fig. 10.13. **a** Chest radiograph in a patient with chronic beryllium disease shows a focal left lower lung nodule (*arrow*), with left hilar enlargement (*arrowhead*). **b** Computed tomography (CT) through the lower lungs confirms an irregular lingular nodule, proven to represent lung cancer. **c** CT through the mediastinum confirms enlarged left hilar and mediastinal nodes (*arrows*)

10.6 Summary

Beryllium exposure occurs in a wide variety of occupations. It may cause acute berylliosis (currently very rare), beryllium sensitization, chronic beryllium disease, or lung cancer. Imaging manifestations of chronic beryllium disease are generally similar to those of sarcoidosis, with nodules, ground glass abnormality, septal thickening, conglomerate masses, and mediastinal or hilar lymphadenopathy.

References

Brauner M, Grenier P et al (1989) Pulmonary sarcoidosis: Evaluation with high resolution CT. Radiology 172:467–471

Brauner M, Lenoir S et al (1992). Pulmonary sarcoidosis: CT assessment of lesion reversibility. Radiology 182:349–354

Cullen MR (2005) Screening for chronic beryllium disease: one hurdle down, two to go. Am J Respir Crit Care Med 171:3–4

Daniloff E, Lynch D et al (1997) Observer variation and relationship of computed tomography to severity of beryllium disease. Am J Resp Crit Care Med 155:2047–2056

Finch GL, Hoover MD et al (1996) Animal models of beryllium-induced lung disease. Environ Health Perspect 104S:973–979

Gevenois PA, Vande Weyer R et al (1994) Beryllium disease: assessment with CT. Radiology 193:283–284

Gottschall EB (2002) Occupational and environmental thoracic malignancies. J Thorac Imaging 17:189–197

Harris KM, McConnochie K et al (1993) The computed tomographic appearances in chronic berylliosis. Clin Radiol 47:26–31

Hooper WF (1981) Acute beryllium lung disease. N C Med J 42:551–553

Iles PB (1981) Multiple bronchial stenoses: treatment by mechanical dilatation. Thorax 36:784–786

Infante PF, Wagoner JK et al (1980) Mortality patterns from lung cancer and nonneoplastic respiratory disease among white males in the beryllium case registry. Environ Res 21:35–43

Maier LA (2002a) Clinical approach to chronic beryllium disease and other nonpneumoconiotic interstitial lung diseases. J Thorac Imaging 17:273–284

Maier LA (2002b) Genetic and exposure risks for chronic beryllium disease. Clin Chest Med 23:827–839

Mancuso TF (1970) Relation of duration of employment and prior respiratory illness to respiratory cancer among beryllium workers. Environ Res 3:251–275

Mancuso TF (1980) Mortality study of beryllium industry workers' occupational lung cancer. Environ Res 21:48–55

Mancuso TF, el-Attar AA (1969) Epidemiological study of the beryllium industry. Cohort methodology and mortality studies. J Occup Med 11:422–434

Muller N, Mawson J et al (1989) Sarcoidosis: Correlation of extent of disease at CT with clinical, functional, and radiographic findings. Radiology 171:613–618

Murdoch J, Muller N (1992) Pulmonary sarcoidosis: changes on followup examination. AJR Am J Roentgenol 159:473–477

Newman L (1994) Beryllium lung disease: the role of cell-mediated immunity in pathogenesis. Dean J, Luster M Munson A (eds) Immunotoxicology and immunopharmacology. Raven Press, New York, pp 377–393

Newman LS, Buschman DL et al. (1994) Beryllium disease: assessment with CT. Radiology 190:835–840

Newman LS, Mroz MM et al (2001) Efficacy of serial medical surveillance for chronic beryllium disease in a beryllium machining plant. J Occup Environ Med 43:231–237

Newman LS, Mroz MM et al (2005) Beryllium sensitization progresses to chronic beryllium disease: a longitudinal study of disease risk. Am J Respir Crit Care Med 171:54–60

Remy-Jardin M, Giraud F et al (1994) Pulmonary sarcoidosis: role of CT in the evaluation of disease activity and functional impairment and in prognosis assessment. Radiology 191:675–680

Sanderson WT, Ward EM et al (2001) Lung cancer case-control study of beryllium workers. Am J Ind Med 39:133–144

Steenland K, Ward E (1991) Lung cancer incidence among patients with beryllium disease: a cohort mortality study. J Natl Cancer Inst 83:1380–1385

Wagoner JK, Infante PF et al (1980) Beryllium: an etiologic agent in the induction of lung cancer, nonneoplastic respiratory disease, and heart disease among industrially exposed workers. Environ Res 21:15–34

Ward E, Okun A et al (1992) A mortality study of workers at seven beryllium processing plants. Am J Ind Med 22:885–904

11 Hard Metal and Cobalt Disease

Johny A. Verschakelen and Benoit Nemery

CONTENTS

11.1 Introduction *257*
11.2 Hard Metal and Cobalt *257*
11.3 Respiratory Effects of the Exposure to Cobalt *258*
11.4 Radiographic and Computed Tomography Appearance of Hard Metal Lung Disease *258*
11.5 Conclusion *260*
References *260*

11.1 Introduction

Hard metal lung disease is a rare form of occupational lung disease that can occur in workers engaged in the manufacture, utilization, or maintenance of tools composed of hard metal (a material composed mainly of tungsten carbide and cobalt) or diamond-cobalt. Clinically, the condition resembles hypersensitivity pneumonitis, with subacute presentations and possible evolution to pulmonary fibrosis. One of the problems when searching the literature on interstitial lung disease caused by hard metal, is that the condition has been labeled differently since its first description in 1940 by Jobs and Ballhausen. The terms hard metal pneumoconiosis, hard metal (lung) disease, cobalt lung, and giant cell interstitial pneumonitis are often used interchangeably (Nemery et al. 1991b).

11.2 Hard Metal and Cobalt

Hard metal is essentially produced by heating tungsten carbide together with cobalt powder at about 1,500°C (Cugell 1992). Additional metals, such as small amounts of nickel, titanium, chromium, and tantalum may also be added according to the desired properties of final product. Paraffin is then added to bind the agents (Coates and Watson 1971). This mixture of powdered metals is then pressed into various shapes and can be grinded, polished, and cut to precise dimensions, which is performed using diamond-coated or carborundum-coated cutting tools. During this process, a variety of coolants and lubricants are used. The resultant product consists of about 80% tungsten carbide, 10–20% cobalt, and minor amounts of the other metals. It is used in manufacturing and industrial activities in which extreme hardness and high temperature resistance is required (Coates and Watson 1971). Such industries include grinding of hard metal cutting tools, armor plating, oil well drilling, and diamond polishing (Cugell 1992).

During the cutting, grinding, and polishing process and because of the aerosolization of the coolants, a fog or mist containing metal particles ranging from 1.2 µm to 1.9 µm is released into the air and is readily inhaled (Coates and Watson 1971; Cugell 1992). In this mist or fog of coolants, cobalt exists mainly in a dissolved or ionized form. When inhaled, it can combine with body proteins and act as a hapten (Cugell et al. 1990; Harding 1950; Kerfoot et al. 1975; Sjogren et al. 1980). Pure metallic cobalt, however, probably presents a lesser health risk because it is not ionized (Hellsten et al. 1976). Nevertheless, it is well known that, although there are several components present in hard metal, cobalt is the component that induces pulmonary disease (Coates and Watson 1971; Cugell 1992; Cugell et al. 1990; Hartung et al. 1982). It was indeed shown that experimental instillation of cobalt in the trachea induces inflammation and fibrosis. In contrast, the instillation of tungsten does not induce inflammatory changes, although synergism may occur (Coates and Watson 1971; Cugell 1992; DellaTorre et al. 1990; Migliori et al. 1994). Observations of lung changes in diamond

J. A. Verschakelen, MD, PhD
Department of Radiology, K. U. Leuven, Herestraat 49, 3000 Leuven, Belgium
B. Nemery, MD, PhD
Research Unit of Lung Toxicology, Laboratory of Pneumology, Herestraat 49, 3000 Leuven, Belgium

polishers who had used high-speed cobalt polishing disks, and who had been exposed to cobalt only, provide additional evidence (Demedts et al. 1984). The fact that tungsten does not provoke a tissue reaction is remarkable because there is a deposition of large amounts of tungsten powder in the lungs (Fairhall et al. 1947; Harding 1950). In fact, tungsten in the tissues may serve as a marker of previous exposure. Cobalt, however, is rarely found in tissues because of its solubility (Coates et al. 1973; Sprince et al. 1988; Verhamme 1973).

11.3 Respiratory Effects of the Exposure to Cobalt

Reactions of the airways and the lungs after exposure to cobalt are relatively uncommon. The reason for this is not clear but can be related to an immunological mechanism or a genetic susceptibility factor, or a combination of both (Nemery et al. 2001a; Potolicchio et al. 1997). In 1940, Jobs and Ballhausen described for the first time signs and symptoms in workers exposed to hard metals, with 8 of their 27 workers showing a reticulonodular pattern on the chest radiograph (Jobs and Ballhausen 1940). During a survey of nearly 2,000 tungsten carbide workers in the United States a few years later, Fairhall et al. noted an increased prevalence of conjunctivitis, rhinitis and bronchitis (Fairhall et al. 1947). Some of their patients had lung involvement similar to what Jobs and Ballhausen had described previously. In 1987, Sprince et al. reported that, among 1,039 tungsten carbide workers, 10.9% had "work related wheeze" and 0.7% had interstitial lung disease (Sprince et al. 1987). A few papers also described the development of a picture of acute and subacute hypersensitivity pneumonitis in hard metal workers (Davison et al. 1983; Sjogren et al. 1980). However, most studies have found no relationship between disease occurrence and length of occupational exposure. Today, generally three forms of respiratory disease are attributed to the exposure to cobalt: (1) a reversible asthma-like airway obstruction, (2) hypersensitivity pneumonitis or alveolitis, and (3) interstitial lung disease with lung fibrosis (Cugell et al. 1990). Each of these reactions can occur separately, but some patients develop airway obstruction and alveolitis simultaneously (Bech et al. 1962). Both airway obstruction and alveolitis usually improve spontaneously when the subject is no longer exposed to cobalt (Coates and Watson 1971; Sjogren et al. 1980). When exposure is continued, irreversible pulmonary fibrosis may develop gradually. In some patients with hypersensitivity pneumonitis or alveolitis and in some patients with early fibrosis, bizarre giant cells in the terminal bronchioles and alveoli may occur. If these are present, the patient is said to have giant cell interstitial pneumonitis (GIP), a feature that is highly suggestive of cobalt exposure (Cugell et al. 1990; Davison et al. 1983; Michetti et al. 1994; Ohori et al. 1989).

The occupational asthma in hard metal workers is probably an allergic response and is characterized by shortness of breath, wheezing, and coughing (Coates and Watson 1971; Davison et al. 1983; Sjogren et al. 1980). In most patients, the airway obstruction develops 4–6 h after exposure, is often worse in the early hours of the evening, and improves on weekends and holidays (Coates et al. 1973; Cugell et al. 1990). As in other types of occupational asthma, there is a latent period of 6–48 months before sensitization occurs and symptoms develop (Cugell et al. 1990). Hypersensitivity pneumonitis can be acute or chronic and is characterized by fever, anorexia, and shortness of breath (Bech et al. 1962; Davison et al. 1983; Sjogren et al. 1980). Symptoms improve when the patient takes sick leave but recur when he or she returns to work. These episodes usually recur and, after about a year, there is a gradual attenuation of the acute episodes while the shortness of breath persists and slowly worsens, indicating that the repeated exposures have led to fibrosis and permanent parenchymal damage. This fibrosis causes the same physiological changes as those caused by other forms of interstitial fibrosis of the lungs. Early symptoms are dry cough, breathlessness, tachypnea and, occasionally, the production of a small amount of mucoid sputum. The transition from hypersensitivity pneumonitis to irreversible fibrosis is gradual, and signs of fibrosis can already occur after a few years, although they usually appear after 10-12 years of exposure (Cugell et al. 1990; Miller et al. 1953; Moschinski et al. 1959). If the fibrosis becomes important, cor pulmonale and pulmonary hypertension can develop.

11.4 Radiographic and Computed Tomography Appearance of Hard Metal Lung Disease

The chest radiograph in a patient with hard metal lung disease is often normal or consistent with an interstitial process but is usually not diagnostic of the disorder. During the attacks of hypersensitivity pneumonitis, a fine reticulonodular pattern can be seen which involves the upper, middle, and lower lung (DEMEDTS et al. 1984; FIGUEROA et al. 1992) (Fig. 11.1). Since occasionally lymphadenopathy is also present, the chest radiographic changes can mimic sarcoidosis (DELLATORRE et al. 1990; RIZZATO et al. 1994). In a few patients, more extensive and bilateral or rarely patchy consolidation have been reported (Fig. 11.1). However, the more characteristic acinar pattern described in patients with farmer's lung is unusual. In most cases, these lung changes disappear slowly when exposure ceases and when the subject stops working promptly, although the lung volume can continue to appear reduced on the chest radiograph. The administration of steroids hastens the roentgenographic improvement. If, on the contrary, the patient is not treated or if the exposure is not terminated, DELLATORRE et al. have shown that these opacities may progress over time (DELLATORRE et al. 1990). Pneumothorax has been described as a rare complication of hard metal lung disease (RUOKONEN et al. 1996).

Due to the rarity of hard metal lung disease, the number of reports describing the thin-section computed tomography (CT) features of this disease is limited. Nevertheless, the pulmonary infiltrates and their distribution pattern are usually better appreciated on a CT examination (MENDELSON et al. 1991) (Fig. 11.2). The thin-section CT appearance may be variable and may mimic sarcoidosis (Fig. 11.3),

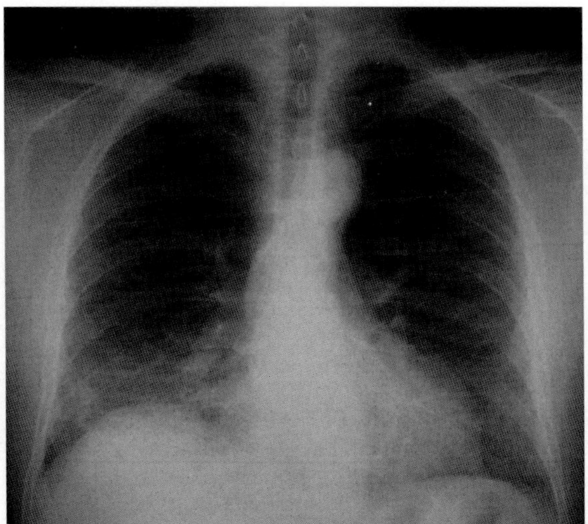

Fig. 11.1. Hard metal lung disease: acute phase. A reticulonodular pattern can be seen in the lower part of both lungs – within the right lower lung some areas of patchy consolidation

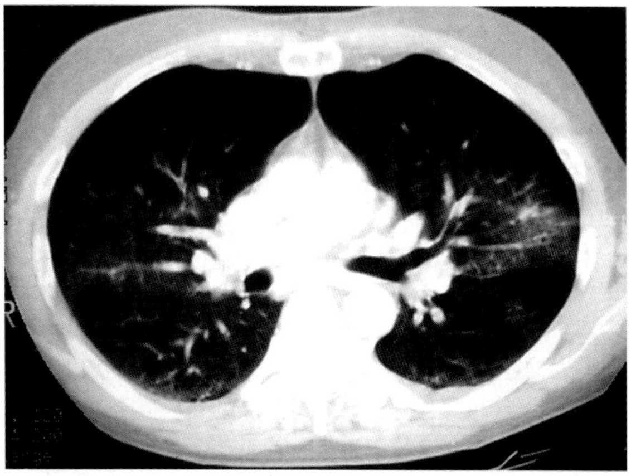

Fig. 11.2. Hard metal lung disease: acute phase. Computed tomography scan shows areas of ground-glass opacity and consolidation

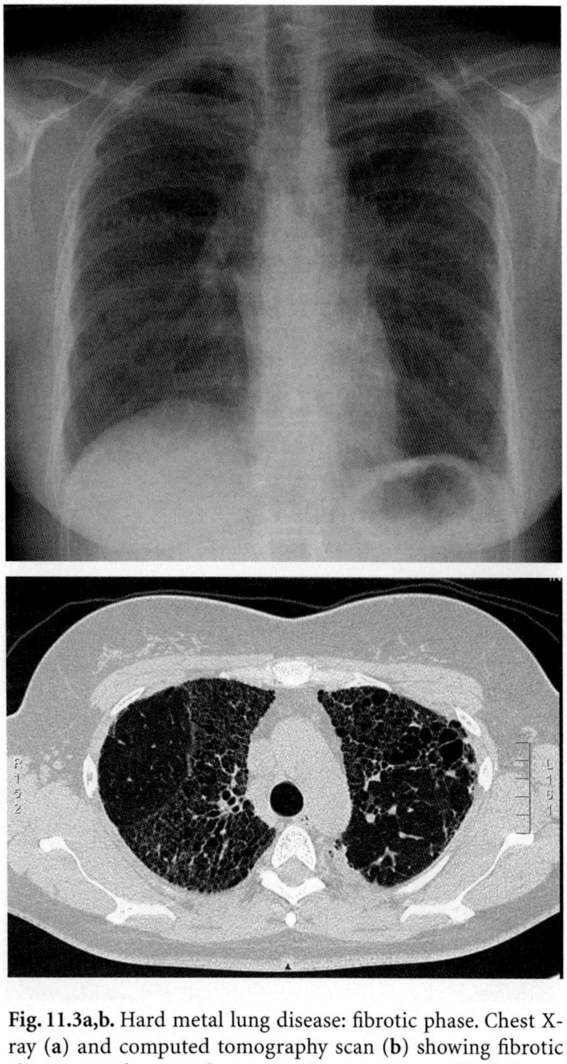

a

b

Fig. 11.3a,b. Hard metal lung disease: fibrotic phase. Chest X-ray (**a**) and computed tomography scan (**b**) showing fibrotic changes predominantly seen in the upper part of both lungs mimicking sarcoidosis non-specific interstitial pneumonia (NSIP), and even usual interstitial pneumonia (UIP) (Fig. 11.4). Gotway et al. described a case of hard metal lung disease in which thin-section CT showed bilateral fine and peripheral reticulation caused by intralobular interstitial thickening, nodular peribronchovascular thickening, traction bronchiectasis, large, peripheral, cystic spaces, and subpleural lines (Gotway et al. 2002). These findings were slightly more prominent in the upper lobes and thus somewhat resembled the distribution pattern of sarcoidosis (Fig. 11.3). In other reports, the primary finding was ground-glass opacity, traction bronchiectasis and reticulation mimicking NSIP (Kim et al. 2001; Lee et al. 2000). Tan et al. described a case of a worker in the tool manufacturing industry who developed peripheral honeycombing in both lungs resembling UIP (Lee et al. 2000; Tan et al. 2000) (Fig. 11.4). Akira reported two cases of histopathologically proven hard metal lung disease in which multifocal, bilateral, fibrotic consolidation and ground-glass opacity were the primary findings (Akira 1995). Lundgren and Oman (1954) reported enlarged hilar lymph nodes, while Mendelson et al. (1991) found an increased density of the mediastinal lymph nodes (Fig. 11.5). Although this author could not detect depositions of metal in these lymph nodes as a cause of this increased density, it was suggested that the presence of dense lymph nodes may offer a means of identifying patients who had significant exposure to dust.

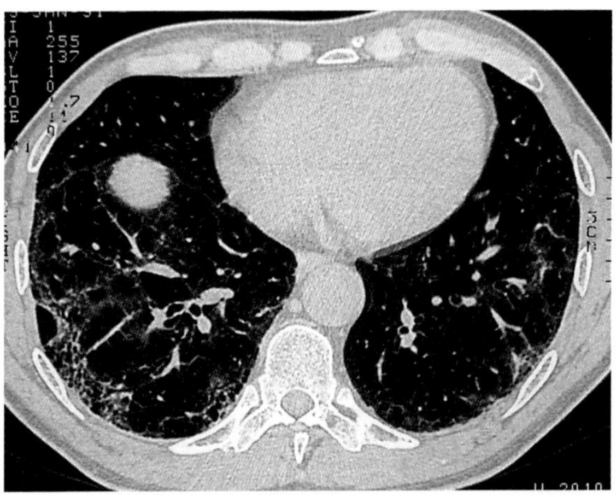

Fig. 11.4. Hard metal lung disease: fibrotic phase. The fibrotic changes are sometimes predominantly seen in the basal parts of the lungs and can mimic usual interstitial pneumonia

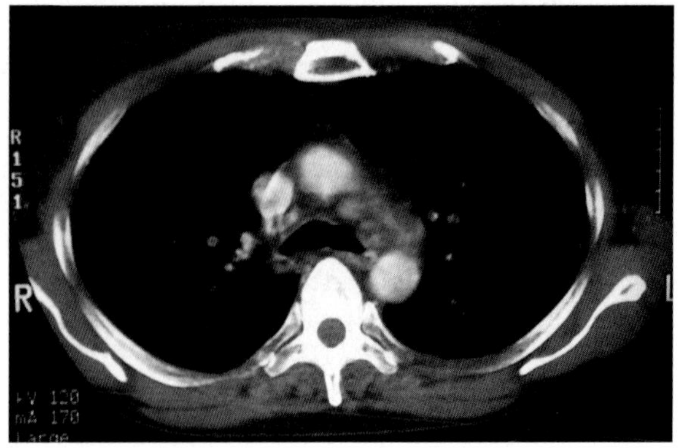

Fig. 11.5. Hard metal lung disease: enlarged lymph nodes. Patient showing enlarged lymph nodes in the aortic pulmonary window. Notice the high density of these lymph nodes, a feature considered suggestive of significant exposure to dust

11.5 Conclusion

Pulmonary involvement resulting from exposure to cobalt is rare and is also, because of the variable and non-specific imaging features, easily missed. However, discovering one of these patterns on a chest radiograph or a CT scan should prompt a search for known associations of these patterns of lung injury, as well as a thorough examination of the occupational history.

References

Akira M (1995) Uncommon pneumoconiosis: CT and pathologic findings. Radiology 197:403-409

Bech AO, Kipling MD, Heather JC (1962) Hard metal disease. Br J Ind Med 19:239-252

Coates EO Jr, Watson JH (1971) Diffuse interstitial lung disease in tungsten carbide workers. Ann Intern Med 75:709-716

Coates EO Jr, Sawyer HJ, Rebuck JW et al (1973) Hypersensitivity bronchitis in tungsten carbide workers. Chest 64:390

Cugell DW (1992) The hard metal diseases. Clin Chest Med 13:269-279

Cugell DW, Morgan WK, Perkins DG et al (1990) The respiratory effects of cobalt. Arch Intern Med 150:177-183

Davison AG, Haslam PL, Corrin B et al (1983) Interstitial lung disease and asthma in hard metal workers: bronchoalveolar lavage, ultrastructural and analytical findings and results of bronchial provocation tests. Thorax 38:119-128

DellaTorre F, Cassani M, Segale M et al (1990) Trace metal lung diseases: a new fatal case of hard metal pneumoconiosis. Respiration 57:248-253

Demedts M, Gheysens B, Nagels J et al (1984) Cobalt lung in diamond polishers. Am Rev Respir Dis 130:130-135

Fairhall LT, Castberg HT, Carrosso NJ, Brinton HP (1947) Industrial hygiene aspects of the cemented tungsten carbide industry. Occup Med 4:371-379

Figueroa S, Gerstenhaber B, Welch L, Klimstra D, Walker Smith GJ, Beckett W (1992) Hard metal interstitial pulmonary disease associated with a form of welding in a metal parts coating plant. Am J Ind Med 21:363-373

Gotway MB, Golden JA, Warnock M et al (2002) Hard metal interstitial lung disease: high-resolution computed tomography appearance. J Thorac Imaging 17:314-318

Harding HE (1950) Notes on the toxicology of cobalt metal. Br J Ind Med 7:76-78

Hartung M, Schaller KH, Brand E (1982) On the question of the pathogenetic importance of cobalt for hard metal fibrosis of the lung. Int Arch Occup Environ Health 50:53-57

Hellsten E, Blomberg M, Henrikson-Enflo A et al (1976) Kobalt. University of Stockholm Institute of Physics, Stockholm, Sweden; report 76

Jobs H, Ballhausen C (1940) Powder metallurgy as a source of dust from the medical and technical standpoint. Vertrauensartz Krankenkasse 8:142-148

Kerfoot EJ, Frederick WG, Domeier E (1975) Cobalt metal inhalation studies on miniature swine. Am Ind Hyg Assoc J 36:17-21

Kim KI, Kim CW, Lee MK et al (2001) Imaging of occupational lung disease. Radiographics 21:1371-1391

Lee KS, Kang KW, Chung MP et al (2000) A case of giant cell interstitial pneumonitis. Notes from the 1999 annual meeting of the Korean Society of Thoracic Radiology. J Thorac Imaging 15:34-35

Lundgren KD, Oman H (1954) Pneumokoniose in der Hartmetallindustrie. Virchows Arch 325:259-284

Mendelson DS, Gendal ES, Janus CL et al (1991) Computed tomography of the thorax in workers exposed to hard metals. Br J Ind Med 48:208-210

Michetti G, Mosconi G, Zanelli R et al (1994) Bronchoalveolar lavage and its role in diagnosing cobalt lung disease. Sci Total Environ 150:173-178

Migliori M, Mosconi G, Michetti G et al (1994) Hard metal disease: eight workers with interstitial lung fibrosis due to cobalt exposure. Sci Total Environ 150:187-196

Miller CW, Davis MW, Goldman A et al (1953) Pneumoconiosis in the tungsten carbide industry. AMA Arch Ind Hyg 8:453-465

Moschinski G, Jurisch A, Reinl W (1959) Die Lungenveränderungen bei Sinterhartmetall-Arbeitern. Arch Gewerbepath 16:697-720

Nemery B, Bast A, Behr J et al (2001a) Interstitial lung disease induced by exogenous agents: factors governing susceptibility. Eur Respir J [Suppl] 32:30s-42s

Nemery B, Verbeken EK, Demedts M (2001b) Giant cell interstitial pneumonia (hard metal lung disease, cobalt lung). Semin Respir Crit Care Med 22:435-447

Ohori NP, Sciurba FC, Owens GR et al (1989) Giant cell interstitial pneumonia and hard-metal pneumoconiosis. A clinicopathologic study of four cases and review of the literature. Am J Surg Pathol 13:581-587

Potolicchio I, Mosconi G, Forni A, Nemery B, Seghizzi P, Sorrentino R (1997) Susceptibility to hard metal lung disease is strongly associated with the presence of glutamate 69 in HLA-DPß chain. Eur J Immunol 27:2741-2743

Rizzato G, Fraioli P, Sabbioni E, Pietra R, Barberis M (1994) The differential diagnosis of hard metal lung disease. Sci Total Environ 150:77-83

Ruokonen E-L, Linnainmaa M, Seuri M, Juhakoshi P, Soderstrom K-O (1996) A fatal case of hard-metal disease. Scand J Work Environ Health 22:62-65

Sjogren I, Hillerdal G, Andersson A, Zetterstrom O (1980) Hard metal lung disease: the importance of cobalt in coolants. Thorax 35:653-659

Sprince NL, Oliver LC, Chamberlain RI et al (1987) Exposure to cobalt and interstitial lung disease in tungsten carbide production workers. Am Rev Respir Dis 135 [Suppl]: A20

Sprince NL, Oliver LC, Eisen EA, Greene RE, Chamberlain RI (1988) Cobalt exposure and lung diseases in tungsten carbide production. Am Rev Respir Dis 138:1220-1226

Tan KL, Lee HS, Poh WT et al (2000) Hard metal lung disease - the first case in Singapore. Ann Acad Med Singapore 29:521-527

Verhamme EN (1973) Contribution to the evaluation of toxicity of cobalt. Cobalt 2:29-32

12 Other Uncommon Pneumoconioses

Masanori Akira

CONTENTS

12.1 Aluminum Pneumoconiosis 263
12.1.1 Prevalence 263
12.1.2 Chest X-Ray 264
12.1.3 Thin-Section Computed Tomography 265
12.2 Welders' Lung 266
12.2.1 Prevalence 266
12.2.2 Chest X-Ray 266
12.2.3 Thin-Section CT 267
12.3 Graphite Pneumoconiosis 268
12.3.1 Prevalence 268
12.3.2 Chest X-Ray 268
12.3.3 Thin-Section CT 269
12.4 Talc Pneumoconiosis 270
12.4.1 Prevalence 270
12.4.2 Chest X-Ray 271
12.4.3 Thin-Section CT 272
12.4.4 Positron Emission Tomography 272
12.5 Kaolinosis 272
12.5.1 Prevalence 272
12.5.2 Chest X-Ray 273
12.5.3 Thin-Section CT 274
12.6 Chemical Pneumonitis 274
12.6.1 Ammonia 274
12.6.2 Nitrogen Dioxide 274
12.6.3 Chlorine 275
12.6.4 Paraquat 275
References 277

12.1 Aluminum Pneumoconiosis

Aluminum is derived from bauxite, an ore that consists of alumina with iron and other minerals. The alumina is extracted from the ore and reduced to metallic aluminum by electrolysis using large pots in the pot room. This process is carried out in large pots. The pot room atmosphere contains not only alumina dust but also a variety of other substances including hydrogen fluoride, sulfur dioxide, metal fumes, cyanide, ozone, and aromatic hydrocarbons. Exposure to aluminum, alumina, and pot room fumes has been putatively associated with diffuse interstitial fibrosis; however, the exact etiological agent of aluminum-induced fibrosis is uncertain (Dinman 1987).

Although exposure to aluminum metal and its oxides in the workplace is very common, pneumoconioses attributable to these agents are rare. In early studies, pulmonary fibrosis in relation to aluminum exposure has been reported almost exclusively in workers involved in bauxite smelting (Shaver's disease) (Shaver and Riddell 1947; Wyatt and Riddell 1948) or in those exposed to finely divided aluminum powders, especially of the flake variety (pyro powder), in the fireworks and explosives industry (Mitchell et al. 1961; Jordan 1961). Subsequently, diffuse interstitial fibrosis has been reported in workers making aluminum oxide abrasives (Bellot et al. 1984; Jederlinic et al. 1990) and in aluminum arc welders (Vallyathan et al. 1982; Herbert et al. 1982).

Desquamative interstitial pneumonia (Herbert et al. 1982), a granulomatous lung reaction (DeVuyst et al. 1987), and pulmonary alveolar proteinosis (Miller et al. 1984), which develop after exposure to fumes from aluminum welding, have been described.

12.1.1 Prevalence

Shaver and Riddell (1947) found 35 cases (10%) of pulmonary fibrosis out of 344 aluminum pot room workers. Studies from Germany revealed that 26% of 628 workers had roentgenographic evidence of pneumoconiosis (Mitchell et al. 1961). In one study, the authors reported that small irregular opacities were observed in 7–8% of 788 male employees of an aluminum production company (Townsend et al. 1988). Jederlinic et al. (1990) found a 1% incidence of interstitial fibrosis in a factory using alumina as an abrasive.

M. Akira, MD
Department of Radiology, Kinki-Chuo Chest Medical Center (former National Kinki Chuo Hospital for Chest Disease), 1180 Nagasone-cho, Sakai City, Osaka 591-8555, Japan

12.1.2 Chest X-Ray

Radiographically and pathologically, aluminum-induced interstitial fibrosis is predominantly upper and mid zonal. The roentgenograms show ground-glass or nodular opacities more pronounced in the upper or middle zones of both lungs and a widening of the mediastinal shadow (Figs. 12.1a, 12.2a). Emphysematous change in the basal lung and displacement of the hila upwards or backwards indicating pulmonary contracture also characterizes the advanced cases (Shaver and Riddell 1947; Edling 1961; Mitchell et al. 1961; De Vuyst et al. 1986). The interstitial changes and honeycombing sometimes shows diffuse distribution (Fig. 12.3a) (Gilks and Churg 1987; Jederlinic et al. 1990).

It is reported in workers employed in the manufacture of alumina abrasives that a man leaving employment of the plant with a negative chest film showed evidence of disease 1 year later (Shaver 1948). Once the disease becomes well established, progression is often rapid, and complete disability may result shortly thereafter.

Aluminum-associated pulmonary fibrosis is associated with a high frequency of spontaneous pneumothorax (Shaver and Riddell 1947; Shaver 1948), which is life-threatening for the patient.

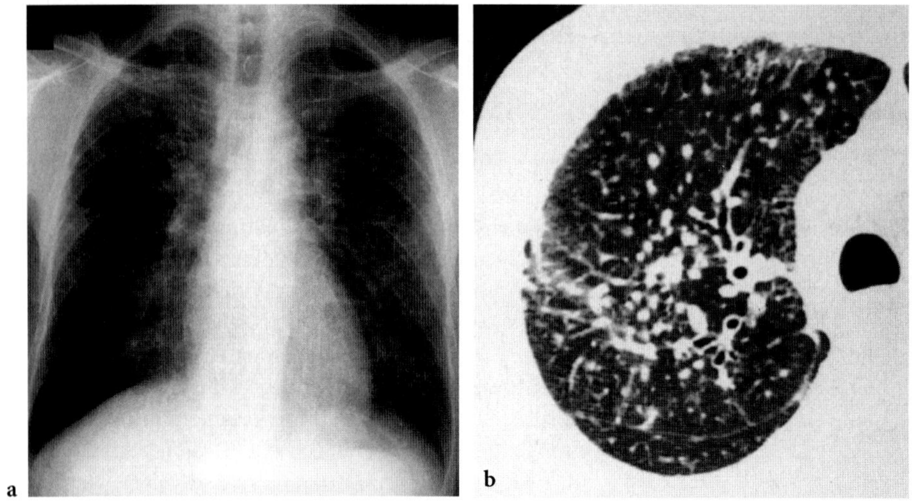

Fig. 12.1a,b. Aluminum pneumoconiosis. (**a**) Numerous small nodules with upper zonal predominance are seen. (**b**) Thin-section computed tomography scan of the same patient shows coalesce of small nodules

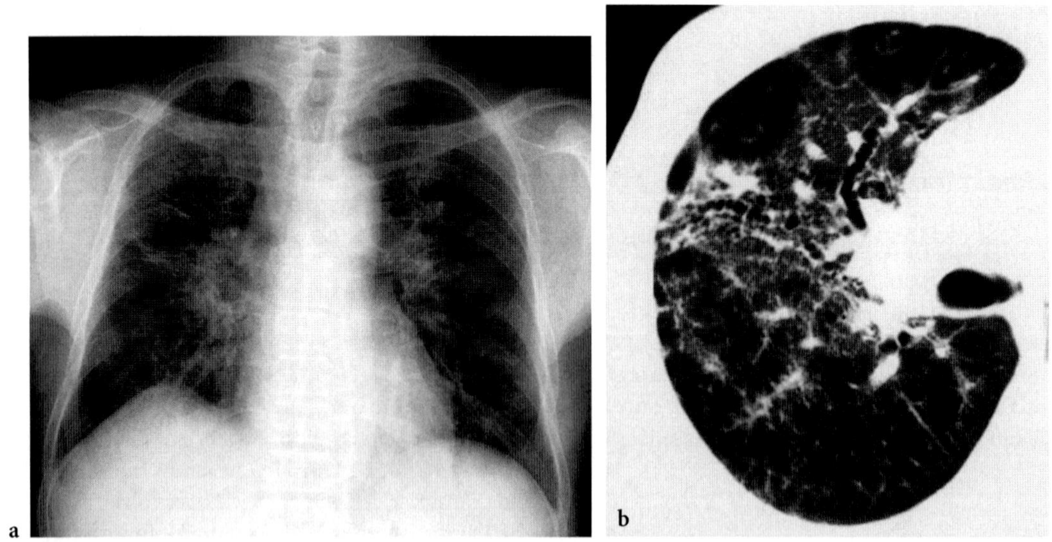

Fig. 12.2a,b. Aluminum pneumoconiosis. (**a**) Fine striations, nodular, and ground-glass opacities more pronounced in the upper and middle lung zones and displacement of the hila upwards are seen. (**b**) Thin-section computed tomography scan of the same patient shows areas of ground-glass attenuation around the bronchovascular bundles and traction bronchiectasis

12.1.3 Thin-Section Computed Tomography

Thin-section computed tomography (CT) findings have several patterns (Figs. 12.1b–12.3b). In one study of six workers, the thin-section CT findings were classified into three forms: predominantly reticular fibrosis; predominantly nodular fibrosis; and upper lung fibrosis. In two patients with predominantly reticular fibrosis, thin-section CT findings were similar to those of usual interstitial pneumonia, and honeycomb formation was found (Fig. 12.3b). In one of these two, the distribution was different from that of IPF in that aluminum-induced interstitial fibrosis had predominantly upper distribution. In one of two patients with predominantly nodular fibrosis, thin-section CT depicted ill-defined centrilobular nodules diffusely throughout both lungs. In the other patient with predominantly nodular fibrosis, thin-section CT findings were similar to those of simple silicosis (AKIRA 1995) (Fig. 12.2b).

Thin-section CT is more sensitive than chest X-rays for detecting the early stage of aluminum dust-induced lung disease. Thin-section CT findings of the early stage in a 40-year-old worker who had worked as a stamper for 14 years in a plant producing aluminum powder were reported. The thin-section CT findings were characterized by small, centrilobular, nodular opacities of up to 3 mm diameter and slightly thickened interlobular septa in all lung sections (KRAUS et al. 2000).

A case with increased CT densities of mediastinal lymph nodes with histologically proven aluminum storage is reported (VAHLENSIECK et al. 2000). The lymph nodes showed increased density on native scans with values of 70–180 HU. Aluminum particles in such patients as well as in animals experimentally exposed to aluminum-containing dust are found in bronchoalveolar lavage, lung tissue, and lymph nodes up to 5 years after stopping the exposure (SNIPES et al. 1983; PEARSON et al. 1986). It is predictable that an aluminum-loaded lymph node results in increased radiographic density due to metallic absorption pattern. Aluminosis is considered as differential diagnosis in patients with increased native CT densities beyond 50 HU (VAHLENSIECK et al. 2000).

a

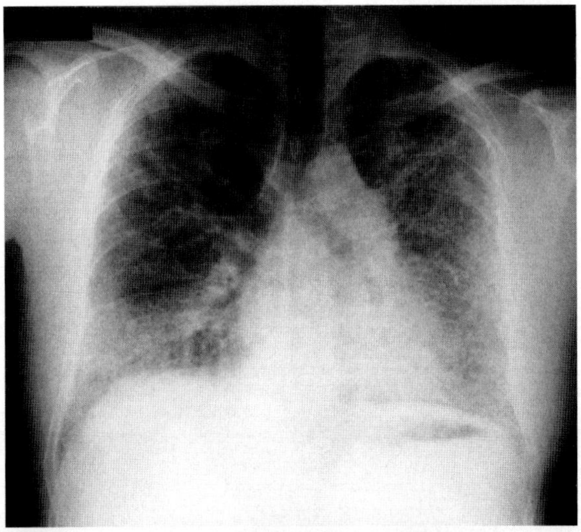

b

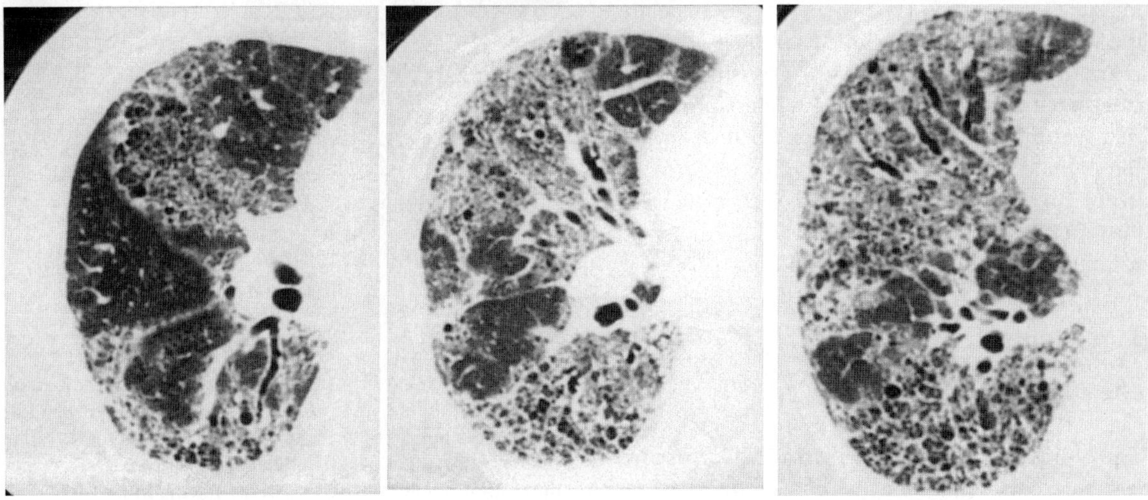

Fig. 12.3a,b. A 52-year-old man with a history of exposure to aluminum for 7 years. (**a**) The chest radiograph reveals reticulonodular opacity, predominantly distributed in the lower lung zones. (**b**) Thin-section computed tomography scans show diffusely distributed reticular hyperattenuation. Traction bronchiectasis and honeycombing are present

12.2 Welders' Lung

Welding is the joining of metal to metal by use of heat and/or pressure. The main fume generated by consumable electrodes is iron oxide. Cadmium, chromium, beryllium, aluminum, titanium, and nickel may also be present. Exposure to welding fumes is known to be a risk factor for chronic respiratory disorders – such as pneumoconiosis, chronic bronchitis, and lung cancer (SFERLAZZA and BECKETT 1991).

Iron oxide is not fibrogenic in human and animal lungs. Some workers exposed to metallic iron or iron oxide fume may also have had significant exposure to other dusts such as quartz, cristobalite, or asbestos, such that siderosis may be complicated by the presence of mixed dust fibrosis or asbestosis (HARDING et al. 1958; GUIDOTTI et al. 1978). However, some authors suggested that the cause of interstitial pulmonary fibrosis seen in some welders did not appear to be coexisting silicosis (FUNAHASHI et al. 1988). HICKS et al. (1983) and HEWITT and HICKS (1983) showed experimentally that nodular fibrosis could be produced with instillation of very large amounts of welding fumes. They concluded that most likely this was a reaction to the iron itself, although other components of the welding fume, such as chromium, nickel, and manganese, also accumulate in the lung.

12.2.1 Prevalence

Welder's pneumoconiosis was first described by DOIG and MCLAUGHLIN in 1936. In one study of 37 arc welders, the radiographic changes were only minimal (ILO category 1, type s, t, p) in the majority of the welders and had developed not only after many years of high but also after low exposure, and ILO category 2 was only found in 4 welders of the high-risk group (SPÁ LOVÁ and KOVAL 1975). A survey of the prevalence of chest radiographic abnormalities in 661 currently employed British electric arc welders found a 7% prevalence of category 0/1 or higher small rounded opacities (ATTFIELD and ROSS 1978).

12.2.2 Chest X-Ray

The typical chest radiographic findings in arc welders' siderosis consist of an increase in the vascular markings and a generalized fine mottling or very fine nodules that are most prominent in the middle third of the lungs in the perihilar regions or in the lower two-thirds of both lungs (Fig. 12.4a). The finely nodular shadows on chest radiographs disappear after removal of patients from occupational exposure (DOIG and MCLAUGHLIN 1948). The micronodules do not reflect reactive fibrosis but, rather, radiopaque accumulations of iron particles that lie within macrophages, aggregated along the perivascular and peribronchial lymphatic vessels. Slight fibrosis may be present, but this is not a prom-

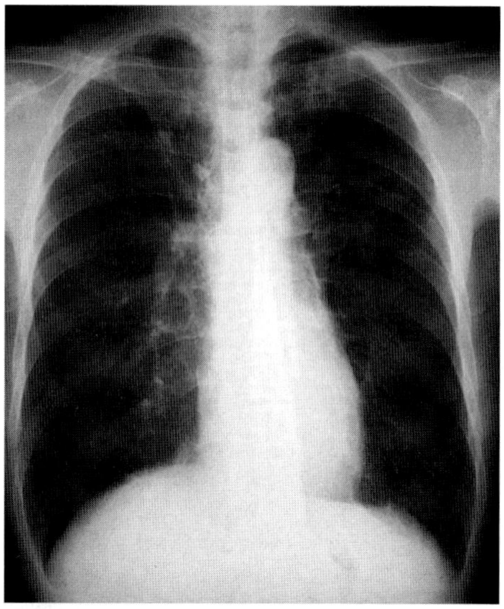

a

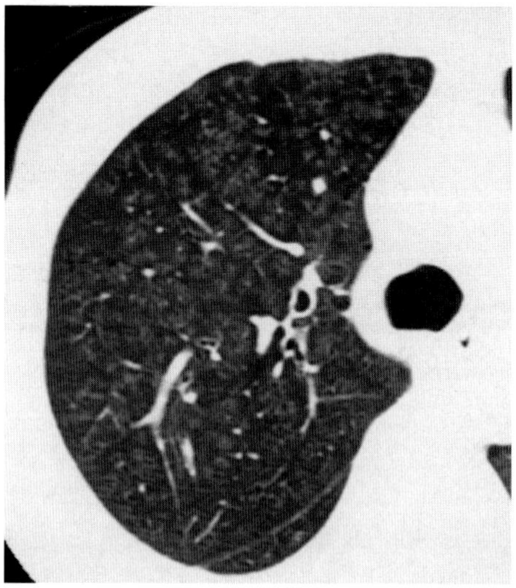

b

Fig. 12.4a,b. Welders' pneumoconiosis. (a) Chest radiograph shows fine nodules that are most prominent in the middle third of the lungs. (b) On thin-section computed tomography, micronodules show centrilobular distribution. The appearance mimics that of hypersensitivity pneumonitis inent feature (Charr 1955; Sander 1967; Guidotti et al. 1978).

However, several authors have reported symptomatic welders with evidence of fibrosis in the lungs (Charr 1956; Meyer et al. 1967; Funahashi et al. 1988). Charr (1956) reported three welders with respiratory disturbances. Their roentgenograms showed exaggeration of linear shadows in the lower half of each lung, compatible with pulmonary fibrosis. The biopsy of the lungs in two revealed fibrosis. Also, both diffuse interstitial fibrosis proceeding to honeycombing and a conglomerative form resembling progressive massive fibrosis are described in arc welders' pneumoconiosis (Morgan 1961; Meyer et al. 1967) (Fig. 12.5a).

12.2.3 Thin-Section CT

The most common CT findings in the arc welders are ill-defined micronodules diffusely distributed in the lung (Akira 1995; Yoshii et al. 2002). Some of the micronodules appear as fine branching lines. In less-affected lung, micronodules show centrilobular distribution. In more-affected lung, gathering of micronodules and fine branching lines form a fine network pattern (Fig. 12.4b, 5b). The micronodules on CT correspond to dust macules, which are collections of dust-laden macrophages surrounding the small airway and vessels (Akira 1995; Yoshii et al. 2002). Emphysema is often seen. There are two patterns of emphysematous change:

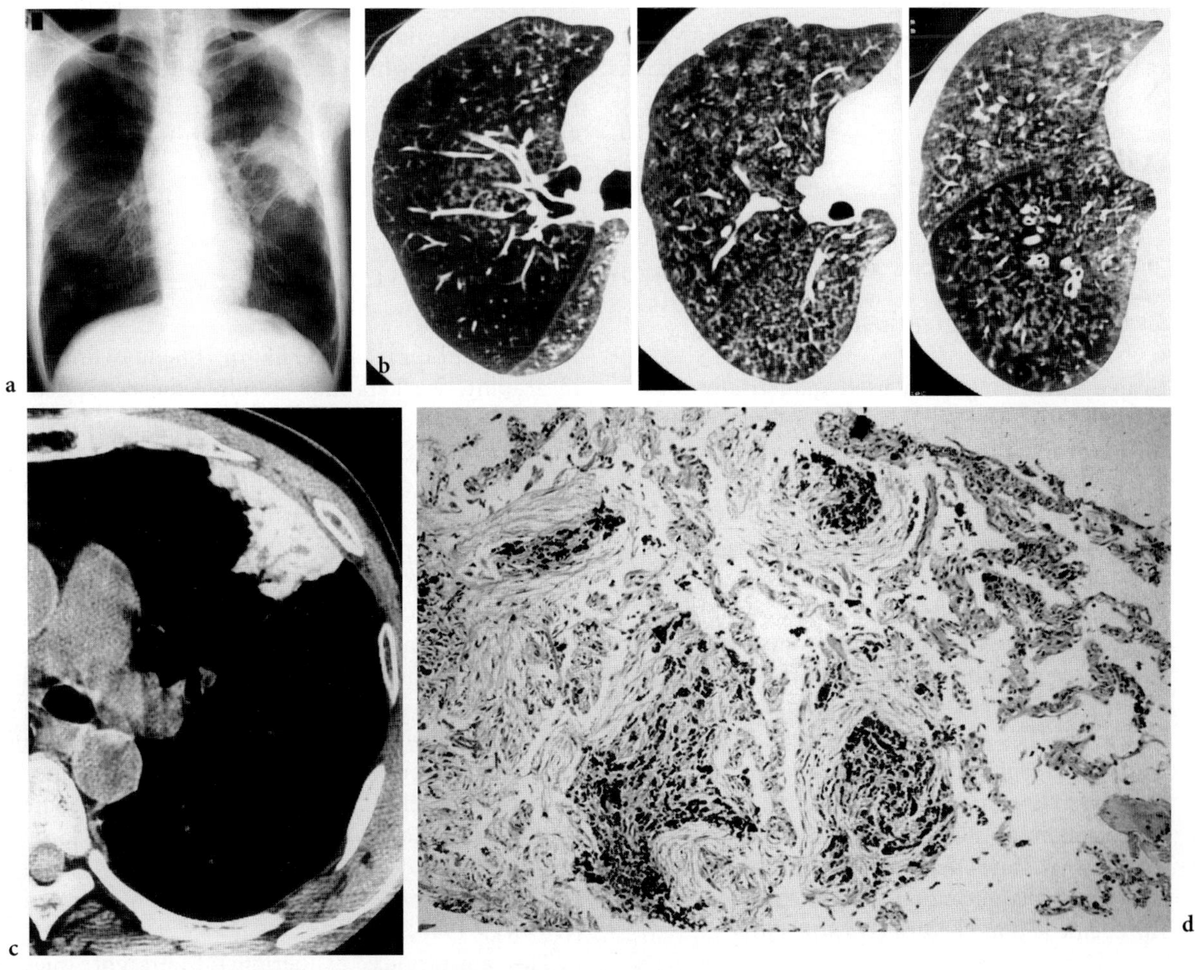

Fig. 12.5a–d. A 60-year-old man employed as an arc welder for 30 years. (**a**) The chest radiograph reveals ill-defined micronodules, most prominent in the middle third of each lung about the hilar regions. Irregularly shaped mass lesion is found in the left middle lung zone. (**b**) Thin-section computed tomography scans show numerous ill-defined micronodules concentrated in the centrilobular regions. In more-affected lung, gathering of micronodules and fine branching areas of increased attenuation create a fine network pattern. (**c**) Viewed at mediastinal windows (level, 35 HU; width, 400 HU), the pulmonary and peripheral mass in the left middle lung zone is seen to contain high-attenuation material. (**d**) The transbronchial biopsy specimen from the mass shows organization with siderosis

centrilobular low attenuating areas with central dot; and focal decreased attenuation distributed multilobularly. Centrilobular emphysema in welders with a smoking history is assumed not to be caused by inhalation of arc-welding fumes. Micronodules also accompany the emphysematous changes, alternatively suggesting the type of focal emphysema commonly seen in coal miners (Akira et al. 1989; Yoshii et al. 2002).

A honeycomb pattern was found in 3 (14%) of 21 arc welders studied by Akira (1995), and fibrotic changes were found in 3 (27.3%) of 11 welder's pneumoconiosis studied by Yoshii et al. (2002). Ground-glass opacity was also seen (Han et al. 2000). In welders, the extent of micronodules seen on thin-section CT showed no significant correlation with the severity of dyspnea or the results of pulmonary function test (Han et al. 2000).

Rarely, is there conglomerate masses with areas of high attenuation (Fig. 12.5c). The mass with areas of high attenuation corresponded histologically to organizing pneumonia with siderosis (Fig. 12.5d) (Akira 1995).

12.3 Graphite Pneumoconiosis

Graphite has long been used industrially for the manufacture of pencils. It is also used extensively for the production of plumbago crucibles, when it is mixed with fire clay; for the manufacture of crucible steel and alloys and for arc-light carbons; for polishing and coating iron articles to prevent rusting; and in an admixture with rubber as an acid-proof coating, and as a pigment and lubricant. Graphite pneumoconiosis is defined as pneumoconiosis in workers exposed to graphite dust at the workplace. Graphite exposure produces roentgenographic and pathological changes similar to those seen in coal workers. The present state of knowledge does not exclude the possibility that analytically pure graphite may cause pneumoconiosis, although the majority of the evidence indicates that pneumoconiosis is a mixed-dust type of lung reaction. Graphite may modify the fibrogenic action of silica (Hanoa 1983).

12.3.1 Prevalence

In clinical and radiographic studies of 415 workers in five collieries, one electrode manufacturing plant, and one milling plant, 24 cases (6%) of pneumoconiosis were found (Parmeggiani 1950). In a study of 71 graphite workers who had been exposed to varying amounts of graphite dust in crucible and graphite mills, 14 (20%) had abnormal roentgenographic patterns interpreted as pneumoconiosis (Müller 1953). According to the findings in a clinical survey of 256 persons employed in the manufacture of carbon electrodes, graphite pneumoconiosis was found in 112 cases (43.8%) of those examined: 70 cases (27.5%) in category 1p, 29 cases (11.4%) in category 2p, and 12 cases (4.7%) in category 3p. After 4 years, the chest radiograms of the workers made progress, 17.9% of them from category 0 to category 1, 17.1% from category 1 to 2, and 30.8% from category 2 to 3 (Okutani et al. 1964). In one study of 344 workers in a large graphite mine in Ceylon, 22.7% of them had radiographic abnormalities, which included small rounded and irregular opacities, large opacities, and significant enlargement of hilar shadows (Ranasinha and Uragoda 1972).

12.3.2 Chest X-Ray

Roentgenographic patterns of pneumoconiosis in graphite workers may simulate those of pneumoconiosis in coal workers, those of anthracosilicosis in coal miners (Fig. 12.6a), or the patterns seen in radiographs of some people with asbestosis (Fig. 12.7a) (Pendergrass et al. 1968). The abnormal patterns include miliary and macronodular opacities, conglomerate and massive lesions of various sizes, emphysema, thickening of the pleura, and distortion of the lung structures. The miliary "snow-storm" pattern can be the final and stationary stage of the pneumoconiosis which will not undergo any further essential change. The extensive abnormal changes seen in roentgenograms of the chest come about quickly in some workers and slowly and late in others. The large opacities may develop by the coalescence of the small lesions shown in the miliary type of reaction (Dunner 1948).

The appearance of peripheral straight lines (Kerley B line) in the lower lobes near the costophrenic sulci occurs in the pneumoconiosis found in graphite workers just as it does in anthracosilicosis and in asbestosis. When massive lesions and emphysema develop, the background nodular pattern may, in some instances, largely disappear.

Serial roentgenograms of the chest made over a period of 5 years or more show that some of the massive lesions migrate toward the midline in posteroanterior radiographs and anteriorly or posteriorly in lateral views (PENDERGRASS et al. 1967). Cysts and cavities are sometimes formed presumably as a result of necrosis secondary to occlusion of the blood vessels supplying the affected area (GLOYNE et al. 1949; DUNNER and BAGNALL 1949).

12.3.3 Thin-Section CT

The common thin-section CT findings of graphite pneumoconiosis include small nodules, interlobular septal thickening, and the prevalence of large opacities (progressive massive fibrosis). Small nodules are classified into two patterns: ill-defined tiny opacities that appear either as fine branching opacities

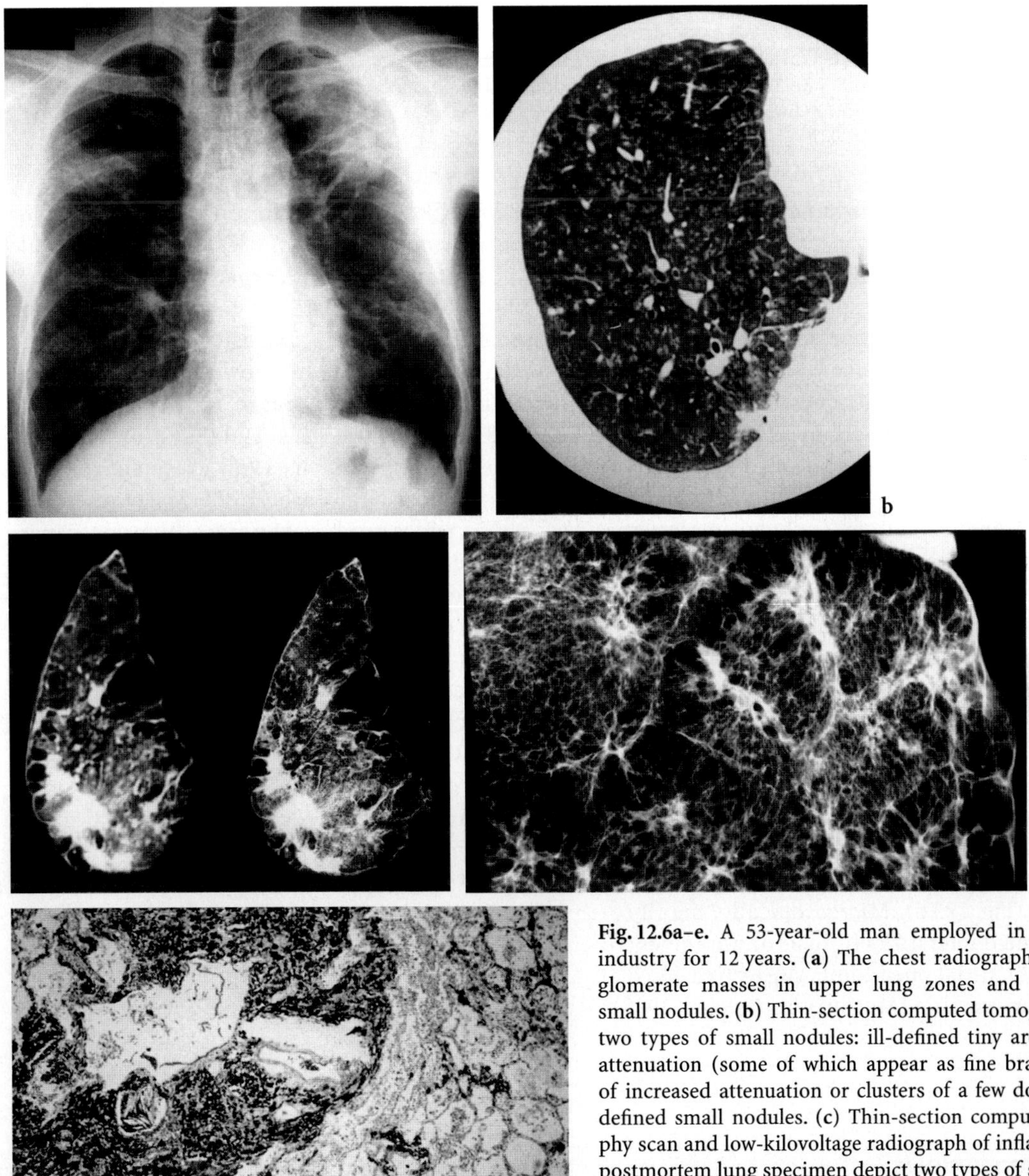

a b c d e

Fig. 12.6a–e. A 53-year-old man employed in the graphite industry for 12 years. (**a**) The chest radiograph reveals conglomerate masses in upper lung zones and disseminated small nodules. (**b**) Thin-section computed tomography shows two types of small nodules: ill-defined tiny areas of hyperattenuation (some of which appear as fine branching areas of increased attenuation or clusters of a few dots) and well-defined small nodules. (**c**) Thin-section computed tomography scan and low-kilovoltage radiograph of inflated and fixed postmortem lung specimen depict two types of small nodules and conglomerate masses. (**d**) Magnified view of postmortem low-kilovoltage radiograph depicts irregular hyperattenuation along the wall of the bronchioles and nodules in a centrilobular location. (**e**) Photomicrograph of lung specimen obtained from **d** demonstrates abundant deposition of anthracotic pigments with mild fibrotic stroma in the centriacinar location a 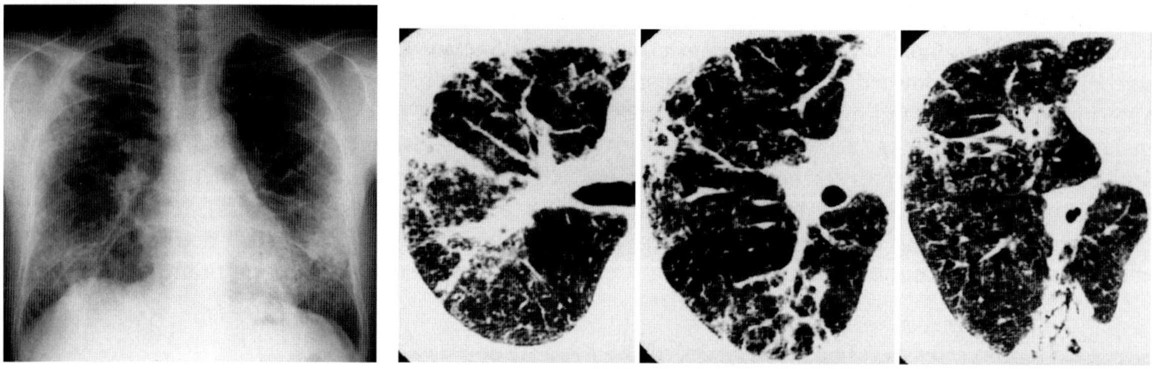 b

Fig. 12.7a,b. A 49-year-old man with a history of exposure to graphite dust for 17 years. (**a**) The chest radiograph reveals coarse reticular opacities throughout both lung fields. (**b**) Thin-section computed tomography scans show prominent peribronchovascular interstitial thickening and intralobular interstitial thickening, as well as a few parenchymal micronodules

or as a few dots clustered together; or well-defined discrete nodules (Fig. 12.6b). Both types of nodules are usually in a centrilobular location. Some nodules are present along interlobular septa or pleural surface. Pseudoplaques, representing macular or nodular lesions along subpleural connective tissue, are sometimes seen in patients with graphite pneumoconiosis. Ill-defined small nodular opacities are abundant, and there are comparably fewer discrete nodules. Bullae are frequently found. Other less common CT manifestations include emphysema, areas of ground-glass attenuation, focal decreased attenuation, and bronchiectasis (Akira 1995).

A thin-section CT–pathological correlation has revealed that ill-defined small nodules corresponded to macular lesions along the walls of bronchioles, which were often dilated, and that the discrete nodules corresponded to larger macular or nodular lesions.

Coarse reticular opacities similar to findings in diffuse interstitial pulmonary fibrosis are a predominant finding in some cases with graphite pneumoconiosis (Fig. 12.7b). Microscopically, the fibrosis is pigmented interstitial fibrosis or unpigmented or mildly interstitial pneumonia suggestive of usual interstitial pneumonia (McConnochie et al. 1988).

12.4 Talc Pneumoconiosis

Talc is used in the ceramic, paper, plastics, rubber, building, paint, and cosmetic industries. Mineralogically, talc is a pure hydrous magnesium silicate with an ideal chemical composition of 63.5% SiO_2, 31.7% MgO, and 4.8% H_2O; but, in practice, substitutions of ions may occur in the mineral lattice, or the talc may be contaminated with other minerals (Gibbs et al. 1992). Findings related to talc exposure can be separated into four principal categories, three forms by inhalation and one by intravenous administration. The first form is caused by talc mined with high-silica-content mineral and that is called talcosilicosis. Findings in this form are identical with those of silicosis. Talcoasbestosis closely resembles asbestosis and is produced by crystalline talc, generally inhaled with asbestos fibers. Pathological and radiographic abnormalities are virtually identical with those of asbestosis, including calcifications and malignant tumor formation. The third form, talcosis, caused by inhalation of pure talc, may include acute or chronic bronchitis as well as interstitial inflammation. Pure talc may also be fibrogenic. The fourth form, due to intravenous administration of talc, is usually associated with abuse of oral medications and production of vascular granulomas (Lockey 1981; Feigin 1986).

12.4.1 Prevalence

The prevalence of pneumoconiosis has been highly related to dust levels observed in the past years, as with other pneumoconioses. In one study of 43 talc workers who had an exposure to talc dust in milling operations for more than 10 years, 16 workers (37%) had roentgenographic findings of reticulonodular infiltrates (Kleinfeld et al. 1965). In one study on 176 workers having worked exclusively in the talc industry, associated with quartz below 3% and no asbestos, 46 suffered from pneumoconiosis (27%) (LEOPHONTE and DIDIER 1990). In a study of 116 miners and millers exposed to talc free of asbestosis and silica, the 12 subjects (10%) had diffuse small rounded or irregular opacities on their chest radiography (WEGMAN et al. 1982).

12.4.2 Chest X-Ray

The various talcs can result in several distinctive radiographic appearances. The nodular pattern consists either of opacities some 3–5 mm in diameter, identical to those of silicosis, or of appearances similar to 'mixed dust fibrosis'. These changes sometimes favor the middle lung fields but may be distributed throughout all zones (Fig. 12.8a). There are large opacities similar to those of silicotic conglomerations or coal progressive massive fibrosis, which may show evidence of cavity formation (JONES et al. 1994) (Fig. 12.9a).

Diffuse linear interstitial patterns are the same as those of asbestosis. Bilateral pleural plaques in the lateral parts of the lower lung fields and diaphragmatic plaques with calcification are sometimes seen. Pleural changes are seen in workers exposed to talc contaminated with asbestos and those free of asbestos (WEGMAN et al. 1982).

Pure talc, when it causes pneumoconiosis, leads to a mixture of rounded (q or r) and irregular (t or u) opacities, which appear in the middle zones and are often perihilar in distribution. The opacities slowly spread both up and down from their perihilar distribution (LEOPHONTE and DIDIER 1990). Exceptionally, very small, widely disseminated opacities (about 2–3 mm in diameter), similar to the miliary lesions of sarcoidosis or tuberculosis, and due to multiple foreign body granulomas, may be seen (TUKIAINEN et al. 1984). Pure talc may also cause acute onset of pulmonary symptoms when very large quantities are aspirated. Such exposure may be accidental and has been documented most often in infants who inhale cosmetic talc (MOFFENSON et al. 1981). Talc is used to promote pleural adhesions in the treatment of spontaneous pneumothorax and recurrent pleural effusions. Pleural instillation of pure talc may result in pleural thickening and fibrosis and may cause significant pulmonary disease if the talc enters the lung (BOUCHAMA et al. 1984).

The radiographic findings of intravenous administration of talc include large, irregular, nodular densities or consolidations in the upper parts of the middle lung fields, which may rapidly progress into large masses or massive consolidations. Widespread irregular nodules may also occur, and loss of pulmonary volume may be permanent. The large mass densities resemble those of massive pulmonary fibrosis in silicosis and anthracosis; they may, however, appear far closer to the hilum than in the latter diseases. Lymph-node enlargement is common and may be massive.

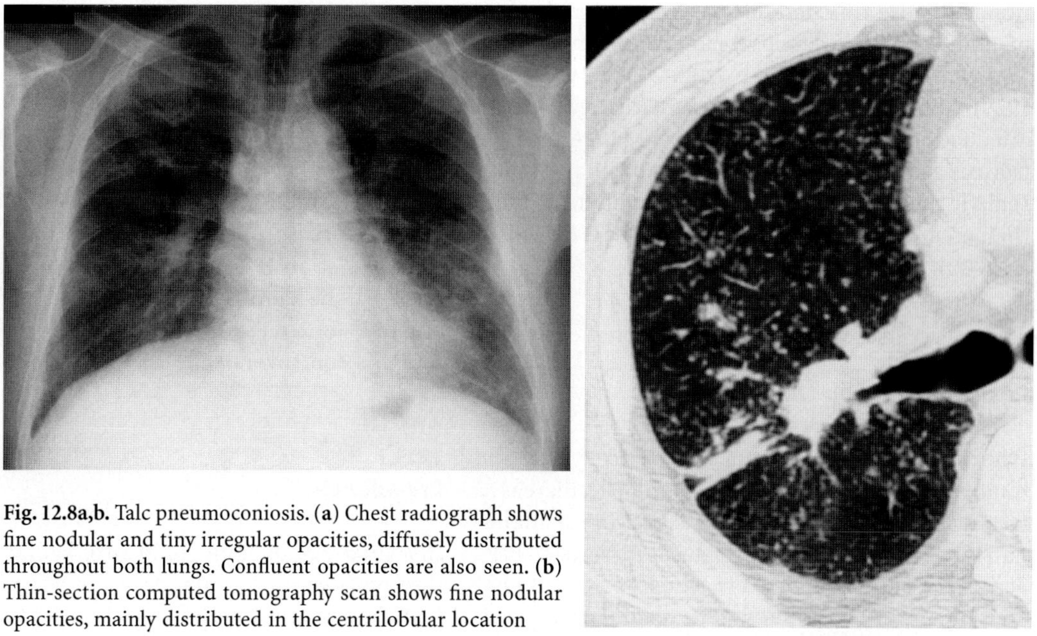

a b

Fig. 12.8a,b. Talc pneumoconiosis. (**a**) Chest radiograph shows fine nodular and tiny irregular opacities, diffusely distributed throughout both lungs. Confluent opacities are also seen. (**b**) Thin-section computed tomography scan shows fine nodular opacities, mainly distributed in the centrilobular location

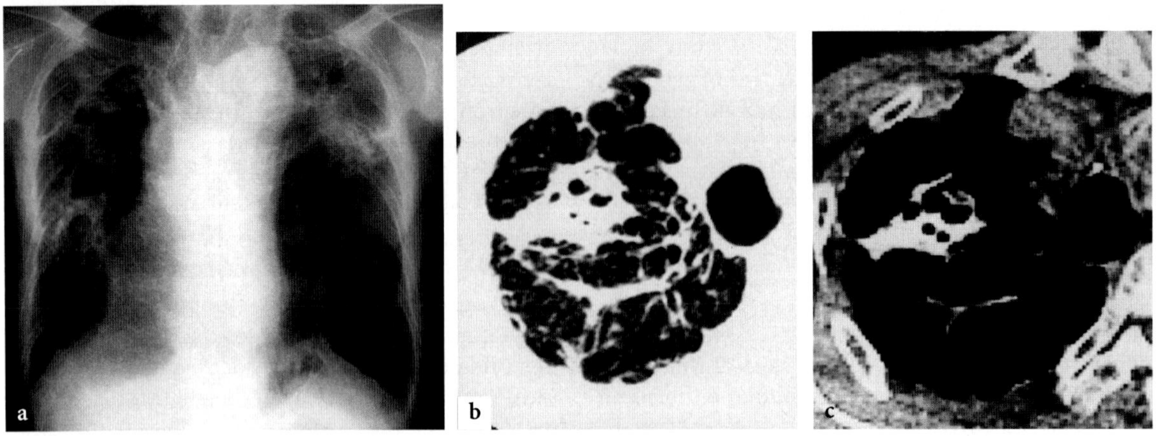

Fig. 12.9a–c. Talc pneumoconiosis. (**a**) Chest radiograph shows large opacities with pulmonary contracture in both lung fields and emphysematous change in the basal lung. Findings resemble those of complicated silicosis. (**b**) Thin-section computed tomography scan shows conglomerated mass. (**c**) When viewed at mediastinal windows (level, 10 HU; width, 300 HU), the mass is seen to contain high-attenuation material

12.4.3 Thin-Section CT

The CT finding of talc pneumoconiosis is fine nodules mainly in centrilobular distribution (Fig. 12.8b) (Akira et al. 1989). Large opacities with areas of high attenuation are often seen (Fig. 12.9b, c). Occasionally, the predominant opacities are of the irregular type and the features are the same as those of asbestosis.

The CT appearances in patients with pulmonary talcosis resulting from chronic intravenous drug abuse include widespread ground-glass attenuation, a diffuse fine nodular pattern, a combination of nodules and lower lobe panacinar emphysema (Padley et al. 1993; Ward et al. 2000; Paré et al. 1989). Confluent perihilar masses with areas of high attenuation similar to that of progressive massive fibrosis are also seen. Lower lobe panacinar emphysema is more common in methylphenidate abusers than in nonmethylphenidate drug abusers (Ward et al. 2000).

12.4.4 Positron Emission Tomography

Fluorine-18 fluorodeoxyglucose positron emission tomography (FDG PET) is being used with increased frequency to aid diagnosis and staging of malignancy. Pleural metastases cause increased FDG activity. A case is reported in which increased FDG activity, presumed to be due to pleural inflammation, was seen at sites where pleural talc had been deposited 10 months earlier after pleurodesis for recurrent pneumothoraces (Murray et al. 1997).

12.5 Kaolinosis

Kaolin is a clay that consists primarily of kaolinite, a nonfibrous silicate of aluminum. It is extremely inactive chemically, is insoluble in water, and has no potential to react as free silica. The name "Kaolin" comes from the Chinese "Kao ling", meaning "high ridge" and is still commonly known as "China Clay". Kaolin is used extensively in a variety of other industries: paper, rubber, ceramics, plastics, adhesives, paint, fertilizers, and insecticides. It is largely accepted in the literature that kaolinosis bears a greater resemblance pathologically to silicosis than to coal-workers' pneumoconiosis (Edenfield 1960; Lapenas et al. 1984). The changes of lungs are due purely to the kaolin content but whether the changes are due to contamination with crystalline silica remains controversial.

12.5.1 Prevalence

In a survey of pneumoconiosis in kaolin workers in the south-west of England, 9% of 553 men studied had abnormal radiographs (Sheers 1964). A study by OLDHAM (1983) found 23% of 1,676 workers to have abnormal radiographs. Of 1,130 workers in the various kaolin plants and mines of Georgia, 44 or 3.7% showed some evidence of pneumoconiosis (EDENFIELD 1960). In these, 2.6% showed X-ray evidence of simple pneumoconiosis, and 1.1% had complicated pneumoconiosis. In two later studies, the prevalence of pneumoconiosis in employees in the Georgia kaolin industry has been reported as 9% (KENNEDY et al. 1983) and 11% (SEPULVEDA et al. 1983).

12.5.2 Chest X-Ray

The most frequent abnormality is the presence of small, rounded opacities generally distributed throughout both lungs (Fig. 12.10a). The nodules measure 1–2 mm in diameter and are quite sharply defined. All zones are usually affected but with an apparent increase at the bases. Less commonly, irregular opacities may be mixed with the rounded opacities, or an irregular pattern may predominate to give a reticulonodular pattern. The opacities of kaolinosis appear to be less dense than those of silicosis, and discernment of the early stages of the reticulonodular pattern may be difficult. Loss of vessel clarity may be a helpful finding in these cases (WELLS et al. 1985).

Complicated pneumoconiosis with large shadows of greater than 1 cm in diameter may occur (Fig. 12.10b). They may develop in any portion of the lung. These fibrotic lesions have been gradually progressive over the years and most are associated with varying degrees of emphysema. The appearances are similar to the progressive massive fibrosis seen in silicosis. There is no associated enlargement of the hilar shadows or of pleural change. As in silicosis, there is usually an obvious background pattern of small nodulation or reticulonodulation on which the large shadows are very spare. One review notes a slower progression in kaolinosis than in silicosis (WELLS et al. 1985).

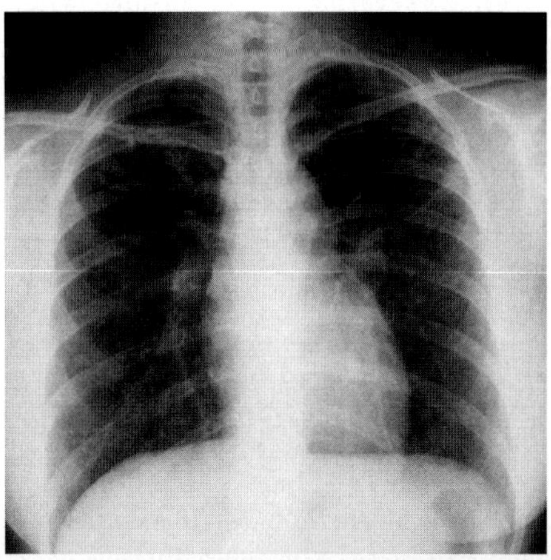
a

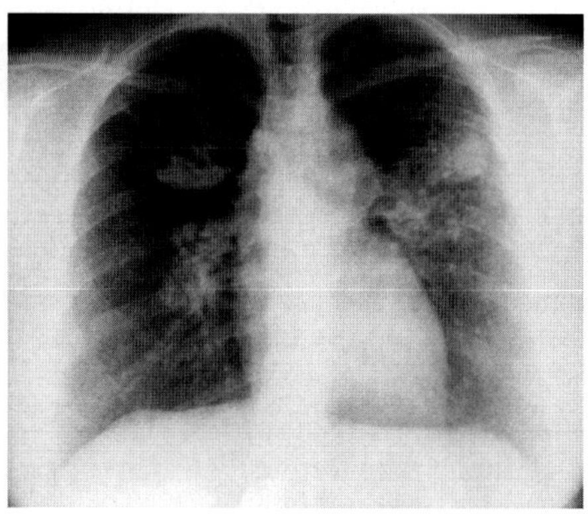
b

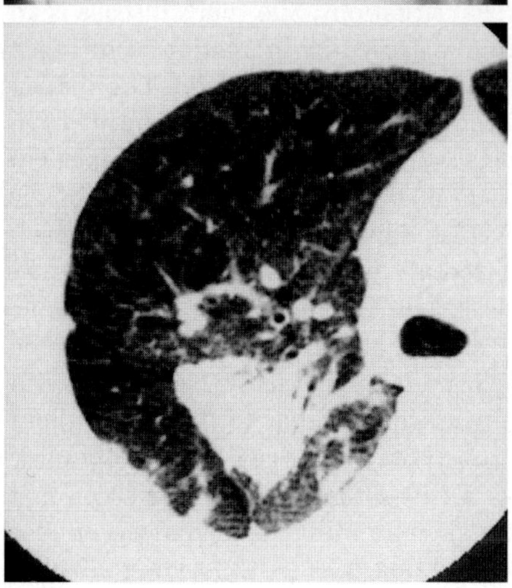
a

Fig. 12.10a–c. Kaolin pneumoconiosis. (**a**) After 7 years as a 'bagger' of dry kaolin, this worker's chest radiograph shows widespread nodulation. (**b**) Radiograph of the same worker 13 years later, showing large shadows of progressive massive fibrosis in both the upper lung zones. (**c**) Computed tomography at the level of Azygos arch shows triangular conglomeration and subpleural nodules

WAGNER et al. (1986) documented that nodular fibrosis appeared to be related to a high quartz content of the dust recovered from the lung; whereas, among those with a high content of kaolin dust in the lungs, interstitial fibrosis was observed. Kaolin workers who inhaled nearly pure kaolin, especially in middle Georgia, appeared to develop primarily small irregular opacities in the mid zones of the lungs (KENNEDY et al. 1983; LAPENAS et al. 1984).

12.5.3 Thin-Section CT

Thin-section CT delineates the changes of the thorax in kaolinosis more than chest radiography. Small nodules distributed mainly in centrilobular regions. The appearance of large opacity resembles that of complicated coal workers' pneumoconiosis or complicated silicosis (Fig. 12.10c). Peripheral emphysema typically occurs with such masses. Unlike with silicosis, hilar and mediastinal lymph node enlargement more than 1 cm in diameter is not usually seen.

12.6 Chemical Pneumonitis

Chemical pneumonitis is caused by exposure to toxic fumes of such gases as sulfur dioxide, ammonia, chlorine, phosgene, oxides of nitrogen, and ozone. Workers in a variety of occupations are exposed to toxic agents in the form of fumes and vapors. A highly soluble gas such as ammonia or sulfur dioxide will be absorbed into the mucus and the tissues in the upper respiratory tract. A less soluble gas such as nitrogen dioxide will reach more peripheral areas of the respiratory tree before being absorbed into the mucous membranes. Inhalation of the toxic agent causes direct irritation and inflammation of the tracheobronchial tree. A large exposure may result in pulmonary edema.

12.6.1 Ammonia

Ammonia is a colorless, highly soluble, extremely irritant alkaline gas with a characteristic pungent odor. Because of its high solubility, ammonia causes chemical burns of eyes, skin, oropharynx, and upper respiratory tract. The severity of the injury is directly related to the concentration of the ammonia and the duration of exposure. Those in the severe group frequently have been overcome by the ammonia and are unable to remove themselves from the area of contamination. They are in severe respiratory distress and have evidence of pulmonary edema (CAPLIN 1941). CLOSE et al. (1980) classified 12 patients exposed to anhydrous ammonia as a result of the same accident into two groups according to history and clinical course. One group of patients who sustained exposure to high concentrations of ammonia over a short period of time manifested upper airway obstruction and required early intubation or tracheostomy. These patients recovered with few pulmonary sequelae. The second group of patients who were exposed to lower concentrations of gas over a prolonged period of time did not manifest upper airway obstruction; however, significant long-term pulmonary sequelae were manifested. Bronchiectasis or bronchiolitis obliterans have developed in several survivors.

The radiographic appearance of ammonia inhalation varies with the severity of the exposure. After severe exposure, radiographs may demonstrate a pulmonary edema pattern. Bronchiectasis developed in several survivors was diagnosed by bronchography (KASS et al. 1972; GURNEY et al. 1991). Thin-section CT scan is more useful for evaluating bronchiectasis and bronchiolitis obliterans than chest radiography.

12.6.2 Nitrogen Dioxide

Nitrogen dioxide may be encountered in a wide variety of industrial situations. Silo filer's disease is an acute lung injury caused by inhalation of nitrogen dioxide in or near an agricultural silo. The sudden death from exposure to silo gas is caused by nitrogen oxide or by asphyxiation. Delayed symptoms begin several hours to days after the episode. The injury is diffuse alveolar damage and pulmonary edema. Patients who recover may pass into a latent period lasting 2–6 weeks, during which time they continue to improve, abnormal clinical and radiographic signs disappear, and then suddenly they relapse with a second acute episode similar to the first without having been re-exposed to the gas. The radiographic appearances consist either of small opacities that have been mistaken for miliary tuberculosis or confluent, ill-defined opacities (BECKLAKE et al. 1957;

DOUGLAS et al. 1989). Little is known about the pathophysiology of this second phase of the disease; MCADAMS (1955) reported finding bronchiolitis obliterans during autopsy of a fatal case. Recovery is usual with prompt treatment with corticosteroid, but irreversible bronchiolitis obliterans seems to have occurred in a few untreated cases (MOSKOWITZ et al. 1964; GALEA 1964; MILNE 1969).

The radiographic features on the acute initial stage vary from normality to typical pulmonary edema (Fig. 12.11). The chest radiographs of patients with pathologically proved bronchiolitis obliterans have shown discrete nodularity with or without confluence (RAMIREZ and DOWELL 1971). Bronchiolitis obliterans may appear as hyperinflation, mosaic pattern, centrilobular nodules, or bronchiectasis on thin-section CT. Expiratory thin-section CT may be useful in the detection of bronchiolitis obliterans.

12.6.3 Chlorine

Chlorine is a heavy irritating gas with a characteristic odor. Chlorine is intermediate in solubility and affects the lower respiratory tract more often than ammonia. Acute exposure of humans and animals to high concentrations of chlorine gas is known to produce bronchiolar and alveolar-capillary damage that is associated clinically with necrotizing bronchiolitis, bronchitis, and pulmonary edema (DAS and BLANC 1993; WILLIAMS 1997). Chest radiographs in patients with significant chlorine exposure usually demonstrate bilateral opacities typical of pulmonary edema. Pulmonary edema may occur almost immediately or be delayed for up to 2 days after exposure (BEACH et al. 1969). Chlorine can also cause irritant-induced asthma and reactive airway dysfunction syndrome (RADS), the latter being defined as an asthma-like condition that arises after a single inhalation of miscellaneous irritant agents (MOORE and SHERMAN 1991; SCHÖNHOFER et al. 1996; LEMIÈRE et al. 1997).

Thin-section CT in patients who are exposed to chlorine gas demonstrates diffuse centrilobular nodular areas of ground-glass attenuation and/or patchy areas of ground-glass attenuation (Fig. 12.12) (AKIRA 2002).

12.6.4 Paraquat

Paraquat is a herbicide that is used throughout the world in agriculture. Paraquat poisonings may be occupational but are often intentional. Most

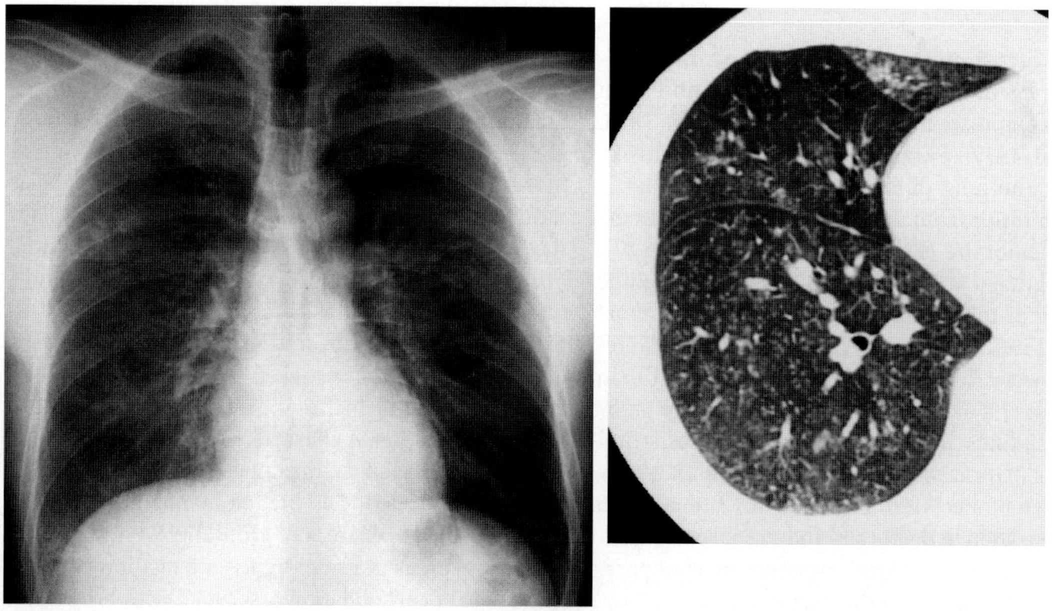

a b

Fig. 12.11a,b. Chemical pneumonitis caused by exposure to nitrogen dioxide. (**a**) Confluent, ill-defined opacities are seen in the peripheral region of right middle lung and the costophrenic angle of right lung. There are also poorly defined fine nodules in the perihilar regions. (**b**) On thin-section computed tomography, centrilobular fine nodules and branching opacities are diffusely distributed throughout the lungs

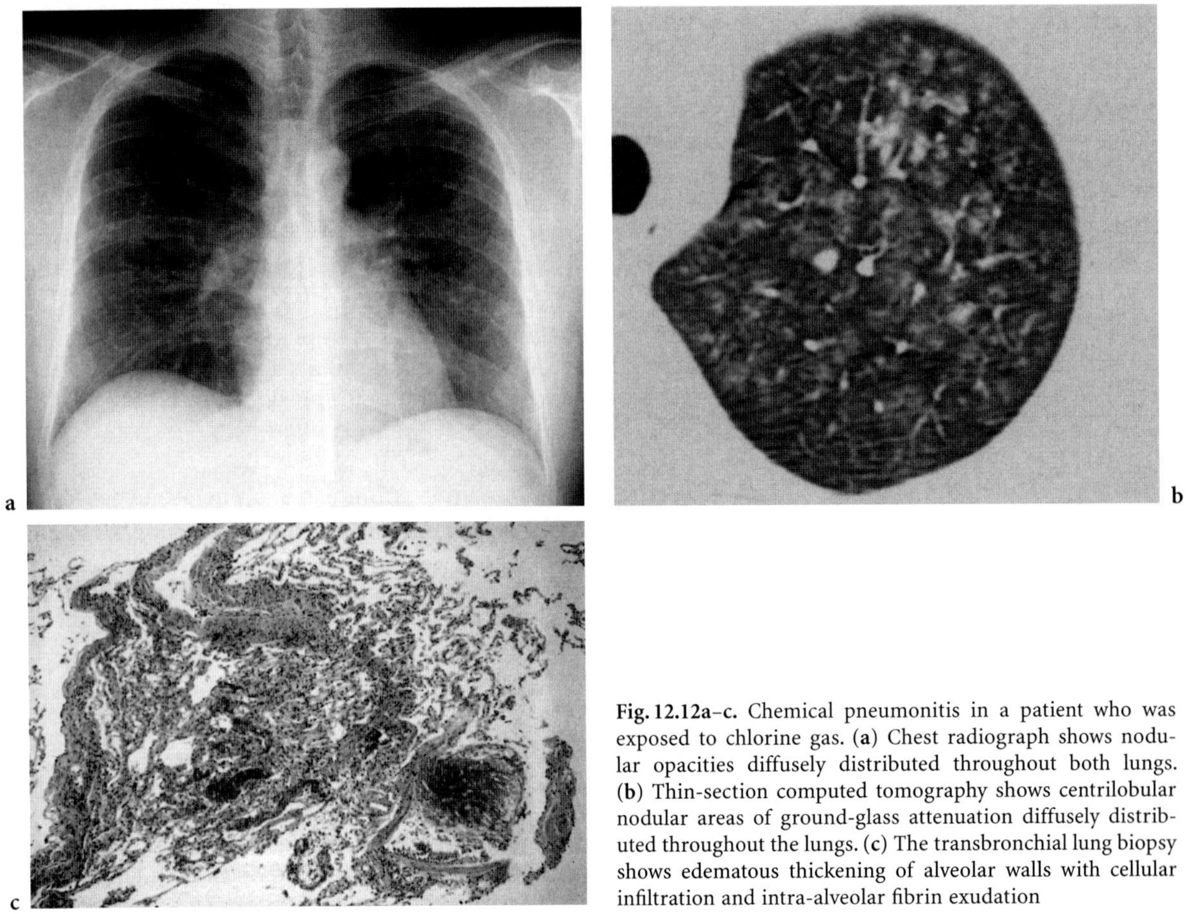

Fig. 12.12a–c. Chemical pneumonitis in a patient who was exposed to chlorine gas. (**a**) Chest radiograph shows nodular opacities diffusely distributed throughout both lungs. (**b**) Thin-section computed tomography shows centrilobular nodular areas of ground-glass attenuation diffusely distributed throughout the lungs. (**c**) The transbronchial lung biopsy shows edematous thickening of alveolar walls with cellular infiltration and intra-alveolar fibrin exudation

instances of paraquat toxicity result from ingestion of the agent, although a fatality resulting from cutaneous exposure has been reported (Jaros 1978; Levin et al. 1979). Paraquat accumulates rapidly in the lungs, and lung damage caused by paraquat is thought to result from oxygen radicals that destroy the cell membrane (Bus et al. 1976; Smith 1987). Early pathological findings in the lung include thickening of the alveolar walls by edema, hemorrhage, and inflammatory cells. Some of the alveoli are filled with fluid and a large amount of fibrin (Bullivant 1966; Mattew et al. 1968). Late pathological findings include pulmonary fibrosis and microcysts (Thurlbeck and Thurlbeck 1976).

Early symptoms after paraquat ingestion are a burning sensation in the throat, abdominal pain, vomiting, and diarrhea. The local corrosive effect of paraquat causes ulcerations on the tongue, buccal mucosa, and the esophagus. Esophageal perforation can lead to death before pulmonary toxicity becomes manifest.

The radiographic appearance of paraquat pneumonitis is nonspecific. They have been reported to be diffuse, coarse, reticulonodular infiltrates (Bier and Osborne 1978; Im et al. 1991). There may be no abnormality. Pneumomediastinum occurs frequently. Im et al. (1991) observed the following three patterns of pulmonary abnormalities in paraquat poisoning on chest radiographs: (1) diffuse air-space consolidation, (2) diffuse cystic and linear shadows, and (3) focal interstitial opacities containing small cysts. The pulmonary abnormalities demonstrated a characteristic time course. Diffuse consolidation appeared in the first 7 days, cystic and linear opacities were seen during the next 7 days, and honeycombing in the lung more than 1 month after paraquat ingestion. A characteristic time course for CT findings in paraquat poisoning of the lung has also been demonstrated. The predominant finding within the first 7 days was areas of ground-glass attenuation. The initial areas of ground-glass attenuation changed into areas of consolidation associated with bronchiectasis and irregular lines. The CT pattern on both initial and follow-up CT scans 7 days or more after paraquat poisoning was consolidation with irregular lines and traction bronchiectasis (Lee et al. 1995).

References

Akira M (1995) Uncommon pneumoconiosis: CT and pathologic findings. Radiology 19 7:403-409

Akira M (2002) High-resolution CT in the evaluation of occupational and environmental disease. Radiol Clin North Am 40:43-59

Akira M, Higashihara T, Yokoyama K et al (1989) Radiographic type p pneumoconiosis: high-resolution CT. Radiology 171:117-123

Attfield MD, Ross DS (1978) Radiological abnormalities in electric-arc welders. Br J Ind Med 35:117-122

Beach FXM, Jones ES, Scarrow GD (1969) Respiratory effects of chlorine gas. Br J Ind Med 26:231-236

Becklake MR, Goldman HI, Boxman AR et al (1957) The long-term effects of exposure to nitrous fumes. Am Rev Tuberc 76:398-409

Bellot SM, van Westrum JAFMS, Wagenvoort CA et al (1984) Deposition of bauxite dust and pulmonary fibrosis. Pathol Res Pract 179:225-229

Bier RK, Osborne IJT (1978) Pulmonary changes in paraquat poisoning. Radiology 127:308

Bouchama A, Chastre J, Gaudichet A et al (1984) Acute pneumonitis with bilateral pleural effusion after talc pleurodesis. Chest 86:795-797

Bullivant CM (1966) Accidental poisoning by paraquat: report of two cases in men. Br Med J 1:1272-1273

Bus JS, Cagen SZ, Olgaard M et al (1976) A mechanism of paraquat toxicity in mice and rats. Toxicol Appl Pharmacol 35.501-513

Caplin M (1941) A ammonia-gas poisoning: forty-seven cases in a London shelter. Lancet 2:95-96

Charr R (1955) Respiratory disorders among welders. Am Rev Tuberc Pulm Dis 71:877-884

Charr R (1956) Pulmonary changes in welders: a report of three cases. Ann Intern Med 44:806-812

Close LG, Catlin FI. Cohn AM (1980) Acute and chronic effects of ammonia burns of the respiratory tract. Arch Otolaryngol 106:151-158

Das R, Blanc PD (1993) Chlorine gas exposure and the lung: a review. Toxic Ind Health 9:439-455

DeVuyst P, Dumortier P, Schandene L et al (1987) Sarcoid-like lng granulomatosis induced by aluminum dusts. Am Rev Respir Dis 135:493-497

Dinman D (1987) Aluminium in the lung: the pyropowder conundrum. J Occup Med 29:869-876

Doig AT, McLaughlin AIG (1936) X ray appearances of the lungs of electric arc welders. Lancet 1:771-774

Doig AT, McLaughlin AIG (1948) Clearing of x-ray shadows in welder's siderosis. Lancet 1:789-791

Douglas WW, Hepper NG, Colby TV (1989) Silo-filler's disease. Mayo Clin Proc 64:291-304

Dunner L (1948) Observations of the development of graphite pneumoconiosis. Br J Radiol 21:182-185

Dunner L, Bagnall DJT (1949) Pneumoconiosis in graphite workers. Br J Radiol 22:573-579

Edenfield RW (1960) A clinical and roentgenological study of kaolin workers. Arch Environ Health 1:392-403

Edling NPG (1961) Aluminium pneumoconiosis. Acta Radiol 56:170-178

Feigin DS (1986) Talc: understanding its manifestations in the chest. AJR Am J Roentgenol 146:295-301

Funahashi A, Schlueter DP, Pintar K et al (1988) Welders' pneumoconiosis: tissue elemental microanalysis by energy dispersive x ray analysis. Br J Ind Med 45:14-18

Galea M (1964) Fatal sulfur dioxide inhalation. Can Med Assoc J 91:345-347

Gibbs AE, Pooley FD, Griffiths DM et al (1992) Talc pneumoconiosis: a pathologic and mineralogic study. Hum Pathol 23:1344-1354

Gilks B, Churg A (1987) Aluminum-induced pulmonary fibrosis: do fibers play a role? Am Rev Respir Dis 136:176-179

Gloyne SR, Marshall G, Hoyle C (1949) Pneumoconiosis due to graphite dust. Thorax 4:31-38

Guidotti TL, DeNee PB, Abraham JL et al (1978) Arc welders' pneumoconiosis: application of advanced scanning electron microscopy. Arch Environ Health 33:117-124

Gurney JW, Unger JM, Dobrey CA et al (1991) Agricultural disorders of the lung. Radiographics 11:625-634

Han D, Goo JM, Im J-G et al (2000) Thin-section CT findings of arc-welders' pneumoconiosis. Korean J Radiol 1:79-83

Hanoa R (1983) Graphite pneumoconiosis. Scand J Work Environ Health 9:303-314

Harding HE, McLaughlin AIG, Doig AT (1958) Clinical, radiographic, and pathological studies of the lungs of electric-arc and oxyacetylene welders. Lancet 23:394-399

Herbert A, Sterling G, Abraham J et al (1982) Desquamative interstitial pneumonia in an aluminum welder. Hum Pathol 13:694-699

Hewitt PJ, Hicks R (1983) An investigation of the effects of inhaled welding fume in the rat. Ann Occup Hyg 16:213-221

Hicks R, Al-Shamma KJ, Lam HF et al (1983) An investiga tion of fibrogenic and other toxic effects of arc-welding fume particles deposited in the rat lung. J Appl Toxicol 3:297-306

Im J-G, Lee KS, Han MC et al (1991) Paraquat poisoning: findings on chest radiography and CT in 42 patients. AJR Am J Roentgenol 157:697-701

Jaros F (1978) Acute percutaneous paraquat poisoning. Lancet 1:275

Jederlinic PJ, Abraham JL, Churg A et al (1990) Pulmonary fibrosis in aluminum oxide workers: investigation of nine workers, with pathologic examination and microanalysis in three of them. Am Rev Respir Dis 142:1179-1184

Jones RN, Weill H, Parkes WR (1994) Disease related to non-asbestos silicates. In: Parkes WR (ed) Occupational lung disorders, 3rd edn. Butterworths, London, pp 536-570

Jordan JW (1961) Pulmonary fibrosis in a worker using an aluminium powder. Br J Ind Med 18:21-23

Kass I, Zamel N, Dobry CA et al (1972) Bronchiectasis following ammonia burns of the respiratory tract: a review of two cases. Chest 62:282-285

Kennedy T, Rawlings W, Baser M et al (1983) Pneumoconiosis in Georgia kaolin workers. Am Rev Respir Dis 127:215-220

Kraus T, Schaller KH, Angerer J et al (2000) Aluminium dust-induced lung disease in the pyro-powder-producing industry: detection by high-resolution computed tomography. Int Arch Occup Environ Health 73:61-64

Kleinfeld M, Messite J, Shapiro J et al (1965) Effect of talc dust inhalation on lung function. Arch Environ Health 10:431-437

Lapenas D, Galc P, Kennedy T et al (1984) Kaolin pneumoconiosis: radiologic, pathologic, and mineralogic findings. Am Rev Respir Dis 130:282-288

Lee SH, Lee KS, Ahn JM et al (1995) Paraquat poisoning of the lung: thin-section CT findings. Radiology 195:271-274

Lemière C, Malo J-L, Boutet M (1997) Reactive airways dysfunction syndrome due to chlorine: sequential bronchial biopsies and functional assessment. Eur Respir J 10:241-244

Leophonte P, Didier A (1990) French talc pneumoconiosis. In: Bignon J (ed) Health related effects of phyllosilicates. NATO/ASI series, vol G.21. Springer, Berlin Heidelberg New York, pp 203-209

Levin PJ, Klaff LJ, Rose AG et al (1979) Pulmonary effects of contact exposure to paraquat: a clinical and experimental study. Thorax 34:150-160

Lockey JE (1981) Nonasbestos fibrous minerals. Clin Chest Med 2:203-218

Mattew H, Logan A, Woodruff MFA et al (1968) Paraquat poisoning: lung transplantation. Br Med J 3:759-763

McAdams AJ Jr (1955) Bronchiolitis obliterans. Am J Med 19:314-322

McConnochie K, Green PHY, Vallyathan V et al (1988) Interstitial fibrosis in coal workers-experience in Wales and West Virginia. Ann Occup Hyg 32 [Suppl 1]:553-560

Meyer EC, Kratzinger SF, Miller WH (1967) Pulmonary fibrosis in an arc welder. Arch Environ Health 15:462-469

Miller RR, Churg AM, Hutcheon M et al (1984) Pulmonary alveolar proteinosis and aluminum dust exposure. Am Rev Respir Dis 130:312-315

Milne JEH (1969) Nitrogen dioxide inhalation and bronchiolitis obliterans. J Occup Med 11:538-547

Mitchell J, Manning GB, Molyneux M et al (1961) Pulmonary fibrosis in workers exposed to finely powdered aluminum. Br J Ind Med 18:10-20

Moffenson HC, Greensher J, DiTomasso A et al (1981) Baby powder - a hazard! Pediatrics 68:265-266

Moore BB, Sherman M (1991) Chronic reactive airway disease following acute chlorine gas exposure in an asymptomatic atopic patient. Chest 100:855-856

Morgan WKC (1961) Arc-welders' lung complicated by conglomeration. Am Rev Respir Dis 85:570-575

Moskowitz RL, Lyons HA, Cottle HR (1964) Silofiller's disease. Am J Med 36:457-462

M ller H (1953) Kann Graphit Staublungenveränderungen hervorrufen? Aerztl Wochenschr 8:1226-1229

Murray JG, Erasmus JJ, Bahtiarian EA et al (1997) Talc pleurodesis simulating pleural metastases on 18F-Fluorodeoxyglucose positron emission tomography. AJR Am J Roentgenol 168:359

Okutani H, Shima S, Sato T (1964) Graphite pneumoconiosis in carbon electrode makers. Proceedings of the XIVth international congress of occupational health, Madrid, Spain, 1963. International congress series no 62. Excerpta Medica Foundation, Amsterdam, vol 2, pp 626-632

Oldham PD (1983) Pneumoconiosis in Cornish china clay workers. Br J Ind Med 40:131-137

Padley SPG, Adler BD, Staples CA et al (1993) Pulmonary talcosis: CT findings in three cases. Radiology 186:125-127

Paré JP, Cote G, Fraser RS (1989) Long-term follow-up of drug abusers with intravenous talcosis. Am Rev Respir Dis 139:233-241

Parmeggiani L (1950) Graphite pneumoconiosis. Br J Ind Med 7:42-45

Pearson GR, Longstaffe JA, Lucke VM et al (1986) Lymphadenopathy in dogs associated with aluminiumsilicate. Vet Rec 19:450-453

Pendergrass EP, Vorwald AJ, Mishkin MM et al (1967) Observations on workers in the graphite industry, part 1. Med Radiogr Photogr 43:70-99

Pendergrass EP, Vorwald AJ, Mishkin MM et al (1968) Observations on workers in the graphite industry: part two. Med Radiogr Photogr 44:2-17

Ramirez RJ, Dowell AR (1971) Silo-filler's disease: nitrogen dioxide-induced lung injury. Long-term follow-up and review of the literature. Ann Intern Med 74:569-576

Ranasinha KW, Uragoda CG (1972) Graphite pneumoconiosis. Br J Ind Med 29:178-183

Sander OA (1967) The nonfibrogenic (benign) pneumoconiosis. Semin Roentgenol 2:312-321

Schönhofer B, Voshaar T, Köhler D (1996) Long-term lung sequelae following accidental chlorine gas exposure. Respiration 63:155-159

Sepulveda MJ, Vallyathan V, Attfield MD et al (1983) Pneumoconiosis and lung function in a group of kaolin workers. Am Rev Respir Dis 127:231-235

Sferlazza SJ, Beckett WS (1991) The respiratory health of welders. Am Rev Respir Dis 143:1134-1148

Shaver CG (1948) Further observations of lung changes associated with the manufacture of alumina abrasives. Radiology 50:760-769

Shaver CG, Riddell AR (1947) Lung changes associated with the manufacture of alumina abrasives. J Ind Hyg Toxicol 29:145-157

Sheers G (1964) Prevalence of pneumoconiosis in Cornish kaolin workers. Br J Ind Med 21:218-225

Smith LL (1987) Mechanism of paraquat toxicity in lung and its relevance to treatment. Hum Toxicol 6:31-36

Snipes MB, Boecker BB, McClellan RO (1983) Retention of monodisperes or polydisperes aluminiumsilicate particles inhaled by dogs and mice. Toxicol Appl Pharmacol 69:345-362

Spá lová M, Koval Z (1975) Pulmonary X-ray and functional findings in electric-arc welders. Int Arch Arbeitsmed 34:231-236

Thurlbeck WM, Thurlbeck SM (1976) Pulmonary effects of paraquat poisoning. Chest 69(S):276-280

Townsend MC, Sussman NB, Enterline PE et al (1988) Radiographic abnormalities in relation to total dust exposure at a bauxite refinery and alumina-based chemical products plant. Am Rev Respir Dis 138:90-95

Tukiainen P, Nickels J, Taskinen E et al (1984) Pulmonary granulomatous reactions: talc pneumoconiosis or chronic sarcoidosis? Br J Ind Med 41:84-87

Vahlensieck M, Overlack A, Müller K-M (2000) Computed tomographic high-attenuation mediastinal lymph nodes after aluminum exposition. Eur Radiol 10:1945-1946

Vallyathan V, Bergeron WN, Robichaux PA et al (1982) Pulmonary fibrosis in an aluminum arc welder. Chest 81:372-374

Vuyst PD, Dumortier P, Rickaert F et al (1986) Occupational lung fibrosis in an aluminium polisher. Eur J Respir Dis 68:131-140

Wagner JC, Pooley FD, Gibbs A et al (1986) Inhalation of china stone and china clay dusts: relationship between the mineralogy of dust retained in the lungs and pathological changes. Thorax 41:190-196

Ward S, Heyneman LE, Reittner P et al (2000) Talcosis associated with IV abuse of oral medications: CT findings. AJR Am J Roentgenol 174:789-793

Wegman DH, Peters JM, Boundy MG et al (1982) Evaluation of respiratory effects in miners and millers exposed to talc free of asbestos and silica. Br J Ind Med 39:233-238
Wells IP, Bhatt RCV, Flanagan M (1985) Kaolinosis: a radiological review. Clin Radiol 36:579-582
Williams JG (1997) Inhalation of chlorine gas. Postgrad Med J 73:697-700
Wyatt JP, Riddell ACR (1948) The morphology of bauxite-fume pneumoconiosis. Am J Pathol 65:447-465
Yoshii C, Matsuyama T, Takazawa A et al (2002) Welder's pneumoconiosis: Diagnostic usefulness of high-resolution computed tomography and ferritin determinations in bronchoalveolar lavage fluid. Intern Med 41:1111-1117

13 Hypersensitivity Pneumonitis

MICHEL WILLIAM BRAUNER, PIERRE-YVES BRILLET, and FRANÇOIS GUILLON

CONTENTS

13.1 Introduction 281
13.2 Pathogenesis 281
13.3 Pathology 282
13.4 Clinical Presentation 282
13.4.1 Symptoms 282
13.4.2 Physical Findings 283
13.5 Investigations 283
13.5.1 Blood Tests 283
13.5.2 Pulmonary Function Tests 283
13.5.3 Bronchoalveolar Lavage and Lung Biopsy 283
13.6 Diagnosis of HP 283
13.7 Specific Etiological Features 284
13.8 Etiology of HP 285
13.8.1 Microorganisms Contaminating Plants 285
13.8.2 Wood and Cork 285
13.8.3 Microorganisms in Laboratories 285
13.8.4 Contamination of the Workplace 285
13.8.5 Substances in Humid Environment 286
13.8.6 Contaminating Substances in Waste Processing and Storage 286
13.8.7 Production of Fertilizers and Compost (Table 13.4) 286
13.8.8 Contact with Antigenic Plant Dust 286
13.8.9 Animal Proteins 286
13.8.10 Chemical Hazards 286
13.8.11 Metallic Dusts 286
13.8.12 Metal Working Fluid 287
13.8.13 Detergents 287
13.8.14 Epoxy Resin 287
13.8.15 Acid Anhydride 287
13.9 Compensation 287
13.10 Occupational Differential Diagnosis 287
13.11 Imaging 287
13.11.1 Chest Radiography 287
13.11.2 Thin-Section CT 288
13.12 Treatment and Prognosis of HP 293
References 293

M. W. BRAUNER, MD
Department of Radiology, UFR SMBH, Université Paris13 et Hôpital Avicenne, 125 rue de Stalingrad, 93000 Bobigny Cedex, France
P.-Y. BRILLET, MD
Department of Radiology, UFR SMBH, Université Paris13 et Hôpital Avicenne, 125 rue de Stalingrad, 93000 Bobigny Cedex, France
F. GUILLON, MD, PhD
Unité de Pathologies Professionnelles et Environnementales, UFR SMBH, Université Paris 13 et Hôpital Avicenne, 125 rue de Stalingrad, 93000 Bobigny Cedex, France

13.1 Introduction

Occupational lung disease comprises a wide variety of disorders caused by the inhalation of dust particles. Hypersensitivity pneumonitis (HP), also called extrinsic allergic alveolitis, is a world-wide, diffuse parenchymal lung disease characterized by an abnormal inflammatory immunological reaction to specific inhaled antigens contained in organic dusts. HP is caused by sensitization to repeated inhalation of organic dusts of plant or animal origin containing antigens or certain chemicals. Farmer's lung (FL) (thermophilic actinomycetes) and bird fancier's lung (BFL) (avian proteins) remain the most prevalent forms of the disease. HP is a complex disease of varying intensity, clinical presentation, and natural history. It is a serious disease, limited to the lung, that can lead to permanent lung dysfunction. Although early phases are reversible, chronic HP leads to irreversible pulmonary fibrosis. All cases of HP have striking similarities among the clinical, pathological and radiological features, regardless of the specific exposure involved (FRASER et al. 1999).

13.2 Pathogenesis

The particles of biological dust are small, less than 5 μm in diameter. Deposition of smaller particles (1 μm or 2 μm) occurs predominantly in the distal air spaces of the lung. A large amount of particles is probably necessary.

HP is characterized by diffuse inflammation of lung parenchyma and airways. There is controversy regarding the mechanisms of the immune response. Both humoral (type III) and cell-mediated (type IV) immune responses seem to play a role in pathogenesis (SALVAGGIO and MILHOLLON 1993). They are mediated by immune complexes and Th1 cells, respectively.

Most patients have specific circulating antibodies (IgG and IgM precipitating antibodies to the antigen); however, approximately 10–50% of asymptomatic persons exposed to the sensitizing antigen also have these antibodies. The pathological response in the lung is probably mainly cell mediated resulting in alveolitis and granuloma formation. A variety of cells (macrophages, neutrophils, and lymphocytes) are involved in the pathogenesis. The alveolitis is neutrophilic at the beginning, then neutrophilic and lymphocytic, and latter lymphocytic. Proinflammatory cytokines and chemokines activate alveolar macrophages, cause an influx of CD8+ lymphocytes into the lungs, facilitate granuloma formation, and promote the development of pulmonary fibrosis. Interferon (IFN)-gamma is essential for the development of HP, and interleukin (IL)-10 appears to modulate the severity of disease. Tumor necrosis factor (TNF)-alpha and tumor growth factor (TGF)-beta have been implicated in development of the pulmonary fibrosis that is seen in chronic HP (Mohr 2004). If the exposure is prolonged, collagen deposition and destruction of the lung parenchyma occur.

13.3 Pathology

The different varieties of HP have similar histological features. In early disease, histological examination shows vasculitis. In the subacute stage of the disease, HP is characterized by alveolitis, bronchiolitis, and granuloma formation. Alveolitis consists of mononuclear cell infiltration of alveoli, alveolar wall, bronchioles, and similar interstitial cell infiltrate. Poorly defined non-caseating granulomas are also frequently observed. The lesions are usually diffuse but most severe in the peribronchiolar areas. Bronchiolitis obliterans with intraluminal inflammatory polyps and organizing pneumonia are often seen in localized areas. Granulomas may progress to fibrosis. Chronic forms also reveal chronic interstitial inflammation and different degrees of fibrosis. It may be mild and patchy, mainly in peribronchial areas or dense and diffuse with honeycombing.

Vourlekis et al. (2002) has reported six cases of HP in which the pathological characteristics of surgical lung biopsies met the criteria for non-specific interstitial pneumonitis (NSIP). HP should be included in the differential diagnosis of NSIP made by lung biopsy. Patients with the histopathological diagnosis of NSIP should be evaluated for possible HP.

13.4 Clinical Presentation

HP is a disease limited to the lung. Three different clinical presentations of HP have been described: acute, subacute or intermittent, or chronic, according to duration of illness (Ashok et al. 2001). Continual exposure may cause an overlapping of phases in the same patient (Remy-Jardin et al. 1993).

Recurrent episodes with infiltrative lung disease should raise the possibility of HP.

Intermittent exposure of susceptible individuals to a high concentration of antigens is accompanied by recurrent episodes of fever, chills, dry cough, and dyspnea, whereas continuous exposure to a lower concentration characteristically results in gradually progressive dyspnea in the absence of systemic symptoms (Fraser et al. 1999).

13.4.1 Symptoms

13.4.1.1 Acute Disease

Acute disease manifests as recurrent episodes. The symptoms appear 4–6 h following heavy exposure to an offending agent. The presentation is characterized by an acute pneumonitis-like illness with fever, chills, dry cough, chest tightness, dyspnea, headache, and malaise. Fine bibasilar crackles are often present. Sometimes, patients may develop acute respiratory failure. Systemic and respiratory symptoms often resolve spontaneously within 12–48 h after cessation of exposure to the antigen.

13.4.1.2 Subacute Disease

Subacute disease manifests as recurrent "pneumonia" or as "chronic bronchitis" with an insidious onset occurring several days to weeks after exposure. Patients may gradually develop a chronic cough, sputum production, dyspnea, anorexia, and weight loss. The disease is insidious in onset and may occur over weeks. Improvement or complete recovery is often obtained if exposure terminated early; otherwise the disease may progress to interstitial fibrosis.

13.4.1.3 Chronic Disease

The chronic presentation is characterized by an insidious onset of productive cough, progressive dyspnea, fatigue, and weight loss. Removing exposure results in only partial improvement and patients may have irreversible lung damage.

13.4.2 Physical Findings

There are no specific findings of HP. Inspiratory basilar crackles or an inspiratory squawk (Earis et al. 1982) may be heard on examination of the chest. Clubbing is observed in patients with long-standing hypoxemia and fibrotic disease.

13.5 Investigations

13.5.1 Blood Tests

No single blood test is specific for the diagnosis. Leukocytosis with neutrophilia may be seen in acute disease. Elevated erythrocyte sedimentation rate, C-reactive protein level, and quantitative immunoglobulin level are often present. Precipitating immunoglobulin G antibodies against the suspected antigen confirms exposure but does not indicate active disease. It is only a marker of exposure. Many patients with clinical disease have no detectable antibodies (lack of appropriate antigen).

13.5.2 Pulmonary Function Tests

Pulmonary function tests reveal a restrictive pattern in early disease. In the acute phase, a reduction in lung volume, carbon monoxide diffusing capacity, and static lung compliance are common. Some patients also show evidence of small airway obstruction.

Pulmonary function tests can show restrictive, obstructive, or mixed defect in late disease. An airway obstruction is frequent in the subacute and chronic phase in combination with restrictive pattern.

In one study of long-term outcome of 33 nonsmoking FL dating back at least 6 years (Lalancette et al. 1993), pulmonary function tests revealed an obstructive profile in 13 subjects, restrictive changes in 1, an isolated decrease in lung diffusion capacity in 3, and normal values in 16. Thin-section CT revealed emphysema in 9 of the patients who had airflow obstruction.

13.5.3 Bronchoalveolar Lavage and Lung Biopsy

A lymphocytic alveolitis is frequently observed (>20%) but non-specific. The proportion of suppressor cytotoxic cells (CD8 lymphocytes) is usually increased, and the CD4/CD8 ratio is usually decreased (less than 1) in the lung lymphocytes. Higher levels of immunoglobulins IgG, TNF-α, and IL-6 may be detected in the bronchoalveolar lavage fluid. Abnormalities in this fluid may be found in asymptomatic individuals with antigen exposure.

Lung biopsy may be indicated in some cases, when the clinical diagnosis is difficult.

13.6 Diagnosis of HP

Although there is no single radiological, physiological, or immunological test specific for HP, the diagnosis can often be suspected on the basis of a compatible temporal relationship between pulmonary symptoms and a history of environmental or occupational exposure (Sharma and Fujimura 1995). The criteria required to make the diagnosis of HP are not clearly defined. However, it has been proposed to confirm HP in patients fulfilling four of the following major criteria and at least two of the following minor criteria (Schuyler and Cormier 1997).

Major criteria:

- Symptoms compatible with HP that appear or worsen within hours after antigen exposure

- Confirmation of exposure to the offending agent by history, investigation of the environment, serum precipitin test, and/or bronchoalveolar lavage fluid antibody
- Compatible changes on chest radiography or computed tomography of the chest
- Bronchoalveolar lavage fluid lymphocytosis
- Compatible histological changes
- Positive natural changes or by controlled inhalational challenge

Minor criteria:

- Basilar crackles
- Decreased diffusion capacity
- Arterial hypoxemia, either at rest or with exercise

Lacasse and coworkers (2003) examined whether a clinical prediction rule might be reliable for making the diagnosis of HP without bronchoalveolar lavage or biopsy. They studied a cohort of 400 patients (116 patients with HP and 284 control subjects). HP was diagnosed on the basis of thin-section computed tomography (CT), bronchoalveolar lavage and, if necessary, surgical lung biopsy. Six significant predictors of HP were identified: (1) exposure to a known offending antigen, (2) positive precipitating antibodies to the offending antigen, (3) recurrent episodes of symptoms, (4) inspiratory crackles, (5) symptoms occurring 4–8 h after exposure, and (6) weight loss. When all six factors were present, the probability of HP was 98%. The rule retained its accuracy when validated in a separate cohort of 261 patients. The authors conclude that the diagnosis of HP can often be made or rejected with confidence without bronchoalveolar lavage or biopsy, especially in areas of high or low prevalence. The strongest single predictor of HP was exposure to a known inciting antigen.

13.7 Specific Etiological Features

Identifying exposure factors is essential for the diagnosis and treatment of HP. Circumstances of exposure, as for quantitative (antigen concentration, duration of exposure) or qualitative aspects (nature of antigen, period and frequency of exposure), are important to consider (Dalphin et al. 1999; Wild and Lopez 2001). History of exposure is a major diagnostic tool which may be easily documented in the workplace. It may concern recurrent symptoms after renewal of the exposure, in the acute form of HP. However, those are not specific manifestations. They are also described in the "organic dust toxic syndrome" (von Essen et al. 1990). In the subacute form, improvement after avoidance of the antigen is relevant evidence. This is sometimes difficult to observe, when the contact is continuous. The time of clinical diagnosis is also an appropriate feature, as most of the farmers take medical advice at the end of the winter, after the stabling period.

Chronic form is usually considered to be a sequelae state. It concerns either interstitial fibrosis with airway restrictive disorder or chronic obstructive pulmonary disease (COPD). In the case of farmer's lung disease (FLD), development of COPD may concern half of the population (Braun et al. 1979; Chaudemanche et al. 2003; Dalphin et al. 1993; Erkinjuntti-Pekkanen et al. 1997). The existence of HP forms discovered only at the phase of chronic lesions (fibrosis or emphysema) is now admitted (Malinen et al. 2003). Thus, in the case of BFL, the only symptoms may be those of chronic bronchitis observed in 10% of cases (Bourque et al. 1989; Depierre et al. 1988).

In chronic HP, the development of either fibrosis or emphysema seems to be related to the nature of exposure. Repeated exposure, as in FLD, seems to be associated with an increased risk of developing emphysema (Cormier et al. 2000; Erkinjuntti-Pekkanen et al. 1998). While continuous and uninterrupted exposure, even at low-levels as in the case of BFL, leads mainly to fibrosis forms.

Exposure characteristics influence clinical features. Hence, proliferation of bronchoalveolar lavage lymphocytes exists in half of asymptomatic exposed subjects (Cormier et al. 1984), as well as for the presence of precipitating antibodies against the antigen (Prior et al. 2001; Roussel et al. 2004). None of those biological findings has a prognostic value (Gariepy et al. 1989).

Using precipitating antibodies requires identification of the exposure and information of the laboratory (Dalphin et al. 1994). A variety of detection methods exist with different sensitivity and specificity. Their normalization is still incomplete (Aberer et al. 2001). The choice of the antigenic panel is therefore essential. Some laboratories are able to test sensitivity specifically against the suspected antigen. The knowledge of some regional antigenic particularities in the FLD may be useful for diagnosis (Roussel et al. 2004).

A variety of antigens, some of them proper to a region, because of weather and/or local agricultural context has been associated with FLD (Table 13.1). This is especially the case for grain workers, swine farmers, and hay packing, storage, and harvesting conditions.

Table 13.1. Antigen-inducing Farmer's Lung Disease (Dalphin et al. 1998)

Family	Suspected antigen
Thermophilic actinomycetes	Micropolyspora faeni (Faenia rectivirgula)
	Thermoactinomyces (T.) vulgaris, sacchari, viridis
	Streptomyces sp.
Micromycetes	Aspergillus (A.) sp. (fumigatus, umbrosus)
	C. albicans
	Penicillium brevicompactu and olivicolor
	Absidia corymbifera
Gram bacteria	Erwinia herbicola
	Rhizopus sp.
	Wallemia sebi
	Eurotium amstelodami

13.8 Etiology of HP

HP results from exposure to a variety of allergens and thus to related occupational exposure.

13.8.1 Microorganisms Contaminating Plants

Microorganisms contaminating plants concern mould spores or actinomycetes developing usually on rotting vegetable products. HP has been associated with thermophilic actinomycetes (*T. vulgaris*, *T. sacchari*) growing in sugar cane (bagasse), malt (barley) (*Aspergillus fumigatus* or *A. clavatus*), paprika dust (*Mocur stolonifa*), pulp, and potatoes (thermophilic actinomycetes, *Aspergillus*). Dry sausage mould or "sausage flower" may also be a source of contamination (Penicillium sp) (Marchisio et al. 1999; Rouzaud et al. 2001). It is also the case with cheese dairy, mainly blue cheese and gruyere (*Penicillium et Acarus siro*). Esparto dust has been reported to induce stipatosis. Esparto grass (*Stipa tenacissima*) is a gramineous plant. Its fiber is used in Spain for the manufacturing of ropes, hemp sandals, rush mats, and also for decorative stucco plates used on walls and ceilings (*A. fumigatus*) (Hinojosa 2001).

13.8.2 Wood and Cork

Wood and cork often induce alveolitis because of their contamination by microorganisms (Table 13.2) (Halpin et al. 1994; Morell et al. 2003).

Table 13.2. Sources of antigen for wood (Dalphin et al. 1998)

Source of antigen	Probable antigen
Maple logs	Cryptostroma corticale
Sequoiosis	Aureobasidium sp.
	Graphium spp.
Oak and other wood	Graphium spp.
	Penicillium spp.
	Paecilomyces sp. (varioti)
	Rhizopus spp.
	Trichoderma koningii
	Alternaria
Cork	Penicillium frequentans
Vine	Botrytis cinerea

13.8.3 Microorganisms in Laboratories

Microorganisms in laboratories concern microbial and mycelial microorganisms encountered in research or clinical laboratories. In the chemical, pharmaceutical or biological industries, units of production of yeast, mould, or fungus may be source of contamination.

13.8.4 Contamination of the Workplace

Contamination of the workplace is mainly due to air conditioners and machine systems or humidifiers and dehumidifiers, encountered in the workplace or home environment (Table 13.3).

Table 13.3. Probable antigens causing hypersensitivity pneumonitis in water-based systems (Dalphin et al. 1998)

Thermophilic actinomycetes (*M. faeni, T. vulgaris, candidus*)
Micromycetes: *A. fumigatus, C. albicans, Alternaria, Fusarium, Penicillium, Aureobasidium pullulans, Cephalosporium acremonium, Acanthamoeba*
Bacteria: *Bacillus subtilis, Pseudomonas* sp., *Cytophaga* sp., *Flavobacterium multivorum, Yersinia pseudotuberculosis, Aerobacterium liquefaciens, Klebsiella oxytoca*

13.8.5 Substances in Humid Environment

Mainly microorganisms, algae, mold developing in water or humid environment such as sauna water (*Aureobasidium* sp.), jacuzzi (*Cladosporium cladosporioides*, *Mycobacterium avium*), sewers or swimming-pools.

13.8.6 Contaminating Substances in Waste Processing and Storage

In the industrial or domestic waste treatment plants, waste collectors are the most exposed to variety of dusts. Measures realized show high levels of microorganisms and vegetable or animal dusts, despite ventilation systems.

13.8.7 Production of Fertilizers and Compost (Table 13.4)

Table 13.4. Sources of antigen exposure in fertilizers and compost (Dalphin et al. 1998)

Source of antigen	Antigen
Fertilizers or manure	Streptomyces albus
Residential compost and horticulture (wood chips for orchids)	Aspergillus sp. Cryptostroma corticale
Moldy compost	Thermophilic actinomycetes (M. faeni, T. vulgaris, Actinobifida dichotomica, Exellospora flexuosa, Thermomonospora alba, curvata, fusca)
	Micromycetes (A. glaucus)

13.8.8 Contact with Antigenic Plant Dust

Grain and flour have been associated with HP. It has been described in flour-mill workers because of contamination with wheat weevils (*Sitophilus*).

Tobacco leaves may also be contaminated (*A. fumigatus*), as well as tea plants.

Mushrooms are themselves antigenic, mainly puffballs and their spores, those of pholiota (*Pholiota nameko*), of Shiitake (Suzuki et al. 2001) or of pleurotus (*Pleurotus florida*).

Algae is another cause of HP either when in direct use (alginic acid) or with cyclohexane (1-3-bis isocyanomethyl) for extraction of alginate from sea-weed for food-processing and cosmetic industries.

13.8.9 Animal Proteins

Avian antigens are the most frequently associated with the development of HP (pigeon breeder's lung). Many antigenic substances are concerned: feather bloom, avian serum (pigeons, chicken, turkey, goose, avian proteins), and excrement (mainly due to pigeon intestinal mucin). Continuous domestic exposure is an aggravating factor (Degracia et al. 1989). Also, contact with sea products is a source of HP: mollusk shell dust (Orriols et al. 1997), arthropod, cochineal. Animal furs are directly and indirectly a cause of contamination (furriers, taxidermists).

13.8.10 Chemical Hazards

Production of pyrethrum (insecticide made from the dried flower heads of chrysanthemums) is a source of HP.

Isocyanate vapors and aerosols in the plastic industry also induce HP. Those highly reactive low molecular weight substances are well documented as a cause of asthma and rhinitis. They are widely used in industry, mainly for production and use of plastic, lacquer, varnish, paint, polyurethane foam and in smelting works. HP has been associated with injection molding operation (Merget et al. 2002; Simpson et al. 1996). However, few cases have been reported. HP-like reaction has been investigated among workers using a resin (based on MDI) in a manufacture of wood-chip boards (Vandenplas et al. 1993) and in other isocyanate workers (Baur 1995).

13.8.11 Metallic Dusts

Zirconium, used in tile works and ceramics, may cause HP as may zinc vapors, mainly used by smelter workers.

Cadmium vapors are known to induce metal-fume fever and may lead to a characteristic pneumonitis (Barnhart and Rosenstock 1984). Their association with HP is not supported (Kelleher et al. 2000).

13.8.12 Metal Working Fluid

In metalworking plants, microbial contaminated water-based metalworking fluid may be associated with HP (*Pseudomonas fluorescens*) (Bracker et al. 2003; Freeman et al. 1998; Gordon 2004).

13.8.13 Detergents

Production and use of detergents containing proteolytic enzymes of bacterial origin may be a source of HP due to inhalation of enzyme vapors (*Bacillus subtilis*) (Tripathi and Grammer 2001).

13.8.14 Epoxy Resin

Few reports have mentioned epoxy resins as being associated with HP but they contain solidifying agent and starting compound, especially acid anhydride (Piirilä et al. 1997).

13.8.15 Acid Anhydride

They are largely used in industry and chemistry and have been associated with asthma and HP (Cartier et al. 1994; Czuppon et al. 1994; Gramer et al. 1994, 1998; Patterson et al. 1982; Zeiss et al. 1982, 1983).

13.9 Compensation

Compensation of HP is based on medical clinical features in association with the exposure to an identified antigenic substance at the workplace. In France, those criteria are specified via an executive order (INRS 2004). In the acute and subacute forms, clinical presentation should at least present clinical symptoms (dyspnea, cough, sputum production) with or without general signs (fever, weight loss) associated with disturbed spirometry and precipitating antibodies or lymphocytosis in bronchoalveolar lavage. In chronic HP, the contribution of chest CT scan is necessary.

13.10 Occupational Differential Diagnosis

Byssinosis is a bronchopathy due to inhalation of cotton dust, generally considered as an occupational asthma, although the immunological mechanism is still discussed. Respiratory syndrome induced by inhalation of nylon dust (Flock worker's lung) is considered different from HP (Kern et al. 2000). Metal fume fever following inhalation of metal fumes (zinc, copper) is an influenza-like reaction with poor respiratory symptoms different from HP.

13.11 Imaging

13.11.1 Chest Radiography

The different varieties of HP have quite similar radiological abnormalities regardless of the organic antigen responsible. The results of chest radiography are abnormal in most patients. It is a diffuse involvement of both lungs. Lymphadenopathy is rarely observed.

In the acute phase, chest radiography may be normal during an early phase, but most often shows diffuse or predominantly basal ill-defined air-space consolidation which reflects alveolar filling by various cells (Fig. 13.1). The air-space disease resolves

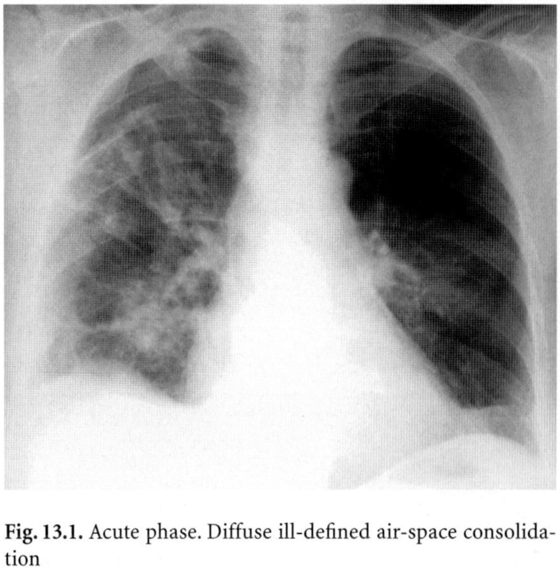

Fig. 13.1. Acute phase. Diffuse ill-defined air-space consolidation

in a few days, and fine nodules are then often visible on radiographs. Nevertheless, striated patchy opacities predispose to development of chronic changes (MONKARE et al. 1985).

During the subacute phase, chest radiography most often shows a nodular or reticulonodular pattern (Fig. 13.2). The most frequent abnormalities are poorly defined small nodules (Fig. 13.3) and ground-glass opacities (Fig. 13.4). These small nodules reflect granulomas, cellular bronchiolitis, alveolitis and interstitial infiltrates. The abnormalities are most severe in the peribronchiolar areas. Even mild degrees of pulmonary involvement may cause severe

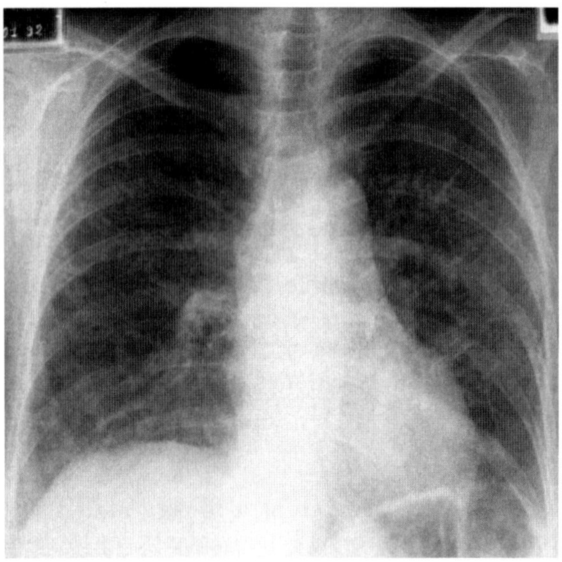

Fig. 13.2. Subacute phase. Reticulonodular pattern

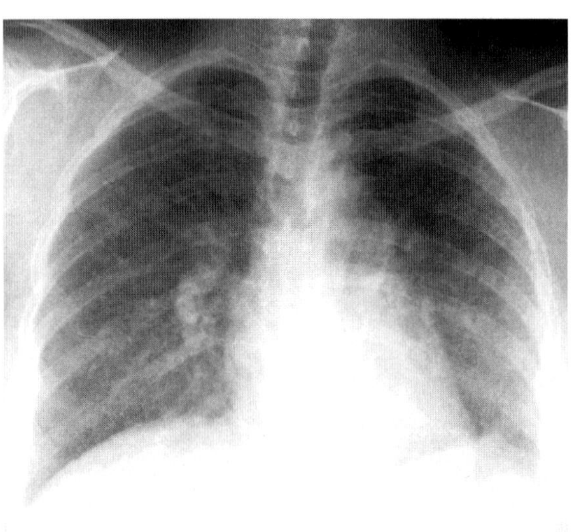

Fig. 13.3. Subacute phase. Diffuse poorly defined small nodules

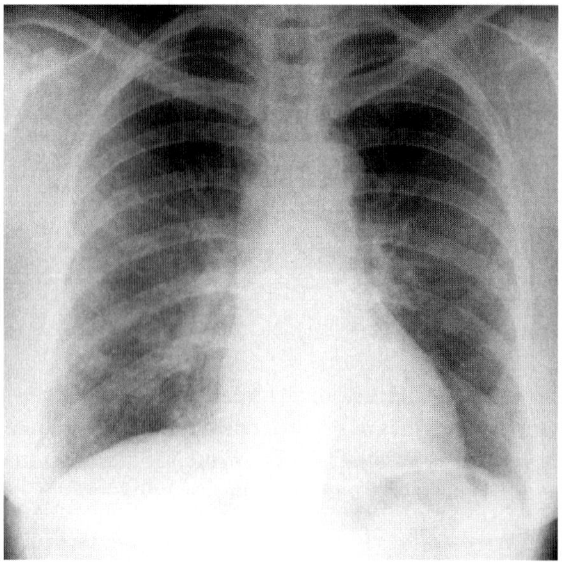

Fig. 13.4. Subacute phase. Ground-glass opacity

impairment of function because of the location of the granulomas within the respiratory bronchioles (GURNEY 1992). The lesions involve mainly the middle and basal lung zones (COOK et al. 1988). In subacute HP, the radiographic abnormalities resolve within a few days or weeks after cessation of antigen exposure. In cases of continued exposure, a diffuse fibrosis appears.

In some cases, chest radiographs are normal, up to 33% in one study (REMY-JARDIN et al. 1993) of BFL. On the contrary, chest radiographs may be abnormal without clinical symptoms.

In the chronic phase, chest radiography most often shows fibrotic changes with loss of lung volume (Fig. 13.5), coarse reticular opacities with sometimes overinflation (Fig. 13.6) of less affected areas, and emphysema. The fibrosis involves predominantly the middle lung zones or shows no zonal predominance. Lung apices and bases are relatively spared (ADLER et al. 1992). This topography of fibrosis is distinct to the subpleural, predominantly basal lesions of idiopathic pulmonary fibrosis and the upper and middle lung zones fibrosis of sarcoidosis. Fibrosis may develop months to years after the initial exposure.

13.11.2 Thin-Section CT

Thin-section CT is more sensitive than chest radiography and may reveal abnormalities in patients with normal chest radiographs (REMY-JARDIN et al.

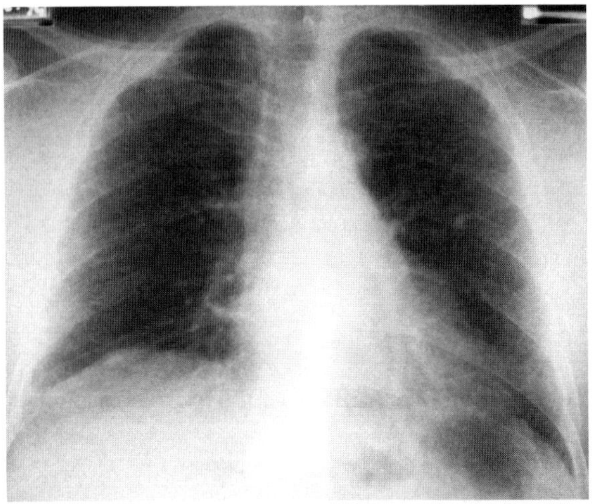

Fig. 13.5. Chronic phase. Fibrotic linear opacities with loss of lung volume

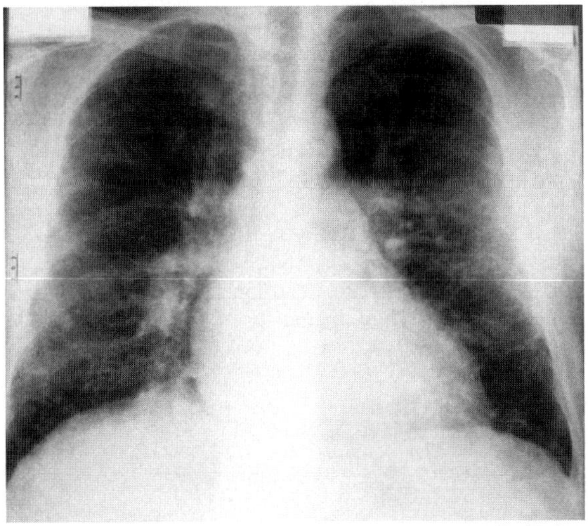

Fig. 13.6. Chronic phase. Coarse reticular opacities with overinflation

1993; Lynch et al. 1992). Thin-section CT can help to determine the specific diagnosis in patients with HP. In a study of 208 patients with various chronic interstitial lung diseases (CILD), including 13 subacute or chronic HP, a confident correct diagnosis was made by combining clinical and radiographic data in 6 and by adding the CT finding to clinical and radiographic data in 10 (Grenier et al. 1994).

Findings in acute HP typically consist of diffuse air-space consolidation. The consolidations may be diffuse or localized in the lower lung zones. Findings in subacute HP consist of patchy (Fig. 13.7 and 13.8) or diffuse (Fig. 13.9) areas of ground-glass attenuation and small centrilobular nodular areas of hyperattenuation. On thin-section CT, the peribronchiolar granulomas result in poorly defined centrilobular nodules (Fig. 13.10) (Silver et al. 1989) and the alveolitis results in patchy or diffuse ground-glass opacities (Coleman and Colby 1988). In the ground-glass pattern, the hazy increase in lung attenuation does not obscure underlying vessels. Ground-glass opacity is the main lesion in HP but also in other subacute or chronic infiltrative lung diseases: desquamative interstitial pneumonia, NSIP, and alveolar proteinosis. The patients with NSIP and alveolar proteinosis have ground-glass attenuation containing reticular opacities.

Sometimes HP has the pathological characteristics of NSIP (Fig. 13.11). The patients with desquamative interstitial pneumonia have often widespread ground-glass opacity indistinguishable from some cases of acute or subacute HP (Lynch et al. 1995).

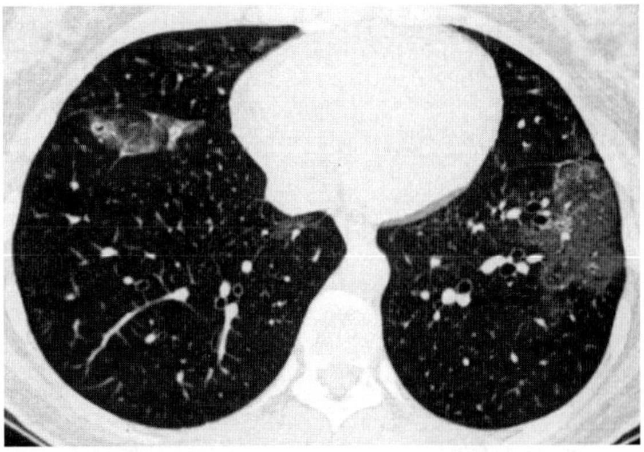

Fig. 13.7. Subacute phase. Patchy ground-glass opacity

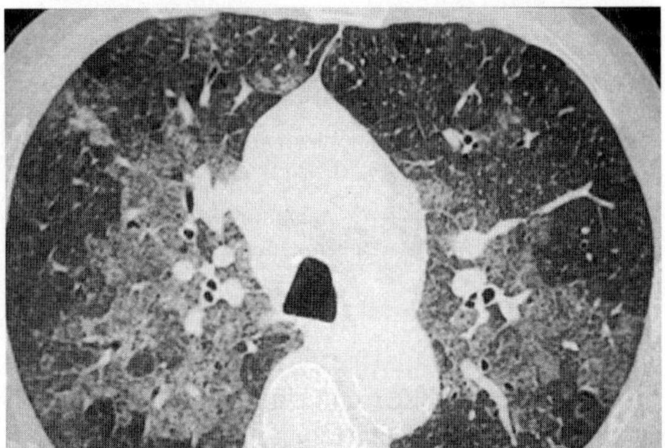

Fig. 13.8. Subacute phase. Geographical ground-glass opacity with some lucent lobules

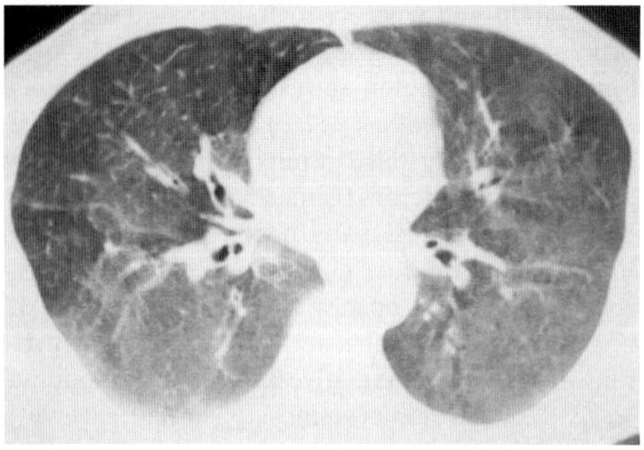

Fig. 13.9. Subacute phase. Diffuse ground-glass opacity

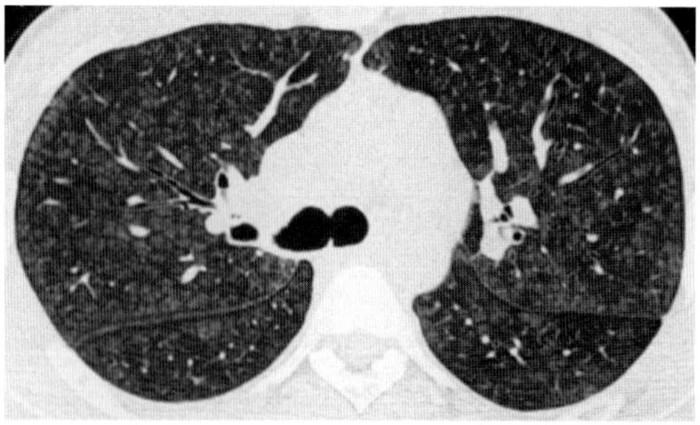

Fig. 13.10. Subacute phase. Poorly defined centrilobular nodules

a

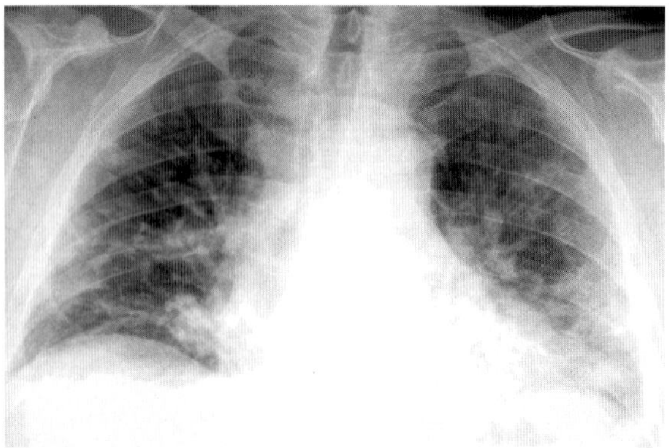

b

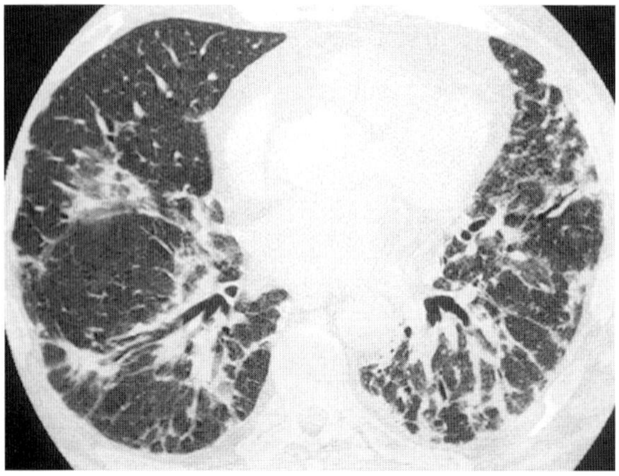

Fig. 13.11a,b. Hypersensitivity pneumonitis with the pathological characteristics of non-specific interstitial pneumonitis

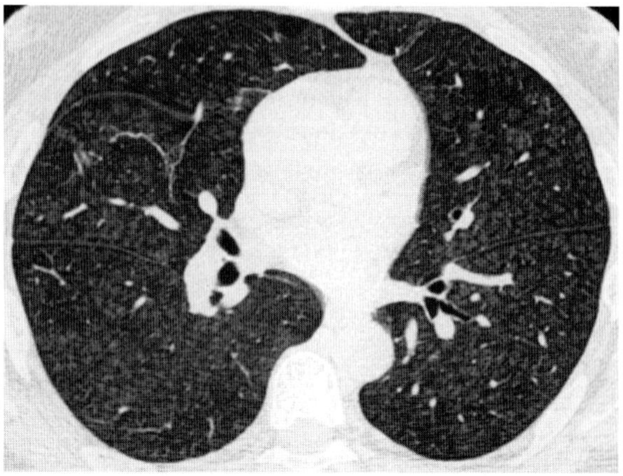

Fig. 13.12. Subacute phase. Centrilobular nodules, the pleural and fissural surfaces are spared

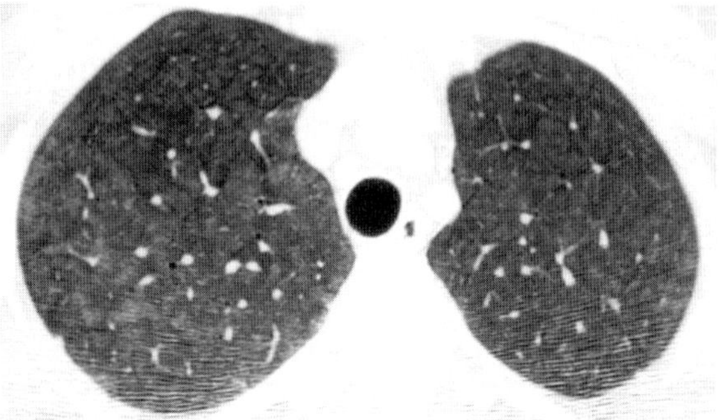

Fig. 13.13. Subacute phase. Diffuse ground-glass attenuation nodules

In the centrilobular pattern, the pleural and fissural surfaces are spared (Fig. 13.12). The nodules of ground-glass attenuation are diffuse (Fig. 13.13), and impacted airways are absent. There is a relationship between the nodules and the visible arterial branches, which are themselves centrilobular structures. Centrilobular nodules may be observed in HP and in other CILD: Langerhans cell histiocytosis, respiratory bronchiolitis, and lymphocytic interstitial pneumonitis, but the majority of patients with centrilobular nodules have HP; and, in the proper clinical context, the thin-section CT appearance is diagnostic if the nodules are correctly assessed (Gruden et al. 1999).

Focal areas of air-trapping on expiratory scans have been reported as common findings. Air-trapping has typically a lobular distribution (Fig. 13.14.a, b). It was observed in 86% of patients by HANSELL et al. (1996). SMALL et al. (1996) reviewed thin-section CT scans in 20 patients with proven subacute HP, 12 of whom also had expiratory scans. On inspiratory scans, 18 patients demonstrated ground-glass opacification, and 14 showed a nodular pattern. Areas of decreased attenuation caused by small airways disease were visible in 15 of 20 patients on inspiratory scans; expiratory scans showed areas of air-trapping in 11 of 12 patients. In a series of 400 consecutive patients with infiltrative lung disease on inspiratory thin-section CT and expiratory images, 14 showed air-trapping on expiratory CT (CHUNG et al. 2001): 6 patients with HP, 5 patients with sarcoidosis, 2 patients with atypical pneumonia and 1 patient with pulmonary edema. In 8 cases, the inspiratory scans showed a combination of patchy or geographical areas of increased attenuation, decreased attenuation, and normal-appearing lung resulting in an appearance that has been termed the "head cheese sign" because of its resemblance to the variegated appearance of a slice of sausage made from mixed meats (CHUNG et al. 2001).

Cystic spaces can be seen in a small proportion of patients with HP (13% in the series of 182 patients of FRANQUET et al. [2003]). The majority of cysts measured less than 15 mm in diameter (Fig. 13.15). The nature of these cystic air spaces is uncertain. It may be that the cysts in HP result from partial bronchiolar obstruction by the peribronchiolar lymphocytic infiltrate. FRANQUET et al. (2003) concluded that ground-glass opacification, focal areas of air-trapping, centrilobular nodules, and cysts, when present, were highly suggestive of the diagnosis of subacute HP. Similar cysts have been reported in patients with lymphocytic interstitial pneumonia. The CT features of lymphocytic interstitial pneumonia are quite similar to subacute HP but the prevalence of lung cysts in subacute HP seems to be considerably lower than in lymphocytic interstitial pneumonia. Lymphocytic interstitial pneumonia nearly always occurs in patients with underlying immunological abnormalities, most commonly Sjögren syndrome, multicentric Castleman disease and acquired immunodeficiency syndrome. It is easier to distinguish HP from other diseases having circumscribed air-containing spaces within the lungs, such as Langerhans cell histiocytosis and lymphangioleiomyomatosis (BRAUNER et al. 1989; LENOIR et al. 1990). Features distinguishing subacute HP from Langerhans cell histiocytosis include the presence of a background of diffuse ground-glass attenuation, ill-defined centrilobular nodules, and areas of air-trapping. HP can also be distinguished from lymphangioleiomyo-

a

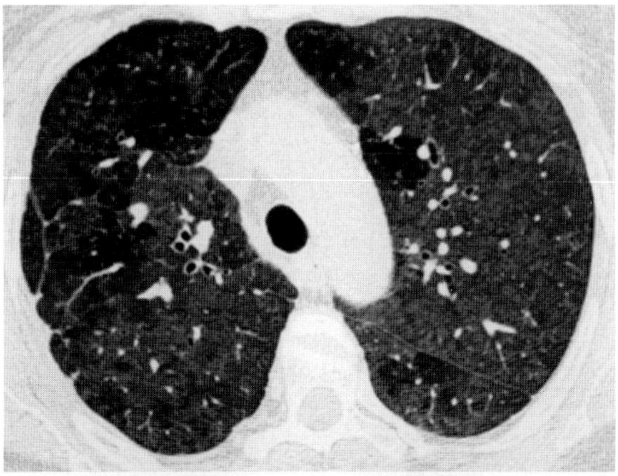

b

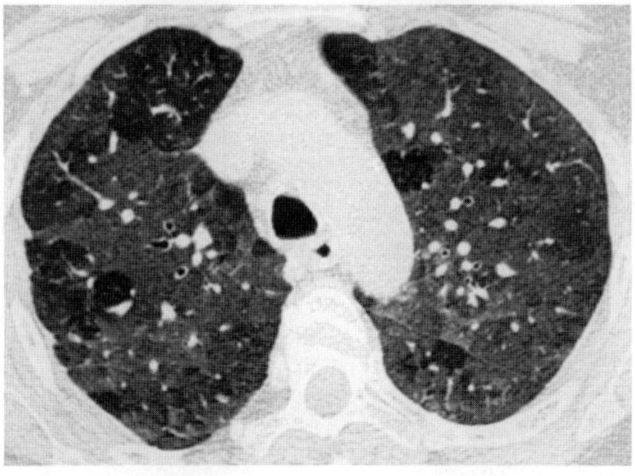

Fig. 13.14. **a** Subacute phase. Ground-glass with focal lucent lobular and non-lobular areas **b** Subacute phase. Focal areas, mainly lobular, of air-trapping on expiratory scan

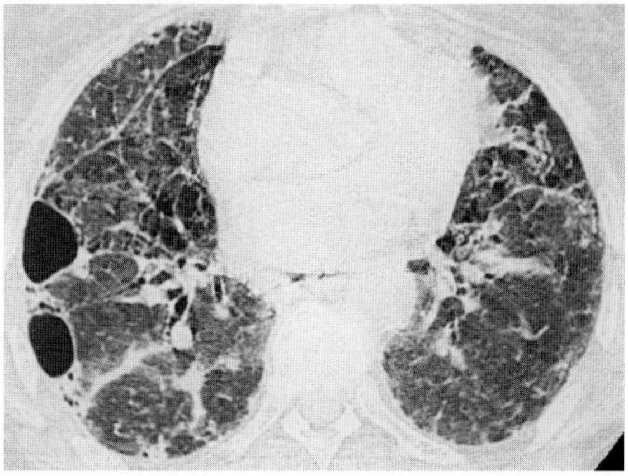

Fig. 13.15. Chronic phase. Fibrotic lesions with cystic spaces

matosis by the presence of centrilobular nodules in the former (Franquet et al. 2003).

Chronic HP is characterized by the presence of fibrosis, although findings of active disease are often present (Remy-Jardin et al. 1993). Fibrosis is characterized by lung distortion (Fig. 13.16) including irregular linear opacities, irregular interlobular septal thickening (Fig. 13.17) (Adler et al. 1992), honeycombing, and traction bronchiectasis (Figs. 13.18 and 13.19).

These abnormalities are often associated with poorly defined small nodules and areas of ground-glass opacities indicative of active disease (Fig. 13.20). The fibrosis can be diffuse but usually involves mainly the middle or lower lung zones. Relative sparing of the lung bases usually allows distinction of this entity from idiopathic pulmonary fibrosis, in which the fibrosis

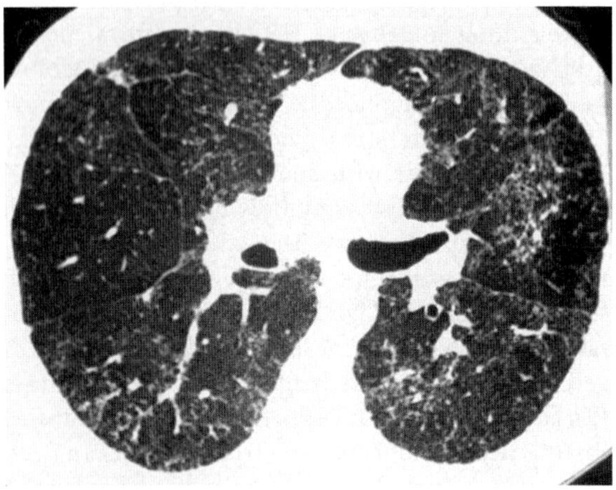

Fig. 13.16. Chronic phase. Slight lung distortion with patchy areas of micronodules

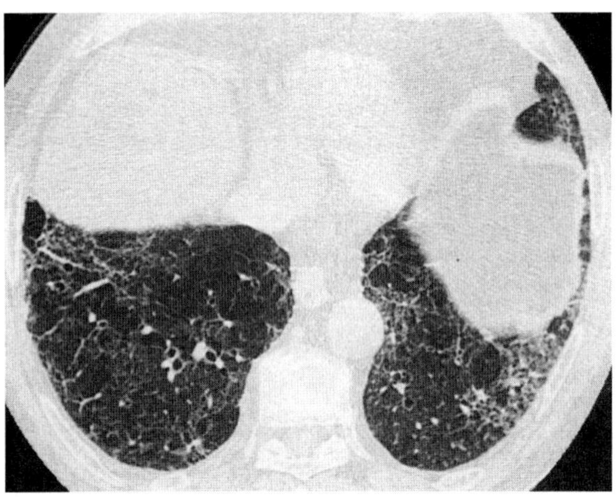

Fig. 13.17. Chronic phase. Irregular linear opacities and irregular interlobular septal thickening

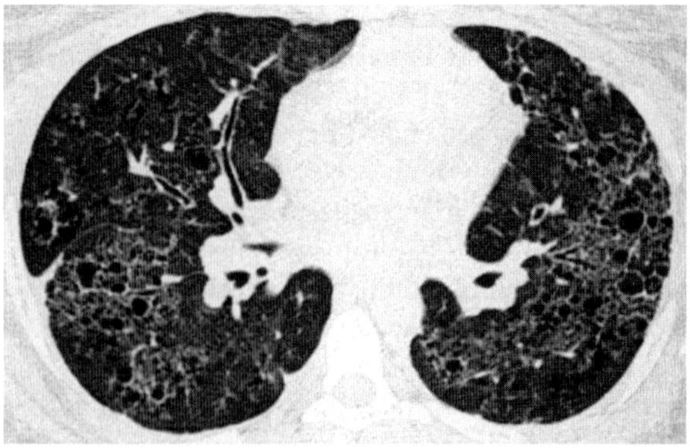

Fig. 13.18. Chronic phase. Honeycombing

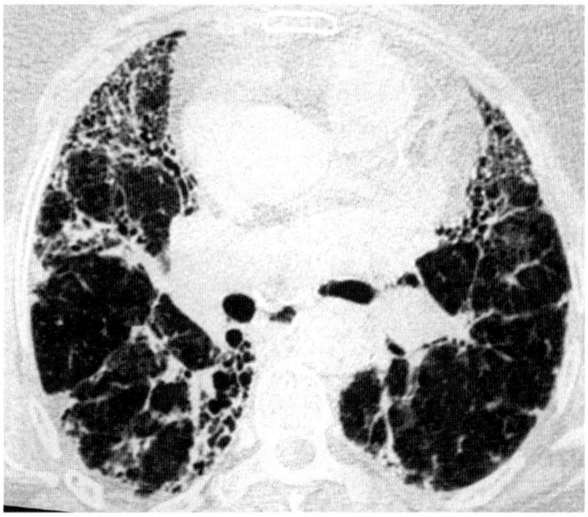

Fig. 13.19. Chronic phase. Honeycombing with linear opacity. Note a traction bronchiectasis in the middle lobe

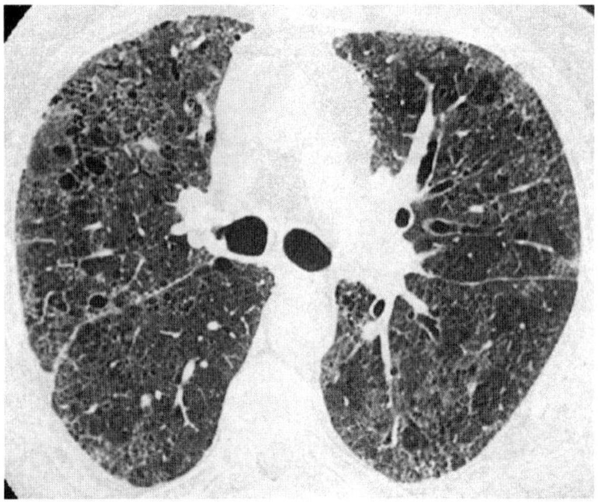

Fig. 13.20. Chronic phase. Reticulations and cysts associated with diffuse ground-glass opacity

usually predominates in the lung bases (Lynch et al. 1995). Malinen et al. (2003) have compared thin-section CT findings of 88 long-term FL patients and 83 matched control farmers with a mean follow-up time of 14 years. Emphysematous, fibrotic, and miliary changes were recorded by means of thin-section CT. Emphysema was found in 20 (23%) FL patients and in 6 (7%) controls (P=0.005). Emphysema in thin-section CT is more common in FL patients than matched control farmers, and the occurrence is increased by recurrences of FL. Emphysematous, fibrous, and miliary changes in thin-section CTs of FL patients are multiform and predominate in the lower parts of the lung.

Thin-section CT findings are often characteristic of HP, however identical findings may be seen in other interstitial lung diseases. Lynch et al. (1995) have compared 27 patients who had HP with 33 patients who had idiopathic pulmonary fibrosis. In 19 of the 27 patients with HP, the disease was chronic, while 8 had acute or subacute symptoms. All diagnoses were confirmed or supported by open lung biopsy. A CT diagnosis was made with a high level of confidence in 39 of 63 patients. In these patients, the CT diagnosis was correct in 35 cases: 23 of 26 patients with a CT diagnosis of idiopathic pulmonary fibrosis and 12 of 13 patients with a CT diagnosis of HP. Of the 19 patients with chronic HP, only 7 had a definite diagnosis of HP based on CT findings. The patients with idiopathic pulmonary fibrosis were more likely than patients with chronic HP to have honeycombing and peripheral or lower lung zone predominance of disease. Thin-section CT can be used to distinguish idiopathic pulmonary fibrosis from HP in most cases. Chronic HP may have findings identical to those of usual interstitial pneumonia.

In conclusion, thin-section CT shows more abnormalities than chest radiographs and assesses better the distribution of lesions. In the subacute phase, the correct diagnosis is often easy using thin-section CT. Centrilobular nodules and areas of ground-glass opacities are reversible lesions. In the chronic phase, the diagnosis may be difficult using thin-section CT. The main lesions are architectural distortion, irregular linear opacities, and honeycombing. They are irreversible (Webb et al. 2001).

13.12 Treatment and Prognosis of HP

In acute and subacute HP, the prognosis is good after cessation of antigen exposure. If the disease is not recognized at an early phase, fibrosis can develop.

Avoidance of organic antigen exposure is the most important factor in the management of HP. Corticosteroids are indicated for the treatment of severe acute and subacute HP and for chronic HP that is severe or progressive. Long-term corticosteroid therapy for the treatment of chronic HP should be considered only if objective improvement in clinical signs, pulmonary function, or radiographic abnormalities is documented (Mohr 2004).

References

Aberer W, Woltsche M, Woltsche-Kahr I, Kranke B (2001) IgG antibodies typical for extrinsic allergic alveolitis – an interlaboratory quality assessment. Eur J Med Res 6:498-504

Adler BD, Padley S, Muller NL, Remy Jardin M, Remy J (1992) Chronic hypersensitivity pneumonitis: high-resolution CT and radiographic features in 16 patients. Radiology 185:91-95

Ashok M, Patel MD, Jay H, Ryu MD, Reed CE (2001) Hypersensitivity pneumonitis: current concepts and future questions. J Allergy Clin Immunol 108:661-670

Barnhart S, Rosenstock L (1984) Cadmium chemical pneumonitis. Chest 86:789-791

Baur X (1995) Hypersensitivity pneumonitis (extrinsic allergic aleveolitis) induced by isocyanates. J Allergy Clin Immunol 95:1004-1010

Bourque SJ, Carter R, Anderson K, Boyd J, King S, Douglas B (1989) Obstructive airway disease in non-smoking subjects with pigeon fanciers' lung. Clin Exp Allergy 19:629-632

Bracker A, Storey E, Yang C, Hodgson J (2003) An outbreak of hypersensitivity pneumonitis at a metalworking plant: a longitudinal assessment of intervention effectiveness. Appl Occup Hyg 18:96-108

Braun SR, Dopico GA, Tsiatis A (1979) Farmers' lung disease: a long-term clinical and physiological outcome. Am Rev Respir Dis 119:185-191

Brauner MW, Grenier P, Mouelhi MM, Monpoint D, Lenoir S (1989) Pulmonary Histiocytosis X:evaluation with HR-CT. Radiology 172:255-258

Cartier A, Vandenplas O, Grammer LC, Shaughnessy MA (1994) Respiratory and systemic reaction following exposure to heated electrostatic polyester paint. Eur Respir J 7:608-611

Chaudemanche H, Monnet E, Westeel V, Pernet D, Dubiez A, Perrin C, Laplante JJ, Depierre A, Dalphin JC (2003) Respiratory status in dairy farmers in France; cross sectional and longitudinal analyses. Occup Environ Med 60:858-863

Chung MH, Edinburgh KJ, Webb EM, McCowin M, Webb WR (2001) Mixed infiltrative and obstructive disease on high-resolution CT: differential diagnosis and functional correlates in a consecutive series. J Thorac Imaging 16:69-75

Coleman A, Colby TV (1988) Histologic diagnosis of extrinsic allergic alveolitis. Am J Surg Pathol 12:514-518

Cook PG, Wells IP, McGavin CR (1988) The distribution of pulmonary shadowing in farmer's lung. Clin Radiol 39:21-27

Cormier Y, Belanger J, Beaudoin J, Laviolette M, Beaudoin R, Hebert J (1984) Abnormal bronchoalveolar lavage in asymptomatic dairy farmers: a study of lymphocytes. Am Rev Respir Dis 130:1046-1049

Cormier Y, Brown M, Worthy S, Racine G, Müller NL (2000) High-resolution computed tomographic characteristic in acute farmer's lung and in its follow-up. Eur Respir J 16:50-60

Czuppon AB, Kaplan V, Speich R, Baur X (1994) Acute autoimmune response in a case of pyromellitic acid dianhydride-induced hemorrhagic alveolitis. Allergy 49:337-341

Dalphin JC, Debieuvre D, Pernet D, Maheu MF, Polio JC, Toson B (1993) Prevalence and risk factors for chronic bronchitis and farmer's lung in French dairy farmers. Br J Ind Med 50: 941-944

Dalphin JC, Toson B, Monnet E, Pernet D, Dubiez A, Laplante JJ (1994) Farmer's lung precipitin in Doubs (a department of France): prevalence and diagnostic value. Allergy 49:744-750

Dalphin JC, Maheu MF, Dussaucy A, Pernet D, Polio JC, Dubiez A, Laplante JJ, Depierre A (1998) Six years longitudinal study of respiratory function in dairy farmers in the Doubs province. Eur Respir J 11:1287-1293

Dalphin JC, Caillaud D, et GERM"O"P (1999) Etiologies des alvéolites allergiques extrinsèques. Références Pratiques Actuelles GERM "O" P, BP Lyon Monchat 69394 Lyon Cedex 03 (http://germop.univ-lyon1.fr)

Degracia J, Morell F, Bofill JM (1989) Time of exposure as a prognostic in avian hypersensitivity pneumonitis. Respir Med 83:139-143

Depierre A, Dalphin JC, Pernet D, Dubiez A, Faucompre C, Breton JL (1988) Epidemiological study of farmers' lung in five districts of the French Doubs province. Thorax 43:429-435

Earis JE, Marsh K, Pearson MG, Ogilvie CM (1982) The inspiratory "squawk" in extrinsic allergic alveolitis and other pulmonary fibroses. Thorax 37:923-926

Erkinjuntti-Pekkanen R, Kokkarinen JI, Tukiainen HO, Pekkanen J, Husman K, Terho EO (1997) Long-term outcome of pulmonary function in farmer's lung: a 14 year follow-up with matched controls. Eur Respir J 10:2046-2050

Erkinjuntti-Pekkanen R, Rytkonene H, Kokkarinene JI, Tukiainen HO, Partanen K, Terho EO (1998) Long-term risk of emphysema in patients with farmer's lung and matched control farmers. Am J Respir Crit Care Med 158:662-665

Franquet T, Hansell DM, Senbanjo T, Remy-Jardin M, Muller NL (2003) Lung cysts in subacute hypersensitivity pneumonitis. J Comput Assist Tomogr 27:475-478

Fraser RS, Müller NL, Colman N, Pare PD (eds) (1999) Inhalation of organic dust. In: Diagnosis of diseases of the chest, 4th edn. Saunders, Philadelphia, pp 2361-2385

Freeman A, Lockey J, Hawley P, Biddinger P, Trout D (1998) Hypersensitivity pneumonitis in a machinist. Am J Ind Med 34:387-392

Gariepy L, Cormier Y, Laviolette M, Tardif A (1989) Predictive value of bronchoalveolar lavage cells and serum precipitins in asymptomatic dairy farmers. Am Rev Respir Dis 140:1386-1389

Gordon TJ (2004) Metalworking fluid the toxicity of a complex mixture. Toxicol Environ Health 67:209-219

Grammer L, Shaughnessy MA, Lowenthal M, Yarnold PR (1994) Risk factors for immunologically mediated respiratory disease from hexadydrophtalic acid. J Occup Med 36:642-646

Grammer L, Shaughnessy M, Kenamore B (1998) Utility of antibody in identifying individuals who have or will develop anhydride-induced respiratory disease. Chest 114:1199-1202

Grenier P, Chevret S, Beigelman C, Brauner MW, Chastang C, Valeyre D (1994) Chronic diffuse infiltrative lung disease: determination of the diagnostic value of clinical data, chest radiography, and CT with Bayesian analysis. Radiology 191:383-390

Gruden JF, Webb WR, Naidich DP, McGuinness G (1999) Multinodular disease: anatomic localization at thin-section CT - multireader evaluation of a simple algorithm. Radiology 210:711-720

Gurney JW(1992) Hypersensitivity pneumonitis. Radiol Clin North Am 30:1219-1230

Halpin DM, Graneek BJ, Turner-Warwick M, Newman Taylor AJ (1994) Extrinsic allergic alveolitis and asthma in a sawmill worker: case report and review of the literature. Occup Environ Med 51:160-164

Hansell DM, Wells AU, Padley SP et al (1996) Hypersensitivity pneumonitis: correlation of individual CT patterns with functional abnormalities. Radiology 199:123-128

Hinojosa M (2001) Stipatosis or hypersensitivity pneumonitis caused by esparto (Stipa tenacissima) fibers. J Invest Allergol Clin Immunol 11:67-72

INRS (2004) Les maladies professionnelles. Guide d'accès aux tableaux du régime général et du régime agricole de la sécurité sociale, 4th edn. Editions INRS ED, Paris, p 835

Kelleher P, Pacheco HO, Newman LS (2000) Inorganic dust pneumonias: the metal-related parenchymal disorders. Environ Health Perspect 108S4:685-696

Kern DG, Khun C, Ely EW, Pransky GS, Mello CJ, Fraire AE, Müller J (2000) Flock worker's lung. Chest 117:251-259

Lacasse Y, Selman M, Costabel U et al (HP Study Group) (2003) Clinical diagnosis of hypersensitivity pneumonitis. Am J Respir Crit Care Med 168:952-958

Lalancette M, Carrier G, Laviolette M, Ferland S, Rodrique J, Begin R, Cantin A, Cormier Y (1993) Farmer's lung. Long-term outcome and lack of predictive value of bronchoalveolar lavage fibrosing factors. Am Rev Respir Dis 148:216-221

Lenoir S, Grenier P, Brauner M et al (1990) Pulmonary lymphangioleiomyomatosis and tuberous sclerosis: comparison of radiographic and high resolution CT findings. Radiology 175:329-334

Lynch DA, Rose CS, Way D et al (1992) Hypersensitivity pneumonitis: sensitivity of high-resolution CT in a population based study. Am J Roentogenol 159:469-472

Lynch DA, Newell JD, Logan PM et al (1995) Can CT distinguish hypersensitivity pneumonitis from idiopathic pulmonary fibrosis? Am J Roentogenol 165:807-811

Malinen AP, Erkinjuntti-Pekkanen RA, Partanen PL et al (2003) Long-term sequelae of Farmer's lung disease in HRCT: a 14-year follow-up study of 88 patients and 83 matched control farmers. Eur Radiol 13:2212-2221

Marchisio VF, Sulotto F, Botta GC, Chiesa A, Airaudi D, Anastasi A (1999) Aerobiological analysis in a salami factory: a possible cas of extrinsic allergic alveolitis by Penicillium camenbertii. Med Mycol 37:285-289

Merget R, Marczynski B, Chen Z, Remberger K, Raulf-Heimsoth M, Willroth PO, Baur X (2002) Haemorrhagic hypersensitivity pneumonitis due to naphtalyne-1,5-diisocyanate. Eur Respir J 19:377-380

Mohr LC (2004) Hypersensitivity pneumonitis. Curr Opin Pulm Med 10:401-411

Monkare S, Ikonen M, Haahtela T (1985) Radiologic findings in farmer's lung. Prognosis and correlation to lung function. Chest 87:460-466

Morell F, Roger A, Cruz MJ, Munoz X, Rodrigo MJ (2003) Suberosis. Clinical study and new etiologic agents in a series of eight patients. Chest 124:1145-1152

Orriols R, Aliaga JL, Anto JM, Ferrer A, Hernandez A, Rodrigo MJ, Morell F (1997) High prevalence of mollusc shell hypersensitivity pneumonitis in nacre factory workers. Eur Respir J 10:780-786

Patterson R, Zeiss CR, Pruzansky JJ (1982) Immunology and immunopathology of triomellitic anhydride pulmonary reactions. J Allergy Clin Immunol 70:19-23

Piirilä P, Keskinen H, Anttila S, Hyvönen M, Pfäffli P, Tuomi T et al (1997) Allergic alveolitis following exposure to epoxy polyester powder paint containing low amounts (<1%) of acid anhydrides. Eur Respir J 10:948-951

Prior C, Falk M, Frank A (2001) Longitudinal changes of sensitization to farming-related antigens among young farmers. Respiration 68:46-50

Remy-Jardin M, Remy J, Wallaert B, Muller NL (1993) Subacute and chronic bird breeder hypersensitivity pneumonitis: sequential evaluation with CT and correlation with lung function tests and bronchoalveolar lavage. Radiology 189:111-118

Roussel S, Reboux G, Dalphin JC, Bardonnet K, Millon L, Piarroux R (2004) Microbiological evolution of hay and relapse in patients with farmer's lung. Occup Environ Med 61:e3

Rouzaud P, Soulat JM, Trela C, Fraysse P, Recco P, Carles P, Lauque D (2001) Symptoms and serum precipitins in workers exposed to dry sausage mould. Int Arch Occup Environ Health 74:371-374

Salvaggio JE, Milhollon BW (1993) Allergic alveolitis: new insights into old mysteries. Respir Med 87:495-501

Schuyler M, Cormier Y (1997) The diagnosis of hypersensitivity pneumonitis. Chest 111:534-536

Sharma OP, Fujimura N (1995). Hypersensitivity pneumonitis: a non infectious granulomatosis. Semin Respir Infect 10:96-106

Silver SF, Muller NL, Miller RR, Lefcoe MS (1989) Hypersensitivity pneumonitis; evaluation with CT. Radiology 173:441-445

Simpson C, Garabrand D, Torrey S, Robins T, Franzblau A (1996) Hypersensitivity pneumonitis-like reaction and occupational asthma associated with 1,3-bis (isocyanatomethyl) cyclohexane prepolymer. Am J Indust Med 30:48-55

Small JH, Flower CD, Traill ZC, Gleeson FV (1996) Air-trapping in extrinsic allergic alveolitis on computed tomography. Clin Radiol 51:684-688

Suzuki K, Tanaka H, Sugawara H, Saito Y, Koba H, Tsunematsu K, Abe S (2001) Chronic hypersensibility pneumonitis induced by Shiitake mushroom spores associated with lung cancer. Intern Med 40:1132-1135

Tripathi A, Grammer LC (2001) Extrinsic allergic alveolitis from a proteolytic enzyme. Ann Allergy Asthma Immunol 86:425-427

Vandenplas O, Leveque J, Cartier A, Grammer LC, Malo JL (1993) Hypersenitivity pneumonitis-like reaction among workers exposed to diphenylmethane diisocyanate. Am Rev Respir Dis 147:338-346

Von Essen S, Robbins RA, Thompson AB, Rennard SI (1990) Organis dust toxic syndrome: an acute febrile reaction to organic dust exposure distinct from hypersensitivity pneumonitis. J Toxicol Clin Toxicol 28:389-420

Vourlekis JS, Schwarz MI, Cool CD, Tuder RM, King TE, Brown KK (2002) Nonspecific interstitial pneumonitis as the sole histologic expression of hypersensitivity pneumonitis. Am J Med 112:490-493

Webb WR, Müller NL, Naidich DP (2001) High-resolution CT of the lung, 3rd edn. Lippincott Williams and Wilkins, Philadelphia, pp 356-366

Wild LG, Lopez M (2001) Hypersensitivity pneumonitis: a comprehensive review. J Invest Allerg Clin Immunol 11:3-15

Zeiss CR, Wolkonsky P, Pruzansky JJ, Patterson R (1982) Clinical and immunologic evaluation of trimellitic anhydride workers in multiple industrial settings. J Allerg Clin Immunol 70:15-18

Zeiss CR, Wolkonsky P, Chacon R, Tuntland PA, Levitz D, Prunzan JJ, Patterson R (1983) Syndromes in workers exposed to trimellitic anhydride A longitudinal clinical and immunologic study. Ann Intern Med 98:8-12

Subject Index

A

Actinolite 21, 117
Air-trapping 80, 86, 291
Airflow obstruction 14, 17, 32, 48, 53, 54, 85, 101, 105, 109, 166, 179, 187, 283
Aluminum 13, 15, 16, 20, 263, 266, 272
Ammonia 70, 274
Amosite 21, 223
Amphibole 21, 26, 116, 123, 223, 231
Anhydride 74, 139, 287
Antimony 13, 72, 116
Ardystil syndrome 73, 74
Asbestos body 22, 25, 86, 117, 118, 125, 215, 224
Asbestos fiber 21, 24, 85, 115, 121, 207, 223, 270
Asbestosis 5, 8, 17, 24, 79, 81, 86, 102, 105, 117, 127, 207–221, 230, 239, 266
Asthma
- occupational 15, 40, 46, 50, 54, 109, 258, 287
Attenuation
- decreased 164, 169, 212, 268, 270, 291
- ground-glass 15, 38, 49, 79, 87, 167, 169, 186, 190, 213, 249, 252, 254, 260, 270, 275, 289
- mosaic 80, 86, 102, 105, 169, 212, 215, 275

B

B Reader 5, 78, 95, 228
Berylliosis 16, 133, 148, 249–256
Beryllium 13, 16, 72, 116, 124, 148, 249–256, 266
Bio-aerosol 31-65, 69
Biopersistence 116, 123
Biopsy
- transbronchial 49, 249
Bird-fancier lung 33, 35
Black spots 119, 224
Bronchiectasis 54, 86, 106, 166, 170, 209, 213, 260, 270, 274
Bronchiolitis 54, 80, 161, 167, 282, 290
- obliterans 38, 73, 274
- respiratory 161, 165, 167, 169, 290
Bronchoalveolar lavage
- cells 36, 69, 134, 165, 283
- mineral analysis 119, 207, 265
Bulla 101, 189, 270

C

Cadmium 16, 55, 68, 72, 106, 108, 266, 286
Caplan's syndrome 18, 20, 152, 188, 204
Cavitation, *see* necrosis 18, 165, 178, 185, 189, 190, 203, 269, 282
Chlorine 70, 275
Chrysotile 21, 26, 116, 123, 223
Cigarette 3, 13, 20, 26, 55, 69, 85, 97, 109, 116, 161–176, 187, 195, 209, 213, 225, 252
Coal worker's pneumoconiosis 6, 17, 85, 87, 95, 185, 188, 195–202, 274
Coalescence 166, 187, 268
Cobalt 15, 72, 105, 116, 125, 257-261
Compensation 74, 78, 81, 93, 117, 196, 204, 210, 215, 228, 247, 287
COPD, *see* airflow obstruction 32, 48, 54, 105, 109, 284
Cotton 42, 45, 52, 55
Chronic obstructive pulmonary disease, *see* COPD
Crosidolite 21, 24, 223, 231
Crow's feet 216, 232

D

Dental technician 15, 116, 250
Diamond 15, 257
Differential diagnosis
- asbestosis versus idiopathic pulmonary fibrosis 86, 117, 207, 209, 215
- auto-immune diseases 151, 154
- berylliosis versus sarcoidosis 16, 149, 250, 254
- COPD 57
- environmental/occupational versus idiopathic 97, 117, 151, 154, 254, 259, 265, 271, 282
- hypersensitivity pneumonitis 36, 39, 40, 169, 282, 288
- inhalation fever 70
- Langerhans' cell histiocytosis 167
- mesothelioma 22, 54, 57, 230, 239, 244
- occupational asthma 54
- organic dust toxic syndrome 49
- pleural effusion 154, 230, 232
- pleural plaque 83, 87, 201, 226, 228
- silicosis 84, 94, 189, 210, 215, 223, 230
Diffusion capacity 24, 37, 69, 73, 103, 111, 149, 187, 217, 232, 283

E

Emphysema 8, 14, 17, 20, 37, 54, 56, 84, 102, 106, 111, 161, 163, 167, 182, 195, 202, 204, 209, 213, 217, 264, 267, 272, 283, 288, 293
Endotoxin 43, 47, 52, 55, 69
Erasmus syndrome 152

Erionite 116, 123, 239
Extrinsic allergic alveolitis, *see* hypersensitivity pneumonitis

F

Farmer's lung 32, 35, 38, 44, 134, 141, 145, 259, 281, 285
Fat
- extrapleural 83, 87, 202, 227, 228, 242
Fever
- Inhalation 42, 45, 68
- Metal fume 42, 68, 286
Fungi 33, 39, 43, 49, 52, 134, 139, 146

G

Granuloma, granulomatous 16, 21, 38, 94, 117, 134, 149, 153, 164, 204, 249, 263, 270, 282, 288
Ground glass, *see* attenuation

H

Hard metal disease 13, 15, 67, 105, 116, 125, 257–261
Honeycombing 15, 24, 79, 86, 165, 208, 211, 215, 252, 260, 264, 267, 276, 282, 292
Humidifier 33, 42, 45, 139, 146, 285
Hypersensitivity pneumonitis 15, 32, 40, 70, 105, 133, 139, 141, 169, 172, 251, 257, 281–295

I

ILO Classification 4, 78, 81, 93-99, 180, 189, 196, 208, 217, 250
Inhalation fever 42, 45, 68
Insensitivity, *see* sensitivity 85, 96
Iron 14, 16, 116, 266, 268
Isocyanate 33, 58, 67, 70, 139, 286

K

Kaolin 21, 116, 178, 272

L

Latency 3, 52, 68, 85, 149, 225, 249
Latex 52, 58, 110, 287
Line
- curvilinear 82, 211, 214
- septal 82, 86, 211, 214
- subpleural curvilinear 82, 211, 214
Lung cancer 3, 16, 26, 79, 88, 161, 217
- asbestos 9, 22, 25, 85, 116, 118, 208, 214
- beryllium 16, 148
- other dusts 16, 26
- silica 20, 188
Lung injury 67–75, 97, 172, 187, 249, 260, 274
Lung volume 8, 10, 24, 38, 39, 48, 59, 74, 96, 101, 105, 109, 111, 119, 165, 187, 217, 232, 259, 283, 287
Lymph node 16, 116, 119, 166, 177, 182, 188, 195, 203, 213, 225, 242, 250, 260, 265, 271
Lymphocyte transformation test 16, 148, 249

M

Man-made mineral fiber 26
Mesothelioma 3, 22, 26, 94, 105, 116, 225, 230, 239–247
Metal fume fever 42, 68, 286
Metal working fluid 33, 105, 287
Mica 21, 116, 178
Micronodule, *see* nodule, *see* opacity
- subpleural 201
Milky spots 224
Mixed dust fibrosis 18, 178, 266, 271
Mortality 3, 51, 254
Mosaic attenuation 80, 86, 102, 105, 169, 212, 215, 275

N

Nodule, *see* opacity
- imaging 15, 79, 84, 94, 95, 109, 162, 165, 167, 169, 177, 180, 182, 184, 187, 196, 210, 226, 244, 249, 265, 266, 267, 269, 272, 274, 288
- pathology 14, 17, 152, 165, 178
Non tuberculous Mycobacterium 35, 286

O

Obstructive lung disease, *see* airflow obstruction 106, 149, 208, 250, 283, 284, *see* COPD
Opacity, *see* nodule
- large 5, 78, 94, 97, 181, 196, 268, 271
- small 3, 78, 94, 97, 180, 196, 204, 274
Organic dust toxic syndrome 32, 37, 42, 45, 68, 284
Overload 116

P

Paraquat 68, 70, 275
Parenchymal band 82, 94, 105, 211, 216, 230, 233
Peak flow 108, 110
Pericardium 224, 239, 244
Pleura
- parietal 23, 104, 116, 119, 127, 201, 223, 230, 241, 246
- visceral 19, 22, 23, 24, 104, 201, 216, 224, 230, 241, 246
Pleural effusion 22, 54, 87, 102, 154, 166, 223, 228, 240, 271
Pleural plaque 7, 22, 83, 94, 104, 119, 127, 209, 213, 216, 223, 242
Pneumonitis
- toxic 49, 70, 73
Pollution 51, 55, 57
Polymers 42, 68, 69
Popcorn worker's lung 74
Precipitating antibodies 33, 38, 40, 282, 284
Progression 96, 166, 180, 196
Progressive massive fibrosis, *see* opacity 9, 17, 18, 88, 109, 178, 196, 201, 267, 272
Provocation test 110
Pulmonary fibrosis
- idiopathic 86, 117, 162, 172, 288, 292

Q

Quartz 19, 55, 116, 124, 180, 200, 266, 270

R

Radiation dose 80, 217, 233
Rare earths 13, 15, 116
Reactive airways dysfunction syndrome 74
Reader variability 5, 78, 95, 96, 228
Refractory ceramic fiber 26, 116, 123
Restrictive lung disease 8, 24, 35, 37, 48, 73, 74, 105, 109, 149, 165, 207, 209, 217, 225, 232, 250, 283
Rheumatoid arthritis 34, 151, 152, 188, 204
Rounded atelectasis 9, 22, 94, 216, 230, 232, 233

S

Sarcoidosis 16, 34, 39, 40, 97, 117, 137, 149, 189, 250, 254, 259, 271, 288
Screening 6, 10, 16, 36, 81, 84, 85, 98, 110, 141, 150, 216, 234, 249
Sensitivity, *see* insensitivity 9, 45, 81, 87, 96, 110, 124, 135, 139, 146, 150, 196, 207, 213, 228, 249, 254, 284
Siderosis 13, 266, 268
Silica 16, 19, 67, 74, 97, 109, 116, 124, 152, 177, 195, 209
Silicate 13, 20, 26, 80, 116, 178, 223, 270, 272
Silicoproteinosis 20, 178
Silicosis 7, 14, 17, 19, 20, 85, 87, 93, 97, 109, 117, 152, 177–193, 196, 199, 209, 266
- acute 13, 20, 21, 32, 38, 79,106, 165, 177, 203
Small airways disease 80, 102, 169, 212, 217, 291
Solvent 68, 70
Spirometry, *see* Lung volume
Stannosis 13
Systematic lupus erythematosus 34, 154, 189

T

Talc 21, 116, 124, 178, 270
Thoracoscopy 118, 224, 230, 247
Tin 13
Transfert factor (DLCO), *see* Diffusion capacity
Translocation 223
Tremolite 21, 117, 127, 223
Tuberculosis 19, 97, 188, 203, 208, 232, 251, 271, 274, 285
Tungsten carbide 15, 125, 257

W

Wall thickening
- bronchial 169, 252
Welder 46, 69, 266

List of Contributors

Masanori Akira, MD
Department of Radiology
Kinki-Chuo Chest Medical Center
1180 Nagasone-Cho, Sakai City
Osaka 591-8555
Japan

Vinicius C. S. Antao, MD, PhD
Division of Respiratory Disease Studies
National Institute of Occupational Safety and Health, CDC
1095 Willowdale Rd – MS 2800
Morgantown, WV 26505
USA

Hiroaki Arakawa, MD
Department of Radiology
Dokkyo University School of Medicine
880, Mibu, Tochigi, 321-0293
Japan

Zelena A. Aziz, MD
Department of Radiology
Royal Brompton Hospital
Sydney Street
London SW3 6NP
UK

Alexander Bankier, MD
Professor, Department of Radiology
Medical University of Vienna
Waehringer Guertel 18–20
1090 Vienna
Austria

Daniel E. Banks, MD
Professor and Head
Department of Medicine
Louisiana State University Health Science Center
1501 King's Highway
P.O. Box 33932
Shreveport, LA 71130 - 3932
USA

Michel William Brauner, MD
Department of Radiology
EA 2363, UFR SMBH
Universté Paris 13 et Hôpital Avicenne
125 rue de Stalingrad
93000 Bobigny Cedex
France

Pierre-Yves Brillet, MD
Department of Radiology
EA 2363, UFR SMBH
Universté Paris 13 et Hôpital Avicenne
125 rue de Stalingrad
93000 Bobigny Cedex
France

Sherwood Burge, MD
Department of Thoracic Medicine
Birmingham Heartlands Hospital
Bordesley Green East
Birmingham B9 5SS
UK

Andrew Churg, MD
Department of Pathology, Room GF227
University of British Columbia
2211 Wesbrook Mall
Vancouver, BC V6T 2B5
Canada

Susan J. Copley, MB.BS, MD, MRCP, FRCR
Consultant Radiologist and Honorary Clinical Lecturer
Radiology Department,
Hammersmith Hospital,
Du Cane Road
London W12 0HS
UK

Jean-Charles Dalphin, MD
Professor, Department of Respiratory Disease
Hôpital Jean Minjoz
Boulevard Fleming
25030 Besançon cedex
France

and

Equipe de recherche SERF (EA 2276)
Faculté de Médecine
place St-Jacques
25000 Besançon
France

Sujal R. Desai, MD, MRCP, FRCR
Consultant Radiologist
Department of Radiology
King's College Hospital
Denmark Hill
London SE5 9RS
UK

Paul De Vuyst, MD, PhD
Professor and Head
Department of Respiratory Medicine
Hôpital Erasme
Université Libre de Bruxelles
Route de Lennik 808
1070 Brussels
Belgium

Pascal Dumortier, PhD
Chest Department – Laboratory of Mineralogy
Hôpital Erasme
Route de Lennik, 808
1070 Brussels
Belgium

Tomas Franquet, MD
Professor, Department of Radiology
Section of Thoracic Imaging
Hospital de Sant Pau
Universidad Autonoma de Barcelona
San Antonio Maria Claret 167
08025 Barcelona
Spain

Pierre Alain Gevenois, MD, PhD
Professor of Radiology
Clinic of Chest Imaging
Department of Radiology
Hôpital Erasme
Université Libre de Bruxelles
Route de Lennik 808
1070 Brussels
Belgium

François Guillon, MD, PhD
Unité de Pathologies Professionnelles et Environnementales
UFR SMBH
Universté Paris 13 et Hôpital Avicenne
125 rue de Stalingrad
93000 Bobigny Cedex
France

David M. Hansell, MD, FRCP, FRCR
Professor of Thoracic Imaging
National Heart and Lung Institute and Division of Investigative Science
Imperial College School of Medicine, London
and
Department of Radiology, Royal Brompton Hospital
Sydney Street
London SW3 6NP
UK

David A. Lynch, MD
Professor of Radiology and Medicine
Department of Radiology, Box A030
University of Colorado Health Sciences Center
4200 East Ninth Avenue
Denver, CO 80262
USA

Nadine Magy, MD, PhD
Department of Internal Medicine
Hôpital Jean Minjoz
Boulevard Fleming
25030 Besançon cedex
France

Benoit Nemery, MD, PhD
Research Unit of Lung Toxicology
Laboratory of Pneumology and
Division of Occupational,
Environmental and Insurance Medicine
K. U. Leuven
Herestraat 49
3000 Leuven
Belgium

Øyvind Omland, MD, PhD
Department of Environmental and
Occupational Medicine
Aalborg Hospital
Aarhus University Hospital and Institute of Public Health
University of Åarhus
University Park Building 260
Vennelyst Boulevard 6
8000 Åarhus C
Denmark

Clara Gaik Cheng Ooi, MD
Department of Diagnostic Radiology
University of Hong Kong
F/4, Block K
Queen Mary Hospital
Pokfulam Road
Hong Kong SAR
China

John E. Parker, MD
Professor and Chief
Pulmonary and Critical Care Medicine
West Virginia University
HSC 4075A-9166
Morgantown, WV 26506-9166
USA

Anna Rask-Andersen, MD, PhD
Department of Medical Sciences,
Occupational and Environmental Medicine
University Hospital
751 85 Uppsala
Sweden

Gabriel Reboux, PhD
Department of Mycology and Parasitology
Hôpital Jean Minjoz
Boulevard Fleming
25030 Besançon cedex
France

Johny A. Verschakelen, MD, PhD
Department of Radiology
K. U. Leuven
Herestraat 49
3000 Leuven
Belgium

MEDICAL RADIOLOGY Diagnostic Imaging and Radiation Oncology

Titles in the series already published

DIAGNOSTIC IMAGING

Innovations in Diagnostic Imaging
Edited by J. H. Anderson

Radiology of the Upper Urinary Tract
Edited by E. K. Lang

The Thymus - Diagnostic Imaging, Functions, and Pathologic Anatomy
Edited by E. Walter, E. Willich, and W. R. Webb

Interventional Neuroradiology
Edited by A. Valavanis

Radiology of the Pancreas
Edited by A. L. Baert, co-edited by G. Delorme

Radiology of the Lower Urinary Tract
Edited by E. K. Lang

Magnetic Resonance Angiography
Edited by I. P. Arlart, G. M. Bongartz, and G. Marchal

Contrast-Enhanced MRI of the Breast
S. Heywang-Köbrunner and R. Beck

Spiral CT of the Chest
Edited by M. Rémy-Jardin and J. Rémy

Radiological Diagnosis of Breast Diseases
Edited by M. Friedrich and E.A. Sickles

Radiology of the Trauma
Edited by M. Heller and A. Fink

Biliary Tract Radiology
Edited by P. Rossi, co-edited by M. Brezi

Radiological Imaging of Sports Injuries
Edited by C. Masciocchi

Modern Imaging of the Alimentary Tube
Edited by A. R. Margulis

Diagnosis and Therapy of Spinal Tumors
Edited by P. R. Algra, J. Valk, and J. J. Heimans

Interventional Magnetic Resonance Imaging
Edited by J.F. Debatin and G. Adam

Abdominal and Pelvic MRI
Edited by A. Heuck and M. Reiser

Orthopedic Imaging
Techniques and Applications
Edited by A. M. Davies and H. Pettersson

Radiology of the Female Pelvic Organs
Edited by E. K.Lang

Magnetic Resonance of the Heart and Great Vessels
Clinical Applications
Edited by J. Bogaert, A.J. Duerinckx, and F. E. Rademakers

Modern Head and Neck Imaging
Edited by S. K. Mukherji and J. A. Castelijns

Radiological Imaging of Endocrine Diseases
Edited by J. N. Bruneton in collaboration with B. Padovani and M.-Y. Mourou

Trends in Contrast Media
Edited by H. S. Thomsen, R. N. Muller, and R. F. Mattrey

Functional MRI
Edited by C. T. W. Moonen and P. A. Bandettini

Radiology of the Pancreas
2nd Revised Edition
Edited by A. L. Baert
Co-edited by G. Delorme and L. Van Hoe

Emergency Pediatric Radiology
Edited by H. Carty

Spiral CT of the Abdomen
Edited by F. Terrier, M. Grossholz, and C. D. Becker

Liver Malignancies
Diagnostic and Interventional Radiology
Edited by C. Bartolozzi and R. Lencioni

Medical Imaging of the Spleen
Edited by A. M. De Schepper and F. Vanhoenacker

Radiology of Peripheral Vascular Diseases
Edited by E. Zeitler

Diagnostic Nuclear Medicine
Edited by C. Schiepers

Radiology of Blunt Trauma of the Chest
P. Schnyder and M. Wintermark

Portal Hypertension
Diagnostic Imaging-Guided Therapy
Edited by P. Rossi
Co-edited by P. Ricci and L. Broglia

Recent Advances in Diagnostic Neuroradiology
Edited by Ph. Demaerel

Virtual Endoscopy and Related 3D Techniques
Edited by P. Rogalla, J. Terwisscha Van Scheltinga, and B. Hamm

Multislice CT
Edited by M. F. Reiser, M. Takahashi, M. Modic, and R. Bruening

Pediatric Uroradiology
Edited by R. Fotter

Transfontanellar Doppler Imaging in Neonates
A. Couture and C. Veyrac

Radiology of AIDS
A Practical Approach
Edited by J.W.A.J. Reeders and P.C. Goodman

CT of the Peritoneum
Armando Rossi and Giorgio Rossi

Magnetic Resonance Angiography
2nd Revised Edition
Edited by I. P. Arlart, G. M. Bongratz, and G. Marchal

Pediatric Chest Imaging
Edited by Javier Lucaya and Janet L. Strife

Applications of Sonography in Head and Neck Pathology
Edited by J. N. Bruneton in collaboration with C. Raffaelli and O. Dassonville

Imaging of the Larynx
Edited by R. Hermans

3D Image Processing
Techniques and Clinical Applications
Edited by D. Caramella and C. Bartolozzi

Imaging of Orbital and Visual Pathway Pathology
Edited by W. S. Müller-Forell

MEDICAL RADIOLOGY Diagnostic Imaging and Radiation Oncology

Titles in the series already published

Pediatric ENT Radiology
Edited by S. J. King
and A. E. Boothroyd

Radiological Imaging of the Small Intestine
Edited by N. C. Gourtsoyiannis

Imaging of the Knee
Techniques and Applications
Edited by A. M. Davies
and V. N. Cassar-Pullicino

Perinatal Imaging
From Ultrasound to MR Imaging
Edited by Fred E. Avni

Radiological Imaging of the Neonatal Chest
Edited by V. Donoghue

Diagnostic and Interventional Radiology in Liver Transplantation
Edited by E. Bücheler, V. Nicolas,
C. E. Broelsch, X. Rogiers,
and G. Krupski

Radiology of Osteoporosis
Edited by S. Grampp

Imaging Pelvic Floor Disorders
Edited by C. I. Bartram
and J. O. L. DeLancey
Associate Editors: S. Halligan,
F. M. Kelvin, and J. Stoker

Imaging of the Pancreas
Cystic and Rare Tumors
Edited by C. Procacci
and A. J. Megibow

High Resolution Sonography of the Peripheral Nervous System
Edited by S. Peer and G. Bodner

Imaging of the Foot and Ankle
Techniques and Applications
Edited by A. M. Davies,
R. W. Whitehouse,
and J. P. R. Jenkins

Radiology Imaging of the Ureter
Edited by F. Joffre, Ph. Otal,
and M. Soulie

Imaging of the Shoulder
Techniques and Applications
Edited by A. M. Davies and J. Hodler

Radiology of the Petrous Bone
Edited by M. Lemmerling
and S. S. Kollias

Interventional Radiology in Cancer
Edited by A. Adam, R. F. Dondelinger,
and P. R. Mueller

Duplex and Color Doppler Imaging of the Venous System
Edited by G. H. Mostbeck

Multidetector-Row CT of the Thorax
Edited by U. J. Schoepf

Functional Imaging of the Chest
Edited by H.-U. Kauczor

Radiology of the Pharynx and the Esophagus
Edited by O. Ekberg

Radiological Imaging in Hematological Malignancies
Edited by A. Guermazi

Imaging and Intervention in Abdominal Trauma
Edited by R. F. Dondelinger

Multislice CT
2nd Revised Edition
Edited by M. F. Reiser, M. Takahashi,
M. Modic, and C. R. Becker

Intracranial Vascular Malformations and Aneurysms
From Diagnostic Work-Up
to Endovascular Therapy
Edited by M. Forsting

Radiology and Imaing of the Colon
Edited by A. H. Chapman

Coronary Radiology
Edited by M. Oudkerk

Dynamic Contrast-Enhanced Magnetic Resonance Imaging in Oncology
Edited by A. Jackson, D. L. Buckley,
and G. J. M. Parker

Imaging in Treatment Planning for Sinonasal Diseases
Edited by R. Maroldi and P. Nicolai

Clinical Cardiac MRI
With Interactive CD-ROM
Edited by J. Bogaert,
S. Dymarkowski, and A. M. Taylor

Focal Liver Lesions
Detection, Characterization,
Ablation
Edited by R. Lencioni, D. Cioni,
and C. Bartolozzi

Multidetector-Row CT Angiography
Edited by C. Catalano
and R. Passariello

Paediatric Musculoskeletal Diseases
With an Emphasis on Ultrasound
Edited by D. Wilson

Contrast Media in Ultrasonography
Basic Principles and Clinical Applications
Edited by Emilio Quaia

MR Imaging in White Matter Diseases of the Brain and Spinal Cord
Edited by M. Filippi, N. De Stefano,
V. Dousset, and J. C. McGowan

Diagnostic Nuclear Medicine
2nd Revised Edition
Edited by C. Schiepers

Imaging of the Kidney Cancer
Edited by A. Guermazi

Magnetic Resonance Imaging in Ischemic Stroke
Edited by R. von Kummer and T. Back

Imaging of the Hip & Bony Pelvis
Techniques and Applications
Edited by A. M. Davies, K. J. Johnson,
and R. W. Whitehouse

Imaging of Occupational and Environmental Disorders of the Chest
Edited by P. A. Gevenois and
P. De Vuyst

Contrast Media
Safety Issues and ESUR Guidelines
Edited by H. S. Thomsen

Virtual Colonoscopy
A Practical Guide
Edited by P. Lefere and S. Gryspeerdt

Springer

MEDICAL RADIOLOGY Diagnostic Imaging and Radiation Oncology

Titles in the series already published

RADIATION ONCOLOGY

Lung Cancer
Edited by C.W. Scarantino

Innovations in Radiation Oncology
Edited by H. R. Withers and L. J. Peters

Radiation Therapy of Head and Neck Cancer
Edited by G. E. Laramore

Gastrointestinal Cancer – Radiation Therapy
Edited by R.R. Dobelbower, Jr.

Radiation Exposure and Occupational Risks
Edited by E. Scherer, C. Streffer, and K.-R. Trott

Radiation Therapy of Benign Diseases
A Clinical Guide
S. E. Order and S. S. Donaldson

Interventional Radiation Therapy Techniques – Brachytherapy
Edited by R. Sauer

Radiopathology of Organs and Tissues
Edited by E. Scherer, C. Streffer, and K.-R. Trott

Concomitant Continuous Infusion Chemotherapy and Radiation
Edited by M. Rotman and C. J. Rosenthal

Intraoperative Radiotherapy – Clinical Experiences and Results
Edited by F. A. Calvo, M. Santos, and L.W. Brady

Radiotherapy of Intraocular and Orbital Tumors
Edited by W. E. Alberti and R. H. Sagerman

Interstitial and Intracavitary Thermoradiotherapy
Edited by M. H. Seegenschmiedt and R. Sauer

Non-Disseminated Breast Cancer
Controversial Issues in Management
Edited by G. H. Fletcher and S.H. Levitt

Current Topics in Clinical Radiobiology of Tumors
Edited by H.-P. Beck-Bornholdt

Practical Approaches to Cancer Invasion and Metastases
A Compendium of Radiation Oncologists' Responses to 40 Histories
Edited by A. R. Kagan with the Assistance of R. J. Steckel

Radiation Therapy in Pediatric Oncology
Edited by J. R. Cassady

Radiation Therapy Physics
Edited by A. R. Smith

Late Sequelae in Oncology
Edited by J. Dunst and R. Sauer

Mediastinal Tumors. Update 1995
Edited by D. E. Wood and C. R. Thomas, Jr.

Thermoradiotherapy and Thermochemotherapy
Volume 1:
Biology, Physiology, and Physics
Volume 2:
Clinical Applications
Edited by M.H. Seegenschmiedt, P. Fessenden, and C.C. Vernon

Carcinoma of the Prostate
Innovations in Management
Edited by Z. Petrovich, L. Baert, and L.W. Brady

Radiation Oncology of Gynecological Cancers
Edited by H.W. Vahrson

Carcinoma of the Bladder
Innovations in Management
Edited by Z. Petrovich, L. Baert, and L.W. Brady

Blood Perfusion and Microenvironment of Human Tumors
Implications for Clinical Radiooncology
Edited by M. Molls and P. Vaupel

Radiation Therapy of Benign Diseases
A Clinical Guide
2nd Revised Edition
S. E. Order and S. S. Donaldson

Carcinoma of the Kidney and Testis, and Rare Urologic Malignancies
Innovations in Management
Edited by Z. Petrovich, L. Baert, and L.W. Brady

Progress and Perspectives in the Treatment of Lung Cancer
Edited by P. Van Houtte, J. Klastersky, and P. Rocmans

Combined Modality Therapy of Central Nervous System Tumors
Edited by Z. Petrovich, L. W. Brady, M. L. Apuzzo, and M. Bamberg

Age-Related Macular Degeneration
Current Treatment Concepts
Edited by W. A. Alberti, G. Richard, and R. H. Sagerman

Radiotherapy of Intraocular and Orbital Tumors
2nd Revised Edition
Edited by R. H. Sagerman, and W. E. Alberti

Modification of Radiation Response
Cytokines, Growth Factors, and Other Biolgical Targets
Edited by C. Nieder, L. Milas, and K. K. Ang

Radiation Oncology for Cure and Palliation
R. G. Parker, N. A. Janjan, and M. T. Selch

Clinical Target Volumes in Conformal and Intensity Modulated Radiation Therapy
A Clinical Guide to Cancer Treatment
Edited by V. Grégoire, P. Scalliet, and K. K. Ang

Advances in Radiation Oncology in Lung Cancer
Edited by Branislav Jeremić

New Technologies in Radiation Oncology
Edited by W. Schlegel, T. Bortfeld, and A.-L. Grosu

Springer

Printing and Binding: Stürtz GmbH, Würzburg